EDITORS

Pierre-Alain Clavien
Michael G. Sarr
Yuman Fong

Atlas of Upper Gastrointestinal and Hepato-Pancreato-Biliary Surgery

Panco Georgiev (*Associate Editor*)

EDITORS

Pierre-Alain Clavien
Michael G. Sarr
Yuman Fong

Atlas of Upper Gastrointestinal and Hepato-Pancreato-Biliary Surgery

Panco Georgiev (*Associate Editor*)

With 950 Illustrations

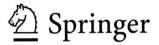 Springer

EDITORS

Pierre-Alain Clavien, MD, PhD
Department of Surgery
University Hospital Zurich
Raemistrasse 100, 8091 Zurich, Switzerland

Michael G. Sarr, MD
Department of Surgery
Division of Gastroenterologic and General Surgery
Mayo Clinic College of Medicine
200 First Street SW, Rochester, MN 55905, USA

Yuman Fong, MD
Department of Surgery
Gastric and Mixed Tumor Service
Memorial Sloan-Kettering Cancer Center
1275 York Avenue, New York, NY 10065, USA

Panco Georgiev, MD (*Associate Editor*)
Department of Surgery
University Hospital Zurich
Raemistrasse 100, 8091 Zurich, Switzerland

Madeleine Meyer (*Staff Assistant*)
Department of Surgery
University Hospital Zurich
Raemistrasse 100, 8091 Zurich, Switzerland

ISBN   978-3-540-20004-8 Springer Berlin Heidelberg New York

Library of Congress Control Number: 2006933609

Springer is a part of Springer Science+Business Media
springer.com

Editor: Gabriele M. Schröder, Heidelberg, Germany
Desk Editor: Stephanie Benko, Heidelberg, Germany
Production: LE-TEX Jelonek, Schmidt & Vöckler GbR, Leipzig, Germany
Illustrations: Jörg Kühn, Heidelberg, Germany
Cover Design: Frido Steinen-Broo, eStudio Calamar, Spain
Typesetting: am-productions GmbH, Wiesloch, Germany
Printing and Binding: Stürtz GmbH, Würzburg, Germany

Printed on acid-free paper   24/3180YL – 5 4 3 2 1 0

Acknowledgments

The creation of an atlas covering the entire scope of upper gastrointestinal and hepato-pancreato-biliary surgery is undoubtedly dependent on a team effort, which is possible only with the support and enthusiasm of many individuals. First of all, an atlas is a series of drawings, which should transmit the appropriate knowledge in an artistic way.
We are deeply indebted to Mr. Jörg Kühn, who so successfully undertook the daunting task of creating an entirely new and exhaustive visual depiction of many upper gastro-intestinal and hepato-pancreato-biliary procedures. His imagination, ingenuity, under-standing of surgical anatomy, and artistic skill have produced what we believe is the definitive rendering of today's upper gastrointestinal and hepato-pancreato-biliary operations.

A very special acknowledgment should go to Panco Georgiev. Panco is a bright young resident, who devoted an incredible amount of time and effort to coordinating and supervising the entire atlas on behalf of the Editors. We are also indebted to Madeleine Meyer, Staff Assistant in the Zurich office, who also put tireless efforts into assisting the Editors in many of their tasks.

Finally, we would like to thank the entire staff at Springer, particularly Gabriele Schröder and Stephanie Benko, as well as Judith Diemer from LE-TeX, who were very supportive from the first idea of this atlas, and maintained their enthusiasm until the end.

Pierre-Alain Clavien
Michael Sarr
Yuman Fong

Preface

Knowledge of anatomy and precise surgical technique remain the foundation of high quality surgery. A knowledgeable surgeon, equipped with excellent theoretical and clinical skills, will only be accomplished when he or she masters the operative techniques of the practice of surgery. The legacy of an academic surgeon or a surgical educator relies in great part on the transmission of his or her surgical abilities. During the last few years, we as surgical educators felt more and more that teaching surgical skills and techniques are compromised due to the plethora of new information dealing with other aspects of surgery. The number of new procedures and techniques developed since the early 1990s, for example, laparoscopic liver resection or Roux-en-Y gastric bypass, although offering obvious advantages for the patients, constitute a real technical challenge for us surgeons. Therefore, possibly more than ever before, surgeons need to acquire sound knowledge about the various surgical procedures and techniques available.

In bringing forth a new surgical atlas, we were motivated by the desire to create a comprehensive and educational atlas focusing on the upper abdomen and emphasizing all details of operative techniques including tricks from experienced surgeons. In view of the availability of many textbooks describing non-technical aspects of surgery, we purposely avoided writing a text addressing the disease processes, but instead concentrated on the operative procedures, which are evolving rapidly. The techniques described are the real message of the atlas. We standardized the text associated with each procedure, covering a list of the most common indications and contraindications, a *step-by-step* description of the procedure, a list of the most common complications, and finally the tricks of the experienced surgeon. We also included an introductory section covering the basic principles of operative surgery including operative accesses, positioning of the patient, and the use of retractors, drains, and staplers. This section, contrary to the specific procedures, was written by residents and junior staff surgeons at the University Hospital of Zurich under the direct supervision of the Editors.

While a surgeon 50 years ago could treat diseases from head to toe, this concept has evolved, and today some degree of specialization is the rule worldwide. Most countries or accrediting authorities are designing various boards for sub-specializations; indeed, after a broad training in general surgery, many young surgeons will move on further into a specific field. Upper gastrointestinal and hepato-pancreato-biliary surgery are emerging as specialized fields of general surgery, including common procedures belonging to the scope of general surgery as well as complex procedures, that should be performed only by specialized surgeons. We opted for a comprehensive approach of upper gastrointestinal and hepato-pancreato-biliary surgery, covering most open and laparoscopic procedures ranging from straightforward procedures such as laparoscopic cholecystectomy to the more complex procedures, such as spleno-renal shunt and liver or pancreas transplantation.

This *Atlas of Upper Gastrointestinal and Hepato-Pancreato-Biliary Surgery* presents illustrations created by a single artist. This approach is key to following a procedure, step-by-step, in a consistent and attractive manner. In selecting contributors from around the world, we sought surgeons who had extensive and recognized experience with the procedure. Most of the contributors are established educators and have successfully mentored many young surgeons.

The *Atlas of Upper Gastrointestinal and Hepato-Pancreato-Biliary Surgery* is subdivided into seven sections, each coordinated by a section editor in a close collaboration with the artist. A balance was achieved in each procedure to highlight the educational message in combination with the art of medical drawing. Based on the personal experience of the expert authors, a few tricks are presented at the end of each procedure. Some procedures, such as those related to portal hypertension, are becoming less popular. This atlas may contribute significantly to saving the accumulating knowledge of these demanding surgical procedures.

The *Atlas of Upper Gastrointestinal and Hepato-Pancreato-Biliary Surgery* is intended for students and residents in surgery and for fellows specializing in upper gastrointestinal and hepato-pancreato-biliary surgery preparing themselves for the operation. At the same time, this atlas will be useful for specialists and general surgeons, who may compare their techniques with the one described herein or find some additional help or tricks when performing rare procedures.

In summary, we believe that the *Atlas of Upper Gastrointestinal and Hepato-Pancreato-Biliary Surgery* is truly a new atlas, new in concept, and new in scope. We hope that specialists as well as surgeons at various levels of training will benefit from this huge effort, combining the work of many experts, a gifted artist, and the publisher.

Pierre-Alain Clavien, Zurich
Michael Sarr, Rochester
Yuman Fong, New York

Contents

Contributors

Takashi Aikou
First Department of Surgery
Kagoshima University School of Medicine
8-35-1 Sakuragaoka, Kagoshima 890-8520, Japan

Christopher D. Anderson
Department of Surgery
Division of Hepatobiliary Surgery and Liver Transplantation
Vanderbilt University Medical Center
Nashville, TN 37232, USA

Gerard V. Aranha
Department of Surgery
Loyola University Medical Center
Maywood, IL 60153, USA

Nicolas Attigah
Department of Surgery
University Hospital Zurich
Raemistrasse 100, 8091 Zurich, Switzerland

Current address:
Department of Vascular Surgery
University of Heidelberg
Im Neuenheimer Feld 110, 69120 Heidelberg, Germany

Michael M. Awad
Department of Surgery
Johns Hopkins Hospital
600 North Wolfe Street
Halsted 614, Baltimore, MD 21287, USA

Daniel Azoulay
Centre Hépato-Biliaire
Hôpital Paul Brousse
University of Paris Sud
12, Avenue Paul Vaillant Couturier, 94800 Villejuif, France

Masamichi Baba
First Department of Surgery
Kagoshima University School of Medicine
8-35-1 Sakuragaoka, Kagoshima 890-8520, Japan

Hans G. Beger
Department of Surgery
University of Ulm
Steinhoevelstrasse 9, 89070 Ulm, Germany

Jacques Belghiti
Department of Hepato-Pancreato-Biliary and Liver Transplantation
Hôpital Beaujon
100, Boulevard du Général Leclerc, 92110 Clichy, France

Richard H. Bell Jr
Department of Surgery
Feinberg School of Medicine
Northwestern University
303 East Chicago Avenue, Chicago, IL 60611–3008, USA

Laurent Biertho
Division of Laparoscopic Surgery
Mt. Sinai Medical Center
Gustave L. Levy Place, 1190 Fifth Avenue, New York, NY 10029, USA

Luigi Bonavina
UO Chirurgia Generale
Istituto Policlinico San Donato
Via Morandi 30, 20097 San Donato Milanese, Milan, Italy

Philip C. Bornman
Department of Surgery
University of Cape Town Health Sciences Faculty
Surgical Gastroenterology Unit, Groote Schuur Hospital
Observatory, 7925 Cape Town, South Africa

Karim Boudjema

Département de Chirurgie Viscérale
Unité de Chirurgie Hépatobiliaire et de Transplantation
Hôpital Pontchaillou
2, Rue Henri-Le-Guilloux, 35033 Rennes , France

Markus W. Büchler

Department of General Surgery
University Hospital of Heidelberg
Im Neuenheimer Feld 110, 69120 Heidelberg, Germany

Christoph Busch

Department of General, Visceral and Thoracic Surgery
University Hospital Hamburg-Eppendorf
Martinistrasse 52, 20246 Hamburg, Germany

Rudolf Bumm

Department of Surgery
Technical University of Munich
Ismaningerstr. 22, 81657 München, Germany

Jean-Pierre Campion

Département de Chirurgie Viscérale
Unité de Chirurgie Hépatobiliaire et de Transplantation
Hôpital Pontchaillou
2, Rue Henri-Le-Guilloux, 35033 Rennes, France

Larry C. Carey

Department of Surgery
University of South Florida College of Medicine
Tampa General Hospital
Tampa, FL 33601, USA

C. Ross Carter

Department of Surgery
Glasgow Royal Infirmary
84 Castle Street, Glasgow G4 OSF, UK

Denis Castaing

Centre Hépato-Biliaire
Hôpital Paul Brousse, 12–14
Av. Paul Vaillant Couturier, 94804 Villejuif Cedex, France

Ravi S. Chari

Department of Surgery
Division of Hepatobiliary Surgery and Liver Transplantation
Vanderbilt University Medical Center
1312 21st Ave South, 801 Oxford House, Nashville, TN 37232, USA

Daniel Cherqui

Digestive Surgery Department
Hospital Henri Mondor
University of Paris XII
51, Avenue du Maréchal de Lattre de Tassigny, 94010 Créteil Cedex, France

Michael A. Choti

Department of Surgery
Johns Hopkins Hospital
600 North Wolfe Street
Halsted 614 , Baltimore, MD 21287, USA

Elie Chouillard

Digestive Surgery Department
Hospital Henri Mondor
University of Paris XII
51, Avenue du Maréchal de Lattre de Tassigny, 94010 Créteil Cedex, France

Pierre-Alain Clavien,

Department of Surgery
University Hospital Zurich
Raemistrasse 100, 8091 Zurich, Switzerland

Chris G. Collins

Department of Surgery
Mercy University Hospital
National University of Ireland
Greenville Place, Cork, Ireland

Kevin C. Conlon
Professorial Surgical Unit
The University of Dublin
Trinity College Dublin
Adelaide and Meath Hospital Incorporating the National Children's Hospital
Tallaght, Dublin 24, Ireland

Felix Dahm
Department of Surgery
University Hospital Zurich
Raemistrasse 100, 8091 Zurich, Switzerland

Michael D'Angelica
Department of Surgery
Hepatobiliary Service
Memorial Sloan-Kettering Cancer Center
1275 York Avenue, New York, NY 10065, USA

Marco Decurtins
Department of Surgery
Kantonsspital Winterthur
Brauerstrasse 15, 8401 Winterthur, Switzerland

Carlos Fernández-del Castillo
Department of Surgery
Massachusetts General Hospital
55 Fruit Street, Boston, MA 02114, USA

Massimo Del Gaudio
Department of Surgery and Transplantation
University of Bologna
Hospital Sant' Orsola-Malpighi
Via Massarenti 9, 40138 Bologna, Italy

Nicolas Demartines
Department of Surgery
University Hospital Zurich
Raemistrasse 100, 8091 Zurich, Switzerland

Current address:
Department of Visceral Surgery
Centre Hospitalier Universitaire Vaudois CHUV
Avenue de Bugnon 46, 1011 Lausanne, Switzerland

Erwin W. Denham
Department of Surgery
Feinberg School of Medicine
Northwestern University
303 East Chicago Avenue, Chicago, IL 60611–3008, USA

Ketan M. Desai
Department of Surgery
Washington University School of Medicine
4940 Parkview, Rm 4449, WUMS Box 8109, St. Louis, MO 63110, USA

Mark Duncan
Department of Surgery
Johns Hopkins Bayview Medical Center
4940 Eastern Avenue, Baltimore, MD 21224, USA

Frederick Eckhauser
Department of Surgery
Johns Hopkins Bayview Medical Center
4940 Eastern Avenue, Baltimore, MD 21224, USA

Hiroto Egawa
Department of Transplant Surgery
Faculty of Medicine
Kyoto University
54 Kawara-cho, Shogoin, Sakyo-ku, Kyoto City, Kyoto, Japan

Claus F. Eisenberger
Department of General, Visceral and Thoracic Surgery
University Hospital Hamburg-Eppendorf
Martinistrasse 52, 20246 Hamburg, Germany

Current address:
Department of Surgery
University Hospital Düsseldorf
Moorenstrasse 5, 40225 Düsseldorf, Germany

Douglas B. Evans

Department of Surgical Oncology
University of Texas MD Anderson Cancer Center
1515 Holcombe Boulevard, Houston, TX 77030, USA

Michael B. Farnell

Department of Surgery
Mayo Clinic College of Medicine
200 First Street SW, Rochester, MN 55905, USA

Hubertus Feussner

Department of Surgery
Technical University of Munich
Ismaningerstrasse 22, 81657 München, Germany

George Fielding

Department of Surgery
Wesley Hospital
451 Coronation Drive, Auchenflower, Brisbane QLD 4066, Australia

Craig P. Fischer

Department of Surgery
University of Texas-Houston
6431 Fannin, MSB 4.294, Houston, TX 77030, USA

Yuman Fong

Department of Surgery
Gastric and Mixed Tumor Service
Memorial Sloan-Kettering Cancer Center
1275 York Avenue, New York, NY 10065, USA

Charles F. Frey

Department of Surgery
University of California
Davis Medical Center
2221 Stockton Boulevard, Sacramento, CA 95817, USA

Michel Gagner

Division of Laparoscopic Surgery
Mt. Sinai Medical Center
Gustave L. Levy Place, 1190 Fifth Avenue, New York, NY 10029, USA

Scott F. Gallagher

Department of Surgery
General Hospital
University of South Florida College of Medicine
12901 Bruce B. Downs Boulevard, Tampa, FL 33612, USA

O. James Garden

University Department of Surgery
Royal Infirmary
51 Little France Crescent, Edinburgh, EH16 4SA, United Kingdom

Karim A. Gawad

Department of General, Visceral and Thoracic Surgery
University Hospital Hamburg-Eppendorf
Martinistrasse 52, 20246 Hamburg, Germany

Panco Georgiev

Department of Surgery
University Hospital Zurich
Raemistrasse 100, 8091 Zurich, Switzerland

Tim Gessmann

Department of Surgery
University Hospital Zurich
Raemistrasse 100, 8091 Zurich, Switzerland

Jean-François Gigot

Department of Digestive Surgery
Saint-Luc University Hospital
Louvain Medical School
Avenue Hippocrate 10, 1200 Brussels, Belgium

Koroush S. Haghighi

Department of Surgery
The University of New South Wales
St. George Hospital
Gray Street, Kogarah, NSW 2217, Australia

Dieter Hahnloser

Department of Surgery
University Hospital Zurich
Raemistrasse 100, 8091 Zurich, Switzerland

Stefan Heinrich

Department of Surgery
University Hospital Zurich
Raemistrasse 100, 8091 Zurich, Switzerland

J. Michael Henderson

Department of Surgery
The Cleveland Clinic Foundation
9500 Euclid Ave/A80, Cleveland, OH 44195, USA

Ronald A. Hinder

Department of Surgery
Mayo Graduate School of Medicine
Mayo Clinic Jacksonville
4500 San Pablo Road, Jacksonville, FL 32224, USA

Stefan B. Hosch

Department of General, Visceral and Thoracic Surgery
University Hospital Hamburg-Eppendorf
Martinistrasse 52, 20246 Hamburg, Germany

Current address:
Department of Surgery
University Hospital Düsseldorf
Moorenstrasse 5, 40225 Düsseldorf, Germany

Scott G. Houghton

Department of Surgery
Division of Thoracic Surgery
Mayo Clinic College of Medicine
200 First Street SW, Rochester, MN 55905, USA

Clement W. Imrie

Department of Surgery
Glasgow Royal Infirmary
84 Castle Street, Glasgow G4 05F, United Kingdom

Jakob R. Izbicki

Department of General, Visceral and Thoracic Surgery
University Hospital Hamburg-Eppendorf
Martinistrasse 52, 20246 Hamburg, Germany

William R. Jarnagin

Department of Surgery
Hepatobiliary Service
Memorial Sloan-Kettering Cancer Center
1275 York Avenue, New York, NY 10065, USA

Johannes Jeekel

Department of General Surgery
Erasmus Medical Center
P.O. Box 2040, 3000 CA Rotterdam, The Netherlands

Sean M. Johnston

Department of Surgery
The Adelaide and Meath Hospital
Dublin, Incorporating the National Children's Hospital
Tallaght, Dublin 24, Ireland

Zakiyah N. Kadry

Department of Surgery
University Hospital Zurich
Raemistrasse 100, 8091 Zurich, Switzerland

Current adress:
Department of Surgery
Division of Transplantation MCH062
The Milton S. Hershey Medical Center
500 University Drive, Hershey, PA 17033, USA

Seiji Kawasaki

Department of Surgery
Hepato-Biliary-Pancreatic Surgery Division
University of Tokyo
7-3-1 Hongo, Bunkyo-ku, Tokyo 113-8655, Japan

Geert Kazemier

Department of General Surgery
Erasmus Medical Center
P.O. Box 2040, 3000 CA Rotterdam, The Netherlands

Marius Keel

Department of Surgery
University Hospital Zurich
Raemistrasse 100, 8091 Zurich, Switzerland

Michael L. Kendrick

Department of Gastroenterologic and General Surgery
Mayo Clinic College of Medicine
200 First Street SW, Rochester, MN 55905, USA

Yvonne Knoblauch

Department of Surgery
University Hospital Zurich
Raemistrasse 100, 8091 Zurich, Switzerland

Wolfram T. Knoefel

Department of General, Visceral and Thoracic Surgery
University Hospital Hamburg-Eppendorf
Martinistrasse 52, 20246 Hamburg, Germany

Current address:
Department of Surgery
University Hospital Düsseldorf
Moorenstrasse 5, 40225 Düsseldorf, Germany

Norihiro Kokudo

Department of Surgery
Hepato-Biliary-Pancreatic Surgery Division
University of Tokyo
7-3-1 Hongo, Bunkyo-ku, Tokyo 113-8655, Japan

Dimitris P. Korkolis

Section of Cardiothoracic Surgery
Yale-New Haven Medical Center
100 York Street, New Haven, CT 06511, USA

Lukas Krähenbühl

Department of Surgery
University Hospital Zurich
Raemistrasse 100, 8091 Zurich, Switzerland

Current address:
Lindenhofspital
Bremgartenstrasse 119, 3012 Bern, Switzerland

J.E.J. Krige

Department of Medicine
University of Cape Town Health Sciences Faculty
Groote Schuur Hospital
Observatory, 7925 Cape Town, South Africa

Asad Kutup

Department of General, Visceral and Thoracic Surgery
University Hospital Hamburg-Eppendorf
Martinistrasse 52, 20246 Hamburg, Germany

Johan F. Lange

Department of General Surgery
Erasmus Medical Center
3000 CA Rotterdam, The Netherlands

Jan Lerut

Department of Digestive Surgery
Saint-Luc University Clinics
Catholic University of Louvain
Avenue Hippocrate 10, 1200 Brussels, Belgium

Mickaël Lesurtel

Department of Surgery
University Hospital Zurich,
Raemistrasse 100, 8091 Zurich, Switzerland

Current address:
Centre de Chirurgie et de Réanimation Digestive
Hôpital Saint Antoine
184, Rue du Fbg Saint Antoine, 75570 Paris Cedex 12, France

Keith D. Lillemoe

Department of Surgery
Indiana University School of Medicine
Indianapolis, IN 46202, USA

Masatoshi Makuuchi
Department of Surgery
Hepato-Biliary-Pancreatic Surgery Division
University of Tokyo
7-3-1 Hongo, Bunkyo-ku, Tokyo 113-8655, Japan

Joseph Mamazza
Department of Surgery and Centre for Minimally Invasive Surgery
St. Michael's Hospital, University of Toronto
30 Bond Street, Toronto, ON M5B, Canada

Oliver Mann
Department of General, Visceral and Thoracic Surgery
University Hospital Hamburg-Eppendorf
Martinistrasse 52, 20246 Hamburg, Germany

Stuart Marcus
Department of Surgery
New York University School of Medicine
530 First Avenue, New York, NY 10016, USA

Kathrin Mayer
Department of Surgery
Davis Medical Center
University of California
2221 Stockton Boulevard, Sacramento, CA 95817, USA

Lucas McCormack
Department of Surgery
University Hospital Zurich
Raemistrasse 100, 8091 Zurich, Switzerland

Current address:
Department of Surgery
Hospital Alemán
Av. Pueyrredón 1640, 1118 Buenos Aires, Argentina

Juan C. Meneu Diaz
Hepatobiliary-Pancreatic Surgery Unit
'Doce de Octubre Hospital'
28041 Madrid, Spain

Miguel A. Mercado
Department of Surgery
Instituto Nacional de Ciencias Médicas y Nutrición
Salvador Zubirán
Vasco de Quiroga No. 15, 14000 Tlalpan, Mexico City, Mexico

Jürg Metzger
Department of Surgery
Chirurgische Klinik A
Kantonsspital Luzern
6000 Luzern 16, Switzerland

Jean-Marie Michel
Department of Surgery
University Hospital Zurich
Raemistrasse 100, 8091 Zurich, Switzerland

Current address:
Department of Surgery
Hôpital Cantonal Fribourg
1708 Fribourg, Switzerland

Frank G. Moody
Department of Surgery
University of Texas Medical School
6431 Fannin, Houston, TX 77030, USA

Frederick A. Moore
Department of Surgery
University of Texas-Houston
6431 Fannin, MSB 4.294, Houston, TX 77030, USA

Almudena Moreno
Elola-Olaso
Department of Surgery
"Doce de Octubre" University Hospital
Avda, Andalucia, KM 5.5, 28041 Madrid, Spain

Enrique Moreno Gonzalez

Department of General Surgery
Digestive Surgery and Abdominal Organs Transplantation
"Doce de Octubre" University Hospital
Avda, Andalucia, KM 5.5, 28041 Madrid, Spain

David L. Morris

Department of Surgery
The University of New South Wales
St. George Hospital
Gray Street, Kogarah, NSW 2217, Australia

Michel Mourad

Department of Kidney and Pancreas Transplantation
University Hospital Saint Luc
Catholic University of Louvain
Avenue Hippocrate 10, 1200 Brussels, Belgium

Markus K. Müller

Department of Surgery
University Hospital Zurich
Raemistrasse 100, 8091 Zurich, Switzerland

Michel M. Murr

Department of Surgery
University of South Florida College of Medicine
C/O Tampa General Hospital
PO Box 1289, Tampa, FL 33601, USA

David M. Nagorney

Department of Surgery
Mayo Clinic
College of Medicine
200 First Street SW, Rochester, MN 55905, USA

Eric Nakakura

Department of Surgery
Johns Hopkins Bayview Medical Center
4940 Eastern Avenue, Baltimore, MD 21224, USA

Shoji Natsugoe

First Department of Surgery
School of Medicine
Kagoshima University
8-35-1 Sakuragaoka, Kagoshima 890-8520, Japan

William H. Nealon

Department of Surgery
University of Texas Medical Branch
Galveston, TX 77555-0544, USA

Yuji Nimura

Division of Surgical Oncology
Department of Surgery
Nagoya University Graduate School of Medicine
65 Tsurumai-cho Showa-ku, Nagoya 466-8550, Japan

Jeffrey A. Norton

Department of Surgery
Stanford University Medical Center
300 Pasteur Drive, Stanford, CA 94305, USA

Marshall J. Orloff

Department of Surgery
University of California San Diego
Medical Center
San Diego, CA 92103–8999, USA

Mark S. Orloff

Department of Surgery
Section of Organ Transplantation
University of Rochester Medical Center
601 Elmwood Ave, Rochester, NY 14627, USA

Susan L. Orloff

Department of Surgery
Section of Hepatobiliary and Pancreas Surgery and Transplantation
Oregon Health Science University
3181 S.W. Sam Jackson Park Road, Portland, OR 97239-3098, USA

Hector Orozco
Department of Surgery
Instituto Nacional de Ciencias Médicas y Nutrición
Salvador Zubirán
Vasco de Quiroga No. 15, 14000 Tlalpan, Mexico City, Mexico

Gerald C. O'Sullivan
Department of Surgery
Mercy University Hospital
National University of Ireland
Grenville Place, Cork, Ireland

Robert Padbury
Department of Surgery School of Medicine
Flinders Medical Research Institute
The Flinders University of South Australia
GPO Box 2100, Adelaide, SA 5001, Australia

Theodore N. Pappas
Department of Surgery
Duke University Medical Center
3479, Durham, NC 27710, USA

Claudio Pasquali
Department for Medical Sciences and Surgery
Universita degli Studi di Padova
Sezione di Semeiotica Chirugica
Ospedale Busonera, 35128 Padova, Italy

Sergio Pedrazzoli
Department for Medical Sciences and Surgery
Universita degli Studi di Padova
Sezione di Semeiotica Chirurgica
Ospedale Busonera, 35128 Padova, Italy

Matthias Peiper
Department of General, Visceral and Thoracic Surgery
University Hospital Hamburg-Eppendorf
Martinistrasse 52, 20246 Hamburg, Germany

Current address:
Department of Surgery
University Hospital Düsseldorf
Moorenstrasse 5, 40225 Düsseldorf, Germany

Alberto Peracchia
Department of Surgery
Centro di Formazione Universitaria
Istituto Clinico Humanitas
Via Manzoni, 56, 20089 Rozzano (MI), Italy

Henrik Petrowsky
Department of Surgery
University Hospital Zurich
Raemistrasse 100, 8091 Zurich, Switzerland

Capecomorin S. Pitchumoni
Department of Surgery
Saint Peter's University Hospital
Robert Wood Johnson School of Medicine
New Brunswick, NJ 08903, USA

Robert J. Porte
Department of Surgery
Section of Hepatobiliary Surgery and Liver Transplantation
University Hospital Groningen
PO Box 30.001, 9700 RB Groningen, The Netherlands

Eric C. Poulin
Department of Surgery and Centre for Minimally Invasive Surgery
St. Michael's Hospital
University of Toronto
30 Bond Street, Toronto, ON M5B, Canada

Bettina Rau
Department of General Surgery
University Hospital of Ulm
Steinhoevelstrasse 9, 89070 Ulm, Germany

Chandrajit P. Raut

Department of Surgical Oncology
University of Texas MD Anderson Cancer Center
1515 Holcombe Boulevard, Houston, TX 77030, USA

Xavier Rogiers

Department of General Surgery
HPB Surgery and Organ Transplantation
Gent University Hospital and Medical School, UZG
De Pintelaan 185 - 2K12 1C, 9000 Gent, Belgium

Alexander S. Rosemurgy II

Department of Surgery
University of South Florida
PO Box 1289, Tampa, FL 33601, USA

Joachim Ruh

Department of General, Visceral and Thoracic Surgery
University Hospital Hamburg-Eppendorf
Martinistrasse 52, 20246 Hamburg, Germany

Barry Salky

Division of Laparoscopic Surgery
Mt. Sinai Medical Center
Gustave L. Levy Place, 1190 Fifth Avenue, New York, NY 10029, USA

Juan M. Sarmiento

Division of Gastroenterologic and General Surgery
Emory University School of Medicine
1440 Clifton Road N.E., Atlanta, GA 30322, USA

Michael G. Sarr

Department of Surgery
Division of Gastroenterologic and General Surgery
Mayo Clinic College of Medicine
200 First Street SW, Rochester, MN 55905, USA

Mitsuru Sasako

Gastric Surgery Division
National Cancer Center Hospital
5-1-1 Tsukiji, Chuo-ku, Tokyo, Japan

Olivier Scatton

Department of Hepato-Bilio-Pancreatic Surgery and Transplantation
Hôpital Beaujon
University of Paris VII
100, Boulevard du Général Leclerc, 92110 Clichy, France

Markus Schäfer

Department of Surgery
University Hospital Zurich
Raemistrasse 100, 8091 Zurich, Switzerland

Christopher M. Schlachta

Department of Surgery and Centre for Minimally Invasive Surgery
St. Michael's Hospital
University of Toronto
30 Bond Street, Toronto, ON M5B, Canada

Wolfgang Schlosser

Department of General Surgery
University Hospital of Surgery
Steinhövelstrasse 9, 89075 Ulm, Germany

Rainer Schmelzle

Department of Oral and Maxillofacial Surgery
(Nordwestdeutsche Kieferklinik)
University Hospital Hamburg-Eppendorf
Martinistrasse 52, 20246 Hamburg, Germany

Uwe Seitz

Department of Interdisciplinary Endoscopy
University Hospital Hamburg-Eppendorf
Martinistrasse 52, 20246 Hamburg, Germany

Markus Selzner

Department of Surgery
University Hospital Zurich
Raemistrasse 100, 8091 Zurich, Switzerland

Current address:
Department of Surgery
Toronto General Hospital
200 Elizabeth Street, Toronto, Ontario M5G 2C4, Canada

Peter Shamamian
Department of Surgery
New York University School of Medicine
530 First Avenue, New York, NY 10016, USA

Bhugwan Singh
Department of General Surgery
Faculty of Health Sciences
Nelson R. Mandela School of Medicine
University of Natal
Congella, South Africa

Hans Sollinger
Department of Surgery
Division of Organ Transplantation
University of Wisconsin School of Medicine
Clinical Science Center - H4,
600 Highland Ave, Madison, WI 53792, USA

Nathaniel J. Soper
Department of Surgery
Northwestern University
201 E. Huren Street, Galter 10-105, Chicago, IL 60611, USA

Cosimo Sperti
Department of Medical Sciences and Surgery
Universita degli Studi di Padova
Sezione di Semeiotica Chirurgica
Ospedale Busonera, 35128 Padova, Italy

Henricus B.A.C.
Stockmann
Department of General Surgery
Erasmus Medical Center
P.O. Box 2040, 3000 CA Rotterdam, The Netherlands

Steven M. Strasberg
Department of Surgery
Section of Hepatobiliary-Pancreatic and Gastrointestinal Surgery
Washington University in Saint Louis
1 Barnes Hospital Plaza, St. Louis, MO 63110, USA

Tim Strate
Department of General, Visceral and Thoracic Surgery
University Hospital Hamburg-Eppendorf
Martinistrasse 52, 20246 Hamburg, Germany

Oliver Strobel
Department of General Surgery
University of Heidelberg
Im Neuenheimer Feld 110, 69120 Heidelberg, Germany

Koichi Tanaka
Department of Transplant Surgery
Faculty of Medicine
Kyoto University
54 Kawara-cho, Shogoin, Sakyo-ku, Kyoto City, Kyoto, Japan

Rebecca Taylor
Department of Surgery
Gastric and Mixed Tumor Service
Memorial Sloan-Kettering Cancer Center
1275 York Avenue, New York, NY 10065, USA

Geoffrey B. Thompson
Department of Surgery
Mayo Clinic College of Medicine
200 First Street NW, Rochester, MN 55905, USA

Benjamin N.J. Thomson
Peter MacCallum Cancer Centre and Royal Melbourne Hospital
Locked Bag 1, A'Beckett Street, Victoria 8006, Australia

L. William Traverso
Department of General, Vascular and Thoracic Surgery
Virginia Mason Medical Center
1100 Ninth Ave, Seattle, WA 98111, USA

John Tsiaoussis
Department of General Surgery
Unit of Gastrointestinal Surgery
University Hospital
Heraklion, Crete, Greece

Gregory G. Tsiotos

Department of General Surgery
Metropolitan Hospital
217 Alexandras Ave, Athens 11521, Greece

Waldemar Uhl

Department of General Surgery
University of Heidelberg
Im Neuenheimer Feld 110, 69120 Heidelberg, Germany

Jean-Nicolas Vauthey

Department of Surgical Oncology
University of Texas MD Anderson Cancer Center
1515 Holcombe Boulevard, Houston, TX 77030, USA

Miranda Voss

Department of Surgery
Duke University School of Medicine
Box 3110, Durham, NC 27710, USA

Andrew L. Warshaw

Department of Surgery
Harvard Medical School
Massachusetts General Hospital
55 Fruit Street, White Building, Boston, MA 02114-2696, USA

David I. Watson

Department of Surgery
Flinders Medical Centre
Bedford Park, South Australia 5042, Australia

Lawrence W. Way

Department of Surgery
University of California
School of Medicine
San Francisco, CA 94143, USA

Stefan Wildi

Department of Surgery
University Hospital Zurich
Raemistrasse 100, 8091 Zurich, Switzerland

Emre Yekebas

Department of General, Visceral and Thoracic Surgery
University Hospital Hamburg-Eppendorf
Martinistrasse 52, 20246 Hamburg, Germany

Tina W.F. Yen

Department of Surgical Oncology
University of Texas MD Anderson Cancer Center
1515 Holcombe Boulevard, Houston, TX 77030, USA

General Principles

Pierre-Alain Clavien
Michael G. Sarr

Introduction

Pierre A. Clavien, Michael G. Sarr

A competent surgeon must be aware of all the general aspects of a surgical procedure to be able to perform specific interventions successfully and expeditiously. The old adage that "exposure, exposure, and exposure" are the three most important factors for the good outcome of a surgical procedure remains true for both open and laparoscopic approaches.

Each procedure must start with careful positioning of the patient prior to wide disinfection of the operative field, draping, and incision. The first chapter covers the various options for positioning of the patient on the operating table and describes the incisions that are available to enter the abdominal cavity. The second chapter focuses on different principles of exposure through the use of various types of retractors, providing examples of the most commonly used retractors. The third chapter addresses the use of mechanical staplers. Currently, staplers are increasingly being used for many open and laparoscopic procedures, and the industry has partnered actively with the surgical field in developing new devices enabling sophisticated maneuvers, often to reach otherwise small and inaccessible areas. Proper knowledge of the general principles of the use and function of mechanical staplers is mandatory for modern surgery, because their misuse may result in devastating complications such as anastomotic leakage or bleeding. Finally, while Billroth claimed more than a century ago that "drainage saves many lives," the use of the "time-honored" surgical drain has changed dramatically, because accumulating studies have shown convincingly that drains are often useless or even harmful in many procedures. Open drains are rarely needed today. The last chapter presents the principles of the various types of drains including a table of "evidence-based" utility of drains for upper abdominal surgery.

These chapters covering the general aspects of surgery were prepared in a simple, yet comprehensive manner. We believe that the didactic and basic information provided in these introductory chapters of the Atlas will be of value for both trainees and specialized surgeons.

Positioning and Accesses

Yvonne Knoblauch, Dieter Hahnloser

Positioning

Correct and stable positioning of the patient is the first step for a successful operation. Safe arm and leg positioning are crucial in preventing pressure lesions, such as ulnar or peroneal neuropathy.

Supine Position

The supine position is used for most abdominal procedures. The arms can be left out (A-1) or kept close to the body (A-2), depending on the type of operation to be performed.
- Anchor the patient's legs and/or ankles with a strap in case tilt is required
- Protect arms with a pillowcase, gauze sponge, or silicone pad
- Avoid traction on the brachial plexus (abduction of the shoulder should be <90°)

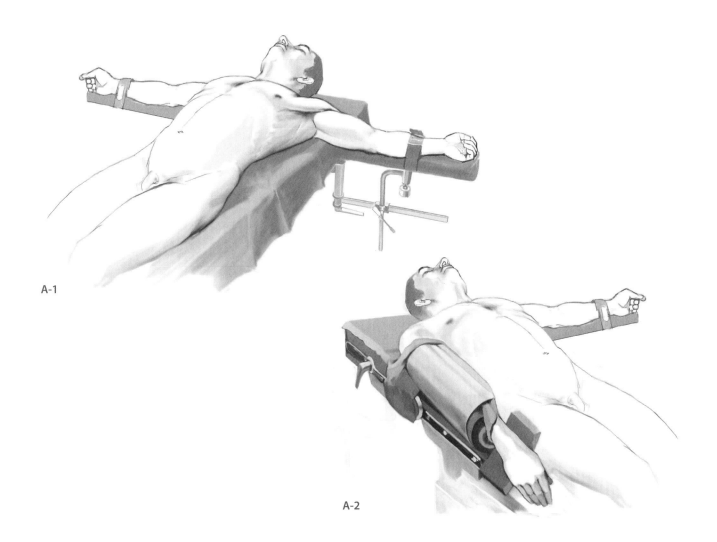

A-1

A-2

French Position

The French position is one possible patient position for a laparoscopic cholecystectomy (the "American" supine position with both arms tucked alongside the body being the other).

- The patient's legs are placed in stirrups or supported under the knee
- Legs need to be placed horizontally or slightly declining to allow free movements with laparoscopic tools
- Avoid any pressure on the peroneal (lateral popliteal) nerve

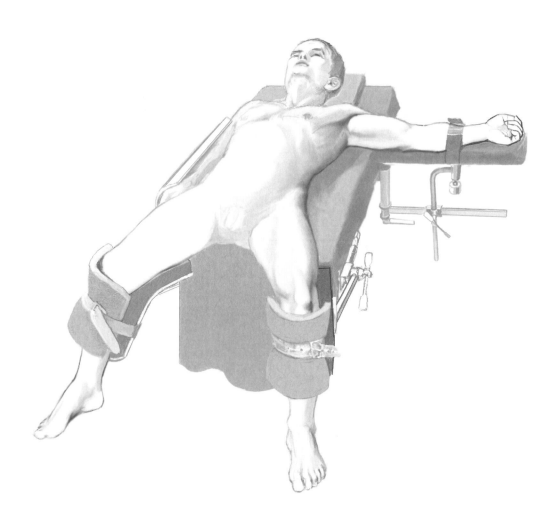

Beach Chair Position

The beach chair position is used for most laparoscopic obesity surgery procedures
- Requires a special weight-bearing table
- The patient is "sitting" on the table
- Avoid any pressure on arms, the brachial plexus, and the peroneal (lateral popliteal) nerve

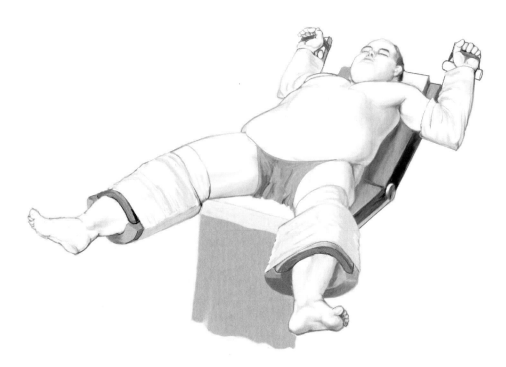

Positioning for Esophageal Surgery

For esophageal resection and reconstruction, several approaches can be used. Depending on the location of the disease and the surgical approach, the positioning is adapted accordingly.

The positions used are:
a) *Supine* position with overextended thoracic spine, the head rotated to the right and extended. The right arm is left out and the left arm is tucked alongside the body (**A**). This position is commonly used for transhiatal esophagectomies enabling:
   - Good exposure of the upper abdomen
   - Good exposure for the cervical anastomosis
b) *Right or left lateral decubitus* (**B**)
   - For the intrathoracic anastomosis
   - Procedures on the upper thoracic esophagus are approached via a right posterolateral thoracotomy, and similar procedures on the lower esophagus are best approached through the same incision on the left side
   - The table is slightly kinked at the thoracic level, further opening the thoracic cavity after thoracotomy
c) *45° lateral decubitus or screw position* (**C**)
   - An advantage is that the abdominal, the thoracic, and/or cervical phase of the procedure can be performed without changing the position
   - For optimal access, the operating table can be tilted
   - The main disadvantage is a more limited exposure

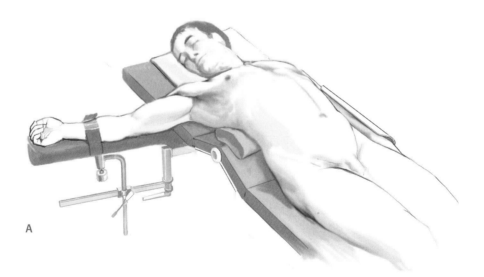

A

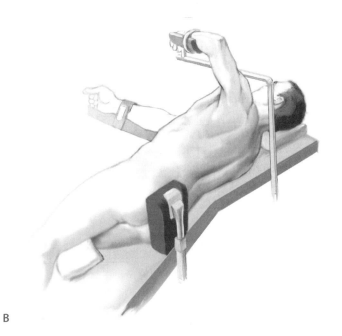

B

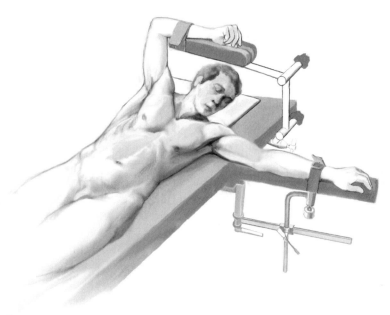

C

Incisions

Abdomen

The choice of the approach for entering the abdominal cavity depends upon:
- The accuracy of the preoperative diagnosis
- The location and extent of the disease
- Previous scars
- The requirement of a possible extension of the incision
- Anatomic structures, such as skin, fascia, muscles, nerves, and blood vessels. The abdominal wall should stay functional. Whenever possible, incisions are placed along the skin split lines, also called the lines of Langer, and muscles and fascia are divided along their fibers

Mark the incision prior to cutting to prevent malpositioning

Midline Incision

The midline incision is the most expedient choice for opening the abdomen and provides unrestricted access, regardless of the patient's size or shape (including exposure of the pelvis). The advantages of a midline incision are:
- Can be extended into a median sternotomy
- Minimal blood loss
- No muscle fibers are divided
- No nerves are injured
- Is suitable for repeated celiotomies
- Offers best exposure in an emergency situation with unclear diagnosis

The Steps
- Place skin incision exactly in the midline, above and below the umbilicus from the tip of the xiphoid to the pubis (extension as needed) (A-1)
- Deflect the incision around the umbilicus to the left or the right. The evasion of the umbilicus on the left side is preferred, because of possible rudimentary umbilical vessels. In general, use the opposite side of the umbilicus if an ostomy is planned
- The scalpel or the cautery can be used all the way
- By pulling the wound, the fat spreads and the midline plane separates down to the fascia (A-2, A-3)
- Apply digital pressure to minimize bleeding
- Incise the fascia with the scalpel or cautery just above or below the umbilicus, as the linea alba is widest around the umbilicus
- Gently lift up the peritoneum with pickups before opening to avoid small bowel lesions (A-4)
- Care to incise the linea alba without exposing the rectus muscles markedly facilitates the closure

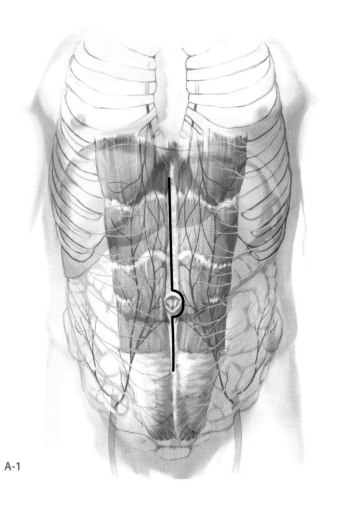

A-1

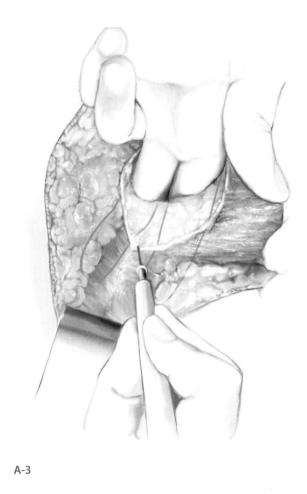

A-3

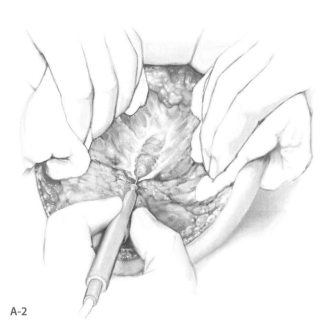

A-2

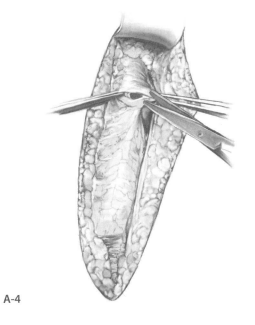

A-4

Subcostal Incision (A-1)

The subcostal incision is usually made for cholecystectomy or common bile duct exploration (right subcostal incision) and for elective splenectomy (left subcostal incision). The major advantage of the subcostal incisions over the upper midline incision are greater lateral exposure and less pain. The disadvantage is that the operation takes longer, because there are more layers to close. The subcostal incision generally heals well with little risk of hernia formation.

The Steps

- Place skin incision two finger breadths below the costal margin. This facilitates closure so that the incision line is not on or over the costal margin
- Incise the anterior and posterior sheet of the rectus muscle. The muscle is cut slowly with the cautery (A-2); care should be taken to ligate or cauterize the inferior epigastric vessels
- Laterally, the fascia of the transverse muscle may need to be cut
- Try not to incise the fascia in the midline, but if necessary, extend the incision medially

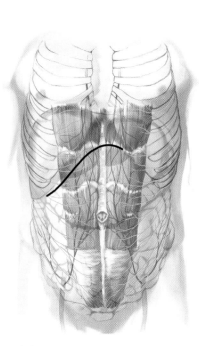

A-1

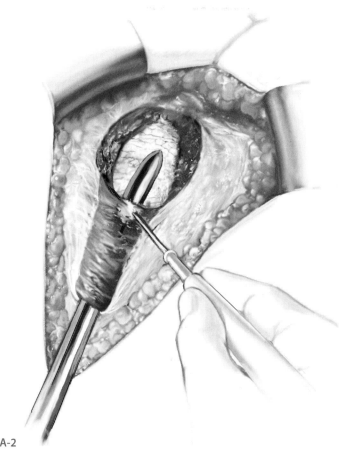

A-2

Bilateral Subcostal Incision

The bilateral subcostal incision is used to access the liver for transplant and major liver resections. Also, most pancreas resections are performed with this incision. The exposure is often helped with a vertical extension to the xiphoid (the so-called "Mercedes star" incision).

The Steps
- Incision of skin and fascia as described above
- For pancreas resections, the incision is generally placed three to four finger breadths below the costal margin
- Mobilization of the liver begins with the division of the falciform ligament (the liver's reflection of peritoneum with the anterior wall)
- Division of the round ligament (a fibrous cord resulting from the obliteration of the umbilical vein), which should be ligated to avoid bleeding, particularly in the presence of portal hypertension
- It is preferable to mobilize the liver prior to the use of stationary retractors to reduce the necessity of frequent repositioning

J-shaped Incision

The J-shaped incision is used most frequently for surgery on the right liver (see page 374). This incision provides a particularly good access to the area between the inferior vena cava and the right hepatic vein. The J-shaped incision can be extended laterally to a thoracotomy for better exposure.

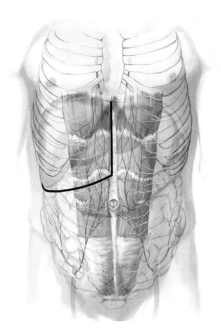

Esophageal Surgery

Like the various positions used in esophageal surgery, there are different incisions used depending on the location of the disease, the level of the anastomosis, and the surgeon's preference. Most of the time, a combination of two or more of the following incisions are used:

a) *Upper midline laparotomy*
   - As described in the previous section on the abdomen
   - Can be combined with a transverse laparotomy for better exposure

b) *Thoracotomy*
   - Anterolateral: skin incision usually in the fourth or fifth intercostal space
   - Posterolateral: skin incision in the seventh intercostal space at the angle of the scapula (A-1). A paravertebral or anterior extension is possible
   - The intercostal muscle is freed from the upper border of the rib (avoids damaging the intercostal nerve and blood vessels, which lie behind the inferior border of the rib) (A-2)
   - The parietal pleura is opened with scissors, and the ribs are separated with a retractor

c) *Cervical incision* (B-1)
   - Incision along the anterior border of the sternocleidomastoid muscle (B-2)
   - Division of the platysma in the direction of the incision
   - The omohyoid muscle (B-3) and, if necessary, the inferior thyroid artery and/or middle thyroid vein are divided to provide clear exposure
   - The sternocleidomastoid muscle and carotid sheath and its contents are retracted laterally, and the trachea and larynx are retracted medially
   - No retractor should be placed against the recurrent laryngeal nerve in the tracheoesophageal groove during the entire cervical phase of the procedure
   - For better exposure, the medial part of the sternocleidomastoid muscle can be cut inferiorly close to the clavicle bone
   - Identification of the flat, decompressed esophagus can be helped by inserting a large tube into the esophagus by the anesthesiologist
   - In patients with a "bull neck" habitus or with osteoarthritis preventing extension of the neck, a partial upper sternal split can provide the prerequisite access to the high retrosternal esophagus

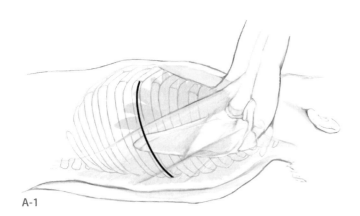

A-1

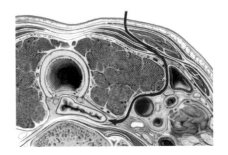

B-1

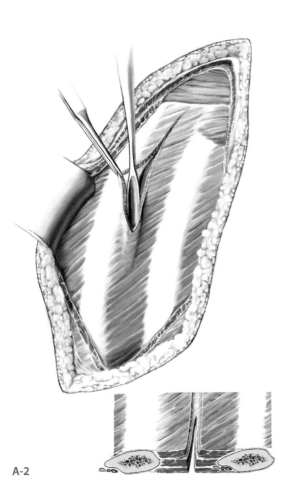

A-2

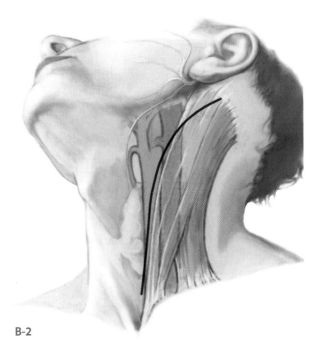

B-2

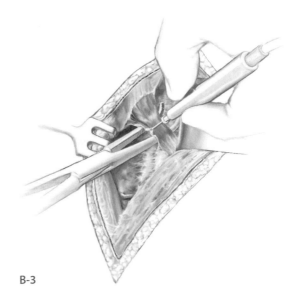

B-3

Laparoscopic Surgery

Establishing Pneumoperitoneum

Pneumoperitoneum can be established using a Veress needle or by an open approach. The open technique is generally preferred, as it minimizes the risks of inherent lesions to the small bowel. However, in obese patients, the Veress needle is used, as the thick subcutis does not allow visualization of the fascia through a 1–2 cm incision.

Gaining Access with a Veress Needle

- Incision of the skin (generally infraumbilical in the midline) and blunt dissection of the subcutaneous tissue
- The fascia is grasped with a hook retractor or a Kocher clamp and is pulled anteriorly (A-1)
- Before inserting the Veress needle, its correct functioning must be checked
- Insertion of the needle at a 90° angle to the abdominal wall. As the needle's spring-loaded safety mechanism crosses the abdominal fascia and then the peritoneum, two clicks are heard and are usually felt
- Verification of the needle's intraperitoneal location by injecting 3 ml of saline with no resistance (A-2) followed by the "hanging drop" test (A-3) (i.e., a drop of saline is placed on the top of the needle, which is sucked into the needle when the abdominal fascia is lifted up)
- Pneumoperitoneum. When a pressure of 13–15 mmHg is reached, the Veress needle is withdrawn, and a sharp-tipped camera trocar is blindly inserted through the same incision

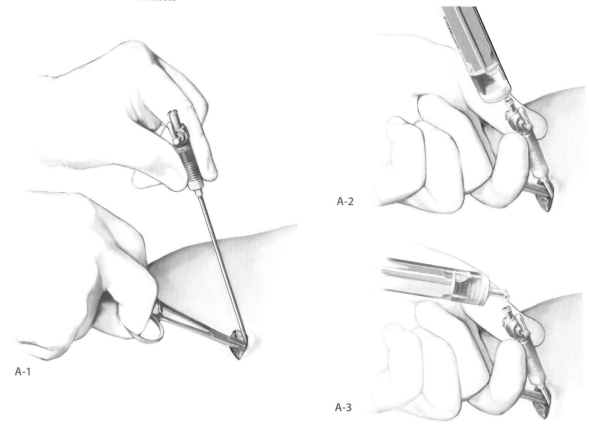

A-1

A-2

A-3

Gaining Access with the Open Technique

- Incision of the skin (generally infraumbilical in the midline) and blunt dissection of the subcutaneous tissue
- Incision of the fascia (1–2 cm) and opening of the peritoneum with scissors (two sutures can be placed to lift up the abdominal wall and to later secure the port) (A-1)
- Entry into the abdominal cavity is easily confirmed by inserting a finger
- A blunt-tipped camera trocar is inserted and fixed with the two sutures if needed (A-2)

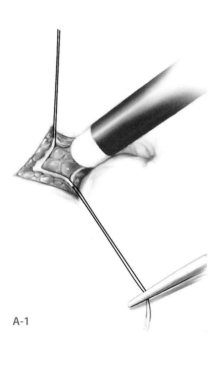

A-1

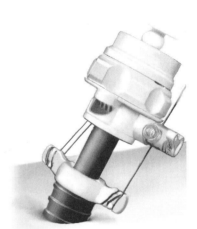

A-2

Placement of Accessory Ports

Selecting the insertion sites of working trocars is dependent on the procedure to be performed and also depends on the surgeon's preference, the patient's body habitus, and the presence or absence of previous scars or intra-abdominal adhesions.

The Steps
- The size of the skin incision must be planned carefully. If the incision is too small, friction will develop between the skin and the port, and greater force will be required for insertion, which will increase the risk of uncontrolled insertion. If the incision is too large, gas may leak and the port may dislocate more easily
- Transillumination of the skin can help to avoid cutting through major blood vessels (A-1)
- The trocar is optimally inserted by holding it between the index and the middle fingers. The shaft of the trocar should also be supported by the opposite hand as the body wall is traversed (A-2)

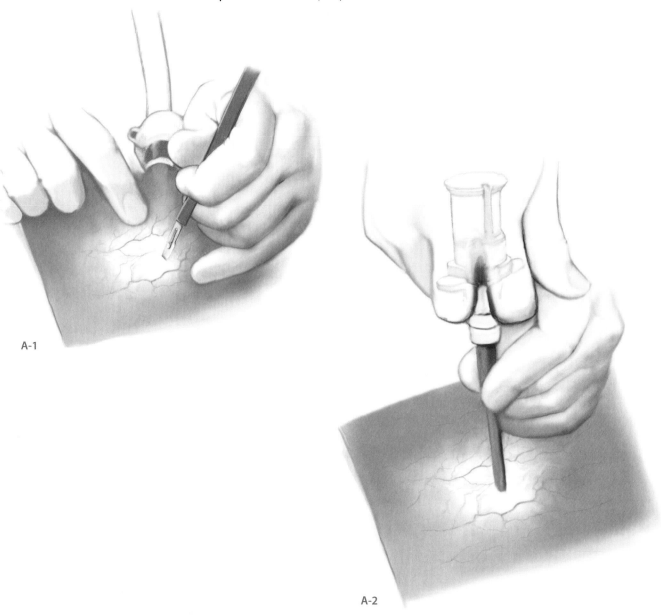

A-1

A-2

Closures

General
- the length of the suture material should be 4:1 to the length of the wound
- avoid excessive tension on the suture closure of the fascial edgestraction as it may compromise vascularization of the wound edges
- below the umbilicus, the posterior fascia (rostral to the smi-circular line caudal to which there is no posterior rectus fascia) and then the anterior fascia of the rectus abdominis muscle can bei closed as separate layers
- Grasp the needle with the tip of the instrument

Midline Laparotomy
- The fascia is closed with a running loop of monofilament, absorbable suture material (e.g., PDS II-1 loop or Maxon-1 loop) with or without inclusion of the peritoneum
- The subcutaneous fatty layer is not closed and subcutaneous drains are rarely needed
- The skin is preferably closed with a running intracutaneous absorbable monofilament suture (e.g., Maxon 5-0) or with staples

Subcostal Incision
- In contrast to the midline laparotomy, the fascia should be closed in two layers

Trocar Wound Closure
- Ports are removed under direct vision with the camera and port sites should be routinely watched for 10s to exclude port site bleeding
- All fascial defects of trocars greater than 5mm are closed with absorbable sutures (e.g., Vicryl 0)
- The skin is closed with interrupted mattress sutures (e.g., Dermalon 4-0) or with staples

Tricks of the Senior Surgeon

- The surgeon should personally check the correct positioning of the patient and the adequate protection of the extremities before draping.
- Marking the incision site before the beginning of the procedure is useful for teaching and prevents malpositioning.
- The incision should always be large enough to guarantee good visualization of the operative fields and to guarantee a safe and efficient operation
- Avoid extensive traction on the wound edges, as it may compromise healing.
- Place trocars carefully according to the operative need and according to the body habitus of the patient (eg. obesity).
- Visualize the port site for at least 10s after removal of the trocar to check for bleeding.

Tim Gessmann, Markus Schäfer

Principles of Surgical Exposure

Introduction

Adequate exposure of the target organ represents a laudable prerequisite of every successful operation. Therefore, it is worthwhile to be equipped with different retractors and to invest enough time intraoperatively to optimize exposure. Basic principles of exposure have recently been challenged by the advent of minimally invasive surgery. However, minimally invasive surgery has only changed the means of surgical access; the procedures performed at the target organs remain largely unchanged. In contrast to open surgery, exposure during laparoscopy is achieved predominantly by patient position and trocar placement. Retractor systems are less important.

Retractor Systems

In general, a retractor system needs to fulfill the following requirements for an ideal surgical exposure:

- Broad, unrestricted view into the abdominal cavity
- Wide access to the target organ
- Illumination provided or enabled
- Stable retraction of the abdominal wall and surrounding organs
- Careful tissue retraction, preventing local ischemia
- Freeing up the hands of the surgeon and assistants
- Adaptability in usage (different patients, different incisions, etc.)
- Various type of accessories to retract the abdominal wall and organs

Hand-held retractors have the main disadvantage of losing „free hands" of the surgical team. Self-retaining retractors are most commonly used to keep open the abdominal and thoracic cavity.

Two types of self-retaining retractors are available:

1. *Closed ring retractors:*
   Ring system retractors are self-stabilizing by the retaining force of the different retracting devices and do not necessarily need to be fixed to the operating table (e.g. Kirschner, **A**). The best exposure is achieved by placing one retracting device strictly opposite to the other. In some systems, stabilization and exposure can further be improved by attaching the ring to the operating table by a rail arm.
2. *Arm retractors:*
   Arm retractors need to be fixed to the operating table. They allow for an asymmetric exposure (e.g. Thompson, **B**).

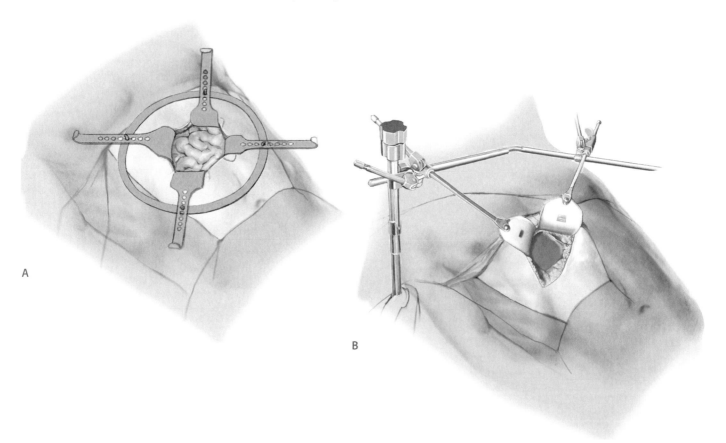

A

B

Overview of Different Self-Retaining Retractors

Thompson (previous page, see figure B)

The basic compounds of this very stable retracting system are the rail arm, the two rods, and the different retracting paddles that are attached to a retaining arm. The Thompson retractor is favored for uni- and bilateral subcostal incisions, which are often used for hepatobiliary procedures, in which most of the retraction required is oriented cephalic and anteriorly. The exposure of the lower abdominal parts is limited. There is a wide range of blades and paddles available as accessories.

Bookwalter (C)

This system has a frame (closed ring) fixed by a rail arm attached to the operating table. Different retracting accessories, such as blades and paddles, are available that can be clamped to the frame. The Bookwalter retracting system is used for both longitudinal and transverse abdominal incisions. Although some training is necessary to achieve a safe installation, fine adjustment is possible in three dimensions. Cleaning and sterilization need substantial effort due to the rather complex single components.

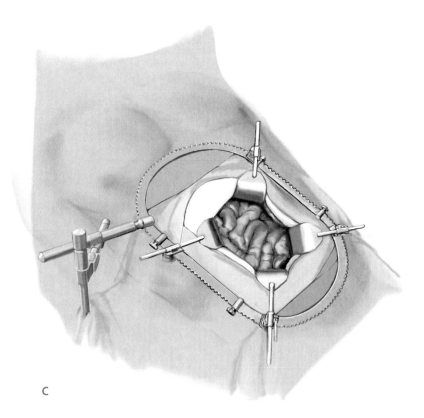

C

Omnitract

Although this retractor system needs precise installation, it offers excellent access for most incisions. The open frame system can easily be completed to a closed ring. This retractor can be used widely for intraperitoneal and retroperitoneal operations. Maintenance and cleaning are not too elaborate. The figure shows longitudinal (A-1) and transverse (A-2) laparotomy using the Omnitract system.

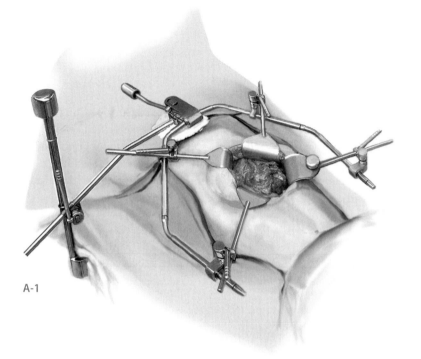

A-1

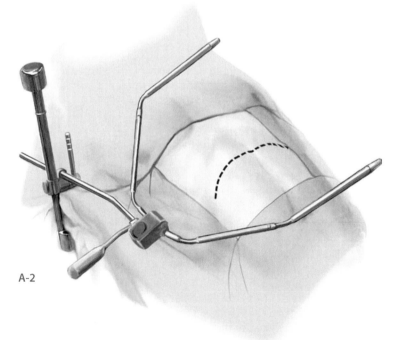

A-2

Rochard

The Rochard retractor (not shown) is a single blade retractor that is mainly used for upper GI surgery. A large semicircular blade retracts the abdominal wall, and is attached to a fixed arm at the operating table. The main disadvantages are the unidirectional tension and the lack of lifting the abdominal wall.

Kirschner, Balfour, O'Sullivan-O'Conner (A, B)

The Kirschner frame (A) and the Balfour retractor (B) are good examples of systems that do not need any form of rail arm. However, retraction is not as stable and tension in the vertical dimension is not possible. They are rapidly usable, readily available, and are preferred when only lateral exposure is desired.

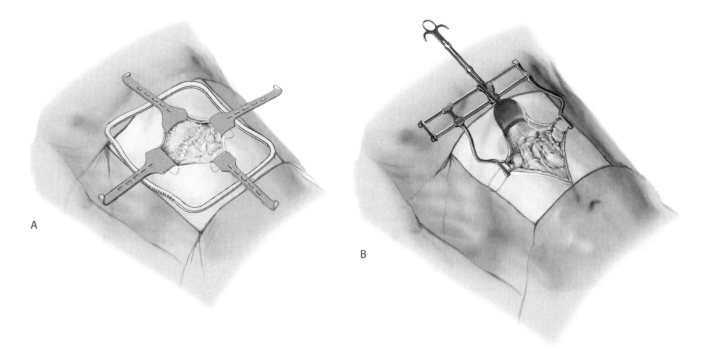

A

B

Recommendation
Many factors and aspects influence the choice of a specific retractor. Some commonly used retractors are compared in *Table* 1. More than one type of retractor should be available to obtain the best possible exposure of the different parts of the abdominal cavity.

Table 1. Comparison of different retractor systems

System	Construction	Installation	Adjustment	Accessories	Maintenance
Bookwalter	Closing ring and fixation	Complex	Three dimensions	+++	Elaborate
Thompson	Arm	Complex	Three dimensions	+++	Elaborate
Omnitract	Arm	Complex	Three dimensions	+++	Elaborate
Rochard	Arm	Complex	Tension only in one direction	+	Elaborate
Kirschner	Closing ring	Quick	Limited	++	Easy
Balfour	Closing ring	Quick	Limited	+	Easy

Retractors in Laparoscopic Surgery

Whereas the abdominal wall is lifted by the pneumoperitoneum, intra-abdominal exposure is achieved primarily by patient positioning and trocar placement. There are several devices that may be used to retract the liver during upper GI operations, such as laparoscopic fundoplication, gastric bypass, or adrenalectomy.

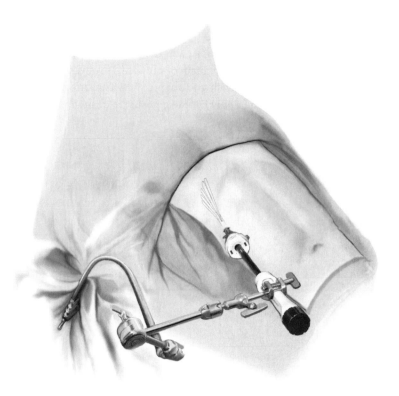

Tricks of the Senior Surgeon

- For optimal use, be familiar with several retractors and have a good knowledge of their individual advantages.
- Slow, incremental retraction prevents rib fractures and postoperative pain.
- Intermittent release of the retraction during long duration operations prevents local ischemic complications.

Surgical Staplers

Nicolas Attigah, Markus Schäfer

Introduction

Stapling devices belong to the standard repertoire of modern gastrointestinal surgery, especially since the successful advent of minimally invasive surgery. Therefore, a thorough knowledge and safe handling of stapling devices need to be acquired early during surgical training.

History

Based on the main principles of mechanical stapling, (Table 1) Hültl from Budapest, Hungary, developed the first linear stapler in 1909 to close the remnant stomach during gastrectomies. The handling of that instrument was hampered by its weight and bulk. Petz, another Hungarian surgeon, and Friedrich and Neuffer from Germany created lighter and more convenient stapling instruments during the 1920s. Driven by the lack of surgeons after World War II, the Russian government encouraged the development of different mechanical devices for linear and circular stapling to help less well-trained surgeons to safely perform standardized surgical procedures, e.g., gastrectomies and bowel resections.

In the 1960s, the American surgeon Ravitch brought those instruments to the United States and focused on their improvement in terms of applicability and reliability. In partnership with industry, preloaded plastic cartridges, double-staggered staple lines, and different lengths of staple lines were developed. Since the mid-1970s, single-patient-use stapling devices have become widespread worldwide.

The success of minimally invasive surgery promoted the development of miniaturized stapling devices during the past decade; such devices are now used routinely in many different operations.

Types of Mechanical Staplers

There are currently three major types of mechanical stapling devices in clinical use for open and laparoscopic surgery. As described in Tables 1 and 2, the principles and prerequisites of mechanical stapling remain largely unchanged.

Table 1. Principles of mechanical stapling

Tissue compression
Tissue stapling using metallic wire as staples
Configuration of the closed staples in B-shape
Staggered positioning of the staple lines

Table 2. Aims of surgical stapling

Creation of an adequate lumen
Preserving adequate tissue vascularization
Preventing tension of adapting tissues
Avoiding leakage and fistula formation
Provision of good hemostasis
Mechanical reliability/uniformity of stapling devices

Linear Stapler or TIA Stapler (Transverse Anastomosis Stapler)

Linear staplers are predominantly used to close the ends of a hollow organ or vessel. They are claimed to give easier access to narrow anatomic sites such as the pelvis. For such applications, linear staplers with articulated heads and flexible shafts have been developed. These staplers normally apply two lines of staples that are staggered to maximize local blood supply. Vascular linear staplers apply three staggered lines of staples to achieve tight closure of the vessel. The staple height is either fixed or, with some brands of stapler, can be "adjusted" during the application. For most applications, the use of a fixed staple height is preferred. Because linear staplers are mainly used to close open organs, they do not include a cutting device.

The length of the stapler lines varies between 30 mm and 90 mm, while the height of individual staples varies from 2.5 mm to 4.8 mm, depending on the tissue to be stapled (e.g., vascular staples = 2.5 mm; staples for normal intestinal tissue = 3.5 mm; for stomach or thicker tissues = 4.8 mm).

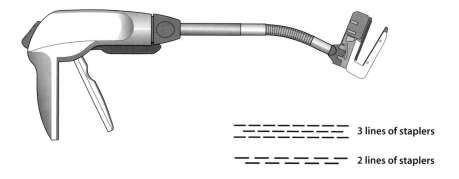

3 lines of staplers

2 lines of staplers

Linear Cutter or GIA Stapler (Gastrointestinal Anastomosis Stapler, A)

These staplers are basically linear staplers with an integrated cutting device. Four staggered lines of staples (two "rows") are applied, and the tissue between the two inner staple lines is transected. The main indications are transecting and stapling closed both ends of a hollow organ (e.g., bowel, bronchus) or vascular structure. In addition, because of the two separate rows of staples, side-to-side anastomoses can be created. The staple height is fixed and must be chosen before using the instrument in accordance to the type of tissue. Different staple sizes and wire diameters are available in preloaded, single-use cartridges.

The length of the staple lines varies between 55 mm and 100 mm for open surgery.

Specially designed linear cutters have been developed for minimally invasive surgery (B). Articulated heads are often used to overcome angulations related to the trocar positioning.

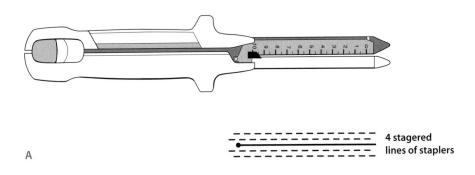

4 stagered
lines of staplers

A

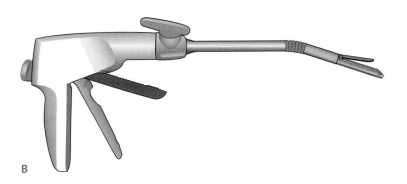

B

Circular Stapler

These staplers apply two staggered circular lines (one "row") of staples. The cutting device transects the tissue inside the staple lines. The staple height is also variable, depending on the tissue thickness. Circular staplers are used mainly for end-to-end and end-to-side anastomoses of the esophagus, stomach, and rectum.

Circular staplers are available with various diameters, ranging from 21 mm to 33 mm. It should be noted that the true (inner) diameter of the created anastomosis is somewhat smaller (range 12.4–24.4 mm). In order to avoid mucosal tears, sizers should be used to estimate the diameter of the respective hollow organ. The anvil must be secured by a proper purse-string suture which is applied intraluminally to create the anastomosis.

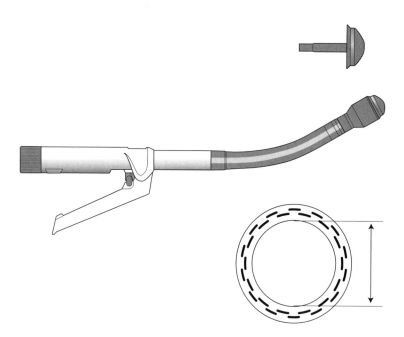

Staples

Design Type of Staplers (Table 3)

The most commonly used staples have a rectangular shape and are preloaded in cartridges. The staples are pushed through the tissue under the pressure created by closing the stapler. Once they reach the anvil, the staples are buckled or bent into the final B-shape. The B-form allows both the firm connection and sufficient vascularization of the adapted tissue. Note that the "height" of the staples after the instrument is "fired" is smaller.

In order to achieve a safe anastomosis or closure, the staple height should be adapted to the thickness of the tissue. The staple height is indicated by different colors of cartridges. The majority of staplers in current use are equipped with a fixed staple height.

The staple height is fixed for linear cutters, whereas linear staplers and circular staplers may have somewhat variable staple heights that can be adapted intraoperatively, according to the type of tissue.

Table 3. Staple characteristics and applications

Cartridge type	Vascular	Standard	Thick
Color	White	Blue	Green
Staple height	Fixed	Fixed	Fixed
Before B formation	2.5 mm	3.5 mm	4.8 mm
After B formation	1.0 mm	1.5 mm	2.0 mm
Applications	Thin tissues	Esophagus	Rectum
	Well-vascularized tissues	Small bowel	Stomach
	Vessels	Large bowel	Bronchus
	Pancreas	Lung	
	Liver		

Technical Aspects

Whereas at the beginning of the stapler era, staples were made of silver and steel, current stapler technology uses titanium. Titanium has better biocompatibility and causes fewer artifacts during CT and MRI. Furthermore, titanium is not affected by static magnetic fields and shows only a minimal temperature rise during MRI. The wire thickness has also been reduced to 0.2–0.3 mm.

Tricks of the Senior Surgeon

- The surgeon must be familiar with the different types of stapling devices. Incorrect handling, not stapler misfunction, remains a major cause of failure.
- Stapling instruments should not be used on ischemic, necrotic, or markedly edematous or inflamed tissue, because tissue closure and anastomosis formation cannot be achieved safely.
- Adjacent adipose tissue from the serosal surface must be removed before firing the stapler.
- To prevent leakage and postoperative peritonitis, every anastomosis must be checked.

Principles of Drainage

Henrik Petrowsky, Stefan Wildi

Introduction

Drains are designated to evacuate intraperitoneal fluid collections. They can be used for diagnostic, prophylactic, or therapeutic purposes. In upper gastrointestinal surgery, diagnostic drains are mainly placed to assess intraperitoneal fluid collections in order to establish a diagnosis. These drains are seldom left in place and are, therefore, of minor importance. In contrast, prophylactic drains placed at the end of an operation are used frequently with two intentions: first, to prevent fluid accumulations which could be harmful (i.e., pancreatic juice or bile) or to evacuate fluid collections that can become infected and lead to the formation of intra-abdominal abscesses; second, prophylactic drains may be used to detect early postoperative complications, such as intra-abdominal bleeding or anastomotic leakage. Sometimes, fluid collections become infected and develop into abscesses; the management of these collections requires therapeutic drainage either by the percutaneous route or by reoperative surgical lavage.

Types of Drain

Drains can be divided into passive and active drains.

Passive Drains

Passive drains, such as the Penrose (A-1) and Easy Flow (A-2) devices, serve to evacuate fluid passively by providing a route of access secondary to the natural pressure gradients, such as gravity flow, muscle contraction, and overflow. The opening in the abdominal wall for these drains should be made large enough, because passive drains are potentially collapsible. Easy Flow drains have intraluminal corrugations to prevent complete collapse (inlay). Passive drains cannot be sealed and are open systems with the potential risk of retrograde infections. The advantages and disadvantages of open and closed-suction drains are outlined in Table 1.

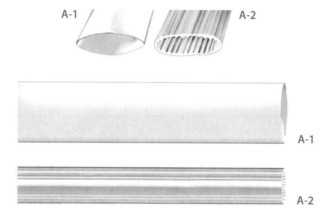

Aktive Drains

Jackson-Pratt (A-1) and Blake (A-2) drains are commonly used radiopaque, silicone products for closed-suction systems. The Jackson-Pratt drain is oval-shaped with numerous orifices and intraluminal corrugations (inlay). The Blake drain has four channels along the sides with a solid core center. In contrast to passive drains, active or suction drains maintain a negative pressure gradient.

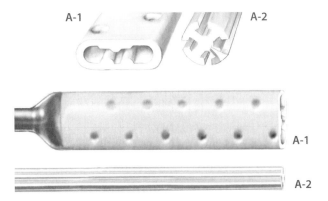

Sump Drains

Sump drains are usually double-lumen tubes with a larger outflow lumen and a smaller inflow "sump" lumen. The larger lumen is connected to a suction system and evacuates intra-abdominal secretions. The smaller lumen serves as a venting tube, allowing air to enter the larger lumen. This principle should help to break the vacuum in the large draining tube, maintaining the drain in a productive state, without the surrounding tissues continually occluding the drainage holes in the tube. Sump drains are often used when large fluid volumes have to be evacuated. The occlusion of the smaller venting tube by tissue debris due to retrograde inflow demonstrates a potential disadvantage of sump drains that occurs especially when the suction is disconnected. Some sump drains have an additional third lumen that allows the instillation of an irrigating solution.

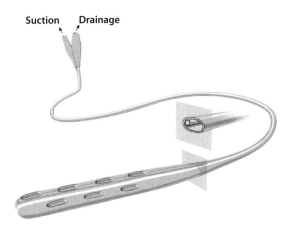

Complete Drainage System

Collapsible devices connected to the drain tubes automatically generate a negative pressure gradient and keep the system "sealed," which is believed to result in a significant reduction of retrograde infections.

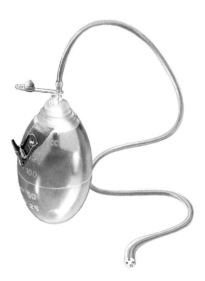

Table 1. Advantages and disadvantages of open and closed-suction drains

	Open drain	Closed-suction drain
Advantages	Generates pathways for bulky or viscous material	Lowers risk of retrograde infection
	Lowers risk of mechanical erosion and pressure necrosis	Accurate measurement of drainage
		Facilitates radiographic studies
		Skin protection from irritating discharge
Disadvantages	Retrograde infection	More vulnerable to obstruction by small tissue fragments or ingrowth of surrounding tissue

Prophylactic Drainage

Drain Orifice

The drain orifice through the skin is created by a penetrating cut with a scalpel (A-1).
A Kelly clamp is inserted into the orifice (A-2) and penetrates the abdominal wall
diagonally (A-3). The hand serves as protection to prevent bowel injury. This technique
creates a tunnel that helps to seal the abdominal cavity after drain removal. After
clamping the drain tip, the Kelly clamp and drain are pulled through the abdominal
wall from inside outwards (A-4). Others prefer to create the tunnel from inside out
and pull the drain into the abdomen. Finally, the drain position
is secured by a non-reactive skin suture, and the drain tube is connected to the suction
device.

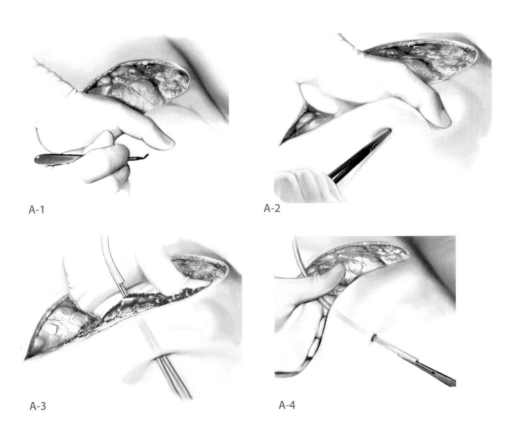

A-1

A-2

A-3

A-4

Prophylactic Drains

Prophylactic drainage after upper abdominal operations is used to evacuate intra-
abdominal fluid that may develop, such as ascites, blood, chyle, bile, pancreatic,
or intestinal juice, that are either harmful/toxic for adjacent tissue or might become
infected. Therefore, drains are placed in spaces that tend to accumulate fluid, such
as the subhepatic (1), right subphrenic (2), left subphrenic (3), and parapancreatic (4)
spaces.

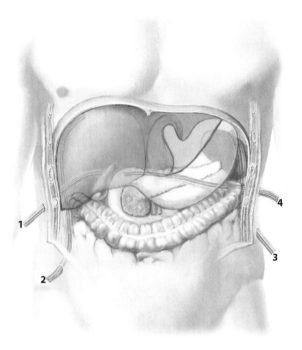

Anastomosis Drains

Another proposed function of prophylactic drainage is the early detection of anastomotic leakage. If drains are to be used near a high-risk anastomosis, it is important that they are not placed in direct contact with the anastomosis, but, rather, with a safety margin in between to prevent drain-related erosions. This principle is illustrated for a biliodigestive anastomosis, where the drain is placed posterior to the anastomosis.

Although the routine use of prophylactic drainage has often been considered as a method to prevent complications, there is growing evidence that this practice may be associated with adverse effects. Retrograde drain infections or drain-related complications are known adverse effects. Several randomized, controlled trials are available investigating the routine use of prophylactic drainage (Table 2).

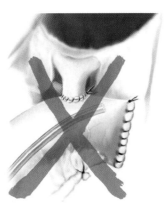 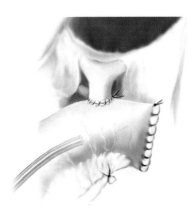

Table 2. Evidence-based recommendations for prophylactic drainage practice

Gastrointestinal surgery	Procedures	Evidence-based recommendation
Hepato-pancreatico-biliary	Hepatic resection without biliodigestive anastomosis	No drain
	Cholecystectomy (open, laparoscopic)	No drain
	Pancreatic resection	No drain[a]
	Biliodigestive anastomosis	NA
Upper GI tract	Esophageal resections	Intrathoracic drain for any approach
	Total gastrectomy	Drain
	Distal gastrectomy	No drain
	Roux-en-Y gastric bypass	NA
	Duodenotomy with omental patch for duodenal perforation	No drain

NA not assessed
[a]Only one randomized controlled trial in pancreatic cancer

Therapeutic Drainage

Predisposed Spaces for Collections

Infected collections, such as abscesses or infected bilomas, are known complications after upper abdominal surgery and require drainage by operative or radiologically guided drain placement. The right subphrenic space (1), left subphrenic space (2), Morison's pouch (3), left subhepatic space (4), and omental sac (5) are anatomic spaces that predispose to abscess development.

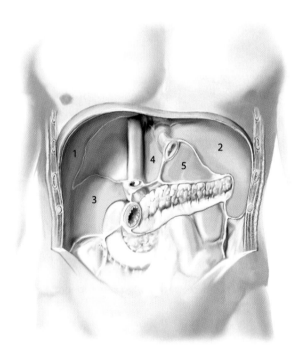

Catheters

The majority of postoperative collections in the upper abdomen are manageable by means of percutaneous drainage by interventional radiologic techniques using standard aseptic technique and local anesthesia. Thereby, collections are drained percutaneously under ultrasonographic or CT guidance using the Seldinger or trocar techniques. This figure illustrates a typical percutaneous drainage catheter, the MAC-LOC (A-1) that can be inserted by the introduction cannula (A-2) or the trocar stylet (A-3). The catheter has large, oval side ports to increase the drainage capability, as well as a radiopaque band that helps to identify the proximal area of the loop. This type of "self-locking" loop catheter has "memory," i.e., the loop at the end can be straightened during insertion by introducing a stylet intraluminally. After the catheter is positioned in place, the stylet is removed, and the loop reforms. This loop prevents displacement of the catheter.

Some fluid collections may require surgical drainage with repeated abdominal lavage and second-look procedures (Table 3).

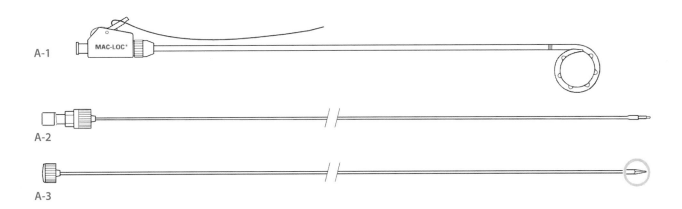

Table 3. Criteria for percutaneous and surgical drainage of infected collections

Percutaneous drainage	Surgical drainage
Unilocular collection/abscess	Multilocular collections/abscesses
Low viscosity of drain fluid	Multiple, non-communicating collections
Drain route not traversing intra-abdominal organs or thorax	High viscosity of drain fluid
	Percutaneous drain route traversing intra-abdominal organs or thorax

Tricks of the Senior Surgeon

- Whenever indicated, always use closed drain systems and keep drains as short as possible to minimize the risk of retrograde infections.
- Place drains near but never in direct contact to the anastomotic sutures to prevent drain-induced erosions or drain-induced anastomotic leaks.
- When drains are not productive, do not rely on them! Drains could be occluded or obstructed by adjacent tissue.
- Try to position intraperitoneal drains such that the drain does not rub against or lie in direct contact with blood vessels or hollow organs in an attempt to prevent drain erosions.

Esophagus, Stomach and Duodenum

Jakob R. Izbicki

Introduction

Jakob R. Izbicki

This section presents the ambitious field of open and laparoscopic surgery in benign and malignant diseases of the esophagus, stomach and duodenum.

Attempts to treat esophageal cancer surgically emerged at the beginning of the twentieth century. Torek successfully resected the thoracic esophagus in 1913, but real progress came as a result of the development of thoracic surgery during and after the Second World War. The concept of extensive lymph node resection in combination with en bloc esophagectomy was proposed by Logan in 1963 but with considerable morbidity and mortality.

However, surgical procedures, pre- and postoperative management and treatment, and prognosis after surgical treatment have improved considerably in the past 3 decades. Expertise of the surgeon and the institution, patient selection, choice and radicality of operation, and pre- and postoperative care are the most important parameters for outcome.

For this reason, the first eight chapters present a comprehensive survey of the different open and laparoscopic surgical procedures, indications, and choice of operation in esophageal cancer. They give clear guidelines as to how and when to operate with regard to the biological characteristics of the tumor. The focus then turns to benign esophageal diseases such as diverticula, strictures, and achalasia.

The following chapters address the techniques of esophago-gastric, subtotal and total gastric resections in benign and malignant diseases, respectively. Four chapters then outline the open and laparoscopic strategies in the case of palliation such as gastroenterostomy and gastrostomy. Next the laparoscopic procedure is described as the gold standard for gastroesophageal reflux, and then the open approach is covered followed by different laparoscopic techniques for hiatal repair in paraesophageal hernia. Another chapter comprehensively covers the available strategies for morbid obesity, and the last chapter in the section deals with the ambitious pancreas-sparing duodenectomy.

The section has been prepared by experts in their surgical fields, and we hope that it will provide the reader with a comprehensive overview of current surgical standards for the various procedures.

Cervical Esophagectomy

Wolfram T. Knoefel, Rainer Schmelzle

Introduction

Cervical esophagectomy for neoplasia includes removal of the cervical part of the esophagus combined with cervical lymphadenectomy and reconstruction by interposition of a free jejunal transplant with microvascular anastomoses.

Resection of a segment of up to 3 cm can be performed with primary anastomosis of the esophagus after adequate mobilization.

Indications and Contraindications

Indications

- Cervical esophageal neoplasia
- Benign esophageal stricture

Contraindications

- Local irresectability (infiltration of larynx, trachea or vertebrae)
- Multifocal lesions
- Distant metastasis
- Florid gastroduodenal ulcer
- Crohn's disease

Preoperative Investigation/Preparation for the Procedure

History:	Risk factors (alcohol, nicotine), previous radiation therapy, concomitant malignancy, Crohn's disease
Clinical evaluation:	Recurrent laryngeal nerve status, cervical lymphadenopathy
Endoscopy:	Esophagogastroduodenoscopy (EGD) to rule out multifocal lesions and gastroduodenal ulcer
CT scan or MRI:	Assessment of stage and resectability (include thorax and abdomen!)
Doppler ultrasound:	Vascular status in the neck
PET scan:	Exclude further lesions
Laboratory test:	SCC antigen, coagulation parameters
Avoid:	Central venous line on the side of anastomoses, wall stents

Procedure

Access

For the cervical part a unilateral or bilateral (U-) incision at the medial margin of the sternocleidomastoid muscle is performed. It extends from the margo inferior of the mandible to the jugulum, where it meets with the contralateral side. For cervical-mediastinal lymph node dissection, the incision is combined with a partial or complete median sternotomy. For harvesting the transplant, a small upper abdominal transverse incision is sufficient.

Exposure

Retraction is performed by hand held retractors of different shapes and sizes according to the anatomy. If available, a self-retaining retraction system will help.

STEP 1   **Preparation of the cervical region**

After transection of the platysma, the sternocleidomastoid muscle is retracted and the omohyoid muscle is divided. Along with the internal jugular vein, the common carotid artery and the vagal nerve are identified along the entire length of the incision and a lymphadenectomy around these structures is performed. This preparation is facilitated by the use of a pair of fine bipolar scissors. The superior thyroid artery can be preserved for reconstruction. From the carotid artery the anterior longitudinal ligament is reached and the posterior dissection of the cervical esophagus is completed under vision. After mobilization of the left (or right) thyroid lobe the recurrent nerve and the parathyroids are identified and preserved. Injuries to the recurrent nerve should be repaired immediately. Autotransplantation of dissected parathyroids should be performed in the forearm if radiation therapy is an option.

Quite frequently a hemithyroidectomy facilitates the further procedure significantly. Now the posterior aspect of the trachea is dissected and after identification of the contralateral recurrent nerve the cervical esophagus is completely mobilized from the hypopharynx to the upper thoracic aperture or below.

Occasionally the identification of important blood vessels can only be guaranteed using intraoperative Doppler ultrasound. Especially following extensive tumor resections of the oropharyngeal region, vast alterations of the typical anatomy must be expected. Injuries of the thoracic duct can lead to the development of persistent fistulas associated with significant fluid loss, protracted by a previous radiotherapy.

In cases of extensive tumor growth that warrant resection, more extensive procedures may become necessary, e.g., larynx or trachea.

Before resection, place retaining sutures on the potential proximal and distal stump.

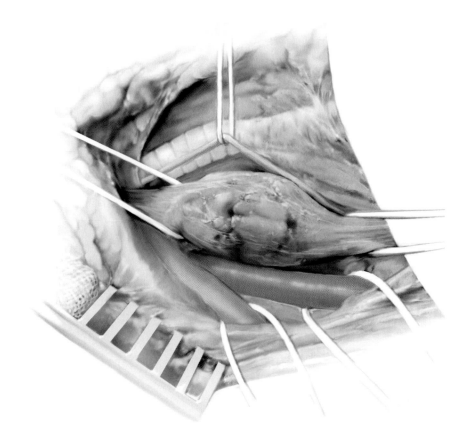

STEP 2

Transection of the esophagus

The cervical esophagus is transected and the nasogastric tube withdrawn to the level of the neck so that the specimen can be removed. Confirm free margins by frozen section on both sides. In case negative margins cannot be achieved, an esophagectomy should be performed.

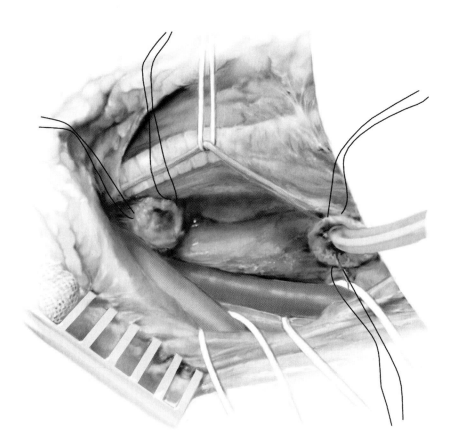

STEP 3	Preparation of the jejunal loop

The jejunal loop is harvested after exploration of the abdominal cavity with sufficient arterial and venous length and lumen. If the mesentery is very thick, a meticulous removal of fatty tissue may enable diaphanoscopy. However, under diaphanoscopy an artery and a vein of sufficient length and lumen are identified. After clamping on the mesenteric side and excision of the graft, the artery is flushed with heparinized saline until the venous outflow is clear.

If the vascular pedicle or one of the vessels are too short, it becomes necessary to harvest a venous or arterial interponate. The primary source for viable venous interponates is the forearm, whereas for the artery the saphenous vein can be employed. Vessels harvested from the arm or foot region are equally suitable for the arterial interponate whereas the saphenous vein, due to its dimension and susceptibility to spasm, proves to be hardly suitable for venous interpositioning and should thus only be reserved for arterial lengthening. At times it is very difficult to differentiate between the artery and the vein in the intestinal flap. To avoid confusing the two, prior to harvesting, the artery or vein should be unmistakably marked.

An end-to-end jejunostomy is performed to reconstruct the bowel, and the abdomen is closed without drainage.

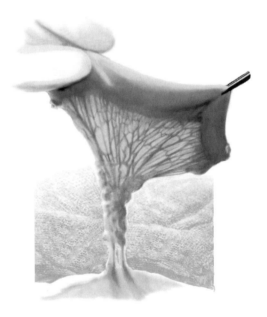

STEP 4   **Vascular anastomoses**

The venous and arterial anastomoses are now performed. First the vein is anastomosed.

Preferably a confluens of the major mesenteric vein with a smaller contributing vein is used on the side of the graft and the internal jugular vein on the other side. The incision in the internal jugular vein should be at least 3–4 mm long. The anastomosis is performed under a magnification of at least ×4, preferably with a microscope. Running sutures with non-resorbable, monofilament material, 7-0 or 8-0, are used. Before closure, the anastomosis is rinsed with heparinized saline.

The vein should only be anastomosed before the artery if an expedient progression of the operation is evident. Should delays occur, e.g., difficulties during the preparation or unforeseen anesthesiological circumstances in conjunction with unstable cardiovascular parameters, the artery should be anastomosed prior to the vein, allowing a perfusion of the intestinal flap with nutrient rich blood until peristalsis returns. If the nature of the delay prevents the anastomoses, the harvested intestinal flap should be stored in moist dressings. If desired, the metabolic rate of the temporary non-perfused flap can be decreased by cooling the flap. Routinely, there is no necessity for the use of organ preservation solutions.

The same technique is used for the artery. The anastomosis can be performed on the superior thyroid artery (often quite small), the thyrocervical trunk or the common carotid artery directly. Rarely other cervical branches like the lingual artery are used.

It is extremely important to avoid kinking and compression especially on the vein during placement of the graft into the neck, and during closure of the neck.

If the vascular reconstruction fails, either a second loop can be harvested or a gastric tube can be fashioned.

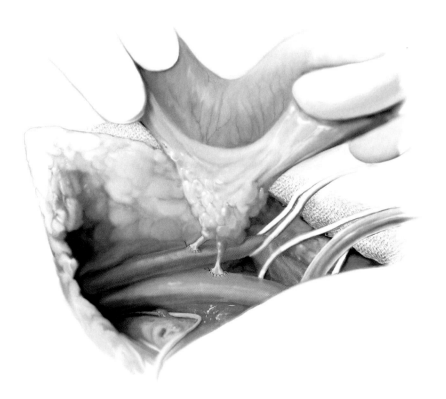

STEP 5

Esophagojejunal anastomoses

After reperfusion an adequate flow is confirmed. Then the lower and finally the upper esophagojejunal anastomoses are performed end-to-end or end-to-side after shortening the graft to an adequate length. These anastomoses are performed using 3-0 or 4-0 absorbable sutures in a single layer. It is important to grasp the entire thickness of the pharynx or esophagus, whereas the stitches in the jejunum are extramucosal. If the anatomy is demanding, e.g., a very low intrathoracic anastomosis, the suture can be performed in an interrupted fashion. The nasogastric tube is then placed through the graft into the stomach.

It is important to implant the graft in an isoperistaltic fashion to facilitate swallowing. Even under optimal conditions, it can take weeks before the graft gains normal transplant function.

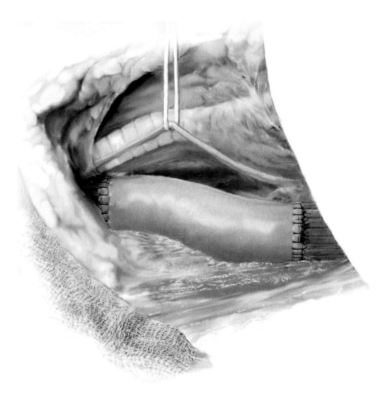

STEP 6

Final aspects

The neck is drained sufficiently from both sides with at least one soft easy flow drain on each side. The neck is closed by loose interrupted subcutaneous and skin stitches.

For the postoperative follow-up, it is advantageous to ensure that parts of the jejunal graft are clinically visible. This can either be achieved by placing a few sutures in a manner such as to allow a division of the covering tissue or by configuring the flap so as to leave parts of the flap uncovered, serving as a "monitor" during the postoperative surveillance. Verification of the blood flow can be performed using Doppler ultrasound. As an adjunct, various tissue probes are available, facilitating the measurement of the oxygen partial pressure.

Standard Postoperative Investigations

- Anticoagulation (PTT 60–70 s)
- Maintain mean arterial blood pressure of 70–80 mmHg
- Monitoring of microcirculation and improved rheology
- Daily Doppler ultrasound
- Regular inspection of the flap on postoperative day 1 every hour

Postoperative Complications

- Venous thrombosis (reoperate immediately)
- Arterial thrombosis (reoperate immediately)
- Necrosis of the transplant (excise and drain by pharyngostomy or reconstruct with gastric tube or colon)
- Salivary leak (drain adequately)
- Lymphatic leak
- Recurrent laryngeal nerve injury
- Esophageal stenosis (dilate by endoscopy) (long term)
- Poor swallowing function (long term)

Tricks of the Senior Surgeon

- Be aggressive to reoperate if vascular status is questionable.
- Avoid kinking of the vein by keeping it short.
- Keep CVP high and perform adequate heparinization to avoid vascular problems.
- Leave the neck open if the jejunum is congested after reperfusion but cover the vessels with tissue.
- If the exposure for vascular reconstruction becomes difficult, perform a hemithyroidectomy.
- Occasionally a partial sternotomy may enable a safer inferior esophageal anastomosis.
- Lymphatic leak can be managed conservatively; only rarely the lymphatic duct must be ligated.
- Exposure can be facilitated by division of the medial head of the sternocleido-mastoid muscle.
- Previous surgery with resection of the internal jugular vein necessitates dissection down to the subclavian vein.

Left Thoracoabdominal Approach for Carcinoma of the Lower Esophagus and Gastric Cardia

Shoji Natsugoe, Masamichi Baba, Takashi Aikou

Introduction

Tumors located aborally to the carina, i.e., Barrett's carcinoma or carcinoma of the esophagogastric junction, may be removed by a left-sided thoracotomy instead of the more usual right-sided access combined with an abdominal approach. The extent of lymphadenectomy is limited to the middle and lower mediastinum.

Indications and Contraindications

Indications

- Tumors of the infracarinal esophagus
- Tumors of the esophagogastric junction

Contraindications

- See chapter on "Subtotal Esophagectomy: Transhiatal Approach"
- High risk patients

Preoperative Investigation/Preparation for the Procedure

- See chapter on "Subtotal Esophagectomy: Transhiatal Approach"

Procedure

Access
- Spiral positioning of the patient with 45° elevation of the left thorax
- Rotating the operating table for the thoracic part/abdominal part

STEP 1   **Thoracotomy**

The skin incision is made obliquely from the epigastrium toward the sixth or seventh intercostal space, and a good exposure of the mediastinum or abdomen can be achieved by rotating the operating table. After 1 cm of costal cartilage is resected, the left side of the chest is opened. Distant and peritoneal metastases should be excluded prior to thoracotomy.

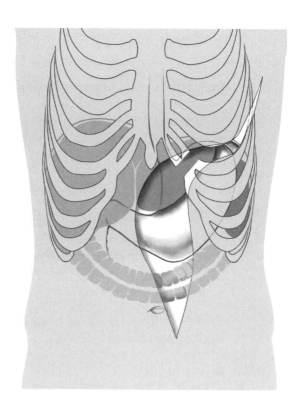

STEP 2   Diaphragmatomy and mobilization of the colon

Para-aortic lymphadenectomy is performed by delivering the splenic flexure into the
chest through an incision in the peripheral diaphragm. The descending colon is then
mobilized down the left paracolic gutter to the base of the sigmoid colon mesentery.
After mobilization of the left kidney from the retroperitoneum as well as pancreas
and spleen, the left renal vein is identified.

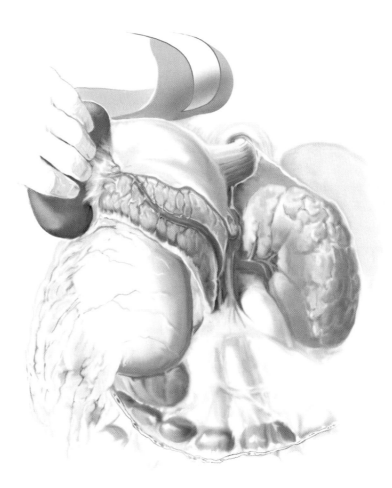

STEP 3   **Para-aortic lymph node removal**

The para-aortic lymph nodes in the left lateral region are then dissected, and the right lateral para-aortic lymph nodes are removed after performing a Kocher maneuver.

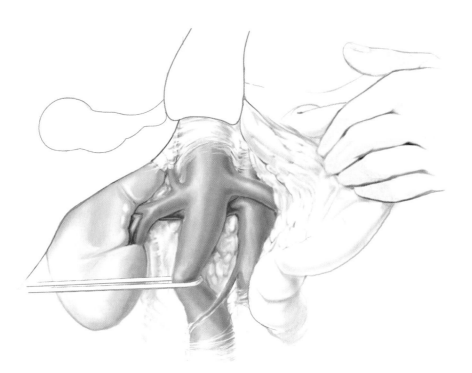

STEP 4   Lymph node removal of the upper abdomen

Lymph nodes of the hepatoduodenal ligament and around the common hepatic artery, left gastric artery and celiac trunk are dissected.

Mobilization of the stomach and transection of the duodenum (see chapter "Total Gastrectomy with Conventional Lymphadenectomy")

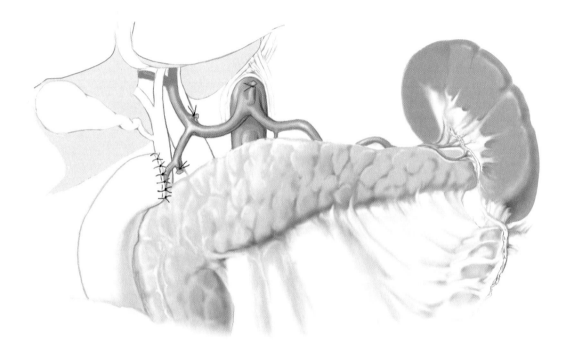

STEP 5   **Lower mediastinal lymph node removal**

Regarding the left intrathoracic approach, the left pulmonary ligament is divided and the mediastinal pleura is opened. The pleura covering the lower thoracic esophagus is incised, allowing the clearance of loose connective tissue together with the lower thoracic paraesophageal, supradiaphragmatic, posterior mediastinal and intradiaphragmatic lymph nodes.

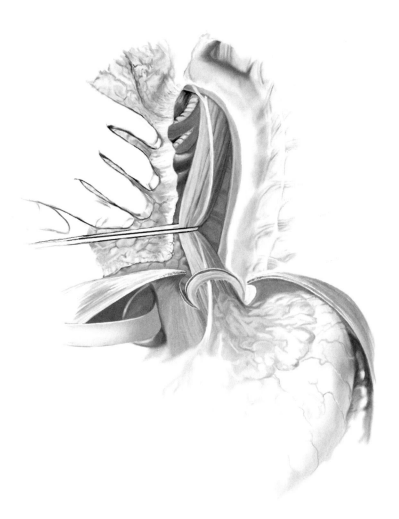

STEP 6

Reconstruction

There are several methods of reconstruction according to the tumor location and extension. Roux-Y reconstruction by using an EEA instrument, as shown here, is an option for performing the esophago-jejunostomy.

See chapter on "Subtotal Esophagectomy: Transhiatal Approach" for standard postoperative investigations and complications.

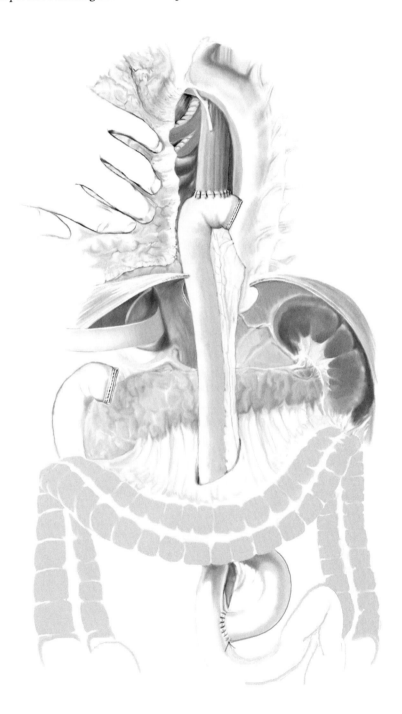

Tricks of the Senior Surgeon

- Kinking of the graft: this is a rare but dangerous complication, due to clinical symptomatic disturbance of the gastrointestinal passage by elongation, which requires surgical intervention and is performed by shortening of the graft.
- If the trachea is injured, use direct suture and pericardial flap.

Subtotal Esophagectomy: Transhiatal Approach

Stefan B. Hosch, Emre F. Yekebas, Jakob R. Izbicki

Introduction

The surgical trauma of the transhiatal approach is less pronounced as compared to a transthoracic approach. On the other hand, the lymphatic clearance is less radical, at least for the mid and upper mediastinum. This is the reason why some surgeons are in favor of the transthoracic approach even for distal adenocarcinoma. Subtotal transhiatal esophagectomy is indicated for benign conditions and for distal carcinoma.

Indications and Contraindications

Indications

- Adenocarcinoma of distal esophagus (>T1 stage)
- Intraepithelial squamous cell neoplasia
- Poor risk patients
- Extensive stricture (stenosis) due to erosion (chemical burns) unresponsive to nonsurgical treatment including bougienage
- Extensive peptic stricture (stenosis)
- Relapse of megaesophagus after surgical repair of cardiospasm combined with peptic strictures and failure of dilatation
- Extensive benign esophageal tumors (exceptional cases, usually local excision)
- Esophageal rupture or iatrogenic perforation with mediastinitis (primary repair not feasible)

Contraindications

- Florid gastroduodenal ulcer
- Infiltration of aorta
- Distant metastasis

Preoperative Investigation/Preparation for the Procedure

History:	Previous gastric or colonic surgery
Risk factors:	Alcohol, nicotine, gastroesophageal reflux disease (GERD), Barrett's esophagus
Clinical evaluation:	Recurrent laryngeal nerve status, cervical lymphadenopathy
Laboratory tests:	CEA, liver function tests, coagulation test
Endoscopy:	Esophagogastroduodenoscopy with biopsy – to exclude gastric infiltration
Colonoscopy	If colonic interposition is likely
CT scanning (thorax + abdomen):	Staging
Abdominal ultrasound:	Staging
Esophageal endosonography:	Staging, r/o aortic infiltration
Bronchoscopy (if tumor is localized in mid-third):	r/o bronchial infiltration
Bowel cleansing	(If colonic interposition is likely)
Respiratory therapy	

Procedure

Access

Upper transverse incision with median extension. Alternatively midline laparotomy.

STEP 1

Laparotomy and inspection of the stomach, distal esophagus, liver and regional lymph nodes

Placement of self-retaining retractor system for exposure of the epigastric region (A).

Mobilization of the left lateral liver by transection of the left triangular ligament. To prevent injury of adjacent structures, a pack is placed under the left lobe of the liver (B).

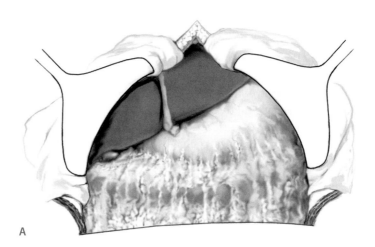

A

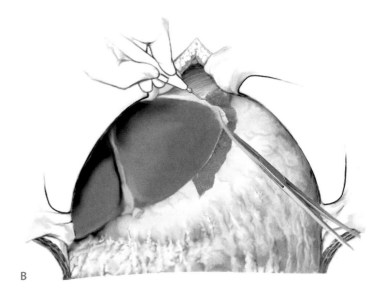

B

STEP 2   **Preparation and mobilization of the stomach with epigastric lymphadenectomy including para-aortic lymphatic tissue**

Dissection of the greater curvature is commenced from below, thoroughly sparing the origin of the right gastroepiploic vessels and the arcade between left and right gastroepiploic vessels up to the level of the splenic hilum (A).

Dissection of the greater curvature is continued towards the spleen. The left gastroepiploic artery is transected directly at its origin at the splenic artery. Transection and ligature of the short gastric vessels is performed, thus mobilizing the fundus and the greater curvature completely. For esophageal carcinoma the parietal peritoneum is incised at the upper pancreatic margin and lymphadenectomy is begun along the splenic artery. The flaccid part of the lesser omentum is dissected. The cranial part of the hepatogastric ligament (hepatoesophageal ligament) is dissected from the diaphragm. An accessory left liver artery with strong caliber should be preserved. In this case the left gastric artery has to be diverted distally to the origin of this accessory liver artery (B).

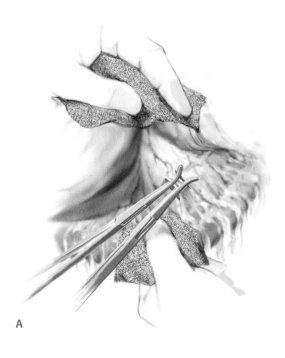

A

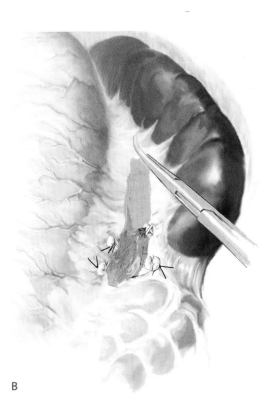

B

STEP 2 (continued)   **Preparation and mobilization of the stomach with epigastric lymphadenectomy including para-aortic lymphatic tissue**

Lymphadenectomy of the hepatoduodenal ligament is performed. Remove all lymphatic tissue around the hepatic artery up to the celiac trunk, of the portal vein and as well as the lymphatic tissue around the common bile duct. Ligature and diversion of the right gastric artery are carried out close to its origin below the pylorus (C-1, C-2).

Transection of the left gastric artery. All lymph nodes along the left gastric artery, the splenic artery, the common hepatic artery, the celiac trunk, and para-aortic lymph nodes are removed (D).

In benign diseases, blunt dissection of the esophagus is performed without lymphadenectomy. The right gastric artery may be ligated below the pylorus.

The blood supply of the gastric tube after preparation is exclusively provided by the right gastroepiploic artery.

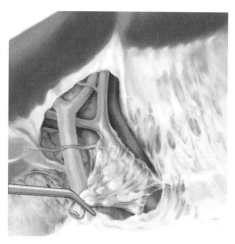

C-1

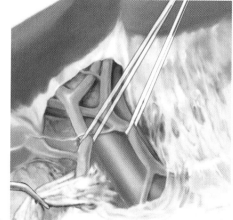

C-2

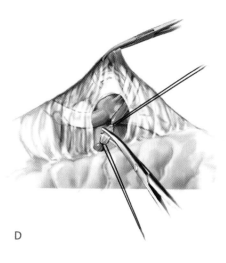

D

STEP 3   **Mobilization of the abdominal part of the esophagus and incision
                                        of the esophageal hiatus**

The lymph node dissection is continued along the celiac trunk to the para-aortic region.
The lymphatic tissue is transposed to the lesser curvature and is later resected en bloc
with the tumor.

For better exposure the diaphragmatic crura are incised with diathermia and the
stumps may be ligated. Blunt mobilization of the esophagus is done with the index
finger. During this maneuver connective tissue fibers between the esophagus, diaphragmatic crua and abdominal aorta must be removed carefully (A).

The abdominal esophagus is mobilized and pulled caudally with a rubber tube.

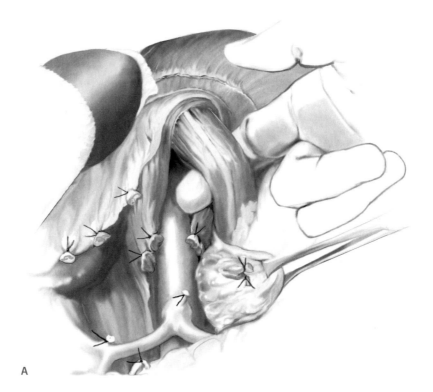

A

Mobilization of the abdominal portion of the esophagus and incision of the esophageal hiatus

The hiatus is incised ventrally following transection of the left inferior phrenic vein between ligatures (B).

Insertion of retractors. The retrocardial lymphatic tissue is removed en bloc with the specimen (C).

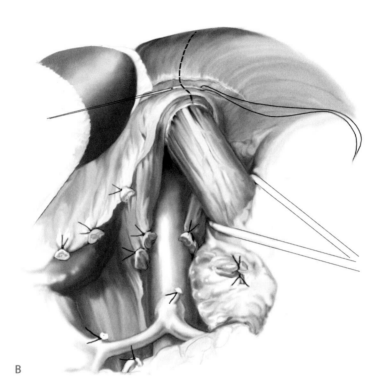

B

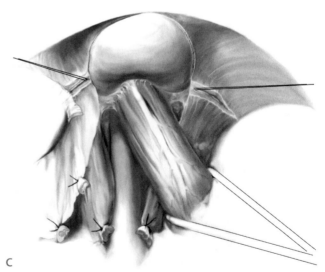

C

STEP 4   **Transhiatal esophageal dissection in the posterior mediastinum including para-aortic lymphadenectomy: mobilization of the distal esophagus**

Dissection of the distal esophagus is performed by detachment of its anterior surface from the pericardium. Infiltrated pericardium can be resected en bloc. Sharp dissection is continued anteriorly up to the tracheal bifurcation and completed by blunt dissection upwards. The trachea and the brachiocephalic trunk are palpable anteriorly. Severe damage of the trachea, the azygos vein, the pulmonary vessels or the aorta, respectively, may occur especially in the case of extensive local tumor growth (A–D).

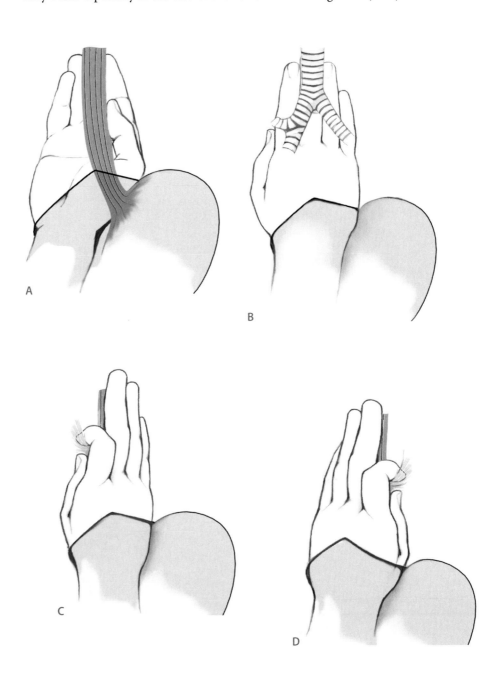

Transhiatal esophageal dissection in the posterior mediastinum including para-aortic lymphadenectomy: mobilization of the distal esophagus

After complete anterior and posterior mobilization, the esophagus is pulled caudally. The ligament like so-called lateral "esophageal ligaments" consisting of branches of the vagus nerves, pulmonary ligaments and esophageal aortic branches should be transsected sharply between clamps (clips may be used alternatively), thus avoiding bleeding, chylothorax or chyloperitoneum (E).

Excision of parietal pleura. In the case of tumor infiltration of the pleura or lung, en-bloc resection of adherent tissue can be performed following enlargement of the diaphragmatic incision if needed (F).

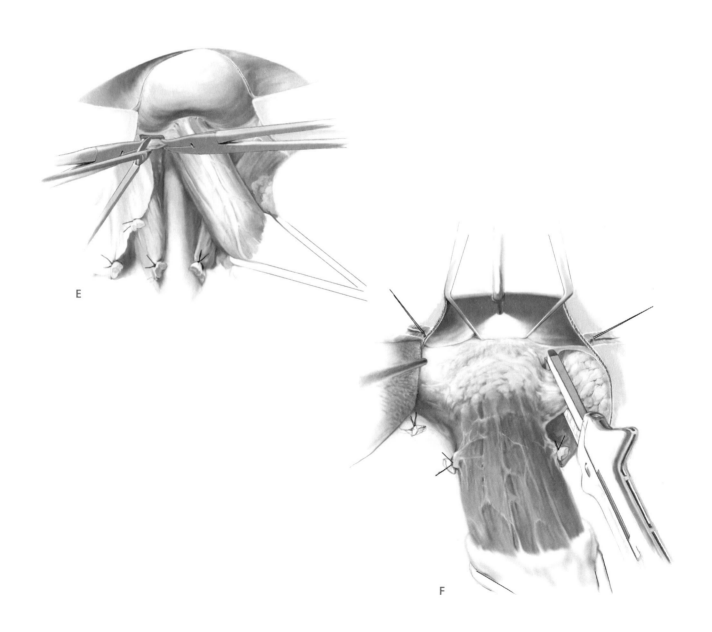

E

F

Transhiatal esophageal dissection in the posterior mediastinum including para-aortic lymphadenectomy: mobilization of the distal esophagus

Further dissection up to the tracheal bifurcation by division of the lateral ligaments. This step includes lymphadenectomy of the posterior mediastinum and posterior to the tracheal bifurcation (G-1, G-2).

For blunt dissection of the esophagus proximal to the tracheal bifurcation, the lateral ligaments should be pulled down and consecutively ligated.

If possible, blunt dissection is completed up to the upper thoracic aperture (H).

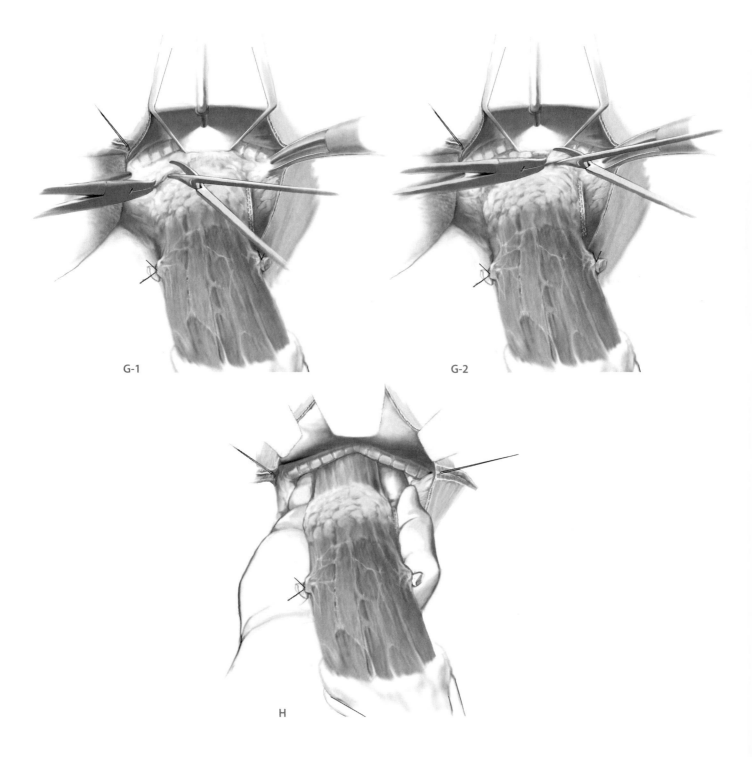

G-1   G-2

H

STEP 5   **Construction of the gastric tube**

Starting at the fundus, the lesser curvature is resected using a linear stapler device.
It follows the direction to the pylorus. Shortening of the gastric tube can be avoided
by stretching the stomach longitudinally (A).

The stapleline is oversewn by seromuscular interrupted sutures. The diameter
of the gastric tube should be 2.5–3 cm following this procedure (B).

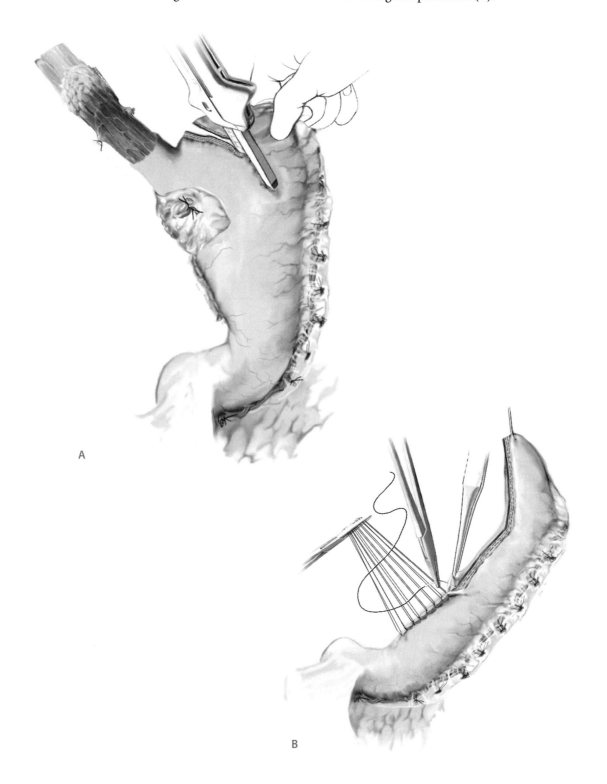

A

B

STEP 6 **Mobilization and dissection of the cervical esophagus; resection of the esophagus**

For better exposure the patient's head is turned to the right. A skin incision is performed along the anterior edge of the sternocleidomastoid muscle. Dissection of the platysma and blunt dissection between the straight cervical muscles and the sternocleidomastoid muscle are done followed by lateral retraction of the sternocleidomastoid muscle. Sharp dissection of the omohyoid muscle enables exposure of the lateral edge of the thyroid, the jugular vein and the carotid artery by retracting the strap muscles medially (A, B).

Displacement of the esophagus using a curved instrument. Dissection of the cervical esophagus and upper thoracic esophagus is completed by blunt dissection with the finger or dissector (C, D). The nasogastric tube is removed. Transection of the esophagus is performed with a stapler (C) or with scissors (E), after ligation of the aboral part of the esophagus. A strong thread or a rubber band is fixed at the aboral stump of the esophagus before the esophagus is transposed into the abdominal cavity. This eases later transposition of the gastric tube to the neck.

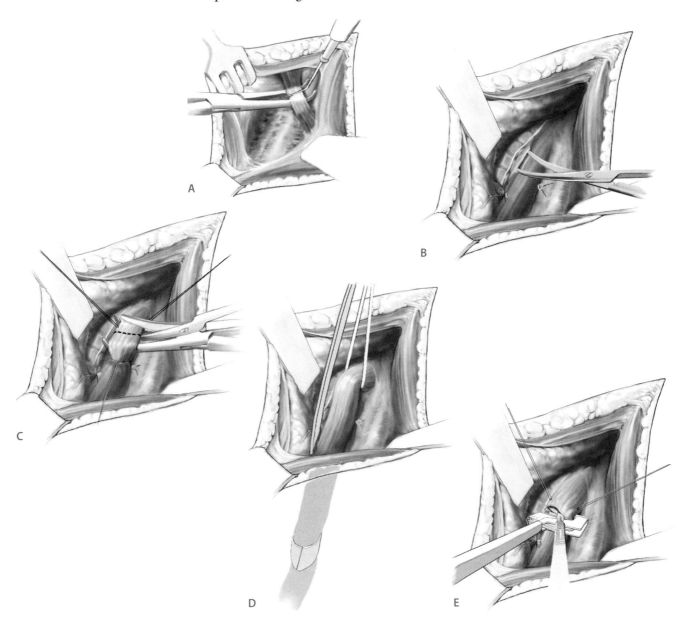

STEP 7   **Reconstruction**

Gastric tube pull-through. In rare cases mobilization of the duodenum may be necessary (Kocher maneuver) to lengthen the gastric tube.

Optional methods of placement (**A, B, C**):

a) Esophageal bed
b) Retrosternal
c) Presternal

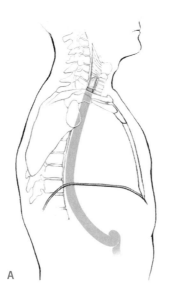

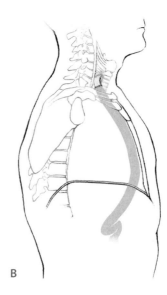

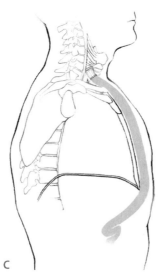

STEP 8	Cervical anastomosis

A two-layer anastomosis of the gastric tube and the esophageal stump is performed. The first seromuscular sutureline is performed in an interrupted fashion (**A**). The protruding parts of the esophagus and the gastric tube are resected (**B**). The second inner sutureline of the posterior wall can be performed as a running suture (**C**). An enteral three-lumen feeding tube is then inserted over the anastomosis and placed into the first jejunal loop for postoperative enteral nutrition (**D**).

The anterior wall is completed with interrupted or running sutures. The second suture of the anterior wall can be performed in a U-shaped fashion. This may provide an inversion of the anastomosis into the gastric tube (**E, F**).

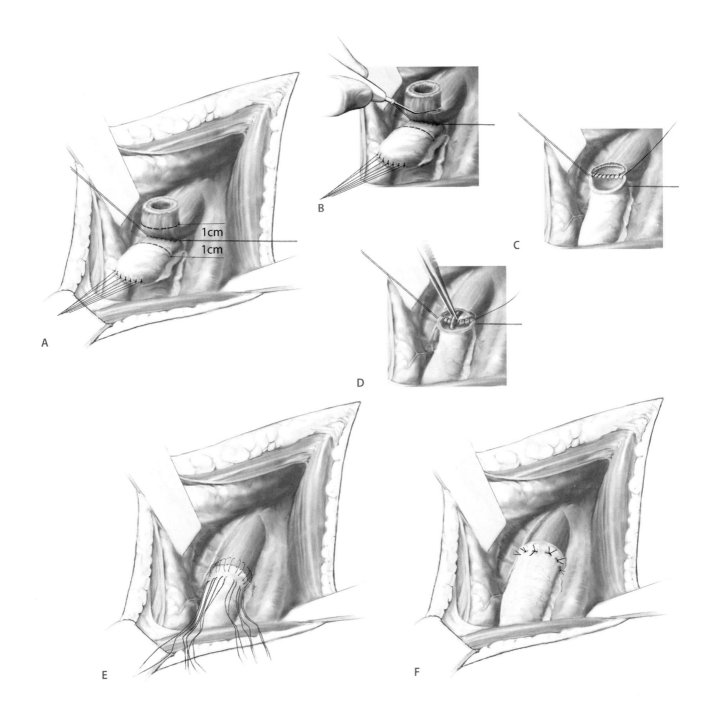

STEP 9   **Final situs**

A soft drainage is placed dorsal to the anastomosis, followed by closure of the skin.
Drainage of the mediastinum is warranted by two soft drains from the abdomen.

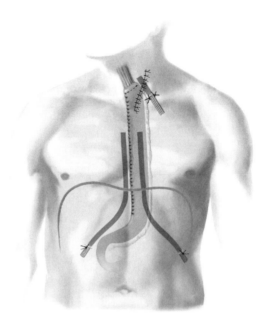

Standard Postoperative Investigations

- Postoperative surveillance on intensive care unit
- "Generous" indication for postoperative endoscopy
- Daily check of the drainage

Postoperative Complications

- Pleural effusion and pneumonia
- Anastomotic leakage
- Necrosis of the interponate
- Injury to recurrent laryngeal nerve (uni- or bilateral)
- Mediastinitis
- Chylus fistula
- Scarring of the esophageal anastomosis with stenosis (long term)

Tricks of the Senior Surgeon

- Mobilization of the duodenum on the one hand may facilitate the placement of a feeding tube. On the other hand, it may include the possibility of shortening the length of the tube to get a better blood supply of the anastomotic region.
- Wide incision of the diaphragm crura provides optimal exposure of the posterior mediastinum to minimize risks of blunt mediastinal dissection.

Subtotal En Bloc Esophagectomy: Abdominothoracic Approach

Stefan B. Hosch, Asad Kutup, Jakob R. Izbicki

Introduction

The goal of this operation is to remove an esophageal cancer with the widest possible lymphatic clearance (two-field lymphadenectomy), which comprises upper abdominal lymphadenectomy and lymphatic clearance of the posterior and mid mediastinum. Reconstruction is accomplished by either gastric tube or colonic interposition.

Indications and Contraindications

Indications

- Thoracic esophageal carcinoma
- Benign stricture, if transhiatal resection is ill-advised (e.g., adherence to trachea)

Contraindications

- See chapter on "Subtotal Esophagectomy: Transhiatal Approach"
- High risk patients

Preoperative Investigation/Preparation for the Procedure

See See chapter on "Subtotal Esophagectomy: Transhiatal Approach".

Procedure

Access
- Patient in left lateral positioning for the thoracic part of the operation
- Anterolateral thoracotomy through the 5th intercostal space (ICS)
- Re-positioning to a supine position (see chapter on the transhiatal approach)
- Upper transverse incision with median extension (see chapter on the transhiatal approach)

STEP 1

Thoracotomy and incision of the pleura along the resection line

Thoracotomy through the 5th ICS with skin incision from the apex of the scapula to the submammarian fold (A).

Two retractors are positioned stepwise. Single left lung ventilation is performed. The mediastinal pleura is incised along the resection line for the en bloc esophagectomy. Incision starts from the pulmonary ligament, circumcising the dorsal part of the right hilum of the lung and along the right bronchus. It follows the right main bronchus at the lateral margin of the superior vena cava up to the upper thoracic aperture. Then the incision line changes direction caudally along the right lateral margin of the spine, down to the diaphragm along the azygos vein. It is of the utmost importance to identify the right phrenic nerve (B).

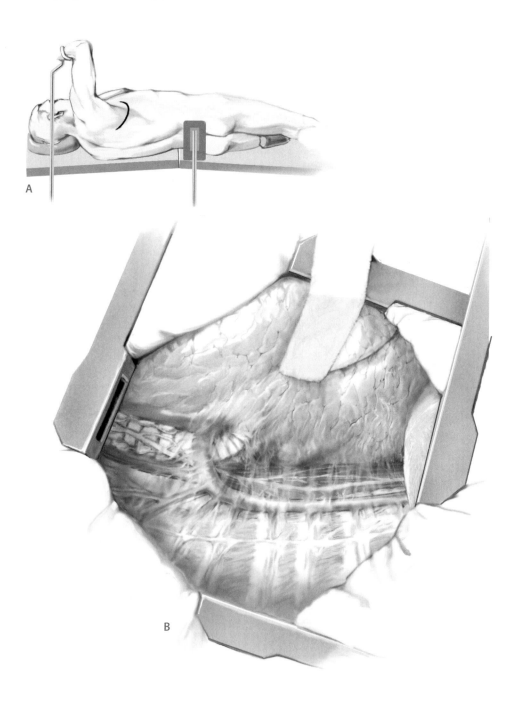

STEP 2	Division of the pulmonary ligament

For exposure of the pulmonary ligament the lung is pushed cranially and laterally. All lymphatic tissue should be moved towards the esophagus. Care has to be taken not to injure the vein of the lower lobe of the right lung.

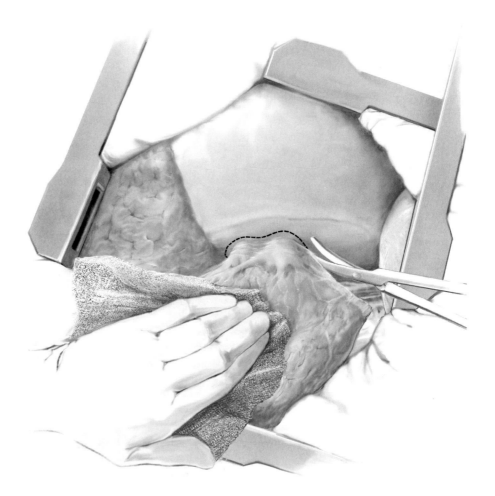

STEP 3   **Ligation of the azygos vein**

The superior vena cava and the azygos vein are dissected. Suture ligation towards the vena cava and ligation of the azygos venal stump are performed.

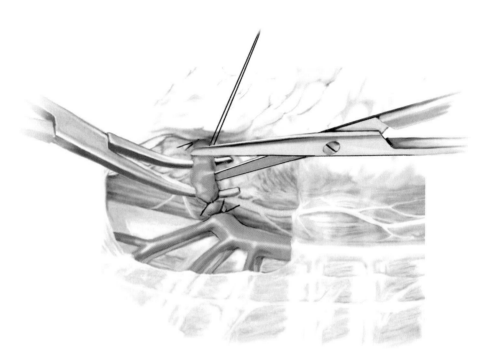

STEP 4   Radical en bloc lymphadenectomy

Lymphadenectomy starts from the superior vena cava up to the confluence of the two vv. anonymae. Dissection of the bracheocephalic trunk and right subclavian artery is followed by dissection of the right vagal nerve and identification of the right recurrent laryngeal nerve. Caudal to the branching of the recurrent laryngeal nerve, the vagal nerve is transected and the distal part is pushed towards the en bloc specimen. Then lymphadenectomy is performed continuously along the dorsal wall of the superior vena cava (A).

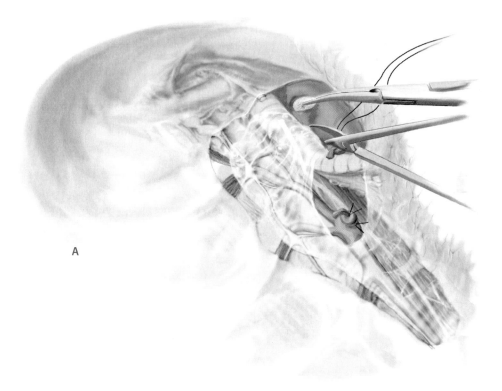

A

Radical en bloc lymphadenectomy

After having completed preparation of the superior vena cava, the trachea and the right- and right-sided main bronchus are completely freed from lymphatic tissue. The pre- and paratracheal fat and lymphatic tissue are dissected towards the esophagus (**B**).

Dissection of the retrotracheal lymph nodes is then performed. Injury of the membranaceous part of the trachea has to be carefully avoided while removing these nodes towards the esophagus (**C**).

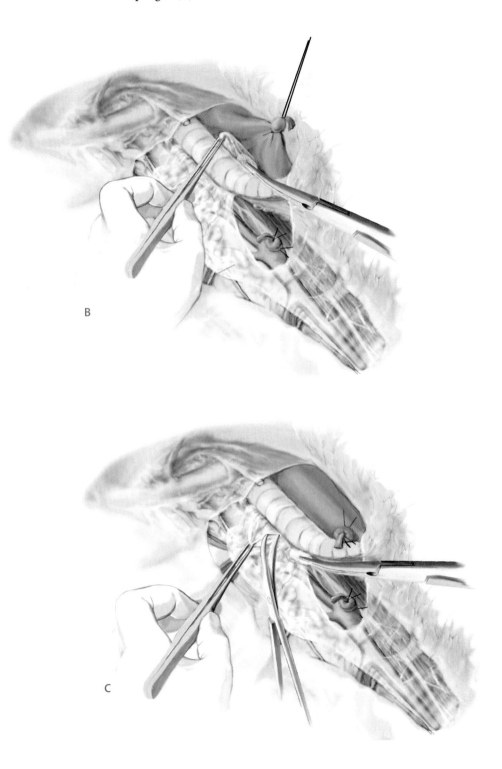

B

C

Radical en bloc lymphadenectomy

Lymph node dissection continues with the upper paraesophageal lymph nodes (D).
    All intercostal veins that drain into the azygos vein are ligated and divided.
Lymphadenectomy of the subcarinal lymph nodes is then performed with dissection
of the left main bronchus (E).

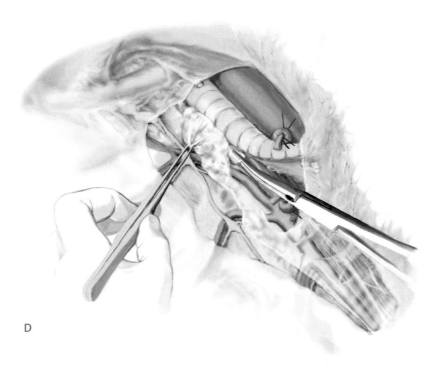

D

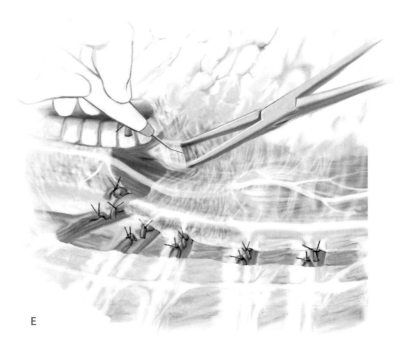

E

STEP 4 *(continued)*   **Radical en bloc lymphadenectomy**

Para-aortic lymphadenectomy is performed. The esophageal branches of the thoracic aorta have to be dissected very carefully and should be ligated with suture ligation (**F**).

Identification and careful dissection of the thoracic duct is done with double ligations directly above the diaphragm and at the level of the main carina (**G**).

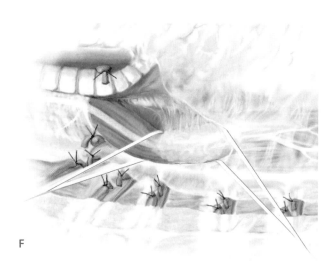

F

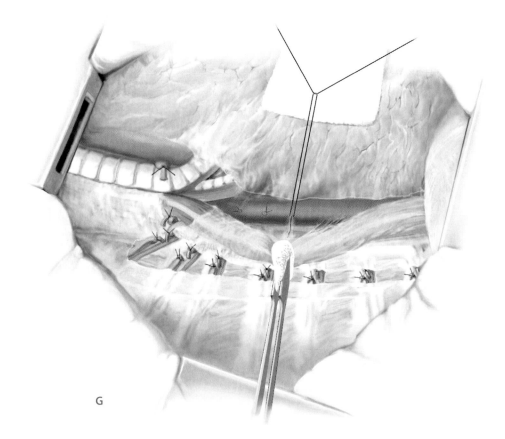

G

STEP 4 *(continued)*

Radical en bloc lymphadenectomy

Mediastinal lymphadenectomy is completed with the removal of the left sided para-aortic and retropericardial lymph nodes, as well as the intermediate and lower lobe bronchus down to the esophageal hiatus (H).

After complete mobilization of the esophageal specimen, thoracic drainage is placed in the right thoracic cavity. After closure of the thoracic incision the patient is repositioned for the abdominal part.

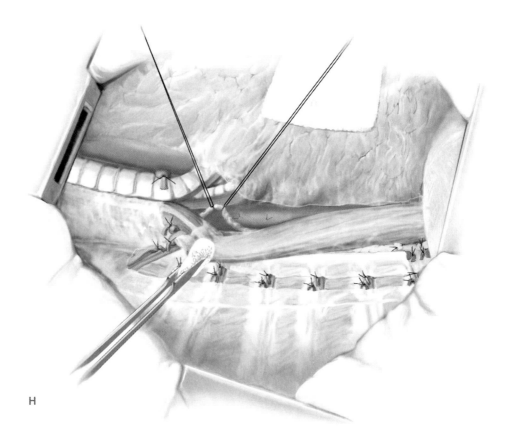

H

For the abdominal and cervical parts: see the transhiatal approach.

Alternatively an intrathoracic anastomosis can be achieved (see chapter on intrathoracic anastomosis).

See chapter "Subtotal Esophagectomy: Transhiatal Approach" for standard postoperative investigations and complications.

Tricks of the Senior Surgeon

- In case R0 resection cannot be accomplished, the retrosternal reconstruction route is preferred.
- If the trachea is injured, use a direct suture and pericardial flap.
- For better exposure of the cervical esophagus, transect the medial head of the sternocleidomastoid muscle.
- Injury of the gastroepiploic arcade directly necessitates colonic interposition.

Abdominothoracic En Bloc Esophagectomy with High Intrathoracic Anastomosis

Asad Kutup, Emre F. Yekebas, Jakob R. Izbicki

Introduction

High intrathoracic anastomosis may be performed without compromising the oncologic requirements alternatively to collar anastomosis for treatment of intrathoracic tumors, i.e., if located distally to the tracheal bifurcation. The benefits of considerably shorter operating times are associated with the risk of developing devastating mediastinitis when anastomotic leakage occurs.

Indications and Contraindications

Indications

- Thoracic esophageal carcinoma
- Long distance peptic stricture, if transhiatal resection is not possible

Contraindications

- See chapter on "Subtotal Esophagectomy: Transhiatal Approach"
- High risk patients

Preoperative Investigation/Preparation for the Procedure

See chapter on "Subtotal Esophagectomy: Transhiatal Approach".

Procedure

Access
- Helical positioning of the patient with 45° elevation of the right thorax and elevated arm
- Turning the table to the patient's supine position for the abdominal part of surgery
- Turning the table to the left for the thoracic part of surgery

STEP 1

See Steps 1–3 and Step 5 of the chapter "Subtotal Esophagectomy: Transhiatal Approach"

STEP 2

See Steps 1–4 of the chapter "Subtotal Esophagectomy: Transhiatal Approach"

STEP 3   **High intrathoracic anastomosis**

Transection of the esophagus is carried out 5 cm below the upper thoracic aperture over a Pursestring 45 clamp. Alternatively the esophagus is transected and a running suture (monofilament, 2-0) is applied as a pursestring suture.

Dilatation of the proximal esophageal stump with a blunt clamp is performed. The anvil of a circular stapler (preferably 28 mm) is introduced into the esophageal stump and fixation is done by tying the pursestring suture.

Mobilization of the gastric tube through the diaphragmatic esophageal hiatus is performed, followed by resection of the apex of the gastric tube. This is usually longer than required. Then introduce the stapler into the gastric tube, and perforation of the wall at the prospective site of the anastomosis with the head of the stapling device (**A**).

In case of limited length of the gastric tube, the stapling device is inserted through a ventral gastrostomy and an end-to-end gastroesophagostomy is performed.

Connection with the anvil is followed by firing of the instrument (**B**).

Check for completeness of the anastomotic rings. The stapler is removed and closure and resection of the protruding part of the gastric tube are done with a linear stapler.

A nasogastric feeding tube is then inserted over the anastomosis and placed into the first jejunal poop for decompression and postoperative enteral feeding. Thoracic drainage is placed in the right thoracic cavity.

Alternatively, this elegant method can be performed in the same manner in the case of colonic interposition after esophagogastrectomy (**C, D**).

STEP 3 *(continued)*

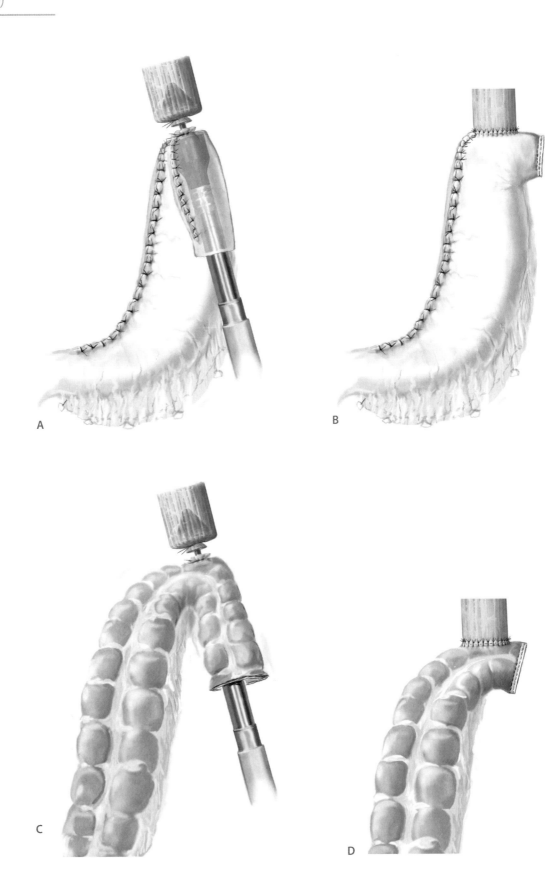

See the transhiatal approach for standard postoperative investigations and complicatons.

Tricks of the Senior Surgeon

- An additional length of the gastric tube is achieved by mobilization of the duodenum (Kocher maneuver). In this way, the end of the gastric tube designated for the anastomosis is located closer to the gastroepiploic pedicle. The improved vascular supply reduces the risk of anastomotic leakage.
- In contrast to cervical esophagogastric anastomosis, in any case of suspected intrathoracic leakage, emergency endoscopy should be done. Even if an insufficiency cannot be definitely visualized, the indication for stenting should be established generously as long as clinical signs suggest a leakage to prevent catastrophic mediastinitis.

Limited Resection of the Gastroesophageal Junction with Isoperistaltic Jejunal Interposition

Asad Kutup, Emre F. Yekebas, Jakob R. Izbicki

Introduction

Limited en bloc resection of the gastroesophageal junction includes complete removal of the esophageal segment with metaplastic mucosa, the lower esophageal sphincter and a part of the lesser gastric curvature and formation of a neofundus. Since even early adenocarcinomas of the distal esophagus (T1b) seed lymph node metastases in up to 20% of patients, removal of the lymph nodes of the lesser curvature, the hepatic and splenic arteries, the celiac trunk, the para-aortal region, and the inferior mediastinum is an essential part of the operation.

In patients with early tumors, staged as uT1a or b on preoperative endosonography or severe dysplasia in the distal esophagus (Barrett's esophagus), a limited resection of the proximal stomach, cardia and distal esophagus with interposition of a pedicled isoperistaltic jejunal segment offers excellent functional and oncological results.

Indications and Contraindications

Indications

- Severe dysplasia in the distal esophagus (Barrett's esophagus)
- Distal adenocarcinoma of the esophagus (stage T1a and b) (UICC 2005)
- For palliative reasons (stenotic tumor with severe dysphagia or profuse hemorrhage in selective patients)

Contraindications

- Esophageal carcinoma staged T2 and more
- Long Barrett's segment above the carina

Preoperative Investigations/Preparation for the Procedure

- Esophagogastroscopy with extensive biopsies
- Endosonography of the esophagus
- Computed tomography of the chest and abdomen
- Abdominal ultrasound
- Pulmonary function test
- Orthograde cleansing of the intestines

Positioning

- Supine position with hyperlordosis

Procedure

Access
- Upper transverse incision with median T-shaped
- Insertion of Rochard retractor to elevate costal margin

| STEP 1 | Exposure of the inferior posterior mediastinum; diaphanoscopy |

The left liver lobe is completely mobilized and the lesser omentum is incised just medial to the anterior and posterior gastric vagal branches. A longitudinal median diaphragmal incision enables exposure of the inferior posterior mediastinum. The distal esophagus is then mobilized including the paraesophageal tissue. The vagal nerves are divided.

Intraoperative esophagoscopy identifies the cranial limit of the Barrett's segment by diaphanoscopy. This also marks the proximal limit of resection.

A lymphadenectomy around the splenic and hepatic artery is performed, the left gastric vein is divided, and the left gastric artery is divided at the celiac trunk. Then the celiac trunk and the para-aortic region above the celiac trunk are cleared from lymphatic tissue (**A, B**).

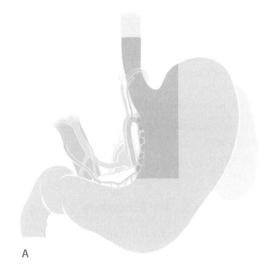

A

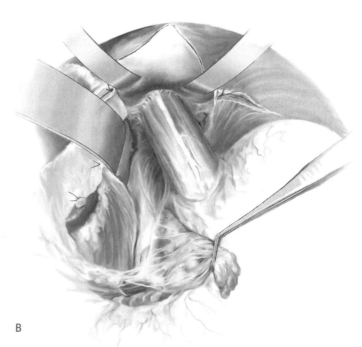

B

STEP 2   **Transection of the esophagus**

Approximately 1 cm proximal to the cranial limit of the Barrett's segment, a pursestring clamp is placed and the esophagus is divided.

Removal of the cardia and lesser curvature is performed by placing multiple linear staplers down to the border between antrum and body. Thus, a neofundus is formed.

In case an advanced tumor stage is encountered, possible extension of the operation including transhiatal esophagectomy or esophagogastrectomy should be performed.

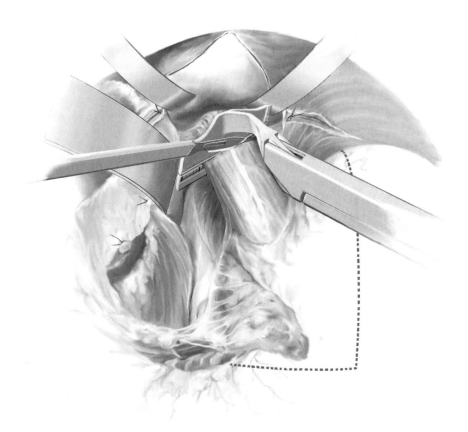

STEP 3   **Transposition of the proximal jejunum segment; esophagojejunostomy**

A 15- to 20-cm-long segment of the proximal jejunum is isolated and is transposed with its mesenteric root to the diaphragmatic region through the mesocolon and behind the stomach. Care has to be taken while dissecting the vascular pedicle of this jejunal interposition to provide adequate length. It is imperative to form an isoperistaltic jejunal interposition which should be pulled up retrogastric and retrocolic. The proximal anastomosis is then performed by a circular stapling device as a terminolateral esophagojejunostomy. The stapler is introduced into the end of the jejunal interponate (A-1).

After firing of the anastomosis, the blind end of the loop is then resected and closed by a linear stapler and then oversewn (A-2).

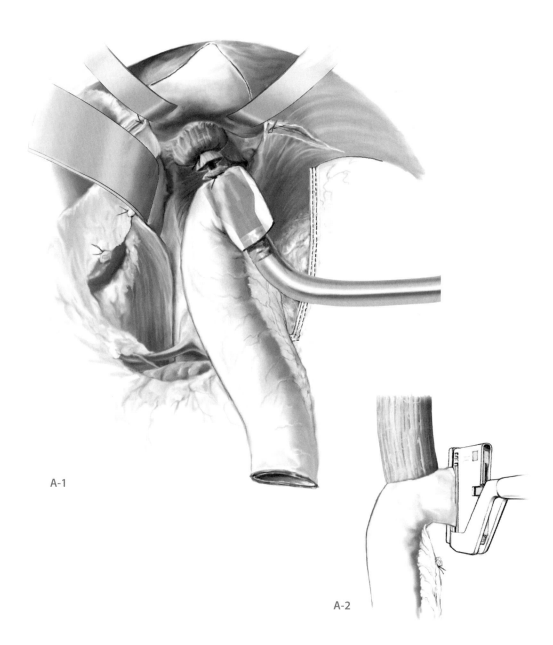

A-1

A-2

STEP 4

Jejunogastrostomy

Close to the base of the neofundus the gastric stapler line is removed over a distance of 3–4 cm and a terminolateral or laterolateral jejunogastrostomy is performed. The remaining gastric suture line is oversewn. A terminoterminal jejunojejunostomy reconstructs the enteric passage. Drainage of the mediastinum is warranted by two soft drains from the abdomen. Finally an anterior and/or posterior hiatal repair is performed.

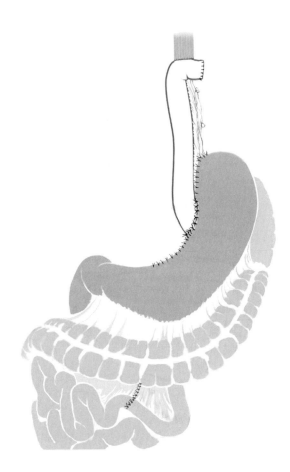

Standard Postoperative Investigations

■ Daily check the drains for insufficiency of the intrathoracic esophagojejunostomy

Postoperative Complications

■ Insufficiency of the esophagojejunostomy or the intra-abdominal anastomosis
■ Mediastinitis
■ Pancreatitis
■ Peritonitis
■ Pleural empyema
■ Necrosis of the transposed jejunal segment
■ Reflux
■ Delayed gastric emptying

Tricks of the Senior Surgeon

■ Intraoperative endoscopy in any case of long-segment irregularities or evidence of multicentric lesions.
■ Insertion of the stapler device through the oral end of the pedicled jejunal segment.

Three-Field Lymphadenectomy for Esophageal Cancer

Masamichi Baba, Shoji Natsugoe, Takashi Aikou

Introduction

Lymphatic drainage from the upper two-thirds of the thoracic esophagus occurs mainly towards the neck and upper mediastinum, although there is also some drainage to the nodes along the left gastric artery. In 1981, the first reported study of three-field lymphadenectomy in Japan noted that 10 of 36 patients with esophagectomy had skip metastases to the neck or abdominal lymph nodes in the absence of associated intra-thoracic spread. In this chapter, we focus on the lymph node dissection of the upper mediastinal and cervical regions.

Indications and Contraindications

Indications

- Tumors of the supracarinal esophagus (>T1m stage)

Contraindications

- Superficial carcinoma (T1m stage)
- Severe comorbidity (heart disease, pulmonary and/or liver dysfunction)
- No evidence of cervical lymph node metastases preoperatively in high risk patients (relative)
- Infracarinal tumors (relative)

Preoperative Investigation/Preparation for the Procedure

- See transhiatal approach
- US+CT scan of the neck
- In locally advanced tumors: primary radiochemotherapy and surgery is done secondarily

Procedure

Access
- Anterior-lateral thoracotomy through the right 5th ICS
- Supine position and T-shaped incision in the neck

STEP 1   **Exposure and lymphadenectomy of the right upper mediastinum**

The arch of the azygous vein is resected, and the right bronchial artery is ligated and
secured at its root to evaluate the tumor for its resectability. This procedure provides a
good exposure of the upper and middle mediastinum. The brachiocephalic and right
subclavian arteries are exposed in order to remove the right recurrent nerve nodes and
right paratracheal nodes followed by carefully ligating the branches of the inferior
thyroid artery (arrow indicates the direction of lymphadenectomy).

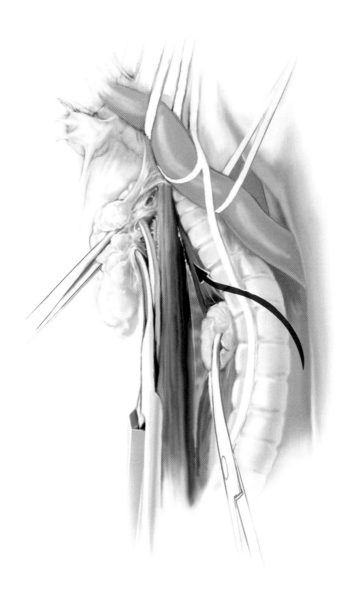

STEP 2   **Transection; resection of the esophagus and completion of lymph node clearance**

After proximal transection of the esophagus at the level of the aortic arch, the left recurrent nerve nodes (left paratracheal nodes) are removed. The middle mediastinal nodes, comprising the infra-aortic, infracarinal, and periesophageal nodes, are cleared in conjunction with the esophagus.

This exposes the main bronchus, the left pulmonary artery, branches of the vagus nerve, and the pericardium. Both pulmonary branches of the bilateral vagus nerves and the left bronchial artery originating from the descending aorta near the left pulmonary hilum are preserved. However, the esophageal branches of the vagus nerves are severed, and the thoracic duct is also removed together with the esophagus.

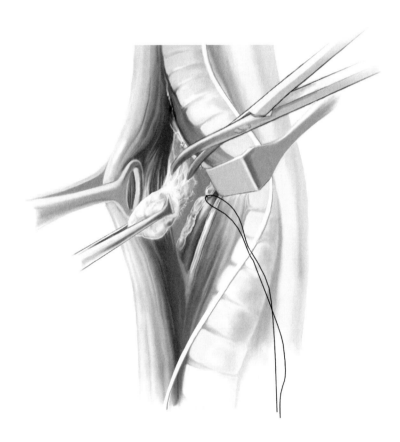

STEP 3   **T-shaped neck incision**

A T-shaped neck incision is made and the sternothyroid, sternohyoid and sternomastoid muscles are divided to the clavicular head and the omohyoid muscle is incised at its fascia. After identification of the recurrent nerve, lymph nodes along this nerve (which are in continuity with the nodes previously dissected out in the superior mediastinum) are dissected. The inferior thyroid arteries are then ligated and divided. The para-esophageal nodes, including the recurrent nerve nodes at the cervicothoracic junction, are classified as either cervical or upper mediastinal nodes, according to their position relative to the bifurcation of the right common carotid and right subclavian arteries.

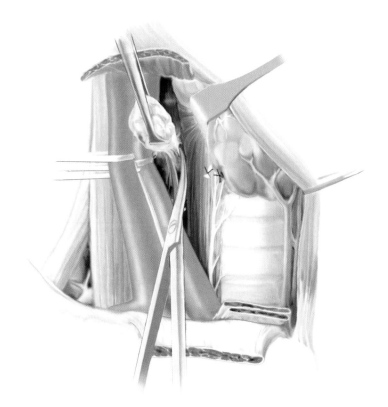

STEP 4   **Cervical lymphadenectomy**

The jugular vein, common carotid artery, and vagus nerve are subsequently identified and divided. On the lateral side, after careful preservation of the accessory nerve, lymph nodes situated lateral to the internal jugular vein are removed. The thyrocervical trunk and its branches and the phrenic nerve are then identified. In this procedure, the cervical nodes (internal jugular nodes below the level of the cricoid cartilage, supra-clavicular nodes, and cervical paraesophageal nodes) are cleared bilaterally (arrow indicates the direction of lymphadenectomy).

See transhiatal approach for standard postoperative investigations and complications.

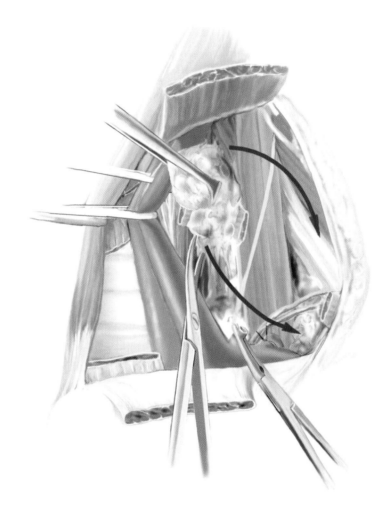

Tricks of the Senior Surgeon

- A better exposure of the upper mediastinum requires transection of the medial head of the sternocleidomastoid muscle and/or partial upper sternotomy.

Minimally Invasive Esophagectomy

Rudolf Bumm, Hubertus Feussner

Introduction

The availability of modern laparoscopic and thoracoscopic techniques as well as videoendoscopy has promoted the development of techniques for minimally invasive esophagectomy. In principle, two techniques have been established and clinically evaluated so far. Thoracoscopic esophagectomy is, in theory, an analog procedure for transthoracic en-bloc esophagectomy, but is in use in only a few centers because it is technically demanding, requires single lung ventilation over extended time periods and has not shown, clinical benefits over conventional open esophagectomy in larger series so far. Radical transhiatal esophagectomy with mediastinoscopic dissection of the esophagus (endodissection) was established in 1990 by Buess and coworkers and clinically tested in our own institution. The method is feasible and safe, and endo-dissection allows for mobilization of the proximal thoracic esophagus under direct vision and enables mediastinoscopic lymph node sampling and reduces peri- and postoperative complications compared to conventional transhiatal esophagectomy.

Thoracoscopic Esophagectomy

Indications and Contraindications

Indications

- Carcinoma of the thoracic esophagus

Contraindications

- Deterioration of lung function (long single lung ventilation)
- Status post-thoracotomy (adhesions)
- Advanced tumors
- Patients older than 65 years (relative)

Radical Transhiatal Esophagectomy with Endodissection

Indications and Contraindications

Indications

- Patients with adenocarcinoma of the distal esophagus (Barrett's carcinoma)
- Age limit: This method can be successfully performed in patients up to the age of 80 years

Contraindications

- Status after thyroid resection or patients in which the cervical esophagus and/or the upper mediastinum may be difficult to access (status after radiation therapy for subsequent oropharyngeal tumors)
- Preoperative detection of enlarged peritumoral or mediastinal lymph nodes (→ transthoracic en bloc resection)

Preoperative Investigations/Preparation for the Procedure

(Re-)endoscopy and (re-)biopsy
Endoscopic ultrasound: UICC T and N categories
Chest X-ray: Distant metastasis?
Abdominal ultrasound: Distant metastasis?
CT scan: Resectability? Enlarged mediastinal lymph nodes?
Risk analysis: Cardiac, lung, liver function, cooperation, zero alcohol intake for several weeks

Procedures

Thoracoscopic Esophagectomy

STEP 1

Positioning and exposure

A double-lumen tube for single lung ventilation is placed by the anesthetist with great care, as the quality of single lung ventilation is crucial for the procedure.

The patient is brought into a left-sided position as for a conventional posterolateral thoracotomy.

Special short and oval trocars for thoracoscopy reduce the danger of intercostal artery bleeding and increase the degree of freedom of instrument handling. The trocar position should be adjusted according to tumor localization, and lung retractors are needed for exposure.

Position of the patient and of the trocars is shown in a patient with esophageal carcinoma adjacent to the tracheal bifurcation.

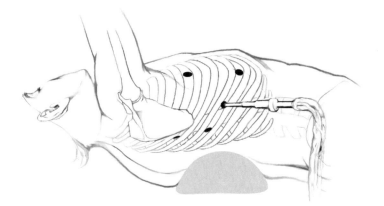

STEP 2   Dissection of the esophagus

The mediastinal pleura is divided and the entire thoracic esophagus is exposed in a
way that the azygos vein is preserved. Then the inferior pulmonary ligament is divided
to the level of the inferior pulmonary vein. A silicone drain is placed around the distal
esophagus to facilitate traction and exposure, and ultrasonic shears are used for dissection of the peri-esophageal tissues, which should remain attached en bloc to the
specimen. The thoracic duct should be sutured with non-resorbable material in order
to reduce the risk of chylothorax, and direct vessels from the aorta should be clipped
to avoid rebleeding.

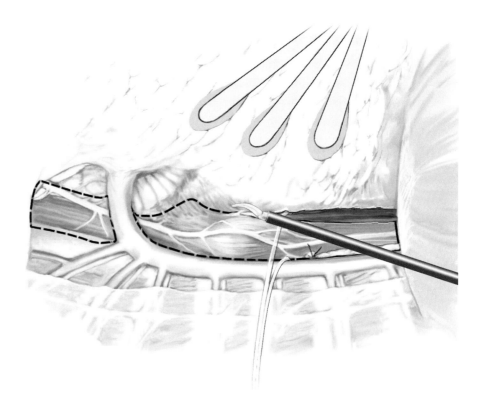

STEP 3	Transection of the esophagus

During dissection of the subcarinal lymph nodes, attention must be paid to avoid injuring the mainstream bronchi. The subcarinal nodes should remain attached en bloc to the specimen.

An Endo GIA II vascular stapler is used to divide the azygos vein. The vagus nerve is divided by ultrasonic shears cephalad to the azygos vein.

Finally, the esophagus is transected at the level of the thoracic inlet with the help of another Endo GIA II stapler magazine. The specimen is removed later through the open hiatus during reconstruction. Alternatively, the esophagus can be divided by stapler distally at the level of the hiatus and removed by one of the port incisions, which should be enlarged to 3–4 cm for this purpose. The operation is completed by inserting a single 26-Fr. chest tube through the camera port, and the other port sites are closed with absorbable running sutures.

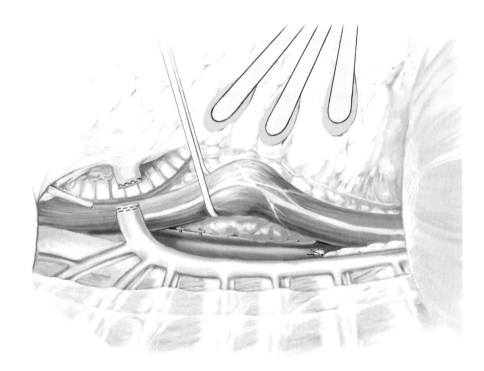

Radical Transhiatal Esophagectomy with Endodissection

STEP 1   **Exposure, preparation and access to the cervical esophagus**

The patient is brought into a supine position and the skin is disinfected. The esophagus should be intubated with a rigid rubber tube. The abdominal wall, the anterior thorax and the left side of the neck must be completely exposed for the two operating teams (abdominal and cervical teams) (A-1).

The cervical incision is made at the anterior edge of the sternocleidomastoideus muscle. The omohyoideus muscle is divided by monopolar electrocautery and the inferior thyroid artery is divided between ligatures. The recurrent laryngeal nerve must be identified and carefully preserved during the next steps of the dissection. The nerve is best located at the point where it undercrosses the inferior thyroid artery. Further dissection of the nerve should be avoided in order to prevent secondary lesions.

The cervical esophagus is mobilized by blunt/sharp dissection and drawn laterally with the help of a silicone tube in order to gain some dissection space between the esophagus and trachea (A-2).

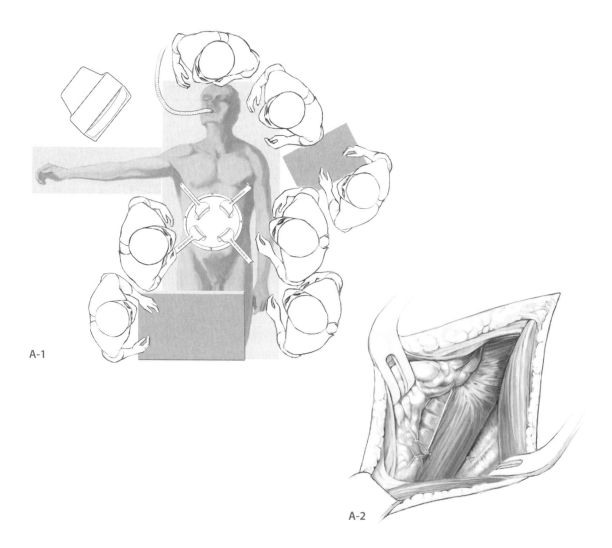

A-1

A-2

STEP 2

Endodissection

The mediastinal endodissector is then assembled and inserted into the upper mediastinum. This instrument features a tissue dilator at the tip, a 15-degree Hopkins fiberoptic device and a working channel for one 5-mm laparoscopic instrument. The tissue dilator is anatomically designed so that it can "ride" on the esophageal surface and opens an anterograde dissection space of 2–3 cm in the mediastinum. The tissue dilator of the mediastinoscope can be freely rotated 360 degrees. For full operation, the mediastinoscope is connected to a video camera, a xenon light source, and a flushing/suction device.

It is normal that the first steps of endoscopic dissection of the retrotracheal space are difficult due to the limited initial vision and the anatomical narrowing of the thoracic inlet. Microinstruments such as scissors, forceps or a coagulation/suction instrument as well as ultrasonic shears can be used through the working channel of the mediastinoscope.

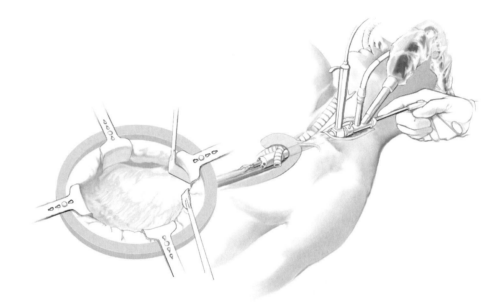

STEP 3   **Endodissection: mediastinoscopic anterior view**

The retrotracheal tissues are divided by pushing the tissue with the coagulation/suction device followed by the application of a short "coagulation" impulse or dissection with ultrasonic shears.

The anterior surface of the esophagus is subsequently dissected until 2–3 cm below the tracheal bifurcation.

We usually identify the left recurrent nerve, both vagal trunks, the tracheal bifurcation and the subcarinal lymph nodes, which can be removed in toto.

By turning the tip of the instrument counterclockwise by 90 degrees, the left surface of the esophagus can be dissected. This is usually the most difficult part of endodissection due to adhesions between esophagus and the left main bronchus. These must be totally divided. Care has to be taken not to divide the longitudinal muscle layer of the esophagus at this point.

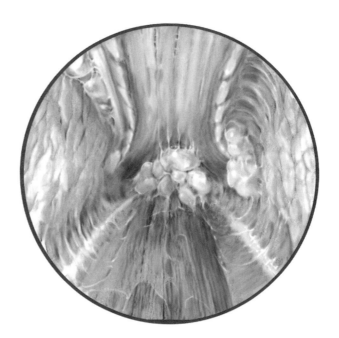

STEP 4

Endodissection: mediastinoscopic posterior view

The back wall and the right surface of the esophagus usually present no major difficulties, and opening of the mediastinal pleura is not usually critical. Finally, the esophagus should be circumferentially mobilized and contact between the abdominal team and the cervical team should be made. The cervical team assists during the phase of en bloc dissection of the infracarinal esophagus by providing light and suction from above. This can be helpful especially in large tumors. Finally, the cervical esophagus is divided by a longitudinal stapler device and retracted into the abdominal cavity. The mediastinal procedure is completed by control of hemorrhage and removal of visible lymph nodes for supplementary staging information.

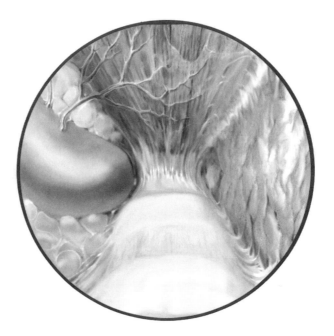

STEP 5
Radical transhiatal esophagectomy with endodissection; dissection of the hiatus and the inferior mediastinum

After abdominal incision (inverse-T laparotomy and self-holding Stuhler's retractors), the hiatus of the patient should be exposed after mobilization of the left lobe of the liver.

When endodissection is nearly completed, the abdominal team widely opens the hiatus by excising portions of the crura of the diaphragm (left adherent to the specimen) and dividing the diaphragmatic vein between clamps. The periesophageal mediastinal lymphatic tissue is dissected from the pericardium and remains adherent to the specimen in "en bloc" fashion. The primary tumor should not be exposed during the operation. Both visceral layers of the pleura may be resected without problems. After complete mobilization of the esophagus by the cervical team and division of the cervical esophagus with a linear stapler, the specimen is retracted into the abdominal cavity. A lymphadenectomy in compartments I and II is always added (A-1, A-2).

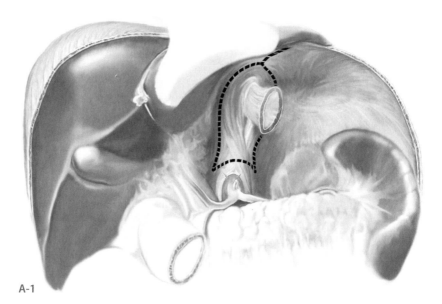

A-1

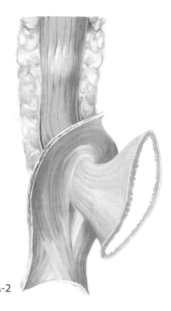

A-2

| STEP 6 | Reconstruction |

Routinely, we reconstruct the gastrointestinal passage by pull-through of a narrow gastric tube in the anterior or the posterior mediastinum. Only in younger patients with good prognosis is a reconstruction with colon accomplished.

See chapter on "Subtotal Esophagectomy: Transhiatal Approach" for standard postoperative investigations.

Postoperative Complications
- Recurrent nerve palsy
- Chylothorax
- Bleeding
- Anastomotic insufficiency

Tricks of the Senior Surgeon

Thoracoscopic Esophagectomy
- Should only be performed with excellent single lung ventilation.
- Convert early in case of bleeding or loss of orientation.
- Suture the thoracic duct with non-resorbable suture material.

Radical Transhiatal Esophagectomy with Endodissection
- Perform endodissection and abdominal approach simultaneously to save time.
- Endodissection: always keep the esophagus in sight to avoid damage to vital mediastinal structures.
- Endodissection: in case of mediastinal arterial bleeding it is better to compress/tamponate than coagulate.
- Do not attempt to dissect the tumor below the tracheal bifurcation. This is better done by the abdominal team through the open hiatus.

Zenker's Diverticula: Open Approach

Claus F. Eisenberger, Christoph Busch

Introduction

The common type of diverticula (Zenker's) is not actually of esophageal origin, but arises from the relatively bare triangle of mucosa located between the inferior pharyngeal constrictors and the cricopharyngeal muscle (Killian's triangle). Zenker's diverticula are 10 times more common than other esophageal diverticula.

Zenker's diverticula are so called false diverticula and are classified according to *Lahey*:

Stage I: No symptoms, local mild inflammation
Stage II: Dysphagia and regurgitation
Stage III: Esophageal obstruction, dysphagia, and regurgitation

Indications and Contraindications

Indications

- Progress over time. Treatment is recommended for patients who have moderate to severe symptoms/complications (pneumonia or aspiration)

Contraindication

- Severe physical constitution

Preoperative Investigations/Preparation for the Procedure

- Clinical examination
- Contrast swallow (water-soluble)
- Upper gastrointestinal endoscopy
- Ultrasound
- Manometry
- A large gastric tube is carefully placed in the upper esophagus

Procedure

Access
The patient is placed in a supine position with the head rotated to the right.

| STEP 1 | Approach |

The approach to the diverticulum for surgical therapy comes through a left cervical incision (most Zenker's diverticula present on this side) at the level of the cricoid cartilage on the anterior aspect of the sternocleidomastoid muscle just above the clavicle. The anatomical overview of the access to the cervical esophagus is given in the figure.

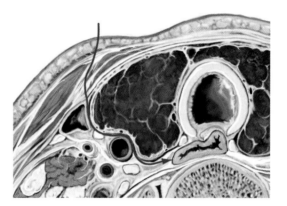

| STEP 2 | Dissection |

Dissection is performed between the medial aspect of the sternocleidomastoid muscle, which is pulled laterally, and the strap muscles by retracting the carotid sheath laterally and preserving the recurrent laryngeal nerve. The omohyoid muscle may be either retracted or transected. The thyroid gland is mobilized and vessels are dissected.

STEP 3   **Mobilization of the esophagus and the diverticulum**

The esophagus is mobilized from the prevertebral fascia, and the diverticulum is evident posterior to the esophagus (a tube may be inserted in the diverticulum for better identification). Large diverticula may extend into the mediastinum, but gentle traction and blunt dissection are sufficient to mobilize even the largest diverticula. The figure shows the anatomy of the cervical diverticula.

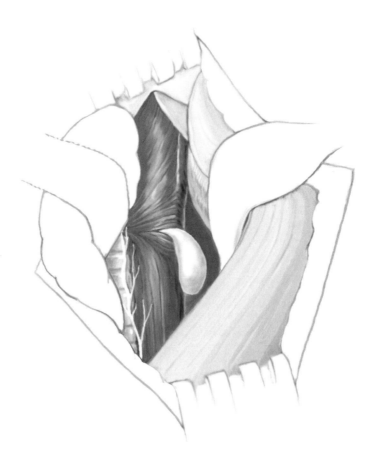

STEP 4   **Preparation of diverticulum**

The neck of the diverticulum is dissected. Gentle traction on the diverticulum exposes
the fibers of the cricopharyngeus muscle. Oral insufflation of air may help to find the
diverticulum. In the figure the anatomical aspects are shown (the vessels are retracted
to the left).

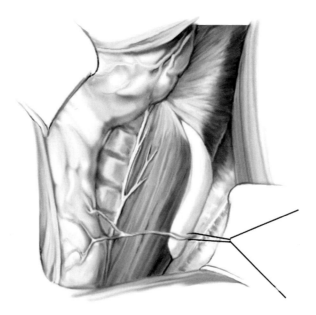

STEP 5   **Myotomy**

The cricopharyngeus muscles are divided and bluntly dissected from the mucosa. Myotomy of the pars transversa and of the upper esophagus is performed.

After myotomy several options exist, depending on the size of the diverticulum.

Small diverticula measuring up to 2 cm virtually disappear after the myotomy is completed and may be left alone or fixed cranially with the apex. They may be inverted and sutured to the prevertebral fascia, which prevents food retention without necessitating creation of a staple line or suture line that is at risk for fistula formation (A).

Larger diverticula are resected with a linear stapler parallel to the esophageal lumen, taking care not to compromise the diameter of the esophagus (B-1, B-2). Alternatively, open resection and closure with a running suture is performed.

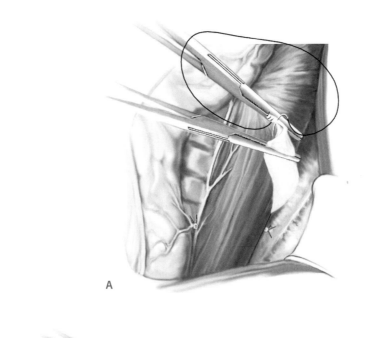

A

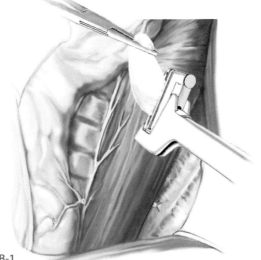

B-1

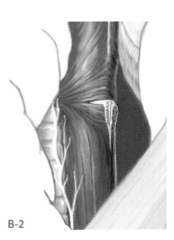

B-2

STEP 6

Closure

A soft Penrose drain is placed at the resection line. The skin is closed after placing only a few subcutaneous sutures.

Standard Postoperative Investigations

- Contrast study of the upper gastrointestinal tract (not routinely performed before starting oral intake).
- Most patients may be started on a liquid intake within hours of the operation.
- The duration of hospitalization has been declining, and may be necessary for 2 or 3 days.
- The drain is left in situ for about 5 days.
- A solid intake should be started after the 5th postoperative day.

Postoperative Complications

- Recurrent laryngeal nerve injury
- Wound infection
- Fistula formation/anastomotic leakage – conservative treatment with drainage and opening of the wound is usually the appropriate treatment.
- Retropharyngeal abscess may require surgical intervention.
- Recurrence rates after resection of a cricopharyngeal diverticulum are low, if the cricopharyngeus muscle has been divided completely.

Tricks of the Senior Surgeon

- Placement of a large gastric tube helps to identify the esophagus and the diverticulum.
- Tension free resection helps to avoid leakage.

Endoscopic Treatment of Zenker's Diverticulum

Uwe Seitz

Introduction

Treatment of Zenker's diverticulum with a flexible endoscope provides an alternative to surgery or the intraluminal approach with a rigid endoscope. The "septum" between the diverticulum and the esophagus is transected, thereby creating a common cavity of esophageal lumen and diverticulum, allowing easier food passage.

Indications

- Feasible in any patient including those not appropriate for general anesthesia

See chapter "Zenker's Diverticula: Open Approach" for contraindications, preoperative investigations, and preparation for the procedure.

Procedure

Intubation of the esophagus is often difficult in patients with a Zenker's diverticulum. A pediatric endoscope should be used to facilitate intubation. If the diverticulum is filled with food, cleaning by using a large channel endoscope should be first performed to avoid aspiration.

After intubating the esophagus, a Savary-Guillard wire is placed in the antrum, the endoscope is withdrawn and a nasogastric tube is placed over the wire through the mouth.

| STEP 1 | Argon-plasma coagulation of the septum |

The nasogastric tube indicates the entrance into the esophagus. This tube provides an excellent anatomical overview and simultaneously protects the esophageal wall during treatment (A).

The septum is treated with argon-plasma coagulation. The advantage of this method over conventional diathermy is the spray-like application. Bleeding from smaller vessels is avoided. In one session 1 cm of the septum is coagulated. The session is repeated after 4 weeks if required (B).

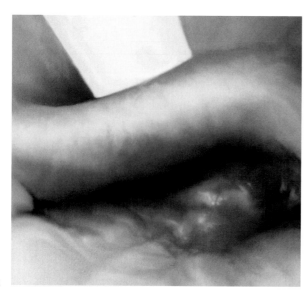

A

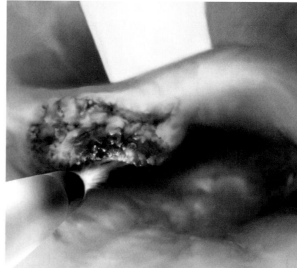

B

STEP 1 *(continued)*   ### Argon-plasma coagulation of the septum

Figure C shows the effect of argon-plasma coagulation at the end of the first session.

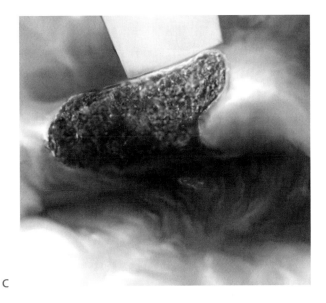

C

STEP 2   ### Needle knife incision

The beginning and the end of a session of needle knife incision are shown. Fibers of the cricopharyngeal muscle are visualized. In our experience the risk of bleeding is higher using the needle knife compared to argon-plasma coagulation, particularly in the first session.

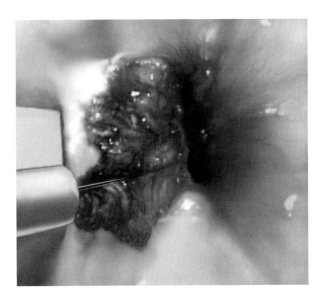

STEP 3   **Residual septum**

Residual septum after successful endoscopic treatment.

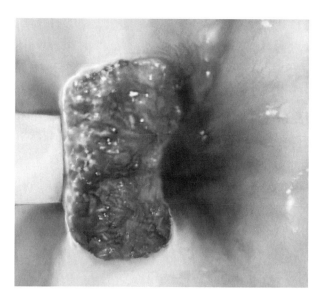

Standard Postoperative Investigations

■ No specific investigations are necessary

Postoperative Complications

■ Bleeding
■ Perforation

Tricks of the Senior Surgeon

■ Control bleeding with hemoclips or injection of diluted epinephrine (1:20,000).

Epiphrenic Diverticula

Chris G. Collins, Gerald C. O'Sullivan

Introduction

An epiphrenic diverticulum is a herniation of a pouch of esophageal mucosa through the musculature of the distal thoracic esophagus within 10 cm of the oesophago-gastric junction. The pathological process is thought to be due to the application of pulsion forces to the mucosa above a functionally obstructing region of abnormal esophageal motility.

In 1804 DeGuise accurately described the symptoms associated with a lower esophageal diverticulum, and in 1898 Reitzenstein provided the first radiological images. Manometry and cinefluorography was used by Cross et al. in 1968 to objectively demonstrate an etiological link between motility disturbance in the distal esophagus and diverticula formation.

Indications and Contraindications

Indications	■ Dysphagia
	■ Pulmonary complications (recurrent pneumonia, aspiration pneumonitis and lung abscess)

Contraindications	■ Asymptomatic diverticula (regular follow-up is advised to detect malignant change or significant enlargement with regurgitation or aspiration)
	■ Ongoing pneumonia or lung abscess (temporary)

Preoperative Investigation/Preparation for the Procedure

Clinical:	Full history and examination.
	Esophagogastroduodenoscopy (EGD): exclusion of associated carcinoma.
	Esophageal manometry: It may be necessary to position the manometry probe distal to the diverticulum in order to accurately define the dysmotility (24-h recordings provide a more accurate diagnosis).
Laboratory:	Routine biochemical profile to out rule any abnormality related to prolonged vomiting or forced fasting such as hypoalbuminia.
Radiology:	Plain chest radiograph.
	Contrast esophagogram (may need rotation to see smaller diverticula).

Broad-spectrum antibiotics are given preoperatively.

Treat complications of the diverticulum (aspiration pneumonia/lung abscess) prior to surgery.

Empty the diverticulum of retained secretions, food, or barium as completely as possible before anaesthesia is induced to reduce the risks of aspiration.

Procedure

Access
- Thoracic approach
- Laparoscopic abdominal approach
- Video-assisted thoracic approach

Thoracic Approach

Access
Standard left posterolateral thoracotomy through the 7th intercostal space (ICS)

STEP 1   **Exposure of the esophagus**

The inferior pulmonary ligament is divided with diathermy to the level of the inferior pulmonary vein and the lung is retracted upward. The mediastinal pleura overlying the esophagus is incised longitudinally to expose the esophagus and diverticulum.

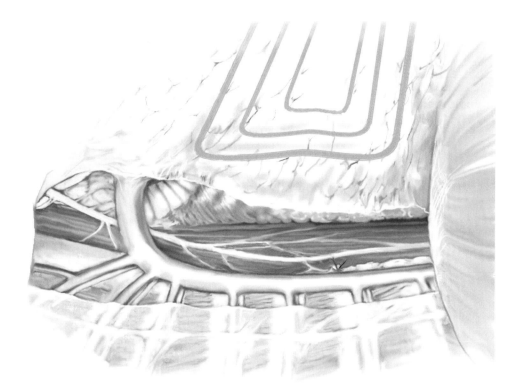

STEP 2

Exposure and resection of the diverticulum

The esophagus is mobilized from its bed sufficiently to allow dissection of the diverticulum, which is most often located posteriorly. The diverticulum is isolated, grasped with a Babcock type forceps, and carefully dissected from its attachments until the entire sac is free and attached to the esophagus only at the neck.

If the diverticulum has a wide neck, a large bougie (60F) is passed down the esophagus, and the diverticulum is then stapled longitudinally using a stapling device (TA) and excised.

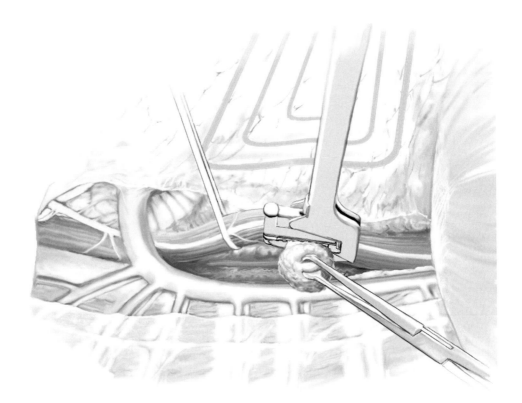

STEP 3

Exposure of the gastro-esophageal junction and myotomy

The muscular layer is closed over the mucosal staple line with interrupted 3-0 sutures.

A 2- to 3-cm incision is made into the abdomen through the phreno-esophageal ligament at the anterior margin of the hiatus along the midlateral border of the left crus. A tongue of gastric fundus is pulled up into the chest. This exposes the gastro-esophageal junction and its associated fat pad. The fat pad is excised.

A longitudinal myotomy is performed along the anterior wall of the esophagus (opposite side to the diverticulum) from approximately 1 cm above the diverticulum extending down for about 1–2 cm into the musculature of the stomach.

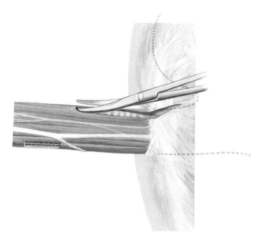

STEP 4

Reconstruction of the cardia

The cardia is reconstructed by suturing the tongue of the gastric fundus to the margins of the myotomy for a distance proximally of 4 cm using interrupted 3-0 Prolene sutures.

A chest tube is left in situ and brought out through a separate intercostal stab wound in the lower thorax.

The chest drain is usually removed 48 h postoperatively, if the lung is completely expanded and there is no evidence of leak or infection.

The nasogastric tube is left on low suction and removed on the third postoperative day.

Patients begin liquid oral intake following nasogastric tube removal, advancing to a full fluid diet as tolerated. Analgesics and anti-emetics minimize nausea and vomiting.

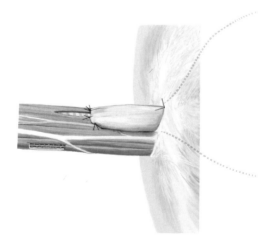

Laparoscopic Procedure

Access and Exposure

- Lithotomy position with 20–30° reverse Trendelenburg ("French position"). The surgeon stands between the legs.
- Pneumoperitoneum is established and five ports inserted.

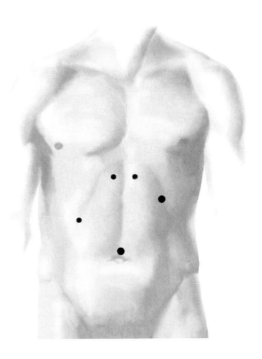

STEP 1

Exposure

The phreno-esophageal ligament is incised using endo-scissors. Dissection begins on the right crus and then moves to the left crus. The right crus is then dissected downward, and the esophagus is encircled with a Penrose drain for traction, via the left subcostal port. The Penrose drain is maintained in position for traction by approximation with a 3-0 endoloop.

Mediastinal dissection is then carried out using blunt instruments and acoustic scalpel, staying close to the esophagus until the diverticular pouch is reached.

STEP 2   **Endoscopy and preparation of the diverticulum**

The endoscope is inserted into the esophageal lumen at the level of the diverticulum. By using insufflation and transillumination, the diverticular pouch is defined to allow safe dissection. The pouch is thoroughly dissected until the neck of the diverticulum is completely clear of all adherent tissue, with care to avoid injury to the pleural sacs.

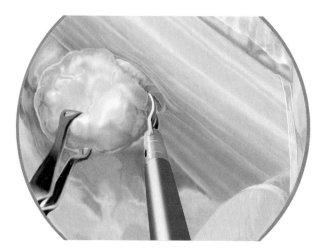

STEP 3   **Resection**

An endoscopic stapling device is introduced through the operative trocar in the left upper quadrant and is advanced to the level of the diverticular neck. The stapler jaws are closed under simultaneous endoscopic control; the endoscope is advanced into the stomach to prevent too much mucosa being excised, and it is then withdrawn. Once this is confirmed, the stapler is fired and mucosal closure is verified. Additional stapler applications may be necessary to completely incise and close the diverticular neck. The pouch is removed and the staple line is inspected using the endoscope.

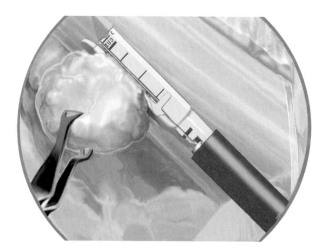

STEP 4

Myotomy

A myotomy is performed on the opposite esophageal wall, with longitudinal and circular muscular fibers divided and the submucosal plane carefully dissected using the acoustic scalpel. The myotomy is extended proximally above the upper limit of the diverticulum and distally for almost 1.5 cm onto the cardia using either acoustic scalpel or endo-scissors.

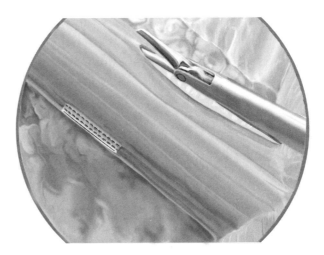

STEP 5

Dor fundoplication

The hiatus is closed posteriorly with two or three interrupted sutures. The anterior wrap is performed by suturing the gastric fundus to the muscular edges of the myotomy (Dor type procedure) and the gastric fundus is also sutured to the superior part of the crura. The fundus is sutured to the right crus and to both the right and left sides of the esophagus.

Video-Assisted Thoracoscopic Approach

Access
Positioning in a right lateral position as for left posterolateral thoracotomy.

The left lung is deflated using a double lumen endotracheal tube. Ports are inserted as follows:
- 10 mm at the 6th intercostal space posterior axillary line for the camera
- 10 mm at the 5th intercostal space at the anterior border of the axillary line for retraction of the lung
- 10 mm at the 3rd intercostal space for working cannula
- 12 mm at the mid-axillary line for working cannula

The procedure is as for the open procedure.

Standard Postoperative Investigations

- A water-soluble *non-ionic contrast swallow* is performed on day 5 postoperatively:
  - To exclude suture line leak
  - To verify the position of the wrap
  - To ensure that no significant obstruction has developed
  - To provide an impression of gastric emptying
- Carbonated beverages and very large meals must be avoided in the early post-operative period

Postoperative Complications

- Early (days to weeks):
  - Hemorrhage
  - Suture-line leak (if symptomatic then proceed to thoracotomy and repair, if asymptomatic then manage conservatively)
  - Pleural effusion
  - Empyema
  - Subphrenic abscess
- Late (months to years):
  - Recurrence of diverticulum. If symptomatic this is managed by open surgery.
  - Gastro-esophageal reflux with stricture (treated by dilatation and anti-reflux medication)
  - Para-esophageal hernia (may require surgical therapy and repair of the hernia)

Tricks of the Senior Surgeon

- Verification of impermeability of the suture line is confirmed using insufflation of air via the gastroscope in conjunction with insertion of saline via the laparoscope.
- Non-ionic contrast media is preferred to Gastrografin for the postoperative swallow as it provides superior images and is less reactive if aspirated or inadvertently leaks into thorax or abdomen.
- Small diverticula may be treated by plication and myotomy.
- Gastric dysparesis. This usually settles with pro-kinetic agents, but may require pyloroplasty.
- Intraoperative upper gastrointestinal endoscopy facilitates transillumination of the diverticulum, safe staple placement as well as suture line evaluation with insufflation.

Techniques of Local Esophagoplasty in Short Esophageal Strictures

Asad Kutup, Emre F. Yekebas, Jakob R. Izbicki

Introduction

Local esophagoplasty is indicated for patients with short esophageal strictures when endoscopic therapies including bougienage and balloon dilatation are not effective.

Indications and Contraindications

Indications

- Short peptic stricture
- Short scarred stenosis

Contraindications

- Suspicion of malignancy

Preoperative Investigations/Preparation for the Procedure

- Esophagogastroscopy with multiple biopsies.
- Special preparation: no peculiarities compared to the previously mentioned operations.
- Anesthesia: endotracheal anesthesia; in case of intrathoracic stenosis, a tracheal tube with the possibility of separate ventilation should be used.

Procedure

Positioning and Access
These depend on the location of the stenosis.
- Collar stenosis: left cervical approach, supination.
- Intrathoracic stenosis: right anterolateral thoracotomy using 4–6th intercostal spaces (ICS).
- Stenosis of the abdominal part of the esophagus: "inverted T-incision" or median laparotomy.

STEP 1

Resection and technique of anastomosis

After resection of the stenotic segment, mobilization of the proximal and distal end of the esophagus restores the basis for reconstruction of the continuity with single layer end-to-end anastomosis in single suture technique. The distance of each suture should be 5 mm. Each stitch should be placed 5 mm distant to the anastomosis.

In stenosis shorter than 1 cm, stricturoplasty according to Heineke Mikulicz should be performed. Therefore a longitudinal esophagectomy is performed using a single layer transverse closure with mattress sutures.

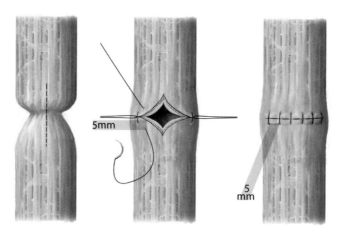

STEP 2

In case of limited stenosis

In stenosis limited to mucosa and submucosa, a transverse transection of the esophageal musculature over the stenosis suffices (A-1). The anterior part of the stricture is resected (A-2). Reconstruction of the continuity of the mucosa and submucosa in the posterior wall area (A-3) is done followed by transverse closure of the anterior wall with single layer mattress sutures (A-4).

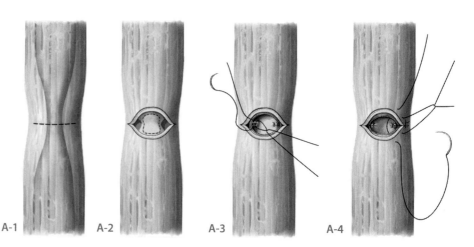

A-1   A-2   A-3   A-4

STEP 3   **In case of prestenotic dilatation**

In case of a prestenotic dilatation of the esophagus, side-to side esophagostomy of the pre- and poststenotic esophageal segment should be performed.

In all local esophagoplasties an intraluminally placed tube (large gastric tube) and abundant external drainage are obligatory.

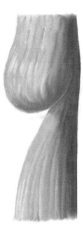 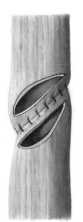 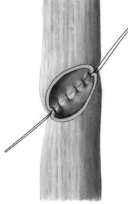

Standard Postoperative Investigations

- Daily check for insufficiency of the esophagoplasty
- If problems occur after removal of the drain, a contrast study with water-soluble contrast is recommended
- In case of early detected insufficiency: esophagoscopy with the feasibility of stenting

Postoperative Complications

- Leakage
- Mediastinitis
- Pleura empyema
- Peritonitis
- Re-stenosis

Tricks of the Senior Surgeon

- In case of caustic ingestions, organs adjacent to the esophagus, i.e., trachea, may be involved. In these instances, preparation of the esophagus has to be performed carefully.

Operation for Achalasia

Luigi Bonavina, Alberto Peracchia

Introduction

In 1913 Heller reported the first esophageal myotomy for achalasia through a left thoracotomy. Over the years, the transabdominal approach has been extensively adopted, especially in Europe. More recently, laparoscopy has emerged as the initial intervention of choice in several institutions throughout the world.

The operation consists of complete division of the two layers of esophageal muscle (longitudinal and circular fibers) and of the oblique fibers at the esophagogastric junction. A further step of the transabdominal procedure is the construction of an antireflux valve, most commonly an anterior fundoplication according to Dor.

Indications and Contraindications

Indications	■ In patients with documented esophageal achalasia, regardless of the disease's stage
Contraindications	■ Not deemed fit for general anesthesia and in those with: ■ Significant co-morbidity ■ Short life expectancy in whom pneumatic dilation or botulinum toxin injection represent a more reasonable therapeutic option ■ Extensive intra-abdominal adhesions from previous upper abdominal surgery can make the laparoscopic approach hazardous

Preoperative Investigation/Preparation for the Procedure

History and clinical evaluation:	Duration of dysphagia, nutritional status
Chest X-ray:	Atelectasis, fibrosis (s/p aspiration pneumonia)
Barium swallow study:	Degree of esophageal dilatation and lengthening
Esophageal manometry:	Non-relaxing lower esophageal sphincter, lack of peristalsis
Endoscopy:	Rule out esophageal mucosal lesions, *Candida* colonization, associated gastroduodenal disease
CT scan and/or endoscopic ultrasound (EUS) in selected patients:	Rule out pseudoachalasia (malignancy-induced)

Insert a double-lumen nasogastric tube 12h before surgery to wash and clean the esophageal lumen from food debris

Short-term antibiotic and antithrombotic prophylaxis

Laparoscopic Procedure

For details on access, see chapter "Laparoscopic Gastrectomy."

| STEP 1 | Exposure |

Incision of the phrenoesophageal membrane. Dissection is limited to the anterior surface of the esophagus and of the diaphragmatic crura to prevent postoperative reflux by preserving the anatomical relationships of the cardia. The cardia is mobilized only in patients with sigmoid esophagus; in such circumstances, it is preferable to reduce the redundancy in the abdomen and to close the crura posteriorly.

| STEP 2 | Heller myotomy |

The Heller myotomy is started on the distal esophagus using an L-shaped hook until identification of the submucosal plane.

The myotomy is extended on the proximal esophagus for about 6 cm using insulated scissors, a Harmonic Scalpel, or Ligasure device.

The myotomy is extended on the gastric side including the oblique fibers for about 2 cm using the L-shaped hook.

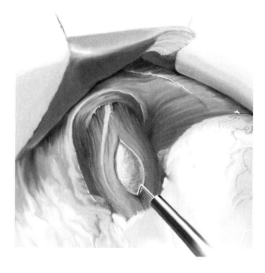

| STEP 3 | Intraoperative endoscopy |

Intraoperative endoscopy aids in evaluating the length of the myotomy, dividing residual muscle fibers, and checking the patency of the esophagogastric junction. This is most helpful in patients previously treated by pneumatic dilation or botulinum toxin injection.

| STEP 4 | Construction of the Dor fundoplication |

The anterior fundic wall is sutured with three interrupted stitches (Prolene for extracorporeal knots, Ethibond for intracorporeal knots) to the adjacent left muscle edge of the myotomy. The most cranial stitch incorporates the diaphragmatic crus.

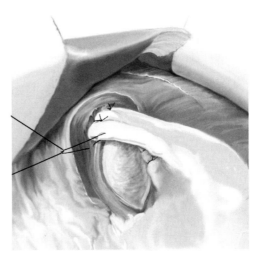

| STEP 5 | Security of the fundic wall |

A more lateral portion of the anterior fundic wall is secured with three interrupted stitches to the right muscle edge of the myotomy and to the left diaphragmatic crus.

Standard Postoperative Investigations

■ Gastrografin swallow on postoperative day 1 to check for esophagogastric transit and absence of leaks

Postoperative Complications

■ Persistent dysphagia
■ Delayed esophageal emptying
■ Recurrent dysphagia
■ Esophagectomy may be required in patients with decompensated sigmoid megaesophagus
■ Gastroesophageal reflux
■ Evidence of stricture may require mechanical dilatation followed by vagotomy and total duodenal diversion
■ Leak after undetected perforation
■ Consider endoscopic stenting and percutaneous CT-guided drainage

Tricks of the Senior Surgeon

■ Once the submucosal plane has been identified, use a pledget swab to create a tunnel before cutting the muscle upward.
■ Bleeding from the muscle edges of the myotomy is self-limiting; it is wise to avoid excessive electrocoagulation and to compress with a warm gauze for a few minutes.
■ Be careful when the endoscope is advanced into the esophagus and past the cardia after the myotomy is performed; the stomach grasper must be immediately released to prevent iatrogenic perforation.

Subtotal Gastrectomy, Antrectomy, Billroth II and Roux-en-Y Reconstruction and Local Excision in Complicated Gastric Ulcers

Joachim Ruh, Enrique Moreno Gonzalez, Christoph Busch

Subtotal Gastrectomy

Introduction

In subtotal gastrectomy, 75% of the stomach is resected. The passage is reconstructed using the proximal jejunum either as an omega loop or as a Roux-en-Y reconstruction.

Indications and Contraindications

Indications

- Gastric carcinoma of the intestinal type in the distal part of the stomach
- Complicated ulcers of the distal part of the stomach and the duodenum

Preoperative Investigations/Preparation for the Procedure

- In gastric carcinoma, the carcinoma should be clearly identified as an intestinal type in histopathological work-up.
- The location of the carcinoma/ulcerative lesion should be clearly identified by means of endoscopy.

Procedure

STEP 1   ### Abdominal incision and mobilization of the stomach

For laparotomy, a transverse epigastric incision should be chosen. In case of inadequate exposure, this incision should be extended with a midline incision. This approach provides adequate exposure up to the gastroesophageal junction. Alternatively, a midline laparotomy is adequate.

Following the exploration of the whole abdomen for metastatic disease in case of gastric cancer, the gastric lesion should be located.

The greater omentum of the stomach is dissected from the transverse colon, exposing the posterior wall of the stomach and opening the lesser sac (**A**).

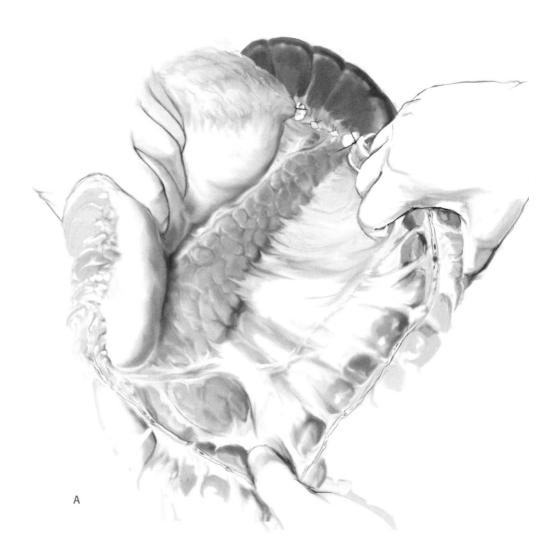

A

Abdominal incision and mobilization of the stomach

The pylorus is freed from adjacent connective tissue (B), and the omentum minus is opened along the minor curvature. Care has to be taken not to overlook a left hepatic artery. The left gastric artery is exposed as well as the coronary vein. Both structures are ligated and transected (C). Thus, the lymphatic tissue along the lesser and greater curvature is included in the specimen. The right gastric artery and vein are ligated and transected as well as the right gastroepiploic artery and vein at the greater curve, preserving the arcade vessels of the proximal part of the stomach.

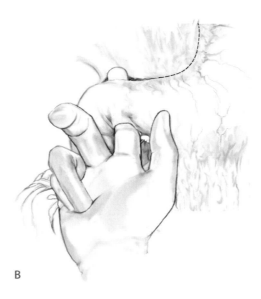

B

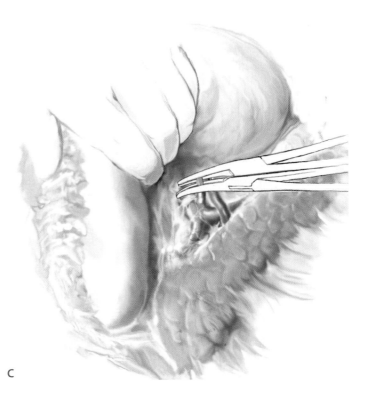

C

STEP 2

Resection

The resection margins are set at the pyloric region about 1 cm distal to the pylorus and the proximal third of the stomach (**A**). The duodenum is divided with the stapler device. It is recommended to make a single layer closure of the gastric incision with a running suture or single stitches. In case a stapler device is used, the serosa should be adapted with seromuscular stitches (**B**). The duodenal stump should be treated with special care, avoiding any tension on the suture line. For its closure, single stitches are used (**C**).

For the gastrojejunostomy, an omega loop, i.e., the Billroth II reconstruction (STEP 1–3), or a Roux-en-Y reconstruction (STEP 1) is used.

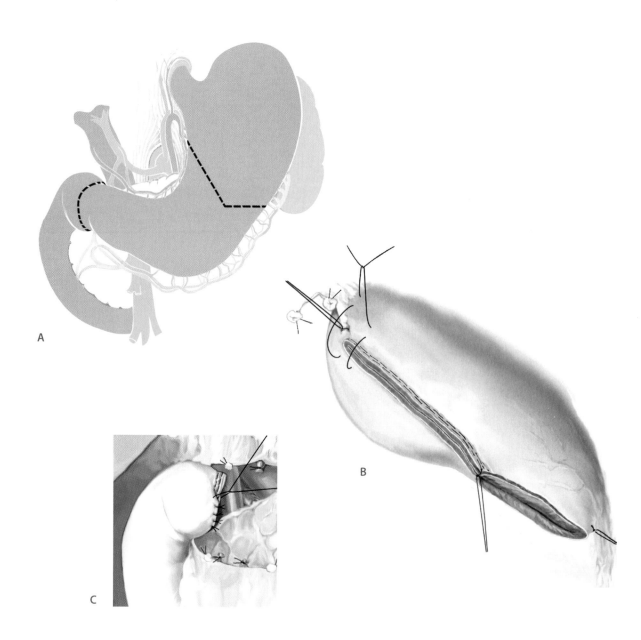

A

B

C

Antrectomy

Introduction

In antrectomy, 25% of the distal part of the stomach is resected.

Indications and Contraindications

Indications

- Complicated duodenal ulcers and ulcers of the prepyloric region. Antrectomy is performed in combination with bilateral truncal vagotomy. This procedure reduces acid secretion by reduction of acetylcholine stimulus of the vagus nerve and gastrin production of the antrum.

Preoperative Investigations

- Endoscopic verification of the lesion
- Exclusion of gastrinoma and hypercalcemia as risk factors
- Exclusion of carcinoma (multiple biopsies)

Procedure

STEP 1   **Mobilization of the stomach and vagotomy**

As in subtotal gastrectomy, the stomach is mobilized and freed from the omentum, and the pylorus is isolated. The vagal trunks are identified on the distal part of the esophagus, with the anterior branch of the nerve lying on the left part of the esophagus, and the posterior branch lying on the back or to the right side of the esophagus (**A**). About 2 cm of each branch is resected, and the nerve ends are ligated (**B**).

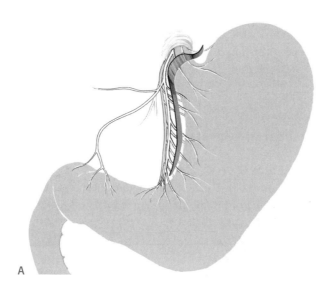

A

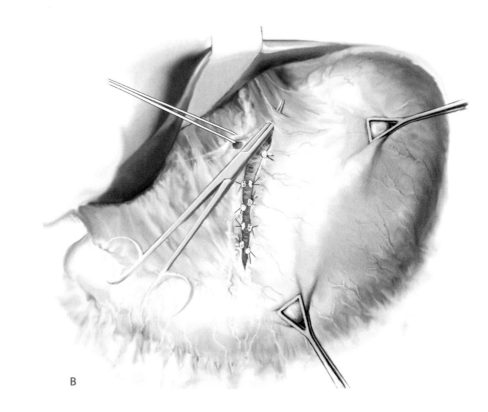

B

STEP 2	**Exposure of the antrum**

The pylorus (see "Subtotal Gastrectomy" STEP 1, Fig. B) and the distal part of the stomach are dissected, ligating the vasculature on the greater and lower curvature. Using a stapling device is the most convenient way to perform the resection.

STEP 3	**Resection margins**

The resection margins are set similar to the subtotal gastrectomy concerning the duodenum (see "Subtotal Gastrectomy" STEP 1). The proximal resection line is placed below the gastroesophageal junction on the lower curvature and in the middle between the fundus and the pylorus at the greater curvature.

STEP 4	**Reconstruction of the passage**

For reconstruction of the passage, the Billroth II (STEP 1–3) or the Roux-en-Y procedure is used (STEP 1).

Billroth II Reconstruction

Procedure

The gastrojejunostomy is done with an omega loop.

STEP 1   **Placement of the omega loop**

Choose a loop of the proximal jejunum that can easily be mobilized to the distal part of the posterior wall of the remnant stomach. The distance of the loop is kept short when a retrocolic route is chosen.

Prepare a small passage in the mesentery of the transverse colon and pull the omega loop through the mesentery. Mind that no tension is exerted on the mesentery when the loop is in place.

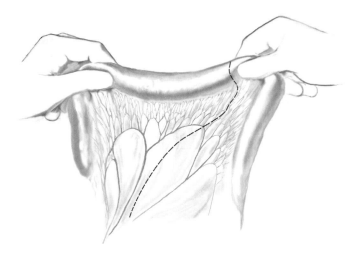

STEP 2

Gastrojejunostomy

Open the closure of the distal gastric remnant and the antimesenteric side of the omega loop. For the backward layer, use single stitches or a running suture (A, B).

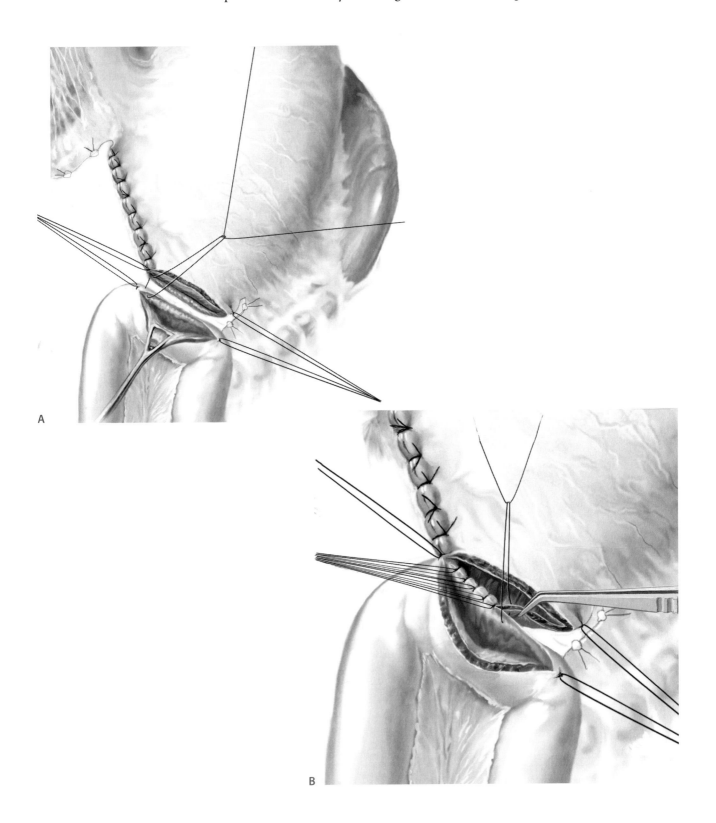

A

B

STEP 2 *(continued)*

Gastrojejunostomy

For the anterior anastomosis, a running inverting suture is adequate. However, a mono-layer with single stitches is also possible as well as the appliance of a stapling device (C). To avoid anastomotic stricture, the gastrojejunostomy should be performed over a distance of 5–6 cm.

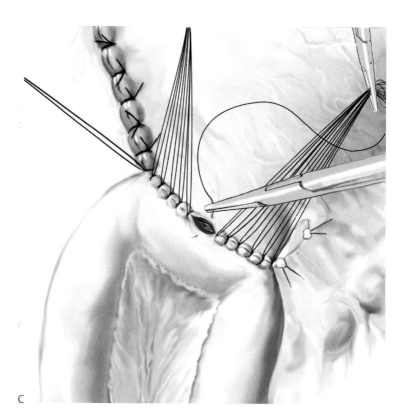

C

STEP 3   **Braun's anastomosis**

Braun's anatomosis is performed as distal as possible (>40 cm) to avoid biliary reflux into the gastric remnant. Side-to-side jejunostomy is done either with single stitches, a running suture, or a stapler device (**A**, **B**, **C**).

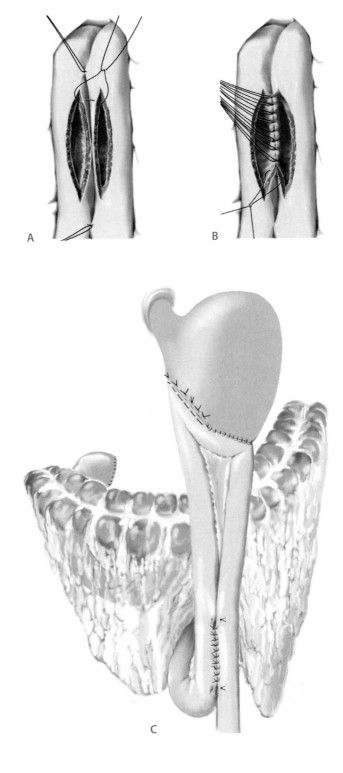

Roux-en-Y Reconstruction

Procedure

STEP 1   **Dissection of the jejunum**

The ligament of Treitz is identified, and the jejunum is dissected about 40–50 cm distal to Treitz' ligament (**A**). For convenience, a stapler device may be used. The blind end of the distal part is closed using a running suture or single stitches. The distal loop is placed side-to-side to the posterior wall of the gastric remnant without exerting any tension on the mesentery. A retrocolic route is preferable. Before performing the anastomosis, the serosa of the jejunal loop is fixed to the serosa of the gastric remnant over a distance of 5–6 cm, thus building the outer layer of the backward suture (**B**).

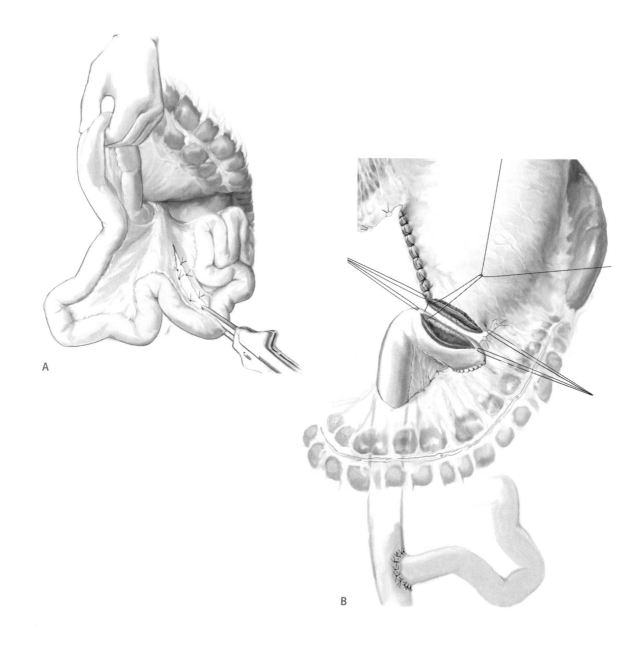

A

B

STEP 2

Gastrojejunostomy

The jejunal loop and the gastric wall are opened along the antimesenteric border using electrocautery, and the posterior part of the anastomosis is done with a running suture representing the inner layer, completed by a running inverting suture on the anterior part of the gastrojejunostomy.

However, single stitches in monolayer technique as well as the appliance of a stapler device are also adequate. The technique is similar to the gastrojejunostomy in the Billroth II reconstruction (STEP 2).

The dissected jejunal loop is anastomosed end-to-side to the distal part of the jejunum 40–50 cm distal to the ligament of Treitz.

Postoperative Investigations

- The gastric tube should be kept until there are no further signs of gastric reflux or gastrointestinal atonia are present. Indwelling drains should be kept until enteral nutrition has been started.

Postoperative Complications

- Short term:
    - Insufficiency of the gastrojejunostomy
    - Insufficiency of the duodenal stump
    - Acute pancreatitis, pancreatic fistula
    - Early dumping syndrome
    - Biliary stricture
- Long term:
    - Biliary reflux
    - Stricture of the gastrojejunostomy
    - Stump carcinoma
    - Late dumping syndrome

Local Excision in the Stomach

Introduction

Ulcers that do not respond to medical treatment, perforation, or bleeding require surgical intervention. In bleeding, an endoscopic treatment is the firstline approach. If bleeding cannot be controlled by endoscopic means, surgical excision is the therapy of choice.

Local excision in the stomach is indicated when the extension of the ulcer allows for readaption without exerting any tension on the anastomosis.

The test for *Helicobacter pylori* and the maintenance of antacid medication are mandatory. Work-up includes gastrin testing and testing for elevated serum calcium levels, both risk factors in complicated ulcers.

Indications and Contraindications

Indications

- Endoscopically uncontrollable bleeding and perforation are indications. for an emergency procedure.

Standard Preoperative Investigations

In Case of Bleeding
- Endoscopy with the identification of the bleeding site: active bleeding is identified by endoscopy or systemic hemoglobin values. Blood pressure and heart rate are recorded.

In Case of Suspected Perforation
- Standard X-ray of the abdomen in upright and left semiprone position
- Gas insufflation via a gastric tube may facilitate the diagnosis in conventional X-ray examination; in case of peritonism without direct evidence of free abdominal gas, a CT scan should be obtained.
- Especially in retroperitoneal perforation of the duodenum, free gas may not be seen in standard X-ray films.

Procedure in Perforated Gastric Ulcers

STEP 1	**Exposure of the ulcerative lesion**

The ulcerative lesion is completely exposed. In case of perforation of the posterior gastric wall, the omentum of the stomach and of the colon is separated, and the omental bursa is exposed (see "Subtotal Gastrectomy" STEP 1, Fig. B).

STEP 2	**Excision of the ulcer**

In case of chronic granulation, the wall of the ulcer is excised longitudally.

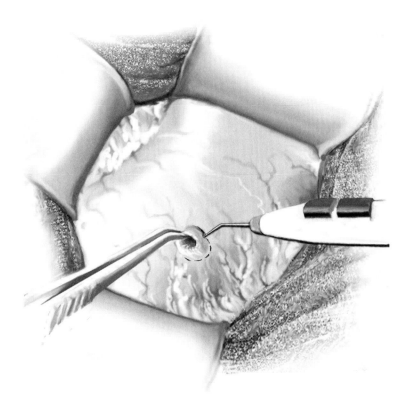

STEP 3

Closure

The ulcer is closed in a crosswise technique by single layer stitches with an absorbable suture. (**A**, **B**).

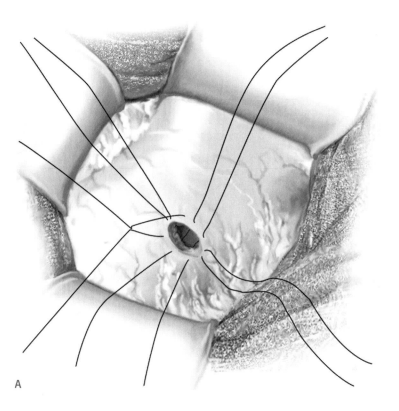

A

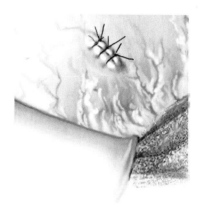

B

Procedure in Bleeding Gastric Ulcers Refractory to Endoscopic Treatment

| STEP 1 | Gastrotomy and exposure of the bleeding site |

In bleeding without perforation, gastrotomy is the exposure of choice.
   Use a longitudinal incision of the anterior gastric wall.

| STEP 2 | Isolation of the bleeding |

In bleeding of the posterior gastric wall, verify that the source of bleeding might arise from an ulceration of the splenic artery. In this case, separate the artery at its origin and ligate it. Additional stitches placed around the ulcer wall on all four sides may help to control bleeding. The use of a non-absorbable suture is preferable. Collaterals maintain blood supply to the spleen, and splenectomy is not required.

| STEP 3 | Closure |

Closure of the incision with the single layer technique.

Local Excision in the Duodenum

Introduction

In complicated duodenal ulcers, local excision is the therapy of choice.

Depending on the localization and the extension, a duodenojejunostomy with a Roux-en-Y reconstruction is indicated. Further, the gastroduodenal artery should be ligated in case of bleeding ulcers.

Indications and Preoperative Investigations

■ These correspond to those in gastric ulcers and bleeding (see "Local Excision in the Stomach" above).

Procedure in Complicated Duodenal Ulcers

Ventral Duodenal Wall

STEP 1   **Exposure of the duodenum**

The duodenum is completely exposed and opened longitudinally.

In case of perforation, the ulcerative lesion is excised.

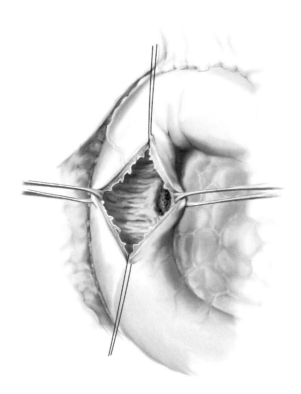

STEP 2   **Closure of the incision**

The incision is closed crosswise using single stitches. Kocher's maneuver may lower the tension to the suture. Mind that the duodenal passage is not compromised. Depending on the extent of the excision, primary closure might not be advisable. In this case, a duodenojejunostomy is required using a Roux-en-Y reconstruction (A-1, A-2, A-3).

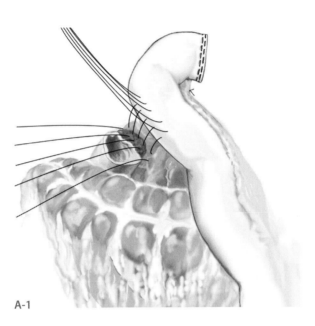

A-1

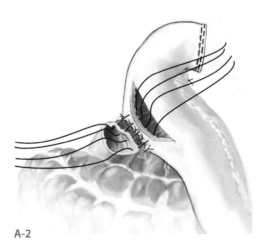

A-2

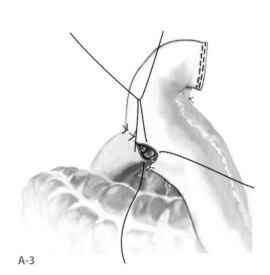

A-3

Posterior Duodenal Wall

STEP 1

Exposure of the duodenum

After exposing the duodenum, Kocher's maneuver is performed, and the posterior wall of the duodenum is completely exposed in case of perforation. In case of bleeding, the anterior wall is opened, and single stitches are placed on all four sides of the ulcerative lesion.

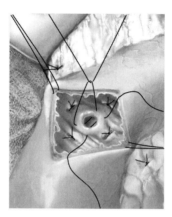

STEP 2

Excision of the ulcerative lesion

The ulceration is excised (see "Local Excision in the Stomach", STEP 2). As a rule, primary closure of the lesion may not be advisable, as mobilization of the posterior duodenal wall is limited. Hence, a duodenojejunostomy is put in place. The gastro-duodenal artery is exposed and ligated at its origin. In case of bleeding ulcers, this step might be taken first, when the bleeding source has previously been identified in gastroduodenoscopy.

Standard Postoperative Investigations

- The clinical course of the patient and the careful daily observation of the drains are the key points in postoperative care.

Postoperative Complications

- Anastomotic leaks and abscess formation
- Peritonitis
- Anastomotic strictures
- Delayed gastric emptying
- Recurrence of bleeding and ulcerations
- Pancreatitis
- Lesion to the pancreatic duct/papilla Vateri with biliary congestion

Tricks of the Senior Surgeon

- When mobilizing the minor curvature of the stomach, bear in mind that an atypical left hepatic artery may be present.
- Take care that the duodenal stump is closed without any tension on the wall. Mobilize the duodenum if required.
- The gastroduodenal artery should be carefully preserved to maintain adequate blood supply to the duodenum in case of Billroth II reconstruction.
- To avoid any biliary reflux, choose an adequate length of the jejunal loop (>40 cm distal of the ligament of Treitz).
- To avoid any stricture of the anastomosis, choose a length of the gastrotomy for the anastomosis of 5–6 cm in gastroenterostomy.
- In case of Roux-en-Y reconstruction, the blind end of the jejunal loop should be kept short to avoid the building of a reservoir within the blind end.
- In case of Billroth II procedure and artificial lesion to the spleen requiring splenectomy, take care that the remnant part of the stomach is adequately supplied with blood as the short gastric arteries arise from the splenic artery. In case of hypoperfusion, resection of the gastric remnant is necessary, and an esophagojejunostomy should be done.

Total Gastrectomy with Conventional Lymphadenectomy

Jürg Metzger

Introduction

In 1884 Connor attempted the first total gastrectomy in humans, reestablishing continuity with an esophagoduodenostomy. His patient did not survive the operation. In 1897 Schlatter carried out the first successful total gastrectomy. In 1892, Roux described a new procedure where the jejunal loop was divided and the distal limb was joined to the esophagus. The proximal limb of the loop was anastomosed to the jejunum some 45 cm distal to the esophagus. A large number of gastric substitutes have been tried over the past century grouped into large and small bowel procedures. Some operations preserve the continuity through the duodenum. Others bypass the duodenal passage. Some procedures include a pouch construction and/or an antireflux modification. Currently, Roux-en-Y reconstruction is still the most widely used procedure after a total gastrectomy.

Indications and Contraindications

Indications	
	■ Adenocarcinomas arising in corpus or fundus of the stomach
	■ Malignant tumors arising in the antrum of the stomach and showing a poor pathohistological diagnosis (low grade tumors, diffuse type, signet-ring)
	■ Zollinger-Ellison syndrome
	■ Mesenchymal tumors (e.g., gastrointestinal stromal tumors, GISTs)
	■ Palliative gastrectomy for severe bleeding

Contraindications	
	■ Peritoneal carcinosis
	■ Penetration into neighboring organs
	■ Child-Pugh C cirrhosis with severe portal hypertension

Preoperative Investigation and Preparation for the Procedure

History:	Cardiac disease, pulmonary disease, gastric outlet function, melena, alcohol, smoking, *Helicobacter pylori* infection, diet, geographic risk, genetic factors
Clinical evaluation:	Nutritional status
Laboratory tests:	Hb, coagulation parameters, tumor markers, albumin
Gastroscopy:	To prove the diagnosis (biopsies), endoscopic ultrasound
CT scan:	Assessment of resectability, distant mestastases
Preparation:	Consider bowel preparation with preoperative signs of involvement of large bowel

Procedure

Access
Midline incision or bisubcostal incision, division of round and falciform ligament

STEP 1

Exposure and exploration of the abdomen with focus on

- Liver metastases
- Peritoneal carcinosis
- Tumor localization and size
- Lymph node enlargement
- Penetration into pancreas, spleen, and transverse colon

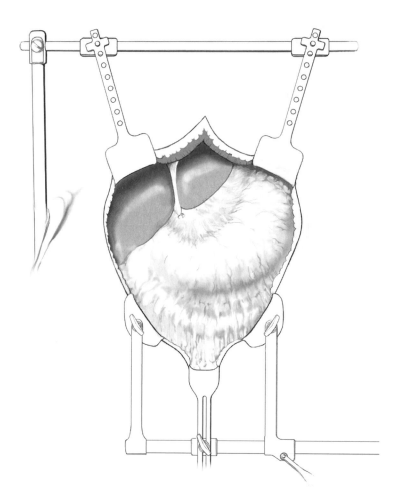

STEP 2   **Separation of the greater omentum from the entire transverse colon**

The entire gastrocolic omentum is separated from the transverse colon by scissors
dissection through the avascular embryonic fusion plane. It is tremendously helpful
to be alert of the difference in texture and color of the fat in the epiploic appendices of
the colon and that of the omentum. Bleeding will be avoided by keeping this important
plane of dissection between these two different structures. The next step is to elevate
the mobilized omentum from the transverse colon and to expose the anterior surface
of the pancreas. As the omentum is mobilized, the venous branch between the right
gastroepiploic and middle colic veins is identified and ligated.

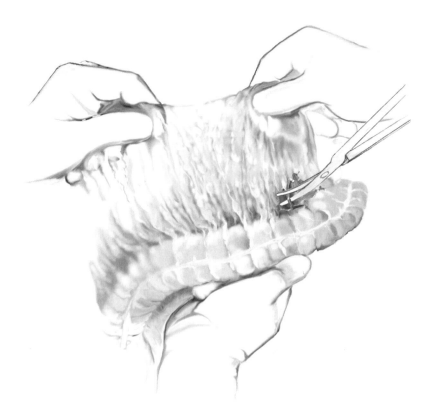

STEP 3   **View of the mobilized left liver lobe and the esophagogastric junction**

Next mobilize the left lobe of the liver unless segments II and III can easily be retracted. The lesser omentum is divided. If present, a replaced left hepatic artery will be identified at this time and should be preserved. An additional liver retractor is used so that the abdominal part of the esophagus is visible. The stomach is then pulled in an inferior direction and the peritoneum and membrana phrenico-esophagea are incised over the esophagogastric junction. Both crura of the diaphragm are identified and cleared. Using a large dissector, the esophagus is separated from the crura and is then encircled by a finger. A rubber band is placed around the esophagus and retained by a clamp. The vagal nerves are divided, which facilitates further mobilization of the distal esophagus.

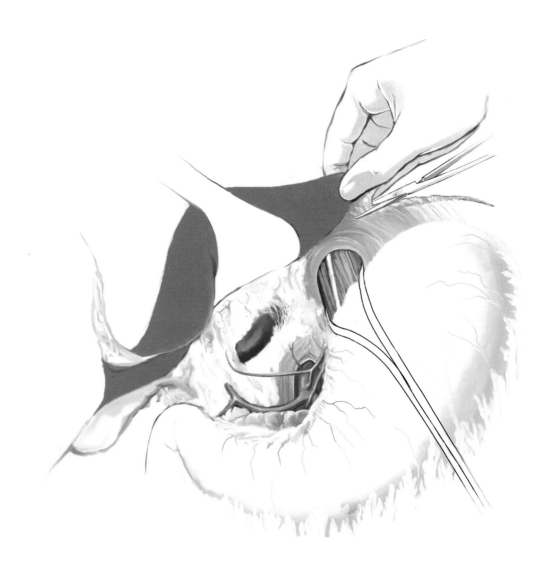

STEP 4   **Mobilization of the greater curvature**

The greater omentum is released from the splenic flexure. The stomach is then gently pulled in an inferior and medial direction and the short gastric vessels are dissected at the point of contact with the greater curvature of the stomach.

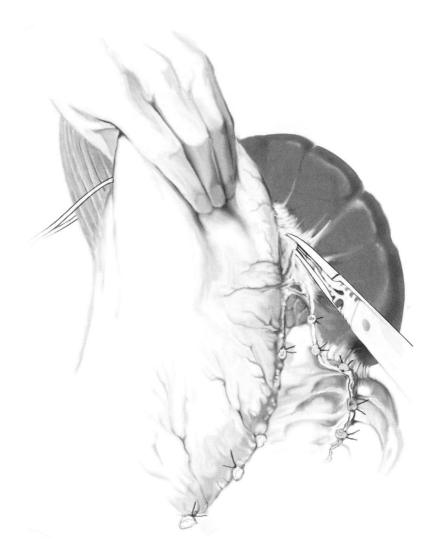

STEP 5

Transection of the duodenum

The right gastroepiploic and the right gastric arteries are divided, and the posterior wall
of the duodenum is freed. Extensive duodenal dissection is not necessary when the
distal antrum is free of tumor. The duodenum is then transected with a linear stapler
1–2 cm below the pylorus. The stapler line is oversewn with a non-dissolvable running
suture. The distal end of the specimen is covered with a gauze, which should be fixed in
place with an additional umbilical tape ligature.

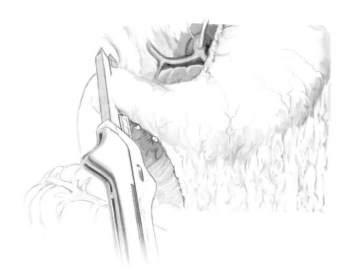

STEP 6

D2 lymphadenectomy

The stomach is now held upwards and to the left, which allows optimal exposure. A D2-compartment lymphadenectomy is carried out. This involves removing all the nodes along the common hepatic artery, nodes behind and within the hepatoduodenal ligament, and nodes along and around the celiac artery, the trunk of the splenic artery and the cranial margin and surface of the pancreas. All the arteries are fully freed of areolar and lymphatic tissue and secured with vessel loops. It is important to clip or ligate all the remaining lymphatic vessels to avoid postoperative lymphorrhea.

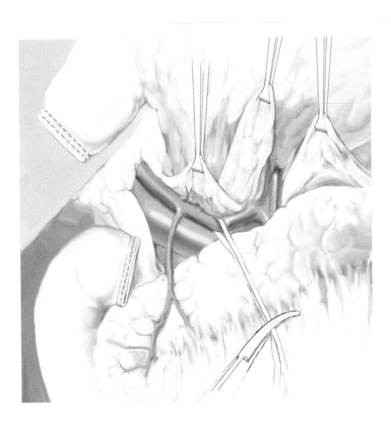

STEP 7   **Division of left gastric vessels**

The left gastric vessels are identified and isolated from adjacent tissues by blunt and sharp dissection and are then ligated and divided. The coronary vein, which is situated just caudal to the artery, is often identified first in the course of dissection.

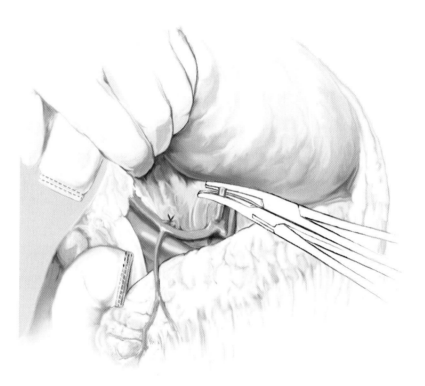

STEP 8	Transection of the distal esophagus

After mobilization of the entire stomach, the esophagus is then divided just above the cardia. A right-angled clamp is placed distal to the lower esophagus and the esophagus is divided by electrocautery. The specimen, which consists of stomach, proximal 2 cm of duodenum, greater omentum and regional lymph nodes, is sent to pathology to confirm the adequacy of the resected margins before reconstruction.

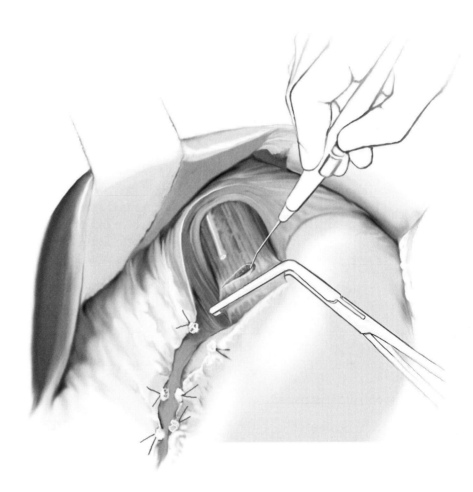

STEP 9   **Roux-en-Y reconstruction**

Preparation of Roux-en-Y jejunal segment: A jejunal loop is elevated about 20–30 cm
beyond the ligament of Treitz (**A-1**). Dissection of the mesentery is facilitated by transillumination. The peritoneum is incised along the resection line. The small bowel is
divided with a linear stapler (**A-2**). To reach a sufficient length of the Roux-en-Y loop it
is sometimes necessary to further divide the main arcades, but it is crucial to preserve
the peripheral arcades.

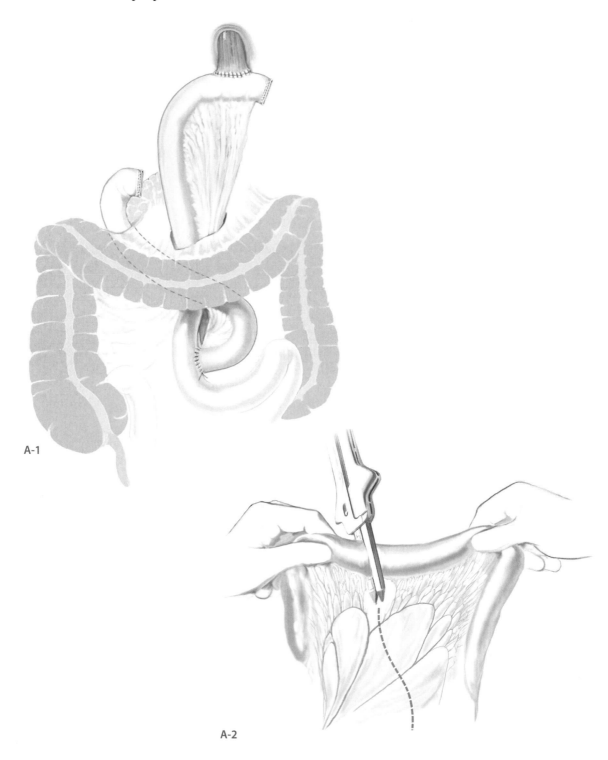

A-1

A-2

STEP 10 **End-to-side sutured esophagojejunostomy**

There are two ways of performing the esophagojejunostomy, suturing either end-to-end or end-to-side. My preference is to use the latter because the end-to-end method carries an increased risk of compromising the circulation at the end of the jejunal loop. It is also easier to match the diameter of esophagus and jejunum in this way. The anastomosis is sutured by hand using a single-layer interrupted suture technique (lift anastomosis).

- An antimesenteric incision is made in the end of the jejunum, its length corresponding to the diameter of the esophagus. To avoid a blind loop syndrome, the incision is made close (1–2cm) to the end of the jejunum closed earlier by the staples and oversewn with a non-dissolvable running suture (A).
- Two corner sutures are inserted and lightly tensioned with Pean forceps. A further stitch is placed midway between the corner stitches on the posterior wall and the back line is completed using full-thickness mattress sutures (B).

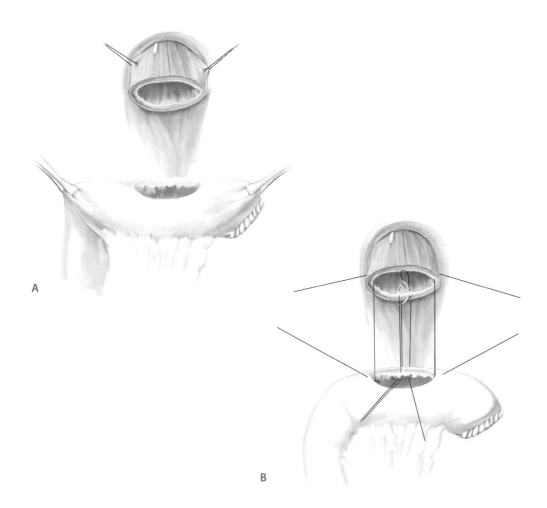

A

B

End-to-side sutured esophagojejunostomy

- The sutures pass from the jejunal lumen outwards through all layers and complete the circuit by passing through the wall of the esophagus from outside to inside. The needle is then turned around and the backstitch picks up only a small bite of mucosa on each side of the bowel lumina. The sutures extend approximately 5–8 mm from the wound margins, depending on the wall thickness, and the gap between the stitches is 4–6 mm (C).
- Threads are then held in a coil fixed to a Kocher clamp on the retractor hook (D).

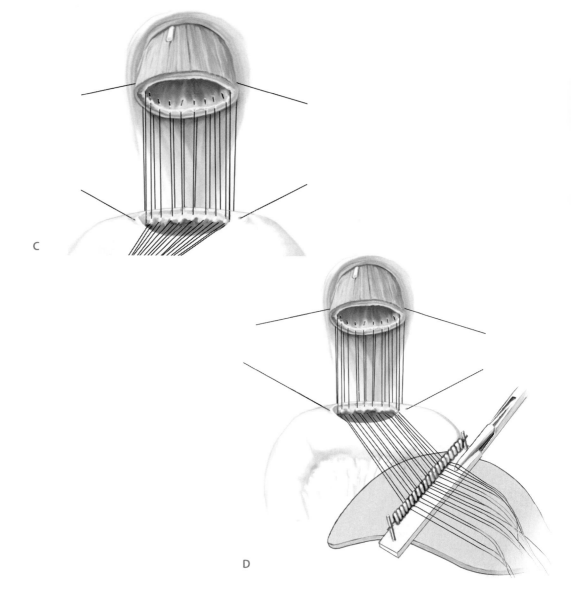

C

D

STEP 10 *(continued)*   **End-to-side sutured esophagojejunostomy**

- After insertion of all backwall stitches, they are then railroaded down to the anastomosis using a wet swab on a stick. It is very important to hold the ends of all threads under firm tension to ease this maneuver (E).
- The anterior wall of the anastomosis is closed with a continuous suture if there is a good view or with interrupted sutures when the view is less satisfactory. The anterior wall anastomosis is also begun at the far corner using an extramucosal stitch on the small-bowel side and a full thickness stitch on the esophagus wall. Before completing the front wall, the gastric tube is led down into the jejunum (F).

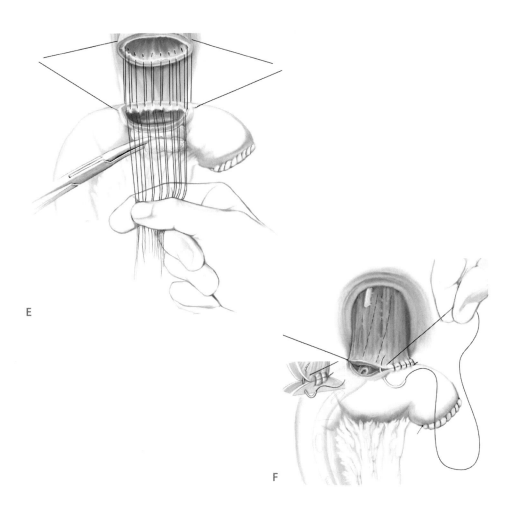

E

F

STEP 11

Reconstruction of the intestine

At a point 50–60 cm below the esophagojejunostomy, an end-to-side jejunojejunostomy is performed using a continuous extramucosal suture technique.

All openings in the mesentery are closed by monofilament suture.

Two drainages are placed behind the esophagojejunostomy and around the duodenal stump.

Standard Postoperative Investigations

- Hemoglobin
- Check daily for clinical signs of infection (anastomotic leak)
- Contrast study of esophagojejunostomy (day 6)

Postoperative Complications

- Short term:
  - Intra-abdominal bleeding
  - Subphrenic abscess
  - Anastomotic leak
  - Pancreatic fistula
  - Duodenal stump leak
- Long term:
  - Weight loss, decreasing nutritional status (reservoir capacity)
  - Diarrhea
  - Dumping syndrome
  - Alkaline reflux

Tricks of the Senior Surgeon

- Ask the anesthesiologist not to introduce a gastric tube before having completed the backwall of the esophagojejunostomy. This may minimize the risk of esophagus spasm.
- Keep the dissection of the short gastric vessels closed to the great curvature of the stomach.
- Secure the duodenal stump (staples row) with a continuous suture.
- Use magnifying glasses to perform the lymphadenectomy.

Total Gastrectomy with Radical Systemic Lymphadenectomy (Japanese Procedure)

Mitsuru Sasako

Introduction

Historically, total gastrectomy with radical lymphadenectomy included distal pancreatectomy and splenectomy and was favored by Brunschwig in 1948. Maruyama modified this procedure by preserving the distal pancreas, so-called pancreas preserving radical total gastrectomy. His initial report was published in Japanese in 1979. Initially he ligated both the splenic artery and vein near their origin, which often caused major congestion of the pancreas tail followed by massive necrosis. The first available English report was published in 1995 and described a modified technique of the original version. There he obtained the splenic vein up to the tip of the pancreas tail to preserve venous return.

The technique of pancreas preserving total gastrectomy with radical systemic lymphadenectomy (D2) by preserving the splenic artery and vein as far as the branching-off of the major pancreatic artery (Sasako's modification) is described.

Indications and Contraindications

Indications

- Gastric carcinoma (T2–T4, M0) involving the upper third of the stomach

Contraindications

- By invasion of the pancreas body or tail or macroscopically evident lymph node metastasis at the splenic artery, an extended total gastrectomy with pancreatico-splenectomy (en bloc resection) should be performed.
- Invasion of the distal esophagus
- Distant metastasis
- Severe cardiopulmonary insufficiency (relative)

Preoperative Investigations/Preparation for the Procedure

See chapter on "Total Gastrectomy with Conventional Lymphadenectomy."

Procedure

Access
Upper median incision or upper transverse incision with median T-shaped extension.

STEP 1   **Exposure**

Laparotomy and inspection are performed of the peritoneum, liver and, after mobilization of the duodenum by the Kocher maneuver, the para-aortic area. After cytological washings out of the Douglas space, one or two Kent type retractors with one or two octopus retractors are inserted for best overall view of the epigastric region, especially the diaphragmatic esophageal hiatus. Excision of the ensisternum is recommended.

Steps of the preparation of the gastrectomy are described in the chapter "Total Gastrectomy with Conventional Lymphadenectomy."

STEP 2   **Omentectomy**

The transverse mesocolon is stretched by the second assistant. Dissection of the greater omentum together with the posterior wall of the omental bursa is performed. It is compromised by two membranes, one continuing to the anterior pancreatic capsule and the other to the posterior duodenopancreatic fascia. Diathermy allows bloodless transection.

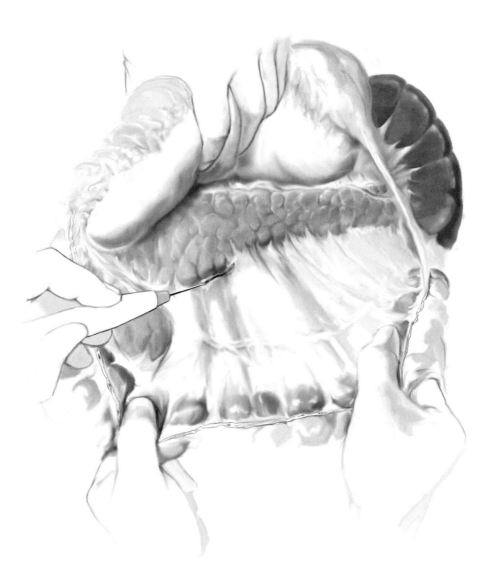

STEP 3   Dissection of infrapyloric lymph nodes

Following the right accessory vein, Henle's surgical trunk can be found. The origin of the right gastroepiploic vein is ligated. Before going on to the third step, the dissection plane should be changed from the posterior to the anterior capsule of the pancreas.

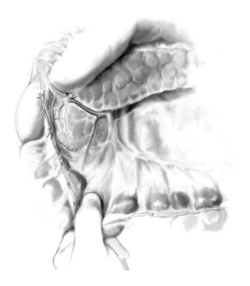

| STEP 4 | Ligation and division of the right gastroepiploic artery |

By dissection of the anterior capsule of the pancreas towards the duodenum, the gastroduodenal artery appears on the anterior surface of the pancreas neck. Following this artery caudally, the origin of the right gastroepiploic artery can be found. After its ligation and division, the gastroduodenal artery should be followed cranially up to the bifurcation of the common hepatic artery.

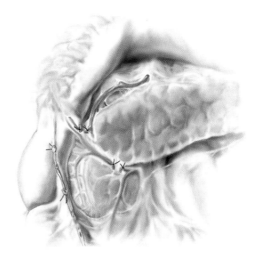

| STEP 5 | Division of the lesser omentum |

Close to the left liver lobe, the lesser omentum is divided from the left edge of the hepatoduodenal ligament towards the esophagus.

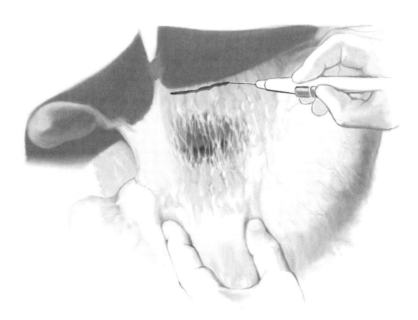

STEP 6

Division of the right gastric artery

The lesser omentum is incised along the hepatoduodenal ligament up to the left side of the common bile duct and caudally to the duodenum. After ligation and division of the supraduodenal vessels, the gastric artery clearly displays in the ligament.

The tissue defined by this incision is dissected from the proper hepatic artery and swept across to the patient's left. The gastroduodenal artery is followed to its junction with the proper hepatic artery, and the latter is cleaned until the origin of the right gastric artery is found and ligated. The dissection to the left of the hepatoduodenal ligament should go deeper than the proper hepatic artery and clear the nodes from the left side of the portal vein.

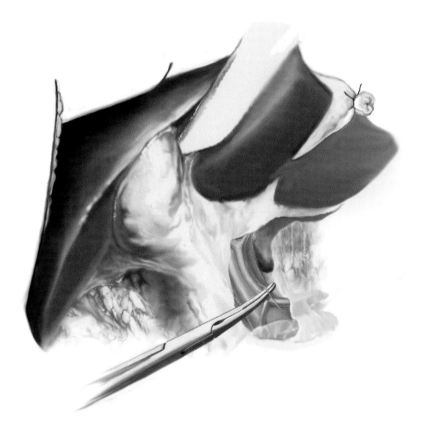

STEP 7 — Dissection of suprapancreatic nodes

Along the superior border of the pancreas the adipose tissue contains many lymph nodes. It is divided from the pancreas and the surface of the common hepatic, splenic, and celiac arteries. These arteries are surrounded by thick nerve tissue. It should be preserved in case of no adherence of suspect lymph nodes. The left gastric vein is visible and therefore ligated and divided. Caudally it crosses the origin of either the common hepatic or splenic artery before entering the splenic vein in about 30–40% of patients. In the majority the left gastric vein passes obliquely behind the hepatic artery to join the junction of the splenic and portal veins.

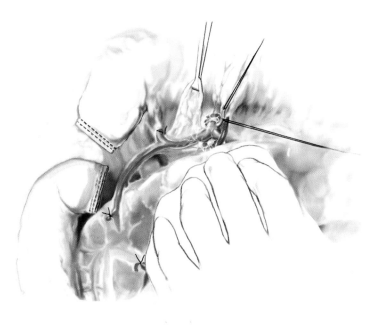

STEP 8 — Dissection around the celiac artery and division of the left gastric artery

The celiac artery is covered by the celiac plexus. All the tissue around these nerve structures is dissected to visualize the celiac and left gastric artery. Ligation and division of the left artery are performed near its origin.

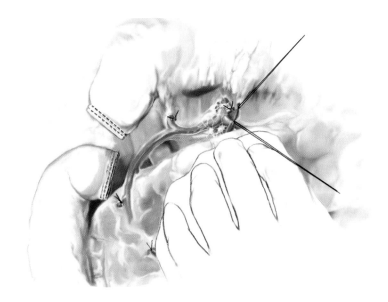

STEP 9   **Mobilization of the pancreas body/tail and the spleen**

View from the patient's feet. To carry out the dissection of the splenic artery and hilar lymph nodes, the pancreas body/tail and spleen should be mobilized from the retroperitoneum, beginning at the pancreas body from the inferior towards the superior border and then towards the tail and spleen. After total mobilization of the spleen, the retroperitoneum is incised lateral of the spleen and divided. The pancreas body/tail and spleen are now completely mobilized for a meticulous dissection of lymph nodes around the pancreas tail.

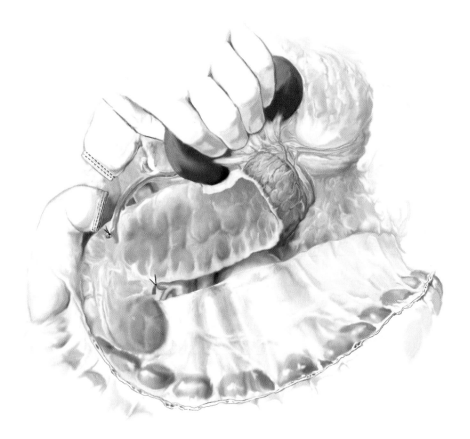

STEP 10   **Division of the splenic artery**

The splenic artery is divided near its origin but more distal in contrast to Maruyama's procedure after branching-off of the great pancreatic artery in Sasako's modification. Sometimes preservation of the tail artery is possible.

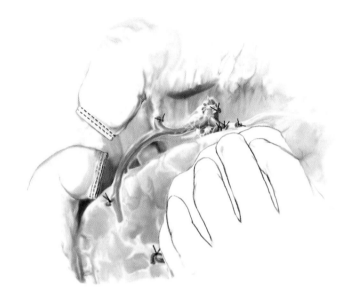

STEP 11   **Dissection of the splenic artery nodes**

The distal portion around the splenic artery is removed from the anterior and posterior way. To avoid venous congestion, the splenic vein should be preserved as distal as possible. If there is a pancreas tail vein at the tip, it should also be preserved.

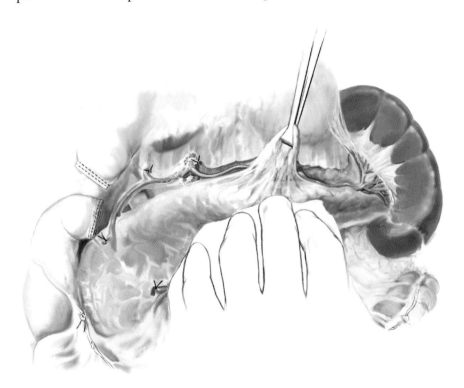

See chapter "Total Gastrectomy with Conventional Lymphadenectomy" for postoperative investigations and complications.

Tricks of the Senior Surgeon

- Avoid transecting the postpyloric duodenum to close to the pancreatic capsule, disabling oversew of the duodenal stump.
- Meticulous dissection of the proper hepatic artery and the splenic artery is mandatory to prevent postoperative pancreatitis.

Transhiatal Esophagogastrectomy

Enrique Moreno Gonzalez, Juan C. Meneu Diaz, Asad Kutup,
Jakob R. Izbicki, Almudena Moreno Elola-Olaso

Introduction

From the pathogenic and therapeutic point of view, adenocarcinomas of the esophago-gastric junction (AEG) should be classified into adenocarcinoma of the distal esophagus (Type I), true carcinoma of the cardia (Type II), and subcardial carcinoma (Type III). In patients with potentially resectable, true carcinoma of the cardia (AEG Type II), this can be achieved by a total gastrectomy with transhiatal resection of the distal esophagus and en bloc removal of the lymphatic drainage in the lower posterior mediastinum and upper abdomen.

Indications and Contraindications

Indications

- Carcinoma of the distal esophagus with involvement of the proximal stomach
- Locally advanced carcinoma of the cardia
- Adenocarcinoma of the proximal stomach with infiltration of the distal esophagus
- Distal esophageal carcinoma after subtotal gastrectomy
- Esophageal carcinoma of the mid or upper third after subtotal gastrectomy (abdominothoracic esophagogastrectomy with cervical or high intrathoracic anastomosis)
- Caustic ingestions

Contraindications

- Active duodenal ulcer
- Severe or irreversible cardiopulmonary insufficiency

Preoperative Investigations/Preparation for Procedure

- Esophagogastroduodenoscopy with histologic diagnosis
- Total colonoscopy to exclude second neoplasm or diverticula in the transposed colon segment
- CT scanning of the thorax and abdomen
- Abdominal sonography
- Esophageal endosonography
- Pulmonary function tests and blood gas analysis
- Echocardiography
- Ergometry and other cardiac investigations if necessary
- Entire orthograde bowel preparation

Procedure

Positioning
■ Supine position with hyperlordosis

Approach
■ Upper transverse incision with median T-shaped
■ Insertion of Rochard retractor to elevate costal margin

STEP 1

Laparotomy

See chapter on "Subtotal Esophagectomy: Transhiatal Approach."

STEP 2

Exposure

After mobilization of the left lateral liver lobe and dissection of the lesser sac close to the liver, the greater omentum is detached from the transverse colon. Lymphadenectomy begins at the basis of the right gastroepiploic vessels.

The peritoneal sheath is incised above the right gastroepiploic vessels. The right epiploic vessels are suture ligated as close as possible to the pancreas without injuring the pancreatic capsule.

STEP 3

Lymphadenectomy: transection of the duodenum

Dissection of the surrounding lymph nodes is performed. For better exposure of these nodes the stomach is held upwards by ventral traction. The lymph nodes at the upper margin of the pancreas are dissected towards the duodenum to facilitate the later en-bloc resection. Injury of the serosa of the duodenum and of the capsula of the pancreas has to be avoided.

The lymphadenectomy of the hepatoduodenal ligament is performed. In addition, the lymph nodes around the origin of the right gastric artery are dissected towards the stomach. The right gastric artery is then ligated at its origin. After circular dissection of the gastroduodenal junction the duodenum is transected 1–2 cm behind the pylorus with a linear stapler device and the stapler suture line is inverted with single sutures (see chapter "Total Gastrectomy with Conventional Lymphadenectomy," STEP 5).

STEP 4

Completion of the lymphadenectomy

The upper margin of the pancreas is now exposed by applying upwards traction to the distal stomach. Lymphadenectomy continues from the hepatoduodenal ligament along the common hepatic artery down to the coeliac trunk. Lymphadenectomy at the splenic artery, the coeliac trunk and the para-aortic space is performed (see chapter "Total Gastrectomy with Conventional Lymphadenectomy," STEP 6).

STEP 5 — Mobilization of the stomach

Traction is applied to the stomach towards the right upper abdomen to expose the origin of the left gastroepiploic artery and the short gastric vessels. These vessels are transected and ligated between clamps. Mobilization of the greater curvature of the stomach is performed up to the gastroesophageal junction. During this step the phrenicogastric ligament has to be transected with electrocautery.

STEP 6 — Transhiatal esophageal resection

See chapter on "Subtotal Esophagectomy: Transhiatal Approach."

STEP 7 — Mobilization of the right colonic flexure

The left lateral peritoneal reflection is finally mobilized by dissection of the peritoneum in the cranial direction. The colicosplenic ligament and the phrenicocolic ligament are ligated and divided using cautery or scissors. Thus, the whole splenic flexure of the colon is mobilized.

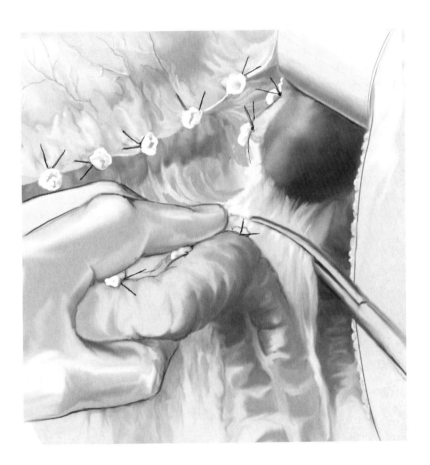

STEP 8   **Mobilization of the sigmoid colon**

Mobilization of the sigmoid colon is facilitated by performing mediocranial traction to expose the embryonic adhesions between the colon and retroperitoneum. Further dissection is done between the mesosigmoid and retroperitoneal fat, taking care of the left ureter and gonadal vessels.

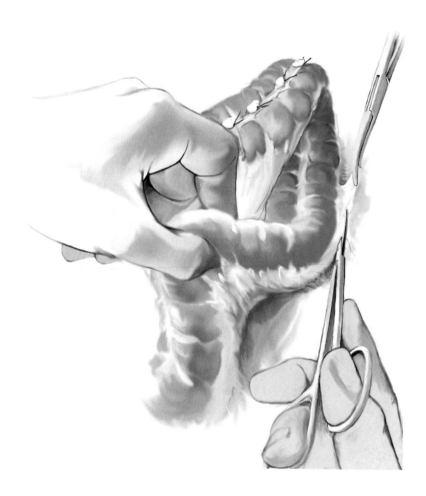

STEP 9	Determination of the essential length

A colonic segment is selected suitable for interposition. The essential length is determined by the following procedure: elevation of the colon in front of the abdominal wall, and measurement of the distance between the abdomen and the angle of the mandible by a suture, fixed at the root of the strongest vessel of the colonic mesentery (A-1, A2). The length of the suture is finally transferred to the colon and the resection margin is marked.

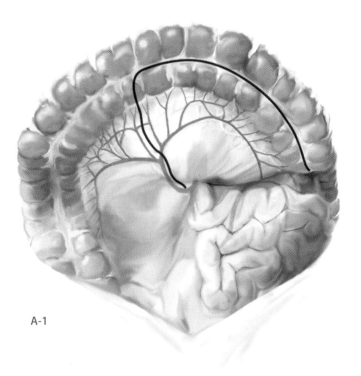

A-1

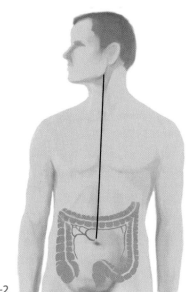

A-2

Determination of the essential length

The black bars show alternative lines for transection of the colon. Resection of bluish margins on the right flexure of the transverse colon between the middle and the right colic artery should be performed under preservation of the paracolic arcades. Following this procedure, a better mobilization of the colonic segment can be obtained. To perform the pharyngocolostomy in carcinomas of the upper third of the esophagus, a fairly long colonic segment is required. Therefore parts of the sigmoid colon have to be used and the first (and probably the second) sigmoid artery has to be ligated close to the inferior mesenteric artery. Prior to dissection of the vessels, a clamp is provisionally applied to prove the sufficiency of the vascular supply. Dark arrows point to the vascular resection margins. The arcade between the right and middle colonic artery should be preserved for a better vascular supply of the colonic segment chosen for interposition (**B**).

Advantages of using the left colonic segment are the following:

1. The more predictably longer length and the smaller diameter of the left colon
2. Adequacy of the vascular pattern due to arteries with larger diameter, instead of vascular supply via several arcades as in the right colon
3. Using an anisoperistaltic colonic segment has no clinical relevance because the nutritional transport follows gravity

The essential advantage of the left colon is the opportunity to obtain a longer colonic segment.

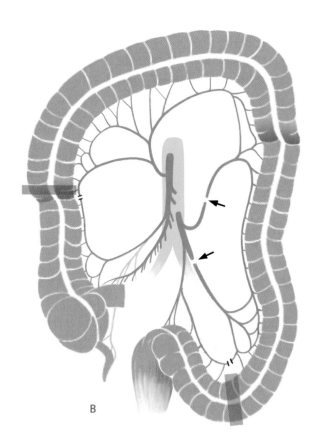

B

STEP 10   **Standard procedure: isoperistaltic reconstruction**

In case of an insufficient vascular supply through the middle colonic artery, the vascular supply can be warranted through the left colonic artery, if a sufficient Riolan's arcade exists.

This approach ensures an isoperistaltic reconstruction (standard procedure). Care has to be taken not to injure the left colic vessels. Therefore preparation has to be done carefully and closely to the wall of the colon, and transection of the descending colon is always done without extensive dissection of the colon using a linear stapler device. The right and middle colonic vessels are dissected close to their origin. A prophylactic appendectomy after total mobilization of the colon is recommended.

An anisoperistaltic colon interposition supplied by the left colonic artery can be performed, if the Riolan's anastomosis is either not present or is insufficient due to previous surgical procedures.

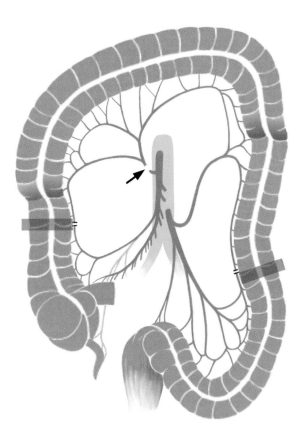

STEP 11   **Anisoperistaltic reconstruction (not standard)**

Preparation of an anisoperistaltic (not standard) colonic segment begins with incision of the peritoneum far from the colon and stepwise preparation of the mesocolon maintaining the paracolic arcades and the middle and left colic vessels. A vascular clamp is provisionally applied across the left colic artery and the sigmoid artery across the provisional colonic transection plane to prove a sufficient arcade of Riolan. If no ischemia occurs after 3 min, the colon interposition can be performed.

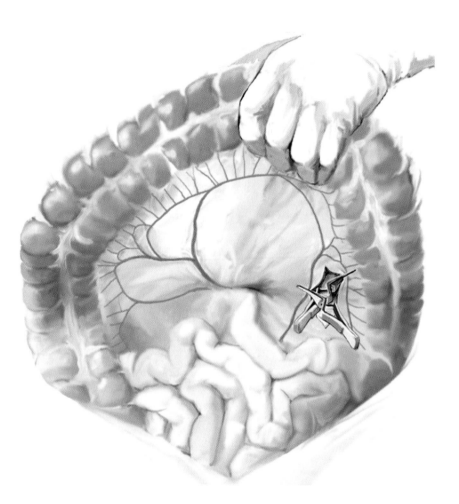

STEP 12

Inadequate vascular supply

In case of an inadequate vascular supply by the left and middle colonic artery, reconstruction of an isoperistaltic colon interposition supplied by the sigmoid artery is possible.

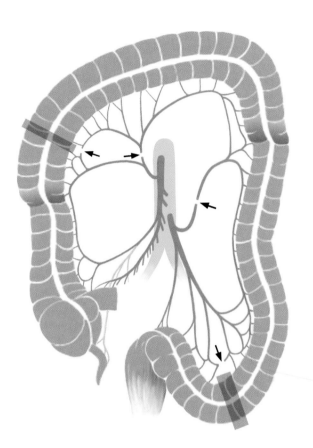

STEP 13   Inadequate vascular supply

In very rare cases no anastomosis is found between the left colonic artery and the first
sigmoid artery. In those cases the main branch of the inferior mesenteric artery can
be used as an anastomosis between the two areas of blood supply. This can only be
accomplished when the distal parts of the sigmoid colon are adequately perfused by
the medial and inferior rectal artery. This has to be checked by temporary clamping.

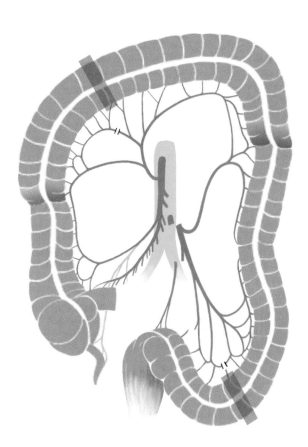

STEP 14

A rare situation

Even after right hemicolectomy (e.g., following complicated right colonic interposition), construction of an anisoperistaltic interposition is possible, if the middle colonic artery has been spared during the first operation. The left colonic artery and the first sigmoid artery are dissected (A). Vascular supply of the interposition comes from the middle colonic artery. Reconstruction is performed with an ileo-sigmoidostomy.

Alternatively, an interposition after right hemicolectomy and after former transection of the middle colonic artery can be performed using the left colon. The blood supply comes from the left colonic artery. The entire sigmoid colon is needed for the purpose of receiving sufficient length for the interposition and all sigmoid arteries have to be dissected (B). The proximal colon segment with poor vascular supply is resected.

If it is impossible to use the left hemicolon for interposition, the right hemicolon can be used to perform the transposition graft.

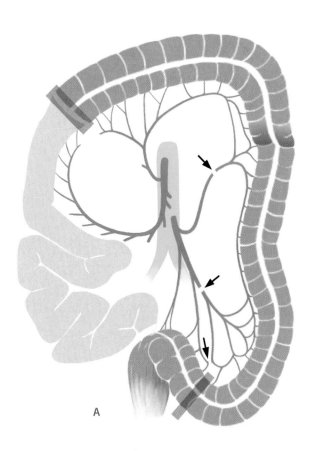

A

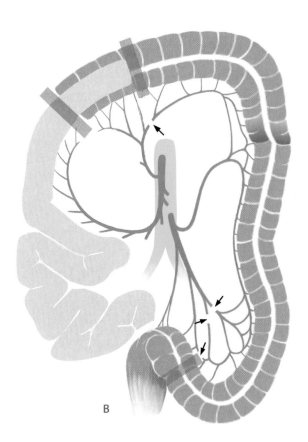

B

A rare situation

Scheme of construction of an isoperistaltic colonic interposition using the right hemicolon and the terminal part of the ileum (C) is illustrated here. The vascular supply comes from the middle colonic artery.

Using the right hemicolon for interposition is burdened by frequent complications leading to poorer postoperative functional results.

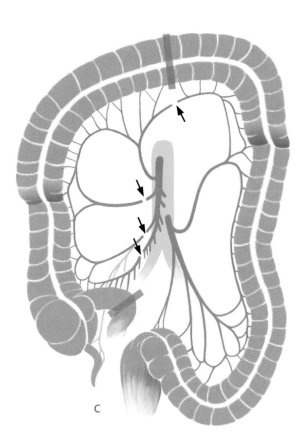

C

STEP 15

Vascular supply of the colonic interposition from the ileocolic artery

Also shown is the preparation of an anisoperistaltic colonic interposition using the right hemicolon, with vascular supply from the ileocolic artery (A).

Adequate length of the right hemicolon enables construction of an isoperistaltic interposition without using the ileocolic portion of the intestine (B). This technique offers several advantages:

- Omission of the terminal ileum, which is prone to necrosis
- Omission of the ileocecal region, which is prone to poor functional results

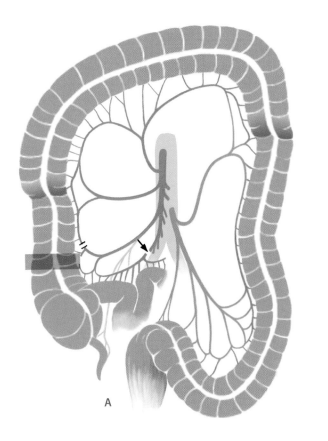
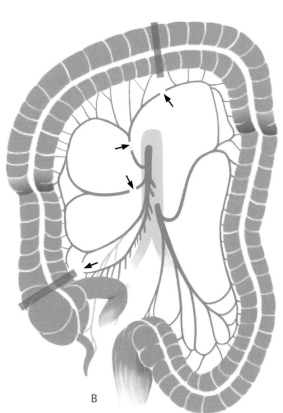

STEP 16   **Preparation of a substernal tunnel**

A blunt opening is made in the substernal cavity by spreading the scissors, while pulling the xiphoid ventrally with a sharp retractor.

After opening the substernal cavity, a substernal tunnel is constructed with an atraumatic clamp.

The sternum has to be pulled continuously, and the endothoracic membrane is to be separated from the sternum. A longitudinal incision along the anterior border of the left sternocleidomastoid muscle is made to expose the cervical esophagus. Blunt preparation with the hand through the substernal tunnel usually leads to rupture of the mediastinal pleura (A-1, A-2, A-3).

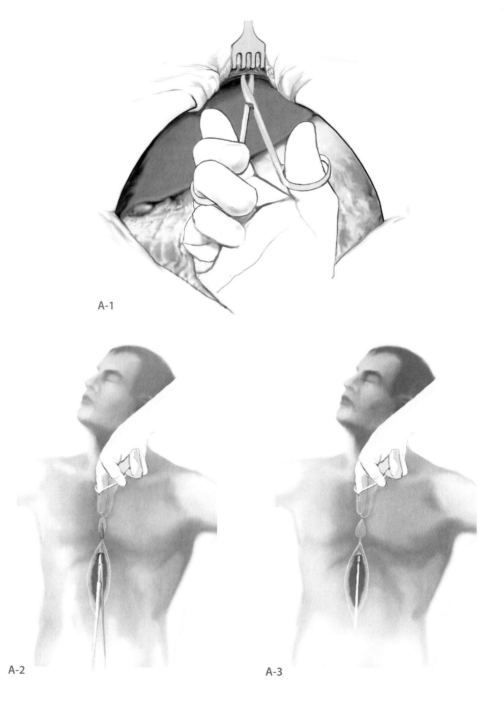

A-1

A-2   A-3

STEP 17   **Completed preparation of the retrosternal tunnel**

In case of tight adhesions to the sternum, these adhesions are dissected sharply with scissors.

Between the corpus and manubrium sterni the substernal fascia is very tightly connected to the sternum. Furthermore, the visceral and parietal pleura are tightly connected in this region. For this reason, very careful, stepwise preparation with a long atraumatic clamp has to be performed, and the preparation should be manually controlled by the substernally introduced finger of the surgeon.

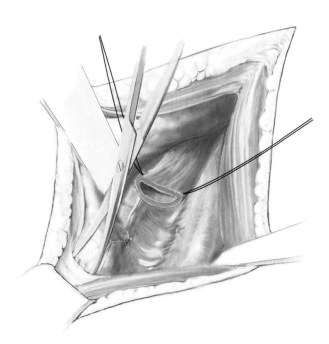

STEP 18   **Pull-through procedure**

For the substernal reconstruction, a long strong suture fixed to a drainage tube can be
used for the pull-through procedure. The suture is tied to the oral end of the colonic
interposition. The colon is transposed in the substernal tunnel to the cervical incision
under a continuous and gentle pull, and the sternum should be pulled upwards with
a sharp retractor during the procedure (A-1, A-2, A-3).

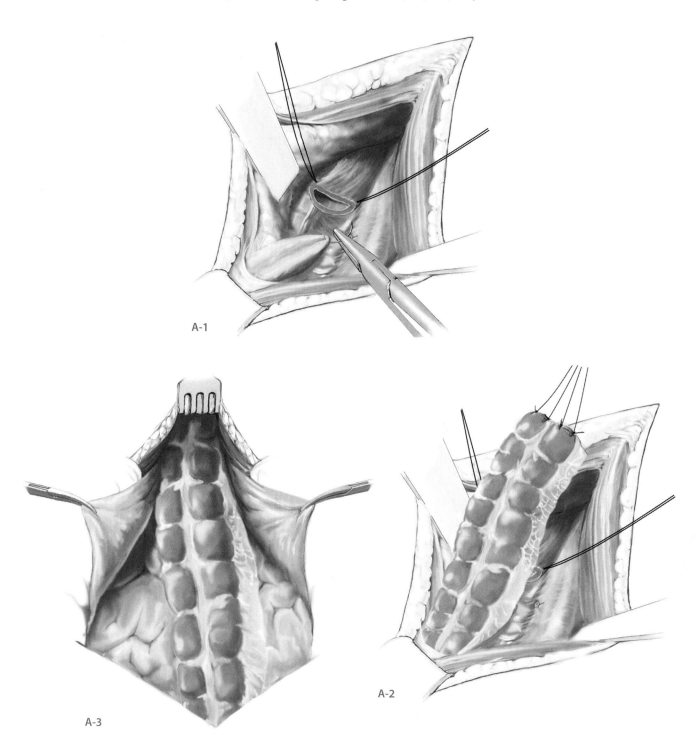

A-1

A-2

A-3

STEP 19   **Posterior mediastinum**

Interposition of the colon through the posterior mediastinum is performed in the bed of the removed esophagus. The posterior mediastinal route of the interposed colon is favorable to the substernal or presternal position because of the shorter distance to the neck. In addition, the posterior mediastinal route prevents kinking of the colon and leads to better functional results. The interposed colon causes hemostasis in the operation field.

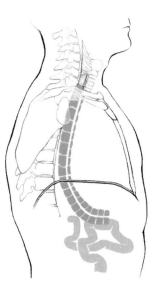

STEP 20   **Terminolateral anastomosis**

If possible, the terminolateral anastomosis should be performed in a double row suture technique.

In case of a different lumen diameter, single stitches and a terminolateral anastomosis can be performed close to the taenia libera.

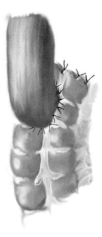

STEP 21

Laterolateral anastomosis

The alternative technique for anastomosis after colonic interposition is a laterolateral colo-esophageal anastomosis performed by a linear stapler.

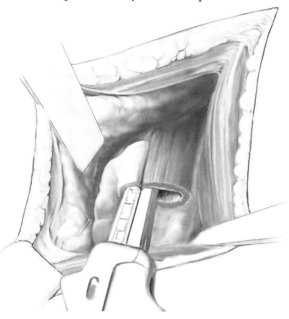

STEP 22

Reconstruction of the intestine

Gastrointestinal continuity is achieved by descendojejunostomy and jejunojejunostomy.
    A caecosigmoidostomy completes the reconstruction. The mesenteric incisions have been closed. The operative site after transposition of the colon and reconstruction is shown.

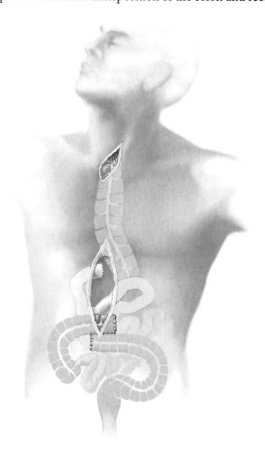

Combined Transhiatal Transthoracic Esophagectomy

Introduction

We reported this technique for the first time in 1980. It uses the concepts acquired in transhiatal dissection in tumors located more superiorly in the cervicothoracic esophagus or in the middle third of the thoracic esophagus, and avoids a "blunt" dissection performed without visual control, which increases the possibility of iatrogenic injury to mediastinal structures. However, at present more and more surgeons favor transhiatal esophagectomy for its technical simplicity and favorable outcome.

Indications and Contraindications

Indication

- Esophageal carcinoma in the mid or upper third after subtotal gastrectomy

Contraindications

See page 189.

Preoperative Investigations/Preparation for Procedure

See page 189.
- Bronchoscopy

Procedure

Access

See chapter on "Subtotal En Bloc Esophagectomy: Abdominothoracic Approach".

STEP 1

Abdominal exposure

The operation begins with a supraumbilical medial laparotomy, and the abdominal viscera and diaphragmatic section are examined (see above), which permits access to the posterior mediastinal space. The mediastinal section is done as for the previous patient, allowing visual control as far as the tracheal branching.

STEP 2

Right anterior thoracotomy

A right anterior thoracotomy is then performed, if possible without costal resection. If the rigidity of the thorax so requires, the anterior arch of the costal vein is removed, and should this prove insufficient, the remaining posterior arch of this rib is resected via the anterior thoracic incision.

STEP 3

Esophageal dissection and mediastinal lymphadenectomy

The ipsilateral mediastinal pleura, which remains in contact with the esophagus, is incised through the anterior thoracic incision. The arch of the azygos vein is incised, enabling the dissection of the cervicothoracic esophagus. To expand the mediastinal lymphadenectomy, this incision is used to dissect the intercostal veins. The trunk of the azygos vein is ligated at the supradiaphragmatic level and associated thoracic duct excision is required by the lymphatic involvement.

During esophageal dissection at the high level of the cervical region, a tracheo-bronchial intubation with a Carlens tube can be used to facilitate access to the esophagus, occluding the right bronchial tube (see Chapter "Abdominothoracic Esophagectomy" STEP 1–3).

| STEP 4 | **Technique of cervical anastomosis** |

See chapter on "Transhiatal Esophagogastrectomy."

| STEP 5 | **Technique of high intrathoracic esophagocolostomy** |

See chapter on "Abdominothoracic En Bloc Esophagectomy with High Intrathoracic Anastomosis."

Standard Postoperative Investigations

See chapter on "Subtotal Esophagectomy: Transhiatal Approach."

Postoperative Complications

Early Postoperative Course
- Pulmonal infections
- Septic complications: subphrenic or intra-abdominal abscess; cervical wound infection
- Anastomotic leak
- Necrosis of the interposition
- Enterothorax

Late Postoperative Course
- Cicatricial strictures of the cervical esophago- or pharyngeo-colostomy, mostly due to anastomotic leak
- Kinking of the interposition
- Mechanical trauma to a subcutaneous graft, which often needs surgical intervention
- Propulsive disorder

Tricks of the Senior Surgeon

- Treatment of the stenosis is performed by bougienage or balloon dilatation. Very rarely is surgical intervention indicated.
- Reasons for necrosis of the interposition are: decrease of circulation due to kinking or compression of the main vessels, hypovolemia, and hypercoagulability. Avoidance is by interposition of a long colonic segment without tension. Optimization of the postoperative hemodynamic and rheologic parameters is necessary.
- Kinking of the interposition is a rare but dangerous complication, which often requires surgical intervention, due to clinical symptomatic disturbance of the gastrointestinal passage by elongation of the interposition. Surgical intervention is performed by shortening of the graft.
- To avoid enterothorax phrenicotomy has to be performed.

Laparoscopic Gastrectomy

Geert Kazemier, Johan F. Lange

Introduction

Laparoscopic resection of the stomach should mimic an open operation as closely as possible. This is applicable to the technique, as well as to the considerations on which the indication is based. Palliative resection for gastric malignancy can be indicated to prevent hemorrhage or obstruction.

Indications and Contraindications

Indications

- Malignant tumors [carcinoma, gastrointestinal stromal tumor (GIST)]
- Benign tumors (e.g., GIST, apudoma)
- Arteriovenous malformations
- Recurrent peptic ulcer disease

Contraindications

- Severe cardiac failure (unable to withstand pneumoperitoneum)
- Sepsis
- Severe coagulopathy
- Morbid obesity (BMI>40) (relative)
- Previous upper abdominal surgery (relative)
- T4 or bulky tumors (relative)

Preoperative Investigation/Preparation for the Procedure

See chapter "Total Gastrectomy with Conventional Lymphadenectomy."

Instrumentation

- Two monitors
- Three 10- to 12-mm trocars, two 5-mm trocars
- One 15-mm trocar (optional) to pass the 60-mm stapler and retrieval bag
- 30° laparoscope
- Unipolar or bipolar coagulation
- Hemostatic device (LigaSure, Ultracision)
- Standard laparoscopic instruments for advanced laparoscopic surgery, including fenestrated clamps and endo-Babcock clamp
- Vascular clip applier
- Endostapler (45–60 mm, with white, blue and green cartridges)
- Liver retractor
- Vessel loops
- Gastroscope (optional, to identify small lesions)
- Retrieval bag

Procedure

STEP 1

Positioning and installations

Positioning:

The patient is placed in the supine position. The surgeon stands between the legs of the patient, the first assistant on the left, the second assistant on the right side of the patient. The scrub nurse is positioned on the right or left hand side of the surgeon (A).

Installation of pneumoperitoneum and inspection of abdominal cavity:

Pneumoperitoneum is installed at the site of the umbilicus. In obese patients, the umbilicus is located more caudally; in these patients the first trocar may be introduced cranially to the umbilicus. In case of malignancy the abdominal cavity is inspected for signs of dissemination to the peritoneum or other organs. To allow for optimal inspection and to create the opportunity to take biopsies, one or more additional trocars are inserted. Inspection of the caudal side of the mesentery of the transverse colon and the region of Treitz ligament can be facilitated by bringing the patient into a Trendelenburg position.

Introduction of trocars (B):

The total number and position of trocars is dependent on the level of resection. The subxiphoidal trocar is only necessary for high resections of the stomach. Introduction of this trocar should be on the left side of the falciform ligament, especially when exploration of the cardia and gastroesophageal junction is necessary.

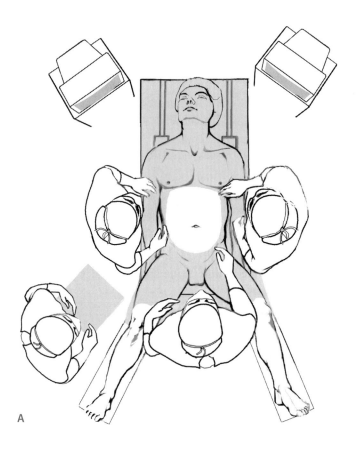

A

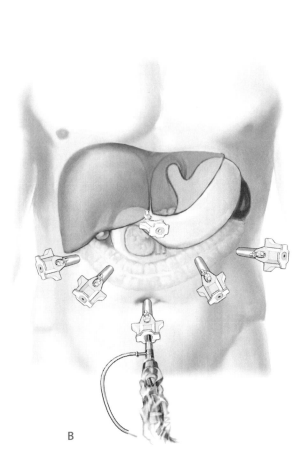

B

STEP 2	**Opening of the lesser sac**

To determine (laparoscopic) resectability of the tumor, opening of the lesser sac is achieved by detaching the greater omentum from the transverse colon by sharp dissection. In case of a benign indication, opening of the lesser sac can be performed more easily by creating a window in the greater omentum, for instance by using Ultracision. Involvement of the pancreas in malignant tumors requires conversion to open resection in most cases. In case of malignancy, once resectability has been established, the lesser sac is opened until the gastrocolic ligament is completely dissected from the hepatic to the splenic flexure.

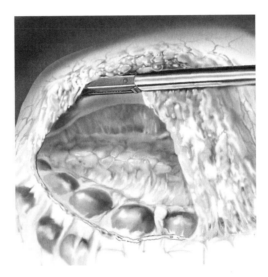

STEP 3	**Resection of benign lesions**

In benign lesions, a stapled wedge resection is performed. Resection is performed under gastroscopic surveillance in case the lesion is not visible on the serosal side of the stomach. The gastrohepatic ligament must be opened if the tumor is located on the smaller curvature of the stomach.

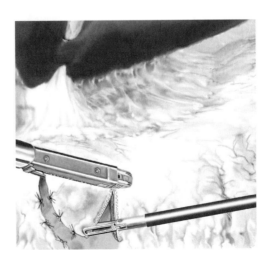

STEP 4   **Transection of duodenum and resection of gastrohepatic ligament**

After detachment of the greater omentum, the right gastroepiploic vessels are identified and secured with clips at the level of the duodenum. Mayo's vein will locate the exact position of the pylorus. Identification of the pylorus can be facilitated by gentle palpation with a clamp in the postpyloric area. Care should be taken not to damage the pancreatic parenchyma as this will result in pancreatitis. Sharp dissection at the posterior side of the postpyloric part of the duodenum creates space to introduce a 45-mm stapling device. A vessel loop can be used to facilitate safe insertion of the stapler. Prior to the closure of the stapler, care should be taken that the vessel loop and vascular clips are not included in the line of stapling (A).

The assistant retracts the liver to allow exposure of the smaller omentum. The gastrohepatic ligament is opened at the level of the hepatoduodenal ligament. The right gastric artery is transected using Ultracision (B). The assistant retracts the liver to allow exposure of the liver hilum. Following the common, proper, and left hepatic artery, the smaller omentum is freed, securing lymph nodes of the pyloric group up to the right pericardial group. This en bloc lymphadenectomy is part of a level D2 resection and is optional. A replaced or aberrant left hepatic artery, originating from the left gastric artery, can be safely dealt with, using clips if necessary. Alternatively this lymphadenectomy can be done after transection of the stomach.

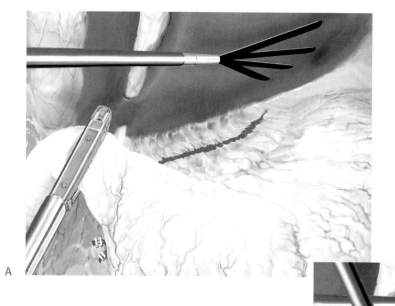

A

B

STEP 5

Securing of left gastric vessels

The posterior aspect of the stomach is freed from the anterior surface of the pancreas by sharp dissection of adhesions. At this stage a vessel loop can be used to allow easier manipulation of the stomach. Cranial to the pancreas the splenic artery is identified in most cases. More cranially, the left gastric vessels are identified and transected with clips or a vascular stapler. Optional D2 lymphadenectomy of the stomach implies truncal lymphadenectomy at this stage.

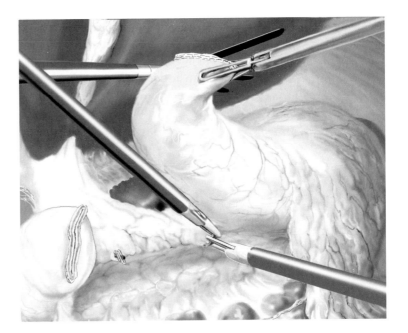

STEP 6   Transection of the stomach

The transection line of the stomach is performed 5 cm orally to the tumor (A). If the tumor cannot be identified adequately on the serosal side of the stomach, intraoperative gastroscopy is mandatory to determine the exact line of transection. Location of the tumor high in the body of the stomach may require opening of the gastrosplenic ligament and securing of short gastric vessels with Ultracision (B).

D2 lymphadenectomy requires resection of lymph nodes of the gastrohepatic ligament and between the hepatic artery. If the nodal clearance has not been performed en bloc, it is feasible to do it at this stage (C).

After transection of the stomach, the specimen is placed in a retrieval bag for safe extraction. Extraction is done through a mini-laparotomy. This laparotomy can be conducted at a cosmetically preferred site (e.g., Pfannenstiehl). Alternatively a midline mini-laparotomy is performed in the upper abdominal region. In the latter option the anastomosis can be done in an open fashion.

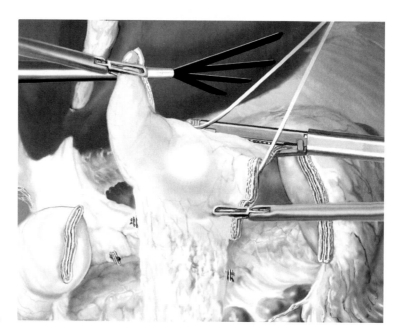

A

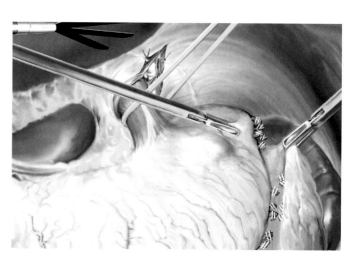

B

STEP 6 *(continued)*   **Transsection of the stomach**

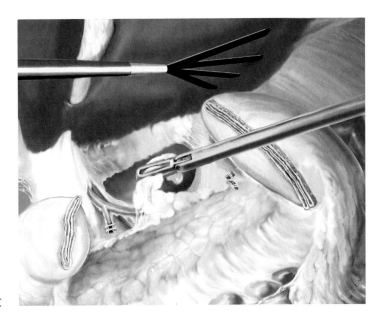

C

STEP 7   **Anastomosis**

Open anastomosis:

Through a small midline laparotomy a standard Billroth II or Roux-en-Y reconstruction can be performed (A).

Laparoscopic anastomosis (Billroth II):

To perform a laparoscopic side-to-side gastrojejunostomy, ligament of Treitz and the proximal jejunum are identified by lifting the transverse colon and tilting the table into a Trendelenburg position (head down). A loop of proximal jejunum is brought up in an antecolic or retrocolic fashion. This loop of jejunum is sutured to the anterior aspect of the stomach remnant with two resorbable, seromuscular stay sutures, approximately 2 cm apart. A stab incision in both the stomach and the jejunum is made with diathermia. Care should be taken that the incision in the stomach is made through all gastric wall layers. The stab incisions are enlarged, and the endostapler is introduced with one blade in the stomach and the other in the jejunum. Subsequently the stapler is fired one or two times, dependent on the size of the cartridges (60 or 45 mm). In case a 60-mm stapler is used, a 15-mm trocar should be introduced (B).

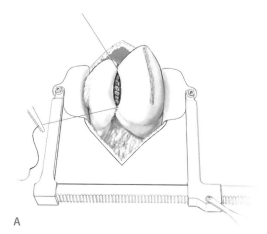

A

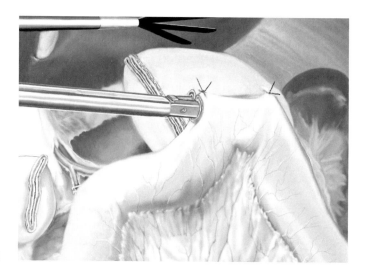

B

| STEP 8 | **Closure of stab incisions** |

The incision that remains in the stomach and the jejunum after firing the endostapler is closed using a single layer resorbable, polyfilament suture. Closure with an endostapler should not be attempted as the anastomosis is easily compromised because it is difficult to ensure inclusion of all tissue of the stomach and jejunum on both sides of the stab incisions in the staple line without narrowing the anastomosis.

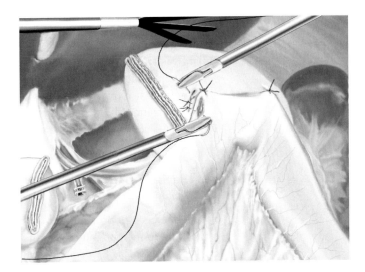

Postoperative Investigations

See chapter "Total Gastrectomy with Conventional Lymphadenectomy."

Postoperative Complications

- Short term:
  - Anastomotic insufficiency (including duodenal stump insufficiency)
  - Acute pancreatitis
  - Chylous ascites (particularly after R2 resection)
- Long term (all indications):
  - Biliary gastritis (particularly after Billroth II reconstruction)
  - Jejunal peptic ulcer disease
- Long term (in case of malignancy):
  - Local recurrence (duodenal stump or resection line of stomach)
  - Distant metastases

Tricks of the Senior Surgeon

- Instead of a vessel loop, a heavy resorbable suture can be used to force the stomach or duodenum into the endostapler. Even if this suture is included in the staple line, this will not compromise your anastomosis.
- In lean patients it is often possible to remove one of the 10- to 12-mm trocars and directly introduce the 60-mm stapler or the retrieval bag, instead of using a 15-mm trocar.
- Suturing is best done with the scope in the middle and two needle holders on either side of the scope with a 60–90° angle between the two needle holders.

Gastroenterostomy

John Tsiaoussis, Gregory G. Tsiotos

Introduction

In this chapter both techniques for gastroenterostomy, the open and laparoscopic approaches, are described in patients with gastric outlet obstruction syndrome.

Indications and Contraindications

Indications

- Palliation of gastric outlet obstruction caused by advanced gastric, duodenal, or periampullary tumor
- Gastric drainage following vagotomy when pyloroplasty is not feasible

Contraindications

- Severe hypoalbuminemia
- Evidence of diffuse metastatic spread, indicating extremely low life expectancy
- Prohibitive comorbidity

Preoperative Investigation/Preparation for the Procedure

History:	Persistent vomiting
Laboratory tests:	Electrolytes, albumin, coagulation parameters
Radiology:	Upper GI contrast study
CT scan:	Assessment of primary disease/condition
Endoscopy:	Assessment of gastric outlet obstruction, periampullary biopsy for tissue diagnosis

A large-bore nasogastric tube is placed the day prior to the operation for gastric decompression and irrigation.

The patient's water and electrolyte balance are corrected preoperatively.

Procedure

Open, Hand-Sewing Technique

Access
Midline incision from xiphoid process to the umbilicus

STEP 1

Preparation of the jejunal loop using the retrocolic route

The gastroepiploic vessels are dissected, clamped, divided and ligated starting about 5 cm proximal to the pylorus and moving 6–7 cm proximally along the greater curvature of the stomach, so this is completely dissected free from the omentum.

The jejunal loop can be brought either anterior to the transverse colon (antecolic), or through a window in the transverse mesocolon (retrocolic). Although a retrocolic gastro-jejunostomy has been considered more prone to obstruction because of its closer proximity to an ever enlarging unresectable periampullary tumor, this has never proved true, especially since patient survival in this context rarely exceeds 6 months. On the other hand, the retrocolic route allows more proximal placement of the jejunal stoma and smoother angles between afferent, efferent loops and stomach in both the coronal and the sagittal planes.

The window (wide enough to allow comfortable sliding of both afferent and efferent jejunal loops) is made in an avascular plane of the mesocolon left to the middle colic vessels. The ligament of Treitz is identified by lifting up the transverse colon, and the jejunal loop is brought up through the mesocolic window in apposition to the greater curvature (now free from omental vessels). The length of the afferent jejunal limb should not exceed 20 cm.

The gastrojejunostomy can be placed either on the anterior (easier and thus preferable) or the posterior gastric wall; the latter has not proved superior in terms of gastric emptying. Then 3-0 silk traction seromuscular sutures are placed, taking into account that the incision in the jejunum will not be made exactly at the antimesenteric border, but at a level closer to its mesentery on the stomal side. This provides for more comfortable lining of the completed anastomosis without any undue angles in the transverse plane. At 5-mm intervals 3-0 silk interrupted seromuscular Lembert sutures are placed and tied to create the posterior outer suture line. Two incisions along the gastric and the jejunal apposite segments are then made. Although the gastric incision should be about 4 cm, the jejunal incision should be a bit shorter, since it always tends to dilate and ends up being realistically longer than initially planned or thought to be.

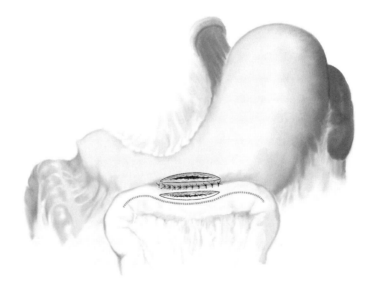

STEP 2   **Technique of anastomosis**

The posterior *full-thickness* inner anastomotic layer is made by two 3-0 PDS running
sutures in an over-and-over fashion starting at the middle of the posterior layer and
moving in opposite directions towards each corner of the anastomosis, where the two
corner traction seromuscular stitches are still present. Then, the two 3-0 PDS running
suture lines continue into the anterior wall of the gastrojejunostomy (again *full-thickness*) using the Connell technique in order to invert all gastric and jejunal mucosa,
which might otherwise protrude out through the anastomosis. Moving from the two
corners towards the middle, the sutures meet and are tied together. The anastomosis is
completed by placing the anterior seromuscular layer with interrupted 3-0 silk Lembert
sutures starting at the corner away from the surgeon and moving towards the surgeon,
so that there are no sutures tangling in the middle of the operative field. These outer
sutures should be first *all* placed and then tied; "tying as we go" will lead to packing of
the serosa towards the inner suture line and thus placement of each successive suture at
an ever increasing distance away from the inner suture line, which may then lead to
entrapment of a lot of seromuscular tissue within the suture lines and protrusion of this
soft tissue mass towards the anastomosis itself with its potential obliteration.

After completion, the anastomosis is brought below the mesocolic window, and the
gastric wall (not the jejunal) is tacked circumferentially on the mesocolon with interrupted 3-0 Vicryl sutures. A drain tube does not need to be placed.

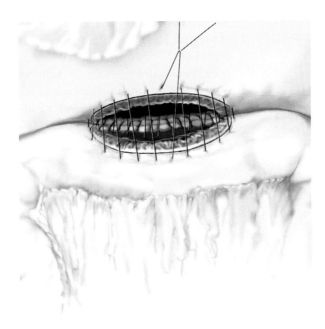

Open Stapling Technique

STEP 1

Stapling technique

The greater curvature is freed from the omentum, the mesocolic window is made and the jejunum and greater curvature are brought to apposition as previously described. Two stab wounds are made with the electrocautery in the greater curvature (12 cm from the pylorus) and at the antimesenteric aspect of the jejunum (20 cm from the ligament of Treitz). Two Allis clamps, incorporating full thickness gastric and jejunal wall, are placed one each in the gastric and the jejunal stab wounds. The cartridge fork of the GIA-60 stapler is inserted in the gastric lumen and the anvil fork into the jejunal lumen (this move is to *push the GIA's jaws* into the lumens, *not to pull* the stomach and jejunum up towards the stapler). With the help and maneuvering of the two Allis clamps, align equal lengths of gastric and jejunal walls on the forks, keep the jejunal mesentery away from the anastomosis, close the instrument and fire. Open the handle of the stapler slowly and slide it out. Inspect the luminal side of the staple line for possible bleeding.

STEP 2

Final reconstruction of the anastomosis

The two Allis clamps are now repositioned to grab the two corners of the GIA staple line and the inner (luminal) anastomotic line is inspected for bleeding. Approximate the gastric and jejunal walls with two additional Allis clamps. Slip the jaws of the TA-55 beneath the Allis clamps incorporating all tissue layers as well as the corner end staples of the GIA staple line within the jaws. The corner ends of the two GIA staple lines should be the two corners of the TA staple line, so that these three staple lines (two from the GIA, one from the TA) form a triangle and the wide patency of the anastomosis is secured. Close the instrument and fire. Use a scalpel to excise the protruding tissue along a special groove on the surface of the stapler. Open the instrument to release the tissue and inspect for bleeding. Three single full-thickness 3-0 silk reinforcing sutures are placed at the three corners of the stapled anastomosis, as these represent the theoretically more "vulnerable" points of the anastomosis, since this is where two staple lines meet and overlap. A drain tube does not need to be placed.

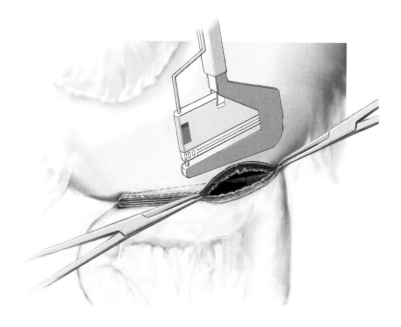

Laparoscopic Technique

| STEP 1 | Positioning |

The patient is placed supine. The senior surgeon stands on the patient's right side and the first assistant on the left. Pneumoperitoneum is established with the Verres needle (by insufflating at a preset pressure of 12–15 mmHg), the 0° or 30° laparoscope is introduced through a supraumbilical 10-mm port, but it can be moved to other ports as needed intraoperatively. Then, two 10-mm trocars and one 12-mm trocar are inserted in the anterior abdominal wall. The table is tilted at a 30° Trendelenburg position and a Babcock forcep (more atraumatic) is used to bring the omentum and transverse colon cephalad to identify the ligament of Treitz.

| STEP 2 | Preparation of the jejunal loop up to the stomach |

The first jejunal loop is identified and approximated to the antrum in an antecolic route. If the retrocolic route is chosen, a window in the transverse mesocolon is made using the harmonic scalpel and the jejunal loop is brought up through it. Two 3-0 silk traction sutures are placed (5–6 cm from each other) to opposite the jejunum (at a distance of 20 cm from the ligament of Treitz) along the greater curvature (at a distance of 5 cm from the pylorus). Two stab incisions are made at the approximated gastric and jejunal walls using the Hook device, one opposite to the other.

| STEP 3 | Technique of anastomosis |

As two graspers are holding the traction sutures on the approximated stomach and jejunum, a 45-mm Endo-GIA stapler is inserted through the 12-mm port. The jaws of the instrument are introduced into the gastric and jejunal lumens. Maneuvering of the suture-holding graspers accommodates stapler insertion. The stapler is closed, fired and eventually removed. The staple line is inspected internally for patency and bleeding.

The common gastric and jejunal opening is closed with full-thickness, running 2-0 Vicryl suture tied intracorporeally. Alternatively, an Endo-TA or an Endo-GIA device can be used for closure of the common gastric and jejunal opening. A drain tube does not need to be placed.

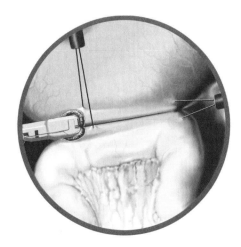

Standard Postoperative Investigations

- Gastrografin upper GI radiograph (when significant nasogastric tube output persists for longer than a week postoperatively)

Postoperative Complications

- Gastric hemorrhage
- Anastomotic bleeding
- Anastomotic leak
- Obstruction (anastomotic or functional)
- Anastomotic stenosis (long term)

Tricks of the Senior Surgeon

- When an antecolic gastrojejunostomy is chosen, the afferent jejunal loop can be kept short by placing the transverse colon as much to the right of the gastrojejunostomy as possible.
- Excessive length of the afferent limb may predispose to "afferent loop syndrome."
- Inadvertent gastroileostomy is not that uncommon! Make sure, especially when a laparoscopic gastroenterostomy is performed, that the appropriate site of the jejunum is used.
- Gastric emptying is based on inherent gastric motor function; not on hydraulic pressure gradients. Thus, placing the anastomosis at the "most dependent" portion of the stomach does not have any scientific merit.
- Place the anastomosis where it lies more comfortably. Provided that there is no kinking, acute angles, or pressure on the efferent and afferent loops, the choice of retrocolic versus antecolic, or distal gastric versus proximal gastric placement of the anastomosis is not so important.

Conventional Gastrostomy (Kader Procedure): Temporary or Permanent Gastric Fistula

Asad Kutup, Emre F. Yekebas

Introduction

Nowadays, gastrostomy has been replaced in most instances by less invasive procedures such as percutaneous endoscopic gastrostomy or feeding tube jejunostomy. However, gastrostomy still does have a place in highly selected instances, e.g., previous gastric surgery, the presence of ascites, or, in some instances, Crohn's disease of the small bowel.

Indications and Contraindications

Indications

- Locally non-resectable and/or metastasized stenosing tumor of the esophagus, gastroesophageal junction, and proximal stomach
- Tumor not passable for endoscope
- Contraindications for endoscopic treatment ("*percutaneous endoscopic gastrostomy*"), i.e., ascites
- Patient unfit for major surgery
- Neurologic disorders (cerebral dysphagia)

Contraindications

- Resectable carcinoma
- Previous major gastric resection/gastrectomy (in this case feeding jejunostomy is the treatment of choice)

Preoperative Investigation/Preparation for the Procedure

History:	Previous upper abdominal surgery, i.e., gastric resection; contraindication for percutaneous endoscopic gastrostomy (PEG)
Clinical investigation:	Exclusion of further obstruction distal to the stomach such as antral and pyloric strictures in cases of caustic burns.

Procedures

Temporary Tube Gastrostomy
(Synonyms: Witzel Procedure, Balloon Catheter Gastrostomy, Kader Procedure)

STEP 1	**Exposure**

Opening of the peritoneal cavity is done through the upper third of the left rectus muscle by a vertical or horizontal incision. Sharp transection of the skin, subcutis, and fasciae should be followed by blunt division of the muscle.

For exposure of the anterior wall of the gastric body, it has to be pulled by clamps or retention sutures anteriorly.

STEP 2	**Preparation and incision of the gastric wall**

Preparation of a purse-string suture with a diameter of about 3 cm usually made at the anterior aspect of the gastric body.

An incision of the gastric wall is made in the center of the purse-string suture, and a tube is inserted with its tip directed to the cardia. After the purse-string suture has been tested for leakage, the suture is tied.

In cases of caustic burns, antral and pyloric irregularities should be excluded by intragastric digital palpation of the poststomal stomach.

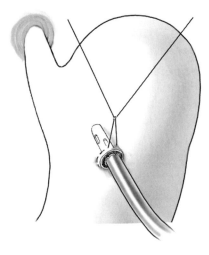

STEP 3	Positioning of the catheter

When inserting a feeding catheter with a diameter of about 1 cm, the tip should be directed to the cardia.

After proper positioning of the catheter with a minimum distance between insertion site and tip of the tube of 5 cm, the purse-string suture is tied.

Check for leaks at the site of the purse-string suture by filling the stomach with liquids.

STEP 4	Gastroplication

A gastroplication sutured with single stitches aborally to the insertion site of the tube is formed. If possible a reinforcing gastroplication of 8 cm aborally to the insertion of the tube in the gastric wall is recommended.

The gastric serosa is fixed with the abdominal wall by drawing the stomach upward and bringing the orifice of the tube distal to the gastroplication to an extraperitoneal location.

The cuff of the tube is then fixed to the skin.

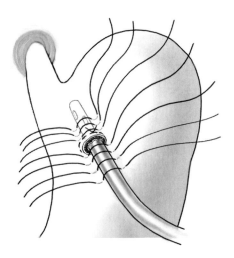

Balloon Catheter Gastrostomy

STEP 1   Exposure

Access to the peritoneal cavity, exposure, and preparation of the anterior aspect of the stomach as described above.

STEP 2   Positioning of the balloon catheter and fixation

After exposure of the anterior wall of the stomach by clamps, a purse-string suture is prepared. In the center of this suture line, the gastric wall is incised. If necessary, the incision is dilated gently and the tube is introduced into the gastric lumen (**A**).

In cases of caustic burns, antral and pyloric irregularities should be excluded by intragastric digital palpation of the poststomal stomach. After proper positioning of the catheter, the purse-string is tied. Sufficiency of the suture line is tested by a filling test. Pulling the catheter to the abdominal wall should not result in ischemia of the peristomal stomach.

Optionally, about four seromuscular interrupted stitches may be appropriate for protection from secondary insufficiency of the purse-string suture, notably when greater amounts of ascites are present (**B**).

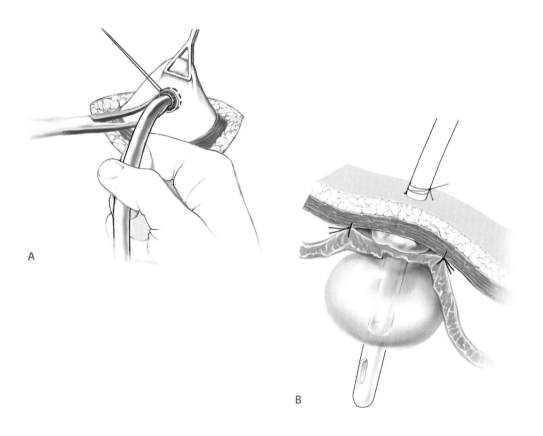

A

B

Permanent Stapled Continent Gastrostomy

STEP 1	Access

Access to the peritoneal cavity and exposure of the stomach as described above.

STEP 2	Creation of a tube

For creation of a permanent reverse gastrostomy, usually the greater curvature is used. The left gastroepiploic vessels represent the vascular pedicle of the tube. After interruption of the right gastroepiploic vessels at the site of the beginning of the tube, the gastrocolic and, if necessary, gastrosplenic ligaments are transected at a safe distance from the left vascular pedicle without compromising the integrity of the gastroepiploic arcade (A).

The basis of the tube is localized at the middle third of the greater curvature. The left gastroepiploic vessels are the vascular pedicle of the gastrostomy.

A sufficient length of the tube is achieved by two to three applications of a linear stapler, depending on the thickness of the abdominal wall. Inversion of the GIA suture lines is done by interrupted or running sutures(B).

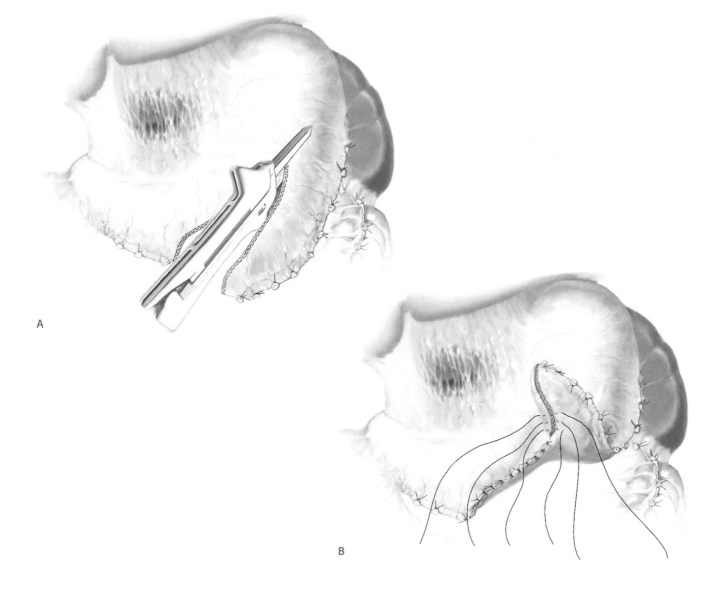

A

B

STEP 3   **Gastroplasty**

A gastroplasty is performed at the site of continuity with the gastric body. This should encircle almost the total circumference of the basis of the tube without compromising its blood supply at the superior aspect of the tube.

Circumferential fixation of the rim of the gastroplication is done by anchor sutures to the wall of the tube. Transabdominal pull-through of the tube is done at the left upper abdomen. Opening of the tube and positioning of the mucosal orifice flush with the skin are done to avoid aggressive gastric mucus secretions that may induce peristomal dermatitis. Stomaplast around the stoma is applied to protect from peristomal problems.

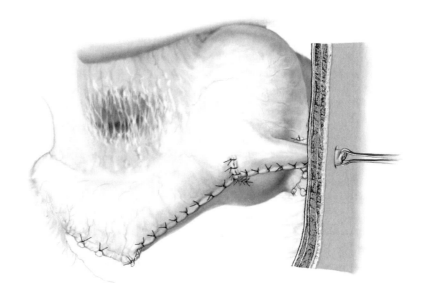

Postoperative Investigations

- Liquid diet feeding 6–12 h following surgery
- Feeding with normal mashed food as soon as evidence for postoperative abnormalities of gastroduodenal clearance has been excluded.

Postoperative Complications

- Postoperative obstruction due to stomal edema
- Insufficiency of the gastrostomy, suture line disruption
- Defective wound healing
- Peritonitis
- Intragastric and intraperitoneal bleeding
- Gastric wall or stomal necrosis

Tricks of the Senior Surgeon

- The continence of the gastrostomy can be enhanced by drawing the tube upward and bringing it to the surface near the costal margin.
- Avoid extreme kinking of the stomal tube by gastroplication and/or anchor sutures of the tube to the gastroplasty. Both may compromise the blood supply of the gastrostomy from the left gastroepiploic vessels.

Percutaneous Endoscopic Gastrostomy

Capecomorin S. Pitchumoni

Indications and Contraindications

Indications

- Failure to thrive
- Poor oral intake
- Dysphagia: mechanical or neurogenic
  Common situations where PEG is required:
- Neurological:
  - Stroke with neurogenic dysphagia
  - Multiple sclerosis
  - Motor neuron disease
  - Cerebral palsy
  - Myotonic dystrophy
- Mechanical dysphagia:
  - Esophageal carcinoma
  - Head and neck malignancy
- Advanced dementia with poor oral intake

Contraindications

- Severe co-morbidity or sepsis
- Expected survival less than 6 weeks
- Abdominal wall infection
- Coagulopathy
- Multiple abdominal surgeries
- Intestinal obstruction
- Partial gastrectomy

Preoperative Investigations/Preparation for the Procedure

- Consent/written advanced directives
- Cardiorespiratory status assessment
- Baseline laboratory parameters

Procedure

| STEP 1 | **Preparation** |

The patient's general condition is reevaluated 24 h prior to and a few hours prior to PEG insertion; acuity of illness could have changed the expected survival.

A single dose of IV antibiotic is administered.

The abdomen is examined for scars/signs of ascites or cellulitis, and the skin over the abdomen is cleaned using povidone iodine.

| STEP 2 | **Esophagogastroduodenoscope** |

The esophagogastroduodenoscope is passed into the stomach.

The stomach is examined to rule out local contraindications, such as tumor, severe erosive gastritis, gastric varices, large ulcer, and outlet obstruction.

| STEP 3 | **Air inflation** |

Inflation of the stomach with air, so that its anterior wall abuts the anterior abdominal wall, pushing away any bowel loops from in between.

STEP 4

Transillumination

Transillumination is attained through the anterior abdominal wall after darkening the room.

The assistant makes a finger impression over the point of transillumination (A).

Failure to transilluminate implies presence of intervening bowel loops, making the procedure unsafe.

This indentation must be clearly visible through the endoscope, which is already positioned facing the anterior abdominal wall (B).

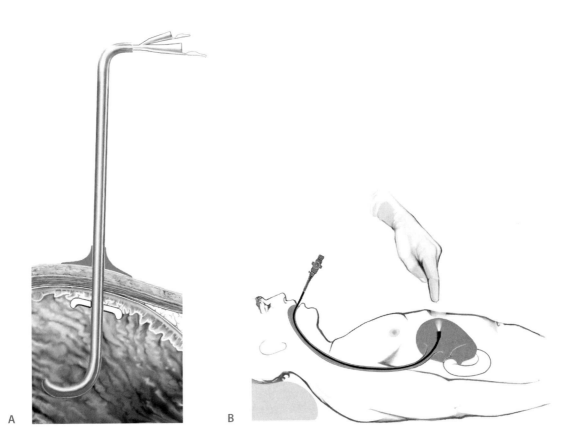

A   B

STEP 5

Local anesthesia

After marking this point on the skin using a blunt tip or marker, the assistant injects a local anesthetic into the skin and makes a shallow 5-mm cut using a scalpel.

An 18G hollow needle is passed through this incision, piercing the gastric wall, thus entering the endoscopic field.

STEP 6

Introduction of a guidewire

The assistant passes a guidewire through the needle.

This is grasped by a snare that is passed through the endoscope.

The scope and the guidewire are pulled out through the mouth as one unit, as the assistant feeds more wire as needed into the stomach.

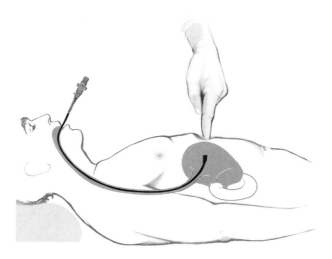

STEP 7

Pull through

The tapering end of the lubricated PEG tube is threaded over the wire and pushed through the mouth into the esophagus and the stomach, while the assistant pulls the wire back through the incision. This is called a "pull" PEG as the assistant *pulls* the PEG out through the anterior abdominal wall by pulling on the wire. As more wire is pulled out, the tapered tip of the PEG tube becomes visible and the process is continued until only about 3–4 cm of the PEG tube remains deep to the skin. The markings on the tube help determine the length.

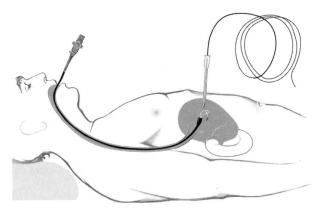

STEP 8

Trimming the length

The tube is trimmed in length, and a feeing port is attached to the tip after anchoring the tube to the anterior abdominal wall using a plastic stopper.

Procedure: "Push PEG"

This procedure is currently less popular.

Alternatively, after withdrawing the needle, a trochar can be passed with a plastic removable catheter around it.

The trochar is then withdrawn, and the feeding tube is passed through the catheter into the stomach.

The catheter is removed, leaving the feeding tube in place, which is then fixed to the abdominal wall. This is called "Push PEG," as it involves *pushing* the feeding tube into the stomach through the abdominal wall incision.

The stopper now approximates the anterior wall of the stomach to the abdominal wall.

Feeding is generally commenced on the following day, after the patient is examined.

PEG Removal

This is only advisable for cases where a well-defined tract has been formed.

Indications and Contraindications

Indications

- The PEG tube is no longer needed (reversal of original indication)
- Worn out tube
- Blocked tube that cannot be cleared by flushing

Percutaneous Removal

STEPS

Identify the type of PEG tube first: a mushroom type will only have one lumen in the tube while a balloon type will have two lumens on sectioning the tube.

"Mushroom" type:

Clean the PEG site and apply lidocaine ointment.

A sustained pull at 90 degrees to the anterior abdominal wall will result in a sudden folding and collapse of the mushroom and the tube "pops" out of the stoma.

Bleeding is uncommon and the stoma closes in 8–48 h.

Balloon type:

Deflate the balloon by using a syringe for the balloon port or by cutting the tube, allowing the water to leak out of the balloon.

Once the balloon is deflated, the tube can be pulled out with no resistance.

Endoscopic Removal

Indication

When percutaneous removal is not possible, e.g., when the balloon cannot be deflated or the "mushroom" PEG tube cannot be pulled out.

STEPS

Upper endoscopy is performed. The PEG tube is snared using a polypectomy snare inside the stomach. (The balloon may need to be deflated using a sclerotherapy needle.)

The tube is cut from the outside using a pair of scissors or scalpel.

The snared end is pulled out along with the endoscope.

Reinsertion

A new balloon-type PEG tube is inserted through the existing stoma and inflated with water. The balloon end is pulled up to the stomach wall and a rubber stopper is applied on the outside to position it snugly against the anterior abdominal wall.

Standard Postoperative Investigations

- Daily check for an adequate approximation of the gastric wall to the abdominal wall to prevent dislocation and peritonitis

Postoperative Complications

- Perforation of esophagus, stomach, transverse colon
- Hemorrhage
- Sepsis: usually detected in 2–3 days
- Clogging of the tube
- Gastrocutaneous fistula
- Gastric ulcer
- Peritonitis
- "Buried bumper syndrome" when the bumper gets buried in the stomach wall
- Distal migration of the tube resulting in gastric outlet obstruction
- An agitated patient may pull the tube out

Tricks of the Senior Surgeon

- Care has to be taken for a necrosis of the gastric wall in case of a too strong approximation by the "mushroom."

Laparoscopic-Assisted Gastrostomy

Tim Strate, Oliver Mann

Introduction

Laparoscopic gastrostomy is an excellent minimally invasive procedure for patients who are unable to swallow and unable to undergo percutaneous endoscopic gastrostomy. The original open method was devised as a feeding tube by Bronislaw Kader in 1896 and modified for minimally invasive technique in the 1990s.

Indications and Contraindications

Indications

- See chapter "Conventional Gastrostomy: Temporary or Permanent Gastric Fistula."

Contraindications

- Ascites
- Previous gastric or major upper abdominal surgery (in this case at least laparoscopic exploration might be feasible)

Preoperative Investigation/Preparation for the Procedure

See chapter "Surgical Gastrostomy: Temporary or Permanent Gastric Fistula."

Procedure

Access
- 3-Trocar technique (2×10-mm and 1×5-mm trocars)
- 10-mm subumbilical trocar
- Pneumoperitoneum of 12 mmHg
- 10-mm trocar in left lower quadrant
- 5-mm trocar in right upper quadrant

Exposure

Exposure and exploration, adhesiolysis if necessary.

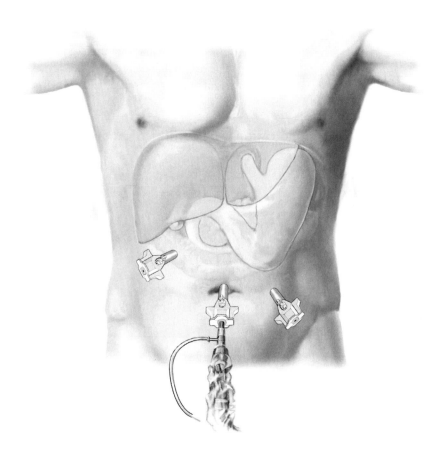

STEP 2

Three full-thickness stitches

Using a straight needle which is brought into the abdomen through the skin at the left hypogastric region, a triangle is created by three full-thickness stitches which allow the catheter system to be introduced under laparoscopic control (stitches: skin-abdominal wall-stomach-abdominal wall-skin).

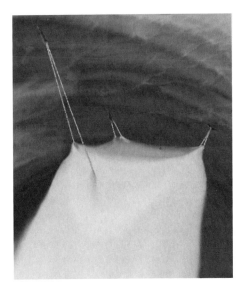

STEP 3

Insertion of the guidewire

A 1-cm stab incision is made in the center of the triangle created by the three sutures which are held under tension. Under laparoscopic vision the anterior stomach wall is punctured by an 18-gauge needle exactly in the center of the triangle. Through the needle a guidewire is inserted into the stomach and a 26-Fr. dilatator with a peel-away sheath is pushed over the guidewire into the stomach percutaneously.

At the end of the procedure the correct placement of the tube is confirmed radiographically.

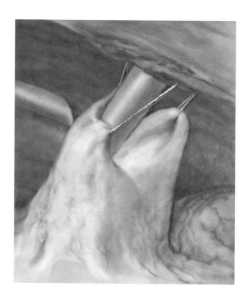

STEP 4   **Introducing the catheter system**

The inner dilatator is removed and a regular 24-Fr. urinary catheter is placed through the remaining peel-away sheath into the stomach. The peel-away sheath is removed. After the balloon of the catheter is inflated, the stomach is pulled against the abdominal wall and the sutures are subcutaneously secured under traction and progressive reduction of the pneumoperitoneum. The catheter is then put under traction for 24h.

See chapter "Conventional Gastrostomy: Temporary or Permanent Gastric Fistula" for postoperative investigations and complications.

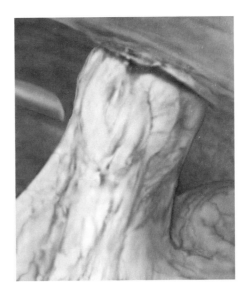

Tricks of the Senior Surgeon

- Exchange the 24-Fr. urinary catheter for a special gastrostomy button device 14 days postoperatively (*see Figure*).
- To avoid dietary deficiencies, patients should be under the supervision of a nutritional specialist.
- In case of contraindications for general anesthesia, the procedure can also be performed under local or regional anesthesia.

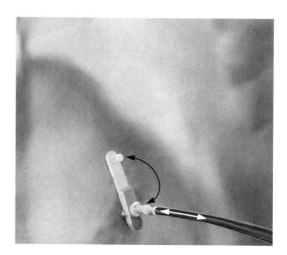

Operation for GERD: Laparoscopic Approach

Ketan M. Desai, Nathaniel J. Soper

Introduction

Laparoscopic antireflux surgery (LARS) has assumed a major role in the treatment of gastroesophageal reflux disease (GERD). The advancement in laparoscopic techniques and instrumentation over the past decade has led to an increase in the number of antireflux operations. Although the operation is fundamentally similar to open antireflux procedures, clear benefits to the laparoscopic approach have been described.

In 1955, Rudolf Nissen reported the efficacy of a 360° gastric wrap through an upper abdominal incision to control reflux symptoms. It was not until 1991 that the first laparoscopic Nissen fundoplication was reported. From that point, acceptance on the part of patients and physicians to proceed with surgical treatment began to grow. Although the minimally invasive approach follows the same surgical principles as the open operation, LARS reduces postoperative pain, shortens the hospital stay and recovery period, and achieves a functional outcome that is similar to that of the open operation.

Indications and Contraindications

Indications

- GERD symptoms (heartburn, regurgitation, dysphagia, chest pain) not controlled by medical therapy
- Volume reflux
- Paraesophageal hernia (PEH) with GERD
- Inability to take acid reduction medication (allergic reaction, poor compliance, cost)
- Preference for surgery (young age, lifestyle choice)

Contraindications

Absolute Contraindications
- Inability to tolerate general anesthesia or laparoscopy

Relative Contraindications
- Previous upper abdominal surgery
- Morbid obesity
- Short esophagus

Preoperative Investigation/Preparation for Procedure

History:	Presence or absence of typical/atypical GERD symptoms, and acid reduction medication use
Upper endoscopy with biopsies:	Evaluation for esophagitis, gastritis, Barrett's metaplasia/dysplasia, hiatal hernia, and strictures
Esophageal manometry for evaluation of eso- phageal motility disorder:	Measurement of esophageal body peristalsis and lower esophageal sphincter (LES) position/length/pressure
24-h pH testing:	Following the cessation of proton-pump inhibitors for >7 days Intravenous antiemetics are administered prophylactically.

Laparoscopic Nissen Fundoplication

Used in >90% of patients with GERD. It can be argued that total (360°) fundoplication is generally not performed in patients with severe esophageal dysmotility.

Procedure

STEP 1   **Operating room and patient setup**

The patient is placed supine with the legs abducted on straight leg boards (no flexion of the hips or knees). An orogastric tube is placed.

The operating room personnel and equipment are arranged with the surgeon between the patient's legs, the assistant surgeon on the patient's right, and the camera holder to the left.

Video monitors are placed at either side of the head of the table and should be viewed easily by all members of the operating team.

Irrigation, suction, and electrocautery connections come at the head of the table on the patient's right side. Special instruments include endoscopic Babcock graspers, cautery scissors, curved dissectors, clip applier, atraumatic liver retractor, 5-mm needle holders, and ultrasonic coagulating shears.

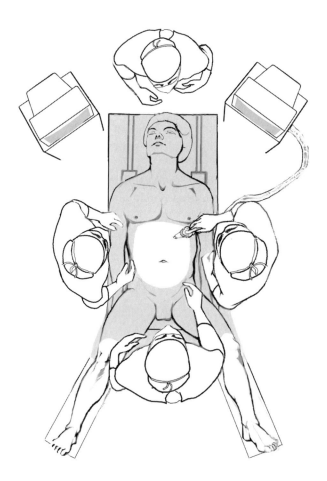

Port placement

Port arrangement should allow easy access to the hiatus and permit comfortable suturing by placing the optics between the surgeon's hands. Access to the abdominal cavity is achieved by either a closed or open technique superior to the umbilicus.

The initial port is placed in the left mid-rectus muscle approximately 12–15 cm below the xiphoid process. Four additional ports are placed under direct vision of the laparoscope. Ports are typically placed in the following locations to optimize visualization and tissue manipulation, and to facilitate suturing: right subcostal, 15 cm from the xiphoid process; a point midway between the first two ports in the right mid-rectus region; in the left subcostal region 10 cm from the xiphoid; and in the right paramedian location at the same horizontal level as the left subcostal trocar (usually 5 cm inferior to the xiphoid process).

The gastroesophageal junction is usually deep to the xiphoid, and from a point 15 cm distant, only half of the laparoscopic instrument must be introduced to reach the hiatus. This distance establishes the fulcrum at the midpoint of the instrument and maximizes its range of motion during tissue manipulation.

With current 5-mm equipment and optics, we generally use only one 10–12 port, for the surgeon's right hand, to allow insertion of an SH needle through the valve mechanism.

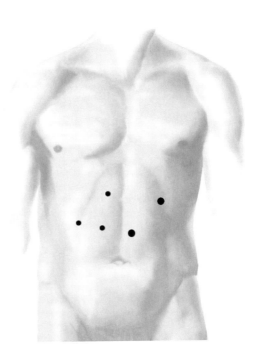

Exposure

Exposure of the esophageal hiatus is facilitated by gravity and maintained by an assistant. Positioning the patient in the reverse Trendelenburg position displaces the bowel and stomach from the diaphragm.

A skilled camera holder and the use of an angled laparoscope (30° or 45°) are important.

The assistant introduces a self-retaining liver retractor through the right subcostal port, and a Babcock grasper is introduced through the right mid-rectus port to pull the stomach and epiphrenic fat pad inferiorly and allow division of the gastrohepatic ligament using the ultrasonic shears. Division of the gastrohepatic ligament is done with preservation of the hepatic branch of the anterior vagus.

The left triangular ligament is not divided but is left to aid in retraction of the liver anteriorly. Next, both the crura and anterior vagus nerve are identified after opening the phrenoesophageal membrane.

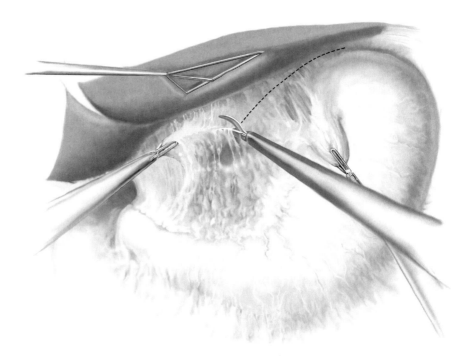

STEP 4

Dissection

If a hiatal hernia is present, it is repositioned into the abdominal cavity with gentle traction after cutting all adhesions to the hernia sac.

The right crus is retracted laterally, and the right side of the esophagus is carefully dissected to visualize the aortoesophageal groove and posterior vagus nerve.

The left crus is similarly dissected from the esophagus and fundus to its point of origin from the right crural leaflet. A "window" is created between the crura and posterior esophageal wall under direct vision from the angled laparoscope (A).

The fundus is then fully mobilized by dividing the proximal gastrosplenic ligament. The short gastric vessels are placed on traction and a window is created into the lesser sac. The short gastric vessels are then divided by serial application of the ultrasonic shears or by clipping and dividing them (B). To fully mobilize the proximal stomach, all posterior retroperitoneal adhesions to the fundus are divided.

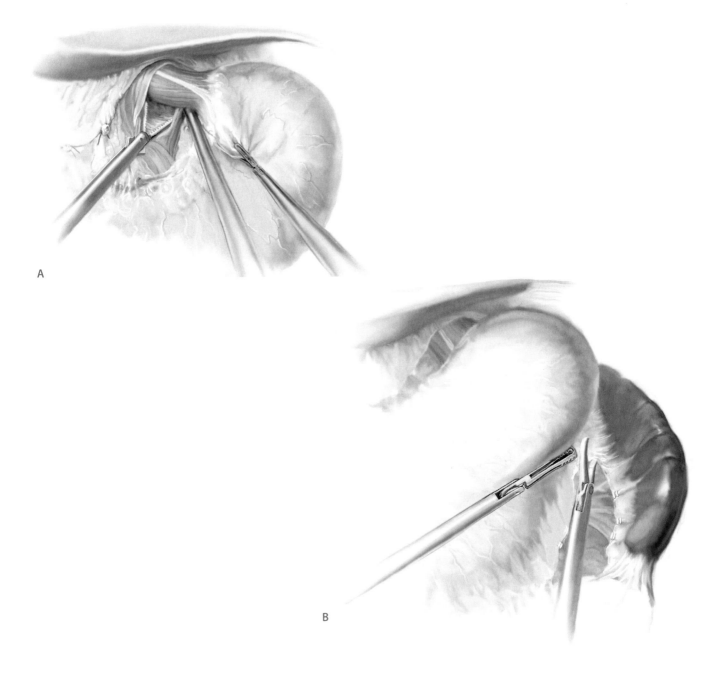

A

B

STEP 5   ### Closure of the hiatal defect

After mobilizing the fundus, a Babcock clamp is passed right to left in front of both crura and behind the esophagus. The Babcock clamp grasps the fundus near the insertion of the short gastric vessels and pulls the fundus left to right around the esophagus. Following the "shoe-shine" maneuver, the fundus should lie in place (**A**). If the fundus springs back around the esophagus, the wrap will be under tension.

The hiatal defect is closed with several interrupted 0-Ethibond sutures (**B**).

Retroesophageal exposure of the crura is gained either by using the mobilized fundus to retract the esophagus anteriorly and to the left, or by placing a Penrose drain around the distal esophagus for retraction. This allows visualization of the retroesophageal space. Approximation of the right and left crura is usually performed posterior to the esophagus, although anterior closure may be appropriate in select cases.

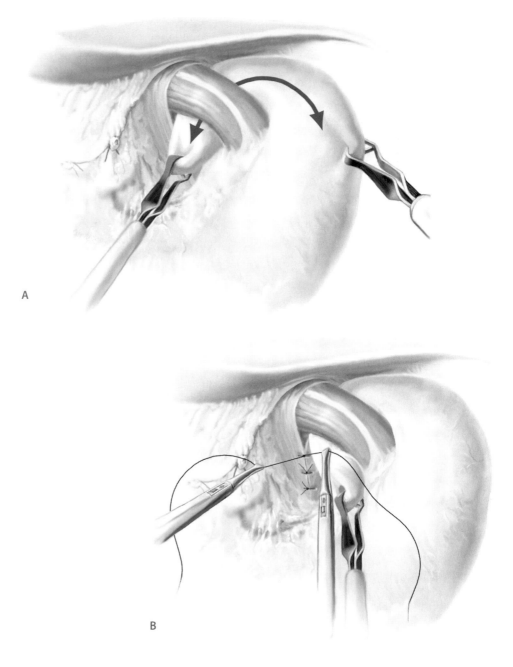

A

B

STEP 6   Fundoplication

The esophagus is serially dilated, and a 50–60 Fr. Maloney dilator is left in place during the creation of the wrap. The dilator calibrates the wrap and prevents excessive narrowing of the esophagus during the actual fundoplication. Dilation must be performed cautiously if the patient has esophageal stricture or severe inflammation. The surgeon should watch the bougie pass smoothly through the gastroesophageal junction. If the bougie appears to be hung up at the gastroesophageal junction, the surgeon can sometimes improve the angulation by retracting the stomach anteriorly or caudally.

With the dilator in the esophagus, the fundus is positioned, and a "short, floppy" Nissen fundoplication is constructed using three interrupted, braided O- or 2-O polyester sutures. Seromuscular bites of fundus to the left of the esophagus, the anterior esophageal wall away from the anterior vagus nerve, and the fundus to the right are all incorporated in the 360-degree fundoplication. The esophageal wall should be incorporated in at least one of the sutures to inhibit slippage of the wrap around the body of the stomach or into the thoracic cavity.

Our practice has been to use extracorporeal knotting techniques, tying square knots and pushing them into position, whereas other surgeons prefer intracorporeal suturing. Regardless, the surgeon should take generous tissue bites and appose the gastric wall without strangulating tissue. Ideally, the wrap should be ≤2 cm in length.

After three sutures secure the fundoplication, additional sutures may be placed from the wrap to the crura for stabilization, although we currently do not perform this step. The esophageal dilator is withdrawn by the anesthesiologist. At this point the Nissen fundoplication is complete.

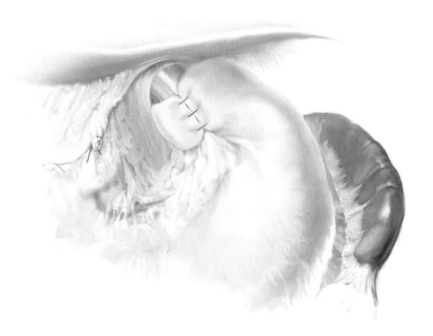

Standard Postoperative Investigations

■ Patients who report unusual abdominal or chest discomfort, GERD related symptoms, or dysphagia should undergo testing (endoscopic, radiological and/or physiologic evaluation).

Postoperative Complications

■ Dysphagia
■ Recurrent GERD symptoms and/or esophagitis
■ Wrap disruption/migration or acute paraesophageal hernia
■ Gas-bloat syndrome

Tricks of the Senior Surgeon

■ Securing the patient to the table using a beanbag will allow steep reverse Trendelenburg positioning for gravity displacement of the bowel and maximum exposure of the gastroesophageal junction.
■ Dividing the short gastric vessels will freely mobilize the fundus.
■ Adequacy of fundic mobilization is checked by releasing the fundus and watching whether the fundus rests in place or recoils under tension.
■ Care should be taken not to create a hypomochlion when performing posterior hiatoplasty.
■ A short, floppy wrap ≤2 cm in length is ideal.
■ A 360-degree wrap is too tight if a 10-mm Babcock clamp does not easily pass under the wrap.

Laparoscopic Partial Fundoplication (Table 1)

Indications and Contraindications

See "Laparoscopic Nissen Fundoplication."

- Procedure of choice for GERD patients with abnormal proximal esophageal motility in order to prevent excessive postoperative dysphagia or gas bloating symptoms (Table 2).

Table 1. Partial fundoplication techniques

Thal	90 degree anterior wrap
Watson	120 degree anterolateral wrap
Dor	150–200 degree anterior wrap
Toupet	270 degree posterior wrap
Belsey Mark IV	270 degree transthoracic anterolateral wrap

Table 2. Indications for partial fundoplications

Primary esophageal motility disorders
    Achalasia (after myotomy)
    Scleroderma

Secondary esophageal motility disorders
    Poor motility secondary to chronic reflux/Barrett's esophagus

Inability to tolerate complete fundoplication
    Dysphagia
    Gas bloating
    Chronic nausea
    Aerophagia
    Revision of obstructing 360 degree wrap

Laparoscopic Toupet Fundoplication

Procedure

- Initial operating room/patient setup, port placement, exposure, dissection, and closure of hiatal defect identical to the procedure outlined in "Laparoscopic Nissen Fundoplication."

Fundoplication

STEP 1

Fixation of the fundus to the left crus

After the leading edge of the fundus is pulled posterior and to the right of the esophagus, the fundus is sutured to the left crus and to the right side of the esophagus over a length of 2–3cm (**A, B**).

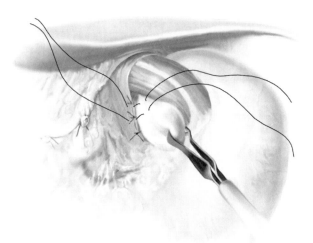

A

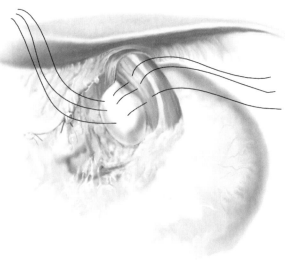

B

STEP 2

Fixation of the fundus to the esophagus and the right crus

The anterior fundus is sutured to the left side of the esophagus over a length of 2cm (A).
The 270-degree fundoplication is secured to the right crus with separate gastrocrural sutures (B).

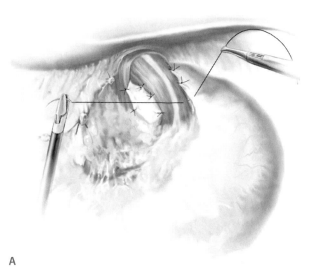

A

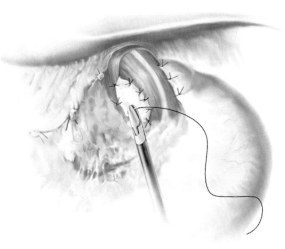

B

Operation for GERD: Conventional Approach

Karim A. Gawad, Christoph Busch

Introduction

The laparoscopic approach to gastroesophageal reflux (GERD) has become the "gold standard" over the past decade. Nevertheless, an open approach may be preferable in patients who have undergone previous open upper abdominal surgery or in cases of recurrent or re-recurrent GERD when revisional laparoscopy may not seem sufficient to definitely treat the disease.

Indications and Contraindications

Indications

- Significant gastroesophageal reflux
- "When a laparoscopic approach is not indicated"
- Recurrent disease following previous open or laparoscopic surgery
- Status postconventional upper abdominal surgery with massive adhesions
- Failure of conservative treatment

Contraindications

- General contraindications for surgery under general anesthesia

Preoperative Investigations/Preparation for the Procedure

See chapter on "Operation for GERD: Laparoscopic Approach."

Procedures

Access

Transverse upper abdominal incision, if required with additional upper midline incision; *alternatively,* left subcostal *or* upper midline incision

Division of the triangular ligament with ligation (cave: accessory bile duct) to expose the esophagogastric junction

Choice of Procedure

- Simple reflux disease (esophagitis up to III):
  - Fundoplication
  - Ligamentum teres (round ligament) plasty
- Complicated reflux disease (esophagitis IV):
  - Fundoplication + dilatation (of florid esophagitis)
  - Fundoplication + parietal cell vagotomy (in gastric hyperacidity) + if necessary dilatation (of florid esophagitis)
  - Fundoplication + parietal cell vagotomy + stricturoplasty (of scarred strictures)
  - Limited resection of the gastroesophageal junction

STEP 1	Mobilization of the distal esophagus and fundus

The distal esophagus is completely dissected and armed with a vessel loop. The gastric fundus is completely mobilized by division of the short gastric vessels in order to form a loose, "floppy" fundoplication.

If ligamentum teres plasty is planned, there is no need for fundic mobilization. Special attention has to be paid to thoroughly preserving the ligament at laparotomy.

In the presence of a hiatal hernia, a posterior hiatoplasty is performed using non-absorbable suture material.

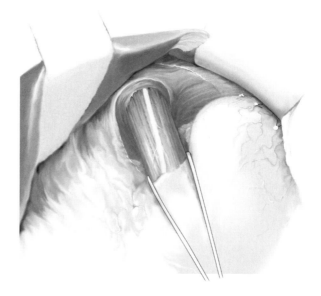

Total ("Nissen") Fundoplication

| STEP 2 | Passage of the fundus |

The mobilized fundus is passed behind the esophagus to the right side so far that it can be easily united with the remaining fundic frontwall in front of the esophagus.

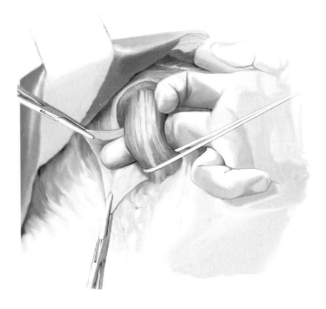

| STEP 3 | Formation of the wrap |

The two cuff-folds are fixed with three, maximally four, non-absorbable sutures. One suture should partially grab the esophageal wall to prevent a telescope phenomenon.

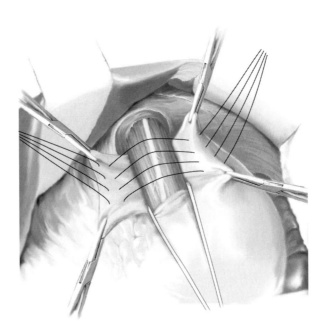

STEP 4   **Anchoring of the wrap**

Finally the fundic cuff is again tested. Two fingers should easily pass the loose wrap around the distal esophagus ("floppy Nissen").

One or two additional sutures can fix the left cuff-fold to the anterior gastric wall in order to prevent slippage (telescope phenomenon).

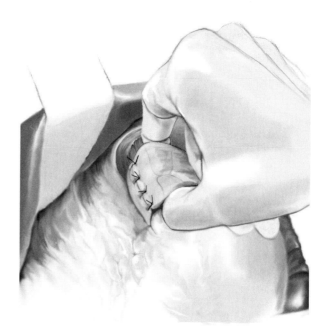

Ligamentum Teres (Round Ligament) Plasty

STEP 1

See above.

STEP 2   **Dissection of the round ligament**

The round ligament is carefully dissected from the abdominal wall and from the liver, respectively. The free end of the ligament is transposed dorsally around the esophagus coming from the right side.

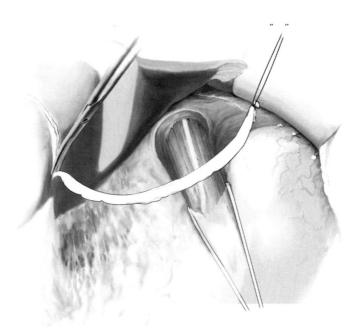

STEP 3   **Fixation to the anterior gastric wall**

The round ligament is then attached to the anterior gastric wall under relative tension
using three or four non-absorbable sutures. Fixation to the anterior aspect of the gastric
corpus is performed.

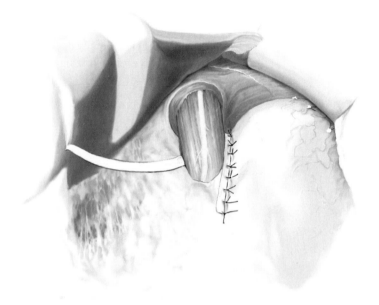

Standard Postoperative Investigations

See chapter "Operation for GERD: Laparoscopic Approach."

Postoperative Complications

- Short term:
  - Esophageal perforation
  - Dysphagia
- Long term:
  - Dysphagia
  - Gas-bloat
  - Recurrent disease

Tricks of the Senior Surgeon

- Perform Nissen fundoplication around a large gastric tube to facilitate formation of a loose "floppy," fundic wrap.
- Use of a self-retaining retractor system will facilitate exposure of the esophagogastric junction.
- Dissection of the short gastrics is not mandatory but will ensure a loose fundoplication, thus preventing postoperative dysphagia.
- Do not dissect the round ligament at laparotomy.

Operation for Paraesophageal Hernia

Jean-Marie Michel, Lukas Krähenbühl

Introduction

Postempski first reported the repair of a wound of the diaphragm in 1889. Ackerlund described different types of paraesophageal hernia in 1926, and the first hiatal hernia repair (fundoplication) was reported by Nissen in 1955. Since then, Nissen fundoplication has gained wide acceptance and is now recognized as the operation of choice for antireflux surgery and, although technically challenging, laparoscopic paraesophageal hernia repair.

The goal of a paraesophageal hernia repair is to bring the stomach (with other organs such as colon, omentum, spleen) and the lower esophagus back into the abdominal cavity, to excise the hernia sac, to approximate crura, to perform a fundoplication in order to prevent gastroesophageal reflux, and finally to perform a gastropexy in order to prevent gastric volvulus.

Indications and Contraindications: Laparoscopy

Indications	■ Symptomatic or asymptomatic Type II and Type III hiatal hernia
Contraindications	**Absolute Contraindications** ■ Gastric incarceration ■ Intrathoracic gastric perforation with Type II or Type III hiatal hernia **Relative Contraindications** ■ Partially fixed paraesophageal hernia ■ Short esophagus

Indications and Contraindications: Laparotomy

Indications

- As for laparoscopy
- Gastric incarceration

Contraindications

Absolute Contraindications
- Intrathoracic gastric perforation with Type II or Type III hiatal hernia

Relative Contraindications
- None

Preoperative Preparation/Preparation for the Procedure

History:	Long-term history of gastroesophageal reflux disease (GERD), symptoms of upper GI occlusion
Upright radiograph of the thorax:	Search for a retrocardiac air-fluid level
Contrast radiographic studies (barium swallow):	Preoperative localization of the gastroesophageal junction, assessment of the type of hernia
Esophageal manometry:	To exclude a motility disorder of the esophagus
Upper endoscopy:	Objective GERD and/or exclusion of gastric ulcer disease
24-h pH monitoring and stationary manometry:	(Facultative) look for GERD and esophageal dysmotility. In type II hernias, 70% of patients have pathologic pH-metry, with up to 100% of patients with type III hernias.
Actively treat dehydration	
Empty the stomach:	Nasogastric tube or immediate preoperative endoscopy
Single-shot antibiotic with second generation cephalosporine	

Procedure

The patient is placed in a modified lithotomy position. The table is placed in a steep reverse Trendelenburg position (French position), with the surgeon standing between the patient's legs, the first assistant on the patient's left, and the camera assistant on the patient's right.

Port Placement

A 10-mm port is placed 5–8 cm above the umbilicus in the midline (open Hasson technique). A carbon dioxide pneumoperitoneum is established (12 mmHg). A 30°-angle laparoscope is mandatory. After exploratory laparoscopy, the next four trocar sleeves are placed under direct vision. A subxiphoid 5-mm port for liver retraction, two working ports: one 5-mm one in the right upper quadrant (UQ), another 10-mm one in the left UQ, and a 5-mm left subcostal port.

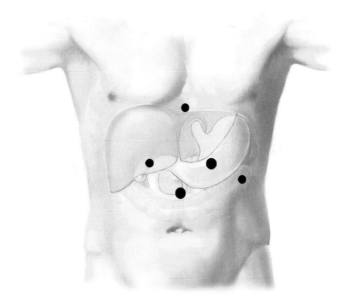

Exposure

To allow free access to the enlarged esophageal hiatus, the left lobe of the liver has to be elevated with a liver retractor.

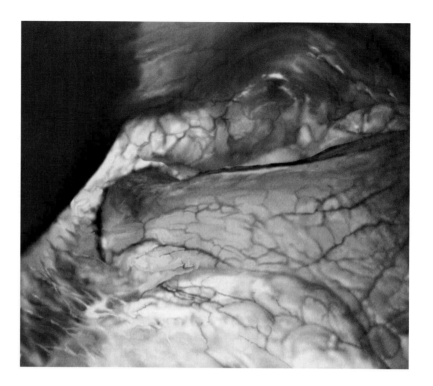

STEP 1

Reduction of herniated stomach

The herniated stomach and the greater omentum are reduced into the abdominal cavity with two Babcock graspers. A nasogastric tube is then introduced to decompress the stomach.

This maneuver is a dangerous step of the procedure with risks of stomach perforation, particularly in case of mechanical obstruction of the stomach (volvulus) with incarceration and gastric wall ischemia.

The spleen, colon, and omentum can also be herniated into the thorax.

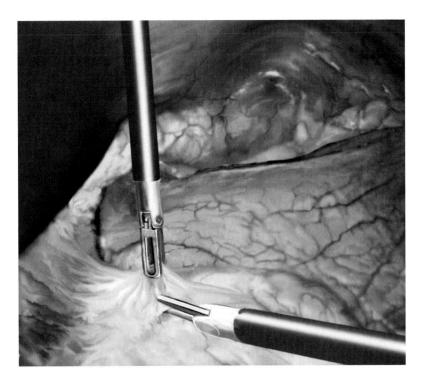

STEP 2   **Exposure of the hiatal hernia**

Open the gastrohepatic ligament after reduction of the hernia content, and expose the right crus of the diaphragm. The hepatic trunk of the vagus nerve and aberrant left hepatic artery should be preserved if possible. The hiatus and the hernia sac are now visible.

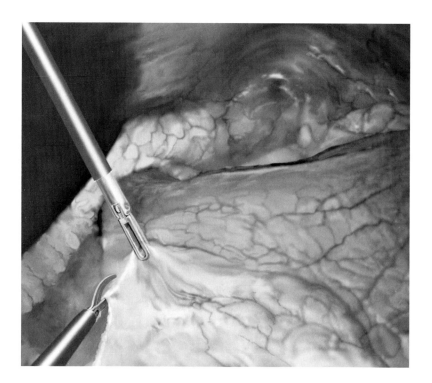

STEP 3

Circular incision of the hernia sac

Start the procedure on the right side and dissect the hernia sac off the right crural edge using the harmonic scalpel (Ethicon Endo-Surgery, Cincinnati, OH, USA). Complete the dissection inferiorly and obtain a good exposure of the junction between the right and left crura, then cranially with the incision of the phrenoesophageal membrane, finally to the left over the left crus. The dissection over the inferoposterior edge of the left crus is difficult at this moment and is best achieved when the hernia sac is completely reduced from the mediastinum.

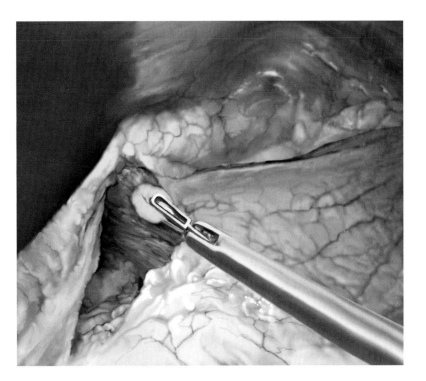

STEP 4

Blunt dissection of the hernia sac

The hernia sac now should be bluntly removed from the mediastinum with complete exposure of the right and left crura (see STEP 3).

During this step anterior and posterior vagal nerves have to be identified and protected; this could be difficult to perform in inflammatory tissue.

It is not rare that the left and/or right pleura can be opened within the mediastinum during blunt dissection, but most of the time a pleural drainage is not mandatory.

Complete the dissection of the inferoposterior edge of the left crus. Pay particular attention to finding the good plane between the esophagus and the body of the left crus, which may sometimes be extraordinarily difficult. It is not necessary to excise the hernia sac.

STEP 5   **Intra-abdominal reduction of the gastroesophageal junction (GEJ)**

The distal esophagus is now completely freed and a Penrose drain has to be placed around the GEJ junction to permit a better retraction in the abdominal cavity.

It is reported that as many as 15% of giant type III paraesophageal hernias will present with a shortened esophagus and have an irreducible GEJ. Adequate mobilization of the esophagus then should be performed as high as possible into the mediastinum. If the reduction remains impossible after this maneuver, the patient will most benefit from a Collis-Nissen gastroplasty, which has been reported to be feasible using a laparoscopic and/or thoracoscopic approach.

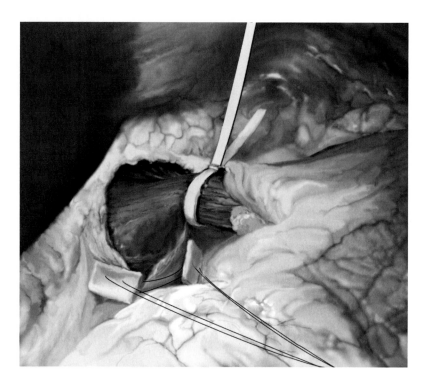

STEP 6   **Closure of the hiatal defect (posterior cruroplasty)**

The hiatal defect is closed with five to six nonabsorbable 2-0 Ethibond mattress sutures placed posteriorly and anteriorly from the esophagus to return the GEJ into the abdomen. The sutures are placed from caudad to cephalad so the hiatus is snug around the esophagus:

The axis of the hiatal hernia has an inferosuperior direction with an angle of about 10% clockwise in the perpendicular plane, and an inferosuperior direction with an angle of about 70% clockwise in the sagittal plane. Thus closure of the hiatal defect must follow the schema represented in A.

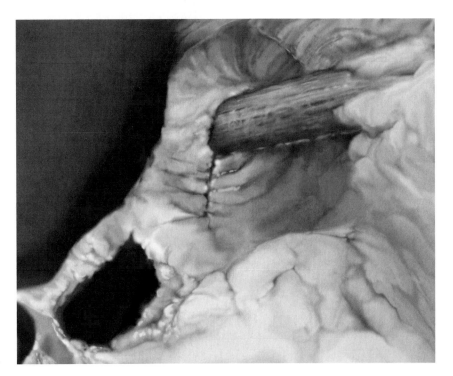

A

Closure of the hiatal defect (posterior cruroplasty)

Sometimes one or two anterior sutures are mandatory to avoid an "S-shape" of the distal esophagus. The inferior edge of the newly created hiatus may produce an external compression leading to dysphagia (B).

Some groups use a prosthetic reinforcement with polytetrafluoroethylene (PTFE) of posterior cruroplasty to reduce the rate of postoperative wrap herniation into the mediastinum.

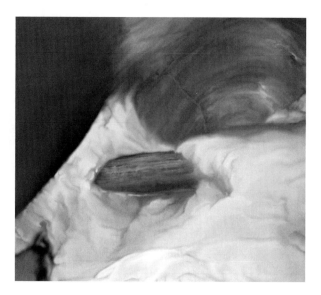

B

STEP 7   **Nissen fundoplication**

Perform a floppy 2-cm three-stitch Nissen fundoplication over a 56F bougie after mobilization of the great curvature (we divide the short gastric vessels). The most cephalad stitch of the fundoplication superficially incorporates the esophagus wall.

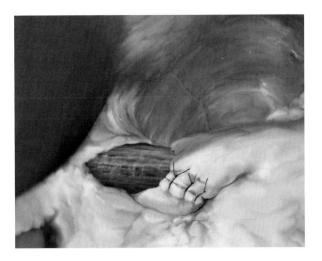

STEP 8   **Anterior gastroplasty**

Perform an anterior gastroplasty with two to three interrupted nonabsorbable 2-0 Ethibond sutures between the greater curvature and the anterior abdominal wall to prevent postoperative intra-abdominal gastric volvulus.

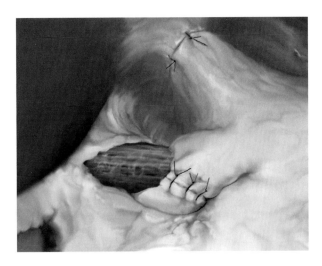

Postoperative Tests

- Resume alimentation the day after surgery
- Obtain a barium esophagogram within 1 month (for follow-up purposes)

Postoperative Complications

- Pneumothorax
- Pleural effusion
- Vagus nerve injury (anterior and posterior bundles)
- Cardiac dysrhythmia
- Pericarditis
- Pneumonia
- Pneumothorax
- Pulmonary embolism

Tricks of the Senior Surgeon

- Use nonabsorbable mattress sutures to perform the posterior cruroplasty.
- At the end of the procedure, perform an anterior gastropexy to avoid postoperative gastric volvulus.

Management of the Duodenal Stump

Matthias Peiper, Wolfram T. Knoefel

Introduction

One of the most serious complications in the postoperative period after gastrectomy is a leakage from the duodenal stump. Historically it has occurred most frequently in Billroth II resections following emergency surgery for duodenal ulcer perforating in the pancreatic head and less frequently after resections for gastric cancer. Causes of duodenal stump suture dehiscence are:

- Technical failure
- Postoperative pancreatitis
- Attempt to close a severely diseased and scarred, edematous duodenal stump
- Blood clots in the duodenal bed leading to infection
- Excessive use of sutures at the stump leading to necrosis

Indications and Contraindications

Indications

- Peritonitis
- Signs of sepsis

Contraindications

- No contraindications in case of emergency

Preoperative Investigations/Preparation for Procedure

- Analysis of abdominal secretion in the drain tube (bilirubin, amylasis, lipase)
- Physical examination
- Abdominal ultrasound
- CT

Procedure

Access
The abdominal cavity is opened through the previous incision.

STEP 1

If the dehiscence is small or barely visible, an omental flap is performed and the area well drained. For some patients, primary suture of the duodenum might be performed. This is usually hand-sewn, though some surgeons prefer the stapler technique.

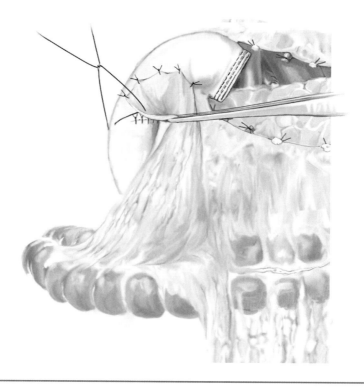

STEP 2

If technically feasible, an end-to-side duodenojejunostomy may be performed using single-layered sutures (Vicryl 3-0).

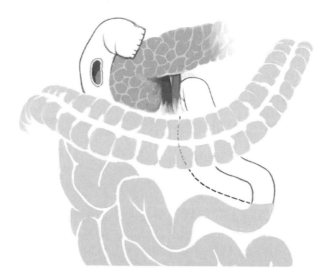

STEP 3

If the duodenum is opened widely and its walls edematous, a primary closure is usually unsuccessful since the sutures will not last. Here it is suggested to insert a Foley catheter into the leak, which may be fixated using a purse-string suture. The catheter shall be completely covered by the greater omentum and externalized using a separate incision. Most fistulas will close spontaneously after 3–4 weeks. An alternative is to cover of the leak by a jejunal loop using the Roux-Y technique.

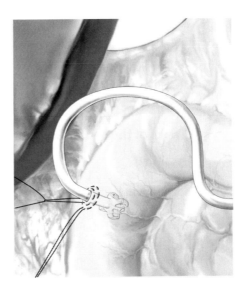

STEP 4

Late suture dehiscences will present usually 2 weeks after (distal) gastrectomy. This course is less dramatic, since postsurgical adhesions lead to a compartmentation of the abdominal cavity. If the drainage is already removed, duodenal juice might drain via the former drainage incision. By using total parenteral nutrition as well as antibiotics, the fistula will close spontaneously. An alternative is the interventional placement of a drainage, such as a Sonnenberg catheter, for optimized drainage of the duodenal fluid.

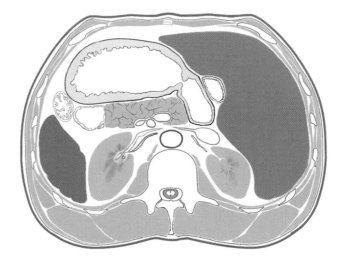

Standard Postoperative Investigations

- Daily check of the abdominal drainage

Postoperative Complications

- Recurrent insufficiency
- Insufficiency of the duodenojejunostomy
- Peritonitis
- Sepsis
- Pancreatitis
- Fistula formation
- Wound infection

Tricks of the Senior Surgeon

- Tissue should not be too edematous. Therefore, the indication for relaparotomy should immediately be established once duodenal stump insufficiency has been diagnosed.
- For some patients, all organ-preserving surgical interventions might not lead to improvement of the patient's condition. As ultima ratio a partial duodenopancreatectomy (Whipple procedure) might be necessary.

Operation for Morbid Obesity

Markus Weber, Markus K. Müller, Michael G. Sarr

Introduction

The prevalence of obesity has increased dramatically over the last several decades worldwide and is currently reaching epidemic proportions. One out of five Americans is currently obese. Morbid obesity, defined as body mass index (BMI) $>40\,kg/m^2$, is associated with many diseases responsible for a high prevalence of morbidity and mortality, such as insulin-resistant diabetes mellitus, hypertension, coronary artery disease, hyperlipidemia, and sleep apnea. These direct weight-related complications eventuate in enormous health care costs. A consensus conference organized by the National Institutes of Health (NIH) in 1991 concluded that surgical therapies offer the best long-term approach for morbid obesity.

Current bariatric surgical procedures are divided into restrictive, malabsorptive, and combined procedures.

- *Restrictive procedures* aim to reduce the volume of oral intake. These include laparoscopic adjustable gastric banding (LAGB) and vertical banded gastroplasty (VBG).
- *Malabsorptive procedures* are designed to reduce caloric absorption by diminishing the absorptive surface for digestion and/or absorption. The most common procedures currently are biliopancreatic diversion (BPD) and duodenal switch with a biliopancreatic diversion (DS/BPD).
- *Combined procedures* utilize both a restrictive and a malabsorptive anatomy and involve primarily the Roux-en-Y gastric bypass (RYGB) (the malabsorptive effect correlates with length of Roux limb).

This chapter addresses the three most commonly performed bariatric procedures. RYGB (A-1) and VBG (A-2) were both considered as being proven effective by the National Institutes of Health consensus conference in 1991. The third procedure, which is widely used in Europe and Australia and is becoming more common in the United States, is LAGB (A-3). Of the three procedures, RYGB has been best documented to produce and maintain long-term weight loss in severely obese patients. All three procedures can be performed by an open or laparoscopic approach. Because of the high incidence of incisional hernia (15–20 %) after open surgery and better patient comfort and acceptance after a laparoscopic approach, increasing numbers of surgeons perform these operations laparoscopically. Therefore, this chapter focuses on the laparoscopic approach with remarks and illustrations on open surgery as well.

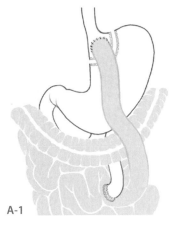

A-1

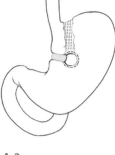

A-2

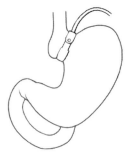

A-3

Indications and Contraindications

Indications

- Patients with ineffective dietary attempts for weight control and
- BMI >40 kg/m^2 or
- BMI >35 kg/m^2 with weight-related comorbidity

Contraindications

- Age <16 and >60 years (these are relative contraindications)
- Obesity history <3 years
- Unacceptable operative risk (e.g., unreconstructable coronary artery disease)
- Active gastric or duodenal ulcer
- Active inflammatory bowel disease
- Chronic infectious disease (e.g., viral hepatitis)
- Portal hypertension
- Pregnancy
- Untreated endocrine disorders
- Severe psychiatric disorders (psychosis, uncontrolled depression, active substance abuse)

Relative Contraindications for Laparoscopic Approach

- Height less than 155 cm
- Multiple intra-abdominal operations
- Previous gastric bariatric procedures

Preoperative Investigations/Preparation for the Procedure

Clinical
- Physical examination (abdominal hernia, former abdominal surgery)
- Phenotype of obesity: androgenic (central obesity) vs gynecoid (peripheral obesity) (note: male/androgene phenotype and BMI >50 associated with increased pre- and perioperative morbidity)
- ECG, pulmonary function tests (if necessary), sleep study if symptoms suggest sleep apnea, and detailed cardiac evaluation if necessary (echocardiography, functional cardiac scintigraphy)

Laboratory
- Nutritional and metabolic parameters
- Hormonal parameters
- Baseline arterial blood gas

Upper GI Examinations
- Gastroscopy in selected patients, esophageal manometry in patients with gastro-esophageal reflux disease if a restrictive procedure is to be performed (VBG, gastric banding)
- Radiology: upper GI studies for reoperative surgery and especially after failed gastric banding (reflux, esophageal dysmotility, pouch dilatation, band penetration?)

Anthropometry/Body Composition (Optional)
- Bioimpedance analysis
- Calorimetry

Psychologic Evaluation
- Exclude psychosis (rare), severe uncontrolled depression, active substance abuse, or borderline personality disorder
- Establish psychiatric care if necessary

Procedures

Roux-en-Y Gastric Bypass

STEP 1   **Positioning of the patient and access**

Laparoscopic approach (A-1):

   The patient is placed in the lithotomy position in steep reverse Trendelenburg tilt with arms positioned upwards. The operating surgeon stands between the legs, first assistant on the left, and the second on the right side of the patient. Two monitors are placed at the head of the bed. Afterwards, six trocars are inserted:

1. One 10/12 mm on the right in the mid-clavicular line distal to the costal arch for the liver retractor
2. One 5 mm right in the mid-clavicular line 15 cm caudal to the costal arch for the grasper and needle driver
3. One 10/12 mm in the midline 15 cm caudal to the xiphoid as the optic port
4. One 10/12 mm in the midline halfway between the xiphoid and umbilicus for the linear cutter, grasper, and ultracision
5. One 10/12 mm on the left in the mid-clavicular line just distal to the costal arch for the linear cutter, grasper, needle holder, and ultracision
6. One 5 mm on the left in the mid-clavicular line 15 cm caudal to the costal arch for the grasper

Open approach (A-2):

   Upper midline incision entering the peritoneal cavity.

   Bariatric retractor (Pilling bariatric retractor, Pilling Co., Ft. Washington, PA) for exposure.

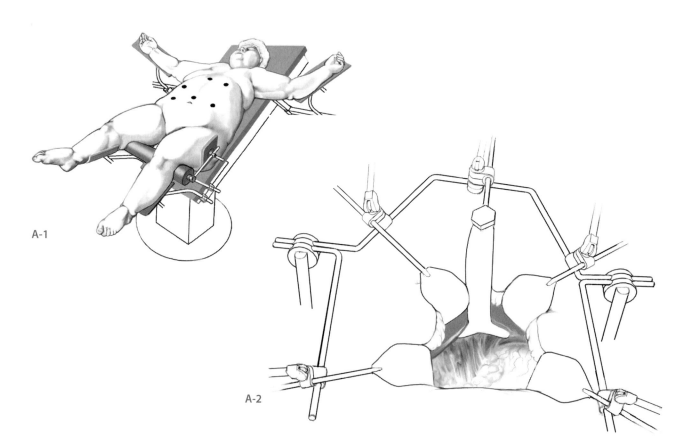

A-1

A-2

STEP 2

Division of stomach and creation of proximal gastric pouch

Laparoscopic approach (A-1):

The left lobe of the liver is retracted with a paddle retractor inserted in the right upper 12-mm port.

A window is created 3–4 cm distal to the esophagogastric junction along the lesser curvature with 5-mm Ultracision shears (Ethicon Endo-Surgery, Cincinnati, OH) close to the gastric wall to avoid injury to the vagus nerves.

Afterwards the stomach is transected with multiple fires of the Endo GIA stapler (U.S. Surgical Co., Norwalk, CT) using a blue cartridge (3.5-mm staples) to create a small proximal gastric pouch of 20 ml. However, be certain to remove any nasogastric tube.

A calibration balloon filled with 20-ml saline can help identify the site of the transection line.

The Endo GIA stapler is first applied once transversely and then vertically 3–4 times, heading to the angle of His until the stomach is completely divided. The dissection of the angle of His before transection is not always necessary, but it may help in difficult exposures or when there is a large fat pad.

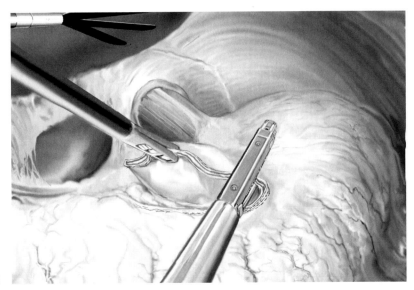

A-1

STEP 2 *(continued)*   **Division of stomach and creation of proximal gastric pouch**

Open approach (A-2):

The first step creates a tunnel from the defect in the gastrohepatic ligament (distal to the left gastric artery) behind the cardia, extending to the left side of the esophagogastric junction.

Two 18-Fr. catheters are passed through the tunnel.

A window 1–2 cm distal to the esophagogastric junction is created along the lesser curve of the stomach and the right end of the catheter is repositioned out of this window; this avoids injury to the neurovascular pedicle along the lesser curve of the stomach.

One end of the catheter is pulled over the end of the anvil of the TA90-B linear stapler (U.S. Surgical Co., Norwalk, CT); the catheter guides the stapler around the gastric cardia.

A second catheter guides a 90-mm linear stapler just distal to the first stapler.

Both staplers are angled in a manner so that a small volume pouch (<15 ml) has a larger surface area of the anterior wall for the anastomosis; both staplers are fired and the cardia between the staple lines is transected. Rostral mobilization of the fat pad of cardia exposes the serosa of the cardia; this allows a very small pouch (<15 ml).

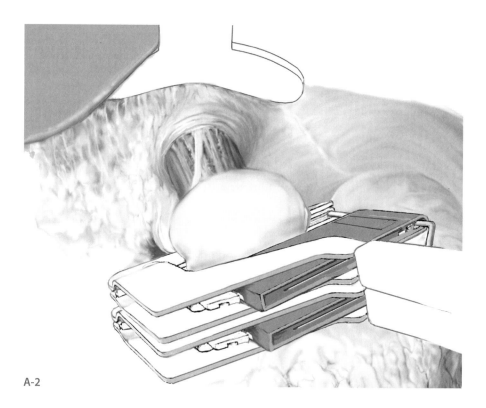

A-2

STEP 3   **Placement of 25-mm EEA anvil into the proximal gastric pouch**

Laparoscopic approach:

Before the anvil of the 25-mm EEA stapler (U.S. Surgical Co., Norwalk, CT) can be inserted, the anvil must be flipped by pushing down the circular blade, and the spring has to be removed to allow an easy flip back (A-1).

The post of the anvil is forced into the proximal end of the 16-Fr. nasogastric tube (end cut off) and fixed in place with 2-0 suture material passed through two holes in the head of the anvil and the hole in the post of the anvil.

The distal end of the nasogastric tube is passed into the oropharynx, down the esophagus, into the gastric pouch, and out of a small gastrotomy made with laparoscopic scissors (A-2). The tube is then pulled into the abdomen with a grasper until the post of the anvil appears through gastrotomy. The nasogastric tube is removed after cutting the suture and tube at the proximal end with Ultracision shears (A-3).

Open approach:

A short (1 cm) cardiotomy is made in the anterior wall of the proximal gastric pouch. The anvil is inserted into the pouch and the cardiotomy is closed around the post of the anvil with a 2-0 polypropylene suture.

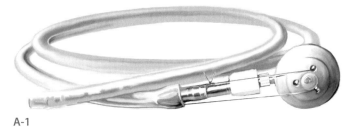

A-1

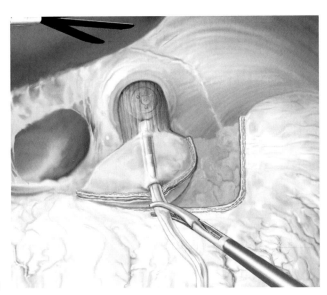

A-2

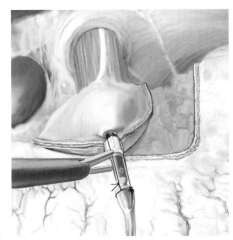

A-3

STEP 4   **Creation of Roux-en-Y limb**

Laparoscopic approach:

The patient is brought into the supine position; the surgeon and first assistant move to the right side of the patient and the camera is inserted through the right upper port after removing the liver paddle.

The transverse colon is lifted up by two graspers inserted through the left-sided cannulas and the ligament of Treitz is identified.

Transection of the jejunum 50 cm distally with 60-mm Endo GIA (white cartridge, 2.5-mm staples minimize staple line bleeding).

Afterwards the mesentery is transected perpendicular to the bowel wall with Ultracision shears or an Endo GIA stapler using white vascular staples (2 mm).

The Roux-en-Y limb is measured (150 cm or 250 cm for superobese patients with BMI >50 kg/m^2).

Fixation of the biliary limb is done with a one stay suture to the Roux-en-Y limb and a jejunojejunostomy is created with a 60-mm Endo GIA stapler using a white cartridge (A-1). The site of stapler insertion is closed with a running 4-0 polydioxanone suture.

The mesenteric defect should be closed with interrupted stitches of non-reabsorbable suture (Ethibond, Ethicon Co., Cincinnati, OH) (A-2) to prevent internal herniation.

The alimentary Roux-en-Y limb is brought antecolic to the proximal gastric pouch, being very careful to avoid a twist in the mesentery; if the omentum is thick and bulky, it can be transected vertically to allow a path for the Roux limb to be brought antecolic. Open approach:

The proximal jejunum is transected about 50–75 cm distal to the ligament of Treitz in an area that both maximizes the blood supply to the proximal aspect of the Roux limb and allows a long transection of the mesentery to gain length. The mesentery is divided by cautery and requires ligation of just one vessel in the arcade that connects the primary feeding vessels from the superior mesenteric artery.

The Roux limb is then brought retrocolic (not antecolic as with a laparoscopic approach) and then antegastric through a wide defect in the gastrocolic ligament.

The defects in the mesocolon and Petersen's hernia (potential infracolic space posterior to the Roux mesentery and anterior to the retroperitoneum) are closed.

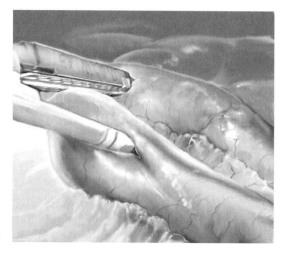

A-1

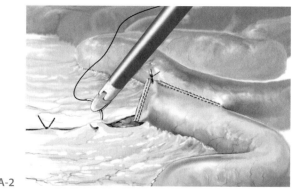

A-2

STEP 5   **Creation of gastrojejunostomy**

Laparoscopic approach:

The end of the Roux limb is opened with Ultracision shears. A 3-cm incision between the two trocars in the left mid-clavicular line allows intraperitoneal introduction of the cartridge of the 25-mm circular EEA stapler. The cartridge head of the EEA stapler is passed into the lumen through the end of the Roux limb and docked with the prong of the anvil (A-1, A-2).

After firing the stapler, the "donuts" are checked carefully; if incomplete, the anastomosis is evaluated by a methylene blue test (150 ml of dilute methylene blue injected through the nasogastric tube into the proximal gastric pouch) after the end of the Roux limb is closed with an Endo GIA stapler using a white cartridge. Closure of any leak is done with a transanastomotic suture.

Even if there is no leak, the gastrojejunal anastomosis is oversewn with three single transmural stitches along the anterior circumference; these sutures reduce tension on the stapled anastomosis. A perianastomotic drain is left routinely and removed postoperatively after a radiographic contrast study confirms the integrity of the anastomosis.

Open approach:

The docking of the cartridge and the anvil post is similar to that for the laparoscopic approach.

The entire anastomotic circumference is then oversewn with interrupted 3-0 silk seromuscular sutures.

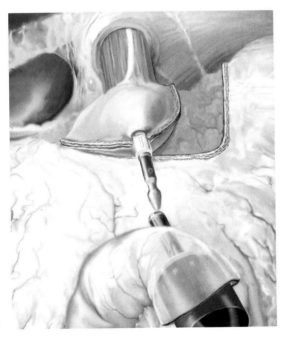

A-1

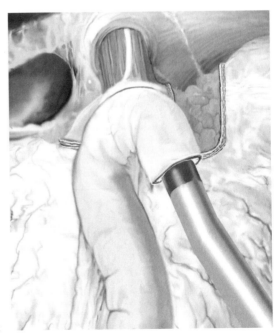

A-2

Vertical Banded Gastroplasty (VBG)

| STEP 1 | Positioning of the patient and access |

VBG can be performed by the open or laparoscopic technique.

A laparoscopic approach is described. The patient and trocars are placed as described for the laparoscopic Roux-en-Y gastric bypass.

| STEP 2 | Placement of anvil of circular stapler |

The gastrohepatic ligament is opened in the avascular window with Ultracision shears to expose the posterior aspect of the stomach.

The optimal position of the anvil is 6–7 cm distal to the esophagogastric junction close to the lesser curvature. It should allow a 32-Fr. tube to pass alongside the lesser curvature; once the optimal site is determined, a straight needle is passed from anterior to posterior through the stomach and a suture tied to the tip of the anvil (**A-1**). This suture will guide the spike of the anvil through the gastric walls.

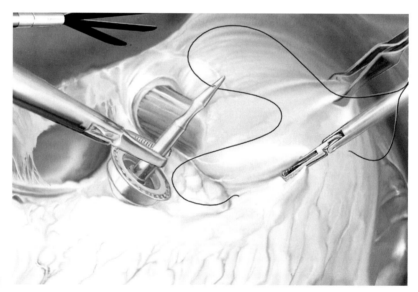

A-1

STEP 2 *(continued)*   **Placement of anvil of circular stapler**

A tight hold of the anvil by a strong grasper is essential. A short incision with electro-cautery where the tip of the anvil will pass helps it to perforate the gastric wall (**A-2**).

The circular stapler cartridge is passed through the abdominal wall, docked with the anvil, and fired, creating the transgastric circular "donut hole" defect in the gastric wall (**A-3**).

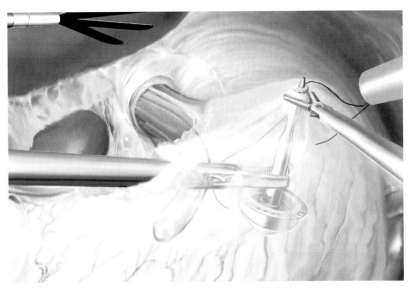

A-2

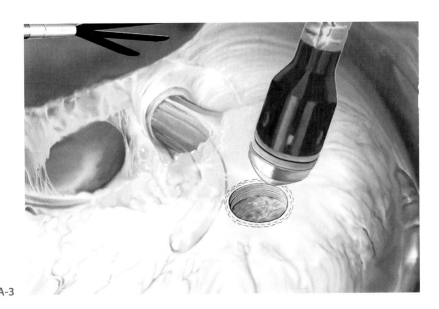

A-3

STEP 3   **Vertical transection of stomach and placement of band**

From this circular defect, the proximal stomach is divided with a 60-mm Endo GIA stapler (blue cartridge) up to the angle of His, staying close to the left side of the calibration tube (A-1).

The 7×1.5-cm band of polypropylene or EPTFE is introduced and wrapped around the outflow (stoma) of the proximal gastric pouch along the lesser curvature.

The circular band is created with three or four interrupted, non-absorbable sutures of 0-nylon (Ethibond) with a 32-Fr. calibration tube in place; the circumference should be 5 cm (A-2).

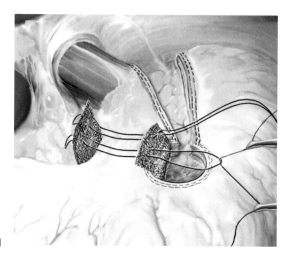

A-1

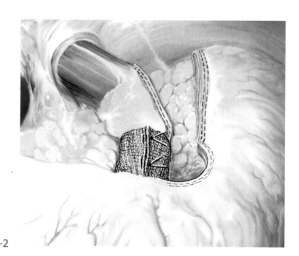

A-2

Laparoscopic Adjustable Gastric Banding (LAGB)

STEP 1   **Positioning of patient and access**

The patient and trocars are placed as described for laparoscopic RYGB; the right lower
5-mm trocar is not necessary for LAGB.

STEP 2   **Determination and creation of pouch size**

A specially designed orogastric balloon calibration tube (Inamed, USA) is inserted;
the balloon is filled with 25 ml saline, and pulled back to wedge itself at the esophagogastric junction.

The dissection begins at the lesser curvature at the largest circumference of the
balloon. The "pars flaccida technique" has less band slippage.

The lesser omentum is entered in the avascular window and the right crus of
the diaphragm identified.

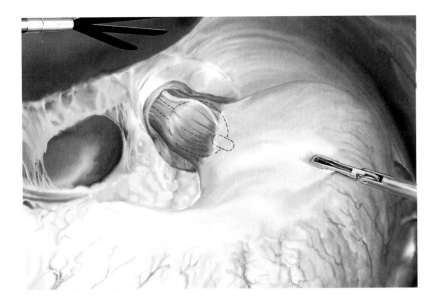

STEP 3   **Retrogastric preparation and band placement**

The retrogastric passage from right to left crus is created by blunt dissection using an articulating "finger" dissector which exits at the angle of His. However, the lesser sac should not be entered during this maneuver. If the lesser sac is entered, retrogastric passage is too far distal along the lesser curvature of the stomach.

The Silicone band is then pulled through the retrogastric tunnel from the left to right side of the stomach, encircling the proximal stomach, anterior vagus nerve, and upper part of the lesser omentum.

The Silastic band is locked around the inflated calibrating catheter and is now inflated with 15 ml saline, which is positioned proximal to the band, thereby determining the size of the proximal pouch. The calibration catheter is deflated but left in place.

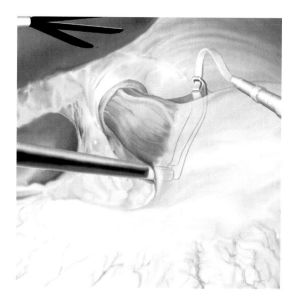

STEP 4   **Band fixation**

The band is fixed in place along the anterior stomach by placing three to five interrupted seromuscular sutures of non-absorbable material, approximating the gastric wall proximal and distal to the band. The left gastric wall distal to the band is fixed to the left crus of the diaphragm.

The procedure is finished by implantation of the reservoir subcutaneously just below the xiphoid, allowing easy access to the port.

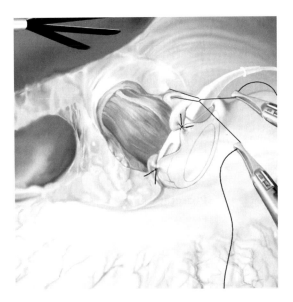

Standard Postoperative Investigations

■ Postoperative surveillance in an intermediate care unit if the patient has sleep apnea or a history of severe cardiac disease
■ Oral liquid diet after routine Gastrografin swallow radiography on the first or second postoperative day if the operative procedure is done laparoscopically
■ Clinical and metabolic follow-up at 2 and 6 weeks and at 3, 6, 9, and 12 months and once yearly thereafter
■ Multivitamin administration routinely, parenteral vitamin B_{12} after RYGB or BPD, and iron supplementation according to the blood tests

Postoperative Complications

General
■ Intra-abdominal bleeding
■ Wound infection
■ Abdominal wound dehiscence
■ Deep vein thrombosis/pulmonary embolism
■ Adhesive small bowel obstruction

Procedure-Specific
■ RYGB:
  – Anastomotic leakage
  – Internal hernia
  – Stenosis at gastrojejunostomy
  – Stomal ulcer/stomal bleeding
  – Afferent (pancreatobiliary) limb obstruction
■ LAGB:
  – Pouch dilatation or band slippage
  – Reservoir infection
  – Band migration into the stomach (late)
  – Band leakage (late)
  – Reservoir/band (balloon) dysfunction
■ VBG:
  – Stricture at the stoma
  – Gastroesophageal reflux
  – Staple line rupture
  – Band erosion into stoma
  – Maladaptive eating disorder

Tricks of the Senior Surgeon

- Creation of pneumoperitoneum with the Veress needle technique avoids a large incision for the first trocar with a subsequent annoying gas leak. The Veress needle should be placed just below (<1 cm) the left costal margin; others prefer the Opti-View trocar.
- Generally a high placement of trocars is recommended, especially the upper two 10/12-mm trocars below the xiphoid and left costal arch.
- The circular EEA staplers for the laparoscopic approach are wrapped with a plastic cover to protect the abdominal wall incision from contact with the contaminated outside of the cartridge of the stapler after intraluminal insertion and firing.
- Conservative weight reduction with dietary measures of 5–10 kg before surgery is believed by some to facilitate technical performance by "shrinking liver size," especially in superobese male patients.

Pancreas-Sparing Duodenectomy

Claus F. Eisenberger, Jakob R. Izbicki, Michael G. Sarr

Introduction

Pancreas-sparing duodenectomy (PSD) is reserved for premalignant lesions of the duodenum and the papilla of Vater, when local excision is not appropriate due to the size or multiplicity of the lesions. PSD involves complete or near complete resection of the duodenum with total preservation of the pancreas. Although the duodenum and the pancreas share the same blood supply, the duodenum may be resected without compromising the viability of the pancreas, but reinsertion of the bile and pancreatic duct into a "neoduodenum" is necessary.

Indications and Contraindications

Indications

- Multiple premalignant lesions of the duodenal mucosa and of the papilla of Vater (e.g., familial adenomatous polyposis syndrome)
- Localized benign or premalignant tumors of the duodenum

Contraindications

- Malignant disease
- Previous surgical procedures of the duodenum, the stomach, or the pancreatic head

Preoperative Investigations

- Gastroduodenoscopy with biopsy
- Endoscopic ultrasonography
- Endoscopic retrograde cholangiopancreatography (ERCP) [alternatively magnetic resonance cholangiopancreatography (MRCP)] for duct anatomy and morphology

Procedure

Exposure of the duodenum

The abdomen is explored via a transverse or midline upper celiotomy. The gallbladder is resected, allowing later passage of a probe to localize the ampulla. The hepatic flexure of the colon is mobilized inferiorly and the lesser sac is opened widely. An extensive Kocher maneuver well to the left of the midline is performed, thus exposing the first through third portions of the duodenum.

Preparation and resection of the duodenum

The ligament of Treitz is incised. The proximal jejunum is then transected with a GIA stapler, after which the mesentery to the proximal jejunum and fourth portion of the duodenum is transected and ligated close to the bowel wall. The freed proximal jejunum is transposed behind the mesenteric root to the right upper abdomen.

The third and fourth portions of the duodenum are detached from the pancreas by meticulous dissection with ligation of these small and fragile mesenteric vessels. This dissection preparation is performed proximally up to the level of the papilla.

Precise localization of the papilla is important to facilitate dissection of the peri-ampullary region. This is accomplished by passing a bile duct probe into the duodenum either via the cystic duct remnant (after cholecystectomy) or a choledochotomy. Retrograde cannulation of the bile duct with a probe via a lateral duodenotomy will also identify the papilla. In the region of the papilla of Vater, the duodenum is dissected carefully from the pancreas, thus exposing the estuaries of the common bile duct and the main pancreatic duct (A).

Next, the extraduodenal bile and pancreatic ducts are transected close to the duodenum. This step is shown in B. If a long common channel (pancreatic and bile ducts) is present and the duodenal disease does not extend past the ampullary region, this common channel can be transected, leaving only one "ductal structure" for reimplantation into the neoduodenum. The pancreatic and bile ducts are intubated separately with two catheters (C).

In the duodenum proximal to the papilla, the pancreas is densely adherent to the duodenum. One can dissect and develop a narrow subserosal plane outside the muscularis propria of the medial wall of the duodenum up to the distal part of the first part of the duodenum where a "duodenal mesentery" becomes present. Alternatively, dissection can also be initiated at the proximal duodenum and continued distally to the papilla. Small vessels are ligated. A careful search for the separate minor pancreatic duct should be made; if found and identified, we recommend suture ligation of this duct. Often, the duct is not identified and thus all vessels and "fibrous" connections to the second portion of the duodenum should be ligated.

The duodenum is transected either 1–2 cm distal to the pylorus if this area is disease-free or directly distal to pylorus. The resected specimen should be sent for pathologic examination with intraoperative frozen section to exclude the presence of invasive malignancy.

Preparation and resection of the duodenum

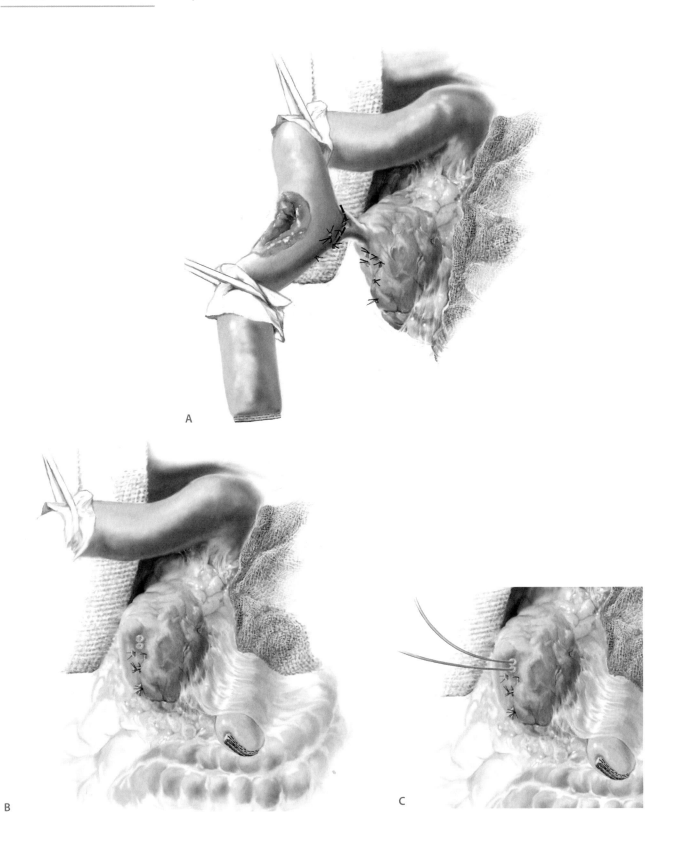

A

B

C

STEP 3   **Reconstruction**

The proximal jejunum which will now become the "neoduodenum" is passed either behind the superior mesenteric vessels or retrorolically through the mesocolon.

The bile and pancreatic duct anastomoses are performed at an equivalent distance from the pylorus as the native papilla. The ducts are implanted into the neoduodenum via a 2-cm enterotomy opposite to the proposed site of reimplantation. The anastomoses are done with interrupted transmural fine (6-0 or 7-0) monofilament resorbable sutures (**A**). Several techniques for ductal reimplantation should be available in the surgeon's armamentarium. If a common channel can be preserved, one anastomosis will suffice. In contrast, if the disease involves the distal ducts and/or ampulla, usually the ductal transection leaves two ducts connected only by the interductal septum. In this situation, a single anastomosis can be fashioned by carefully including both ducts into the anasto-mosis (**B-1**). If the ductal transection leaves two individual ducts without preservation of the interductal septum (an unusual situation), the best approach is to sew together the adjoining walls of the ducts using 6- or 7-0 absorbable suture material and then reim-plant the joined ductal structures as one anastomosis (**B-2**).

The pancreatic stent is passed through the neoduodenum via a hollow needle, thus creating a long submucosal tunnel, and is passed percutaneously through the abdominal wall. The access enterotomy is closed transversely, and the pancreatic stent is left in situ, to be removed 4–6 weeks after surgery.

Gastrointestinal continuity is reestablished by end-to-end anastomosis of the neoduodenum with either the proximal duodenum or pylorus with a single layer of interrupted sutures. A t-tube is inserted in the common bile duct. Soft drains are placed behind the neoduodenum. The complete reconstruction is shown in **C**.

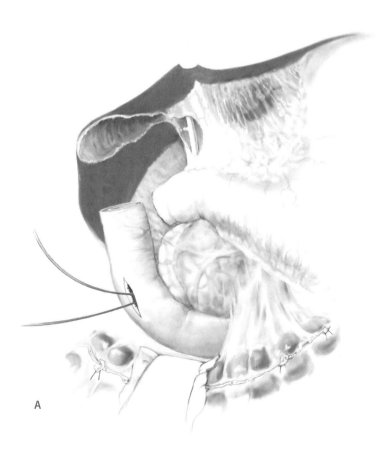

A

Reconstruction

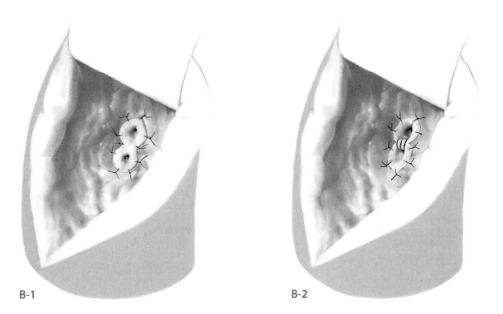

B-1   B-2

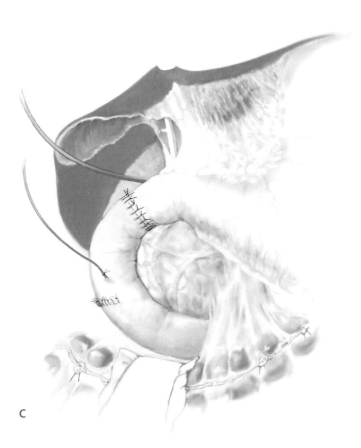

C

Standard Postoperative Investigations

- T-tube and pancreatic duct drain are left in-situ for 6 weeks postoperatively
- T-tube cholangiography is performed prior to removal

Postoperative Complications

- Pancreatic duct drain or t-tube dislocation
- Pancreatic and/or biliary fistula
- Anastomotic dehiscence
- Pancreatitis
- Cholangitis
- Anastomotic strictures

Tricks of the Senior Surgeon

- Fixation of the pancreatic duct drain by a resorbable stay suture at the "neo-papilla."
- Tension-free anastomoses are mandatory; sometimes it is necessary to use an excluded jejunal interponate.

Liver

Pierre-Alian Clavien

Introduction

Pierre-Alain Clavien

Liver surgery was considered until the early 1980s as a "heroic" field of medicine associated with much blood loss, and high patient morbidity and mortality. With such a reputation only life-threatening conditions were usually referred for liver surgery. As surgeons acquired a better understanding of surgical anatomy and physiology, a better understanding of peri- and intraoperative management, and importantly formal training periods in this field, hepatic surgery began to enjoy rapid expansion and high credibility among colleagues and patients. Today, liver surgery is one of the most complex and successful areas of medicine with the availability of a variety of highly sophisticated procedures for many indications including complex liver resection or transplantation of only one part of the liver from a living donor.

The first chapter presents a comprehensive approach to the terminology of liver anatomy and resection (Brisbane 2000 terminology), according to an international effort including leaders from all continents. The next three chapters present available techniques for vascular exclusion, parenchyma dissection and the "hanging" maneuver, which may enable better exposure for anatomic resections. The hepatic surgeon must be familiar with all these techniques, which may be of great help in many difficult situations. Then, the focus turns to formal anatomic and non-anatomic liver resections, including laparoscopic approaches, which are gaining increasing popularity. As liver resection is often not possible due to local difficult situations (poor liver reserve or location of a tumor) or poor general condition of the patient, alternative techniques are presented including cryosurgery, radiofrequency ablation and selective intra-arterial chemotherapy. Benign and infectious cysts require particular strategies, which are well covered in two separate chapters. A chapter also comprehensively covers the available strategies for liver trauma in the modern area of "damage control injury." The last six chapters cover various aspects of liver transplantation from organ procurement, to partial living or cadaveric orthotopic liver transplantation, as well as auxiliary liver transplantation.

While there is no substitute for experience in performing complex surgical procedures, we hope that this section, prepared by worldwide experts, will clarify standards and limitations for surgeons in performing hepatic surgery.

Terminology of Liver Anatomy and Resections: The Brisbane 2000 Terminology

Steven M. Strasberg

In 1998 at its meeting in Berne, Switzerland, the Scientific Committee of the International Hepato-Pancreato-Biliary Association (IHPBA) established a Terminology Committee to deal with the confusion in terminology of hepatic anatomy and liver resections (see below: members of the committee). The recommendations of the Terminology Committee were presented to the Scientific Committee at the biannual meeting of the IHPBA in Brisbane, Australia, in 2000. These recommendations, consisting of a new terminology termed *The Brisbane 2000 Terminology of Liver Anatomy and Resections,* were unanimously accepted by the Scientific Committee of the IHPBA and were presented to the membership as the official terminology of the IHPBA. The terminology was published in the official journal of the IHPBA in 2000. The terminology shown below is based on the hepatic artery and bile duct (Figures 1–3). A terminology based on the division of the portal vein was added as an addendum.

The terminology is presented as a set of four figures. The liver is divided in the tables into successive orders. The following notes serve as a guide to the tables.

Note 1

Couinaud segments are indicated in short form as Sg1–9 (e.g., Sg6).
Comment: Sg is chosen rather than S to avoid confusion of segment with section or sector. Arabic numerals are chosen rather than Roman numerals because many non-Western nations do not use Roman numerals.

Note 2

Anatomical and surgical terms are *underlined*. Explanatory terms and notes within the figures are in *italics.*

Note 3

Wherever the word "**OR**" (uppercase, bold) appears in the table it indicates equally acceptable terminology; e.g., "*right hemiliver*" **OR** "*right liver.*" The choice is that of the user. Wherever the word "**or**" (lowercase, bold) appears in the table or these notes it indicates that the first choice is preferred but that the second is acceptable; e.g., "*right trisectionectomy*" **or** "*extended right hepatectomy.*" The choice is up to the user but the first term is the preferred term. The reason in this case is as follows. As some use the adjective "extended" to indicate any degree of extension of a resection over the midplane, which in some cases is less than a whole section, the terms in the table containing the word "extended," while acceptable, are less preferred.

Note 4

When segment 1 is resected as part of a procedure, it should be stated as in the following example: "left hemihepatectomy with resection of segment 1" **or** "left hemihepatectomy extended to segment 1."

Note 5

It is always correct to refer to any resection by its segments. For instance, "right hepatectomy" and "resection Sgs 5–8" are equally acceptable. "Left lateral sectionectomy" and "resection Sgs 2, 3" are equally acceptable.

Reference

Terminology Committee of the International Hepato-Pancreato-Biliary Association: SM Strasberg (USA), J Belghiti (France), P-A Clavien (Switzerland), E Gadzijev (Slovenia), JO Garden (UK), W-Y Lau (China), M Makuuchi (Japan), and RW Strong (Australia).
The Brisbane 2000 Terminology of Liver Anatomy and Resections. HPB 2:333–339, 2000

Anatomical Term	Couinaud segments referred to	Term for surgical resection	Diagram (pertinent area is shaded)
Right Hemiliver **OR** *Right Liver*	*Sg 5–8(+/Sg1)*	*Right Hepatectomy* **OR** *Right Hemihepatectomy* (stipulate +/-segment 1)	
Left Hemiliver **OR** *Left Liver*	*Sg 2–4 (+/-Sg1)*	*Left Hepatectomy* **OR** *Left Hemihepatectomy* (stipulate +/-segment 1)	

Border or watershed: The border or watershed of the first order division which separates the two hemilivers is a plane which intersects the gallbladder fossa and the fossa for the IVC and is called the "midplane of the liver".

Fig 1. Nomenclature for first order division anatomy and resections

Anatomical Term	Couinaud segments referred to	Term for surgical resection	Diagram (pertinent area is shaded)
Right Anterior Section	Sg 5,8	Add (-ectomy) to any of the anatomical terms an in *Right anterior sectionectomy*	
Right Posterior Section	Sg 6,7	*Right posterior sectionectomy*	
Left Medial Section	Sg 4	*Left medial sectionectomy* OR *Resection segment 4* (also see Third order) OR *Segmentectomy 4* (also see Third order)	
Left Lateral Section	Sg 2,3	*Left lateral sectionectomy* OR *Bisegmentectomy 2,3* (also see Third order)	

Other "sectional liver resections

	Sg 4–8 (+/-Sg1)	*Right Trisectionectomy* (preferred term) or *Extended Right Hepatectomy* or *Extended Right Hemihepatectomy* (stipulate +/-segment 1)	
	Sg 2, 3, 4, 5, 8 (+/-Sg1)	*Left Trisectionectomy* (preferred term) or *Extended Left Hepatectomy* or *Extended Left Hemihepatectomy* (stipulate +/-segment 1)	

Border or watershed: The borders or watersheds of the sections are planes referred to as the *right and left intersectional planes.* The left intersectional plane passes through the umbilical fissure and the attachment of the falciform ligament. There is no surface marking of the right intersectional plane.

Fig 2. Nomenclature for second order division anatomy and resections, based on bile ducts and hepatic artery

Anatomical Term	Couinaud segments referred to	Term for surgical resection	Diagram (pertinent area is shaded)
Segments 1-9	*Any one of Sg 1 to 9*	*Segmentectomy* (e.g. segmentectomy 6)	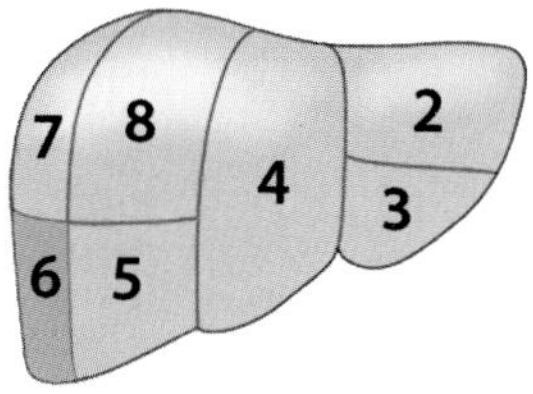
2 contiguous sements	*Any two of Sg 1 to Sg 9 in continuity*	*Bisegmentectomy* (e.g. bisegmentectomy 5,6)	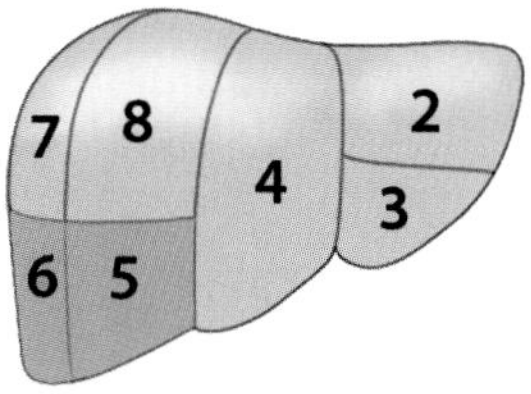

For clarity Sg.1 and 9 are not shown. It is also acceptable to refer to ANY resection by its third-order segments, eg. right hemihepatectomy can also be called resection Sg 5–8.

Border or watershed: The borders or watersheds of the segments are planes referred to as intersegmental planes.

Fig 3. Nomenclature for third order division anatomy and resections

Anatomical Term	Couinaud segments referred to	Term for surgical resection	Diagram (pertinent area is shaded)
Right Anterior Sector **OR** *Right paramedian Sector*	*Sg 5,8*	Add (-ectomy) to any of the anatomical terms as in *Right anterior sectorectomy* **OR** *Right paramedian sectorectomy*	
Right Posterior Sector **OR** *Right lateral Sector*	*Sg 6,7*	*Right posterior sectorectomy* **OR** *Right lateral sectorectomy*	
Left Medial Sector **OR** *Left Paramedian Sector*	*Sg 3,4*	*Left medial sectorectomy* **OR** *Left paramedian sectorectomy* **OR** *Bisegmentectomy 3,4*	
Left Lateral Sector **OR** *Left Posterior Sector*	*Sg 2*	*Left lateral sectorectomy* **OR** *Left posterior sectorectomy* **OR** *Segmentectomy 2*	

Right anterior sector and Right anterior section are synonyms. Right posterior sector and Right posterior section are synonyms. Left medial sector and Left medial section are NOT synonyms and are NOT exchangeable terms. They do not describe the same anatomic areas. Left lateral sector and Left lateral section are also NOT synonyms and are NOT exchangeable terms.

Border or watershed: The borders or watersheds of second-order division based on PV are called right and left intersectoral planes. These have no surface markings.

Fig 4. (Addendum) Nomenclature for alternative second order division, based on portal vein

Techniques of Liver Parenchyma Dissection

Mickaël Lesurtel, Pierre-Alain Clavien

Parenchyma dissection of the liver may cause complications including blood loss, hematoma, infection, bile leakage and liver failure. Various surgical techniques have been developed for careful and safe dissection of the liver parenchyma to prevent intraoperative and postoperative complications.

The aim of this chapter is to give an overview of the techniques and devices frequently used to perform parenchyma dissection of the liver, including:

- Kelly clamp and bipolar forceps
- Water jet dissection
- Ultrasonic dissection
- Ultrasound cutting
- Dissecting sealer

Preparation of Parenchyma Dissection

The liver capsule is incised with diathermy on the resection line. For a better exposure, two stay sutures (2-0 silk) can be placed at the inferior margin of the liver, one on each side of the resection line. These stay sutures are used to lift up the liver and the resection line. Care should be taken not to pull and tear the liver parenchyma, leading to bleeding.

To prevent unnecessary liver ischemia, the Pringle maneuver for continuous or intermittent inflow occlusion is applied individually depending on the intraoperative surgical situation. Indeed, except for the Kelly clamp, the other techniques were developed to avoid use of the Pringle maneuver and to minimize risk of liver ischemia.

Kelly Clamp and Bipolar Forceps

A small clamp (Kelly) is used to crush parenchyma between its blades in order to isolate vessels and bile ducts (A-1, A-2). Fine branches of Glisson's tree or tiny tributaries of hepatic veins (<3mm) are coagulated using a bipolar forceps and are cut by scissors (A-3). Bipolar forceps cautery is equipped with a channel for water dripping, which prevents adhesion of debris to the cautery blades. Bigger identified vessels or bile ducts (>3mm) are ligated or clipped on the remnant liver slice before cutting. The alternative is to use clips only to secure vessels and bile ducts.

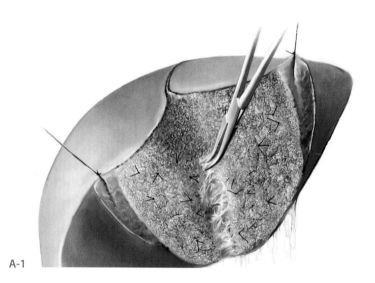

A-1

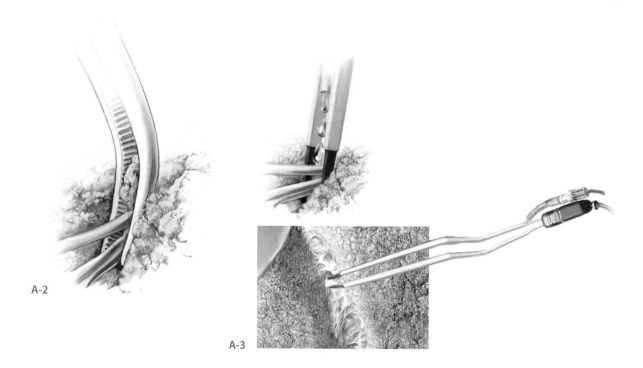

A-2

A-3

Water Jet Dissection (Helix Hydro-Jet, Erbe)

With this device the liver parenchyma is dissected by a jet of water (A-1). Saline is pressurized by high pressure pump and is conducted by a high pressure hose to the nozzle. Here the pressure is converted into kinetic energy. For liver parenchyma, pressures of 30–50 bar should be used. The soft liver tissue is washed off the more resistant vessels and bile ducts (A-2). The applicator should be used in direct contact with the tissue and moved like a paintbrush. It can be used in combination with suction and with an electrosurgical unit. Vessels and bile ducts are isolated and can be secured using bipolar forceps, clips or ligatures as with the Kelly clamp. They can then be transected under controlled conditions.

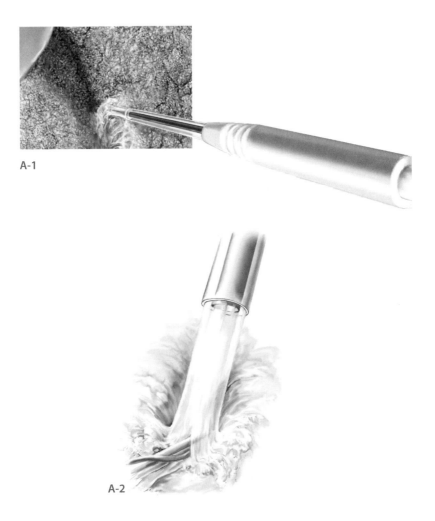

A-1

A-2

Ultrasonic Dissection
(Cavitron Ultrasonic Surgical Aspirator; Dissectron, Integra NeuroSciences)

The principle of ultrasonic dissection is a cavitational effect which occurs at the tip of the vibrating rod of the device. The handpiece delivers ultrasonic vibration and provides simultaneous aspiration and irrigation (A-1). The ultrasonic probe divides parenchymal cells (because of their high water content) by the cavitational effect with less injury to structures with a high content of fibrous tissue, e.g., bile ducts and blood vessels (A-2). Once skeletonized by the probe, these elements are then clipped, ligated or coagulated as with the other techniques. Additional electrocoagulation functions are optionally available. The ultrasonic and high frequency currents can be activated simultaneously to divide and coagulate vessels, ducts and nerves.

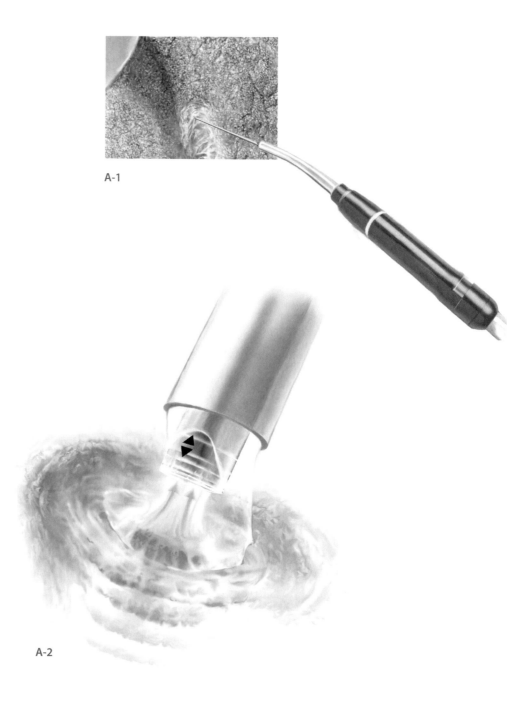

A-1

A-2

Ultrasound Cutting (Ultracision, Ethicon Endo-Surgery)

The ultrasound cutting system includes an ultrasound generator with a foot switch, a reusable handle for the scalpel, and the cutting device with scissors. The electrical energy provided by the generator is converted into mechanical energy by the handpiece through a piezoelectric crystal system. The blade or tip of the instrument being used vibrates axially with a constant frequency of 55,500 Hz (A-1, A-2). The longitudinal extension of the vibration can be varied between 25 and 100 µm in five levels, by adjusting the power setting of the generator. The cutting derives from a saw mechanism in the direction of the vibrating high-frequency blade. The intracellular generation of vacuoles (cavitation) brings about the correct dissection of the liver parenchyma. Blood vessels up to 2–3 mm in diameter are coagulated on contact of the tissue with the vibrating metal. For coagulation of larger vessels, exertion of pressure between blades for 3–5 s is required. Especially in the periphery, the harmonic scalpel allows the liver parenchyma to be divided without causing bleeding, bile leakage or trauma. It is especially used for laparoscopic dissection because of its speed of action and ease of use. However, its use in the depth of the liver may lead to vascular injury, especially to hepatic veins. That is the reason why, in depth, larger vessels should be secured with clips or sutures.

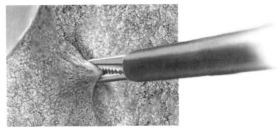

A-1

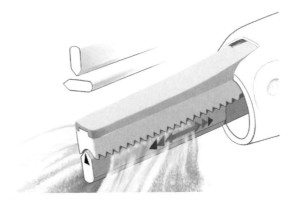

A-2

Dissecting Sealer (TissueLink)

The TissueLink dissecting sealer uses proprietary technology to coagulate and seal tissue to provide hemostasis before and after transection. It delivers radiofrequency (RF) energy through a conductive fluid (saline) to coagulate and seal tissue (A-1, A-2). The saline couples the RF energy into tissue and cools the tissue so that the temperature never exceeds 100 °C. The result is hemostasis via collagen shrinking without the tissue desiccation, smoking, arcing, and char of conventional electrosurgery. The dissecting sealer can be connected to the same standard RF generator that is used for standard electrocautery. The dissecting sealer is applied directly to the target tissue. It is important to maintain constant contact with the liver and move the device in a "painting" motion to ensure effective application of energy. Vessels less than 5 mm in diameter encountered through skeletonization can be completely coagulated within 10 s and can thereafter be transected. Larger vessels should be secured by clips or sutures.

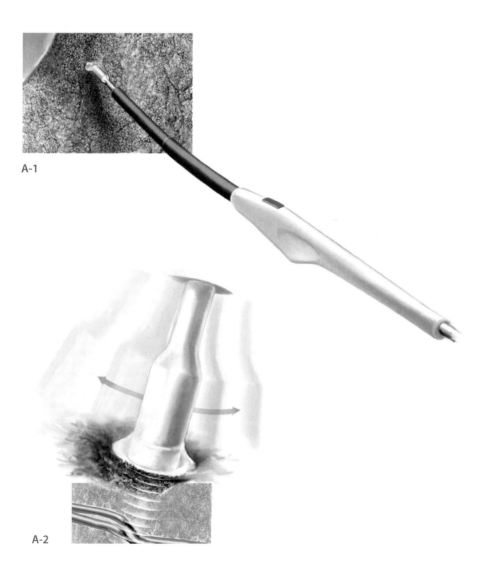

A-1

A-2

Tricks of the Senior Surgeon

- The different devices can be used in the same intervention as they may offer different and cumulative advantages.
- During laparoscopic liver resection, the harmonic scalpel is useful because it can coagulate and divide the hepatic parenchyma during the same application, avoiding changing instruments.
- During parenchyma dissection, whatever the techniques used, central venous pressure must be kept low to minimize blood loss.
- Regardless of the device used, inflow occlusion should be used loosely in case of significant bleeding during transection.

Techniques of Vascular Exclusion and Caval Resection

Felix Dahm, Pierre-Alain Clavien

Vascular exclusion techniques in liver surgery include continuous inflow occlusion (Fig. 1A) (first described by J.H. Pringle in 1908), intermittent inflow occlusion (Fig. 1B) (first described by M. Makuuchi in the late 1970s), and ischemic preconditioning (Fig. 1C) and (continuous) total vascular exclusion. The use of inflow occlusion varies considerably among centers – some use it routinely, while others use it only exceptionally. When using inflow occlusion, a low central venous pressure (CVP) (<3 mm Hg) needs to be maintained to reduce bleeding. The effect of a low CVP associated with a Pringle maneuver can be equivalent to total vascular exclusion. Total vascular exclusion, on the other hand, can lead to cardiovascular instability by reduced cardiac preload, and adequate volume loading with a high CVP (>10 mm Hg) needs to be maintained. A venovenous bypass is sometimes used in this setting.

Table 1. Maximum safe duration (min) of hepatic inflow occlusion with different techniques

	Normal liver	Cirrhotic liver
Continuous inflow occlusion	60	30
Ischemic preconditioning	75	?
Intermittent clamping	>90	>60

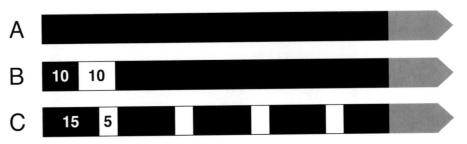

Figure 1. Ischemia periods are drawn in black, reperfusion in white

Indications and Contraindications

Indications

- Reduction of blood loss during parenchymal dissection
- Dissection in proximity of major vascular structures
- Tumor invading vena cava or all hepatic veins, central hepatectomy (for total vascular exclusion)

Contraindications

- Technical reasons (adhesions, etc.)
- Cardiac failure (for total vascular exclusion)

Intraoperative Complications

- Splenic rupture (exceptional) – remove clamps and attempt conservative management of splenic rupture. If not possible, proceed with splenectomy.
- Cardiovascular instability (in total vascular exclusion) – ensure adequate fluid loading, open clamps, consider venovenous bypass.

Procedures

Pringle Maneuver (= Inflow Occlusion)

A right-angle clamp is passed under the hepatoduodenal ligament to allow a Mersilene band to be placed around it (A). A red rubber catheter is passed over the band. It is then pushed downwards as a tourniquet to occlude the ligament, and clamped in place (B). The time of inflow occlusion should now be noted. An alternative technique is to place a vessel clamp on the hepatoduodenal ligament (C). We prefer the tourniquet because it is mobile and does not get in the way when performing the hepatectomy. Another alternative is to selectively clamp portal venous and arterial branches when a dissection of the structures in the hepatoduodenal ligament has been performed, e.g., for cholangiocarcinoma.

Total Vascular Exclusion

Before total vascular exclusion can be performed, the liver needs to be completely mobilized as for a liver transplantation (see chapter "Orthotopic Liver Transplantation").

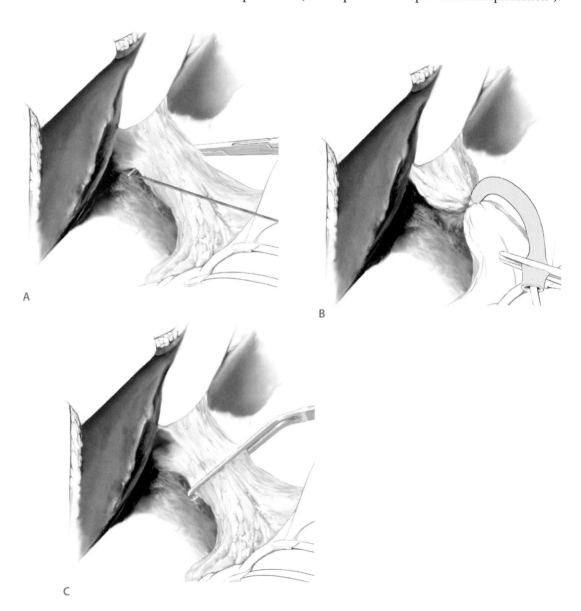

STEP 1

The hepatoduodenal ligament is dissected and the tourniquet is placed around it without closing, as described for inflow occlusion.

STEP 2

The infrahepatic vena cava is prepared on its right and left side for 2–3 cm. The right adrenal vein needs to be identified and transected through ligatures (A).

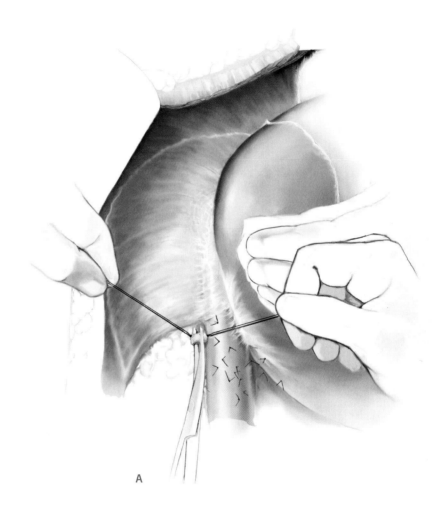

A

STEP 2 *(continued)*

A finger is passed under the cava from the right to the left, and the connective tissue is dissected on the finger with electrocautery (B-1). A large right angle is then passed under the infrahepatic vena cava (B-2), and isolated with a Mersilene band (B-3), which is then pulled through a catheter as when performing inflow occlusion (tourniquet technique as in the Pringle maneuver, see above).

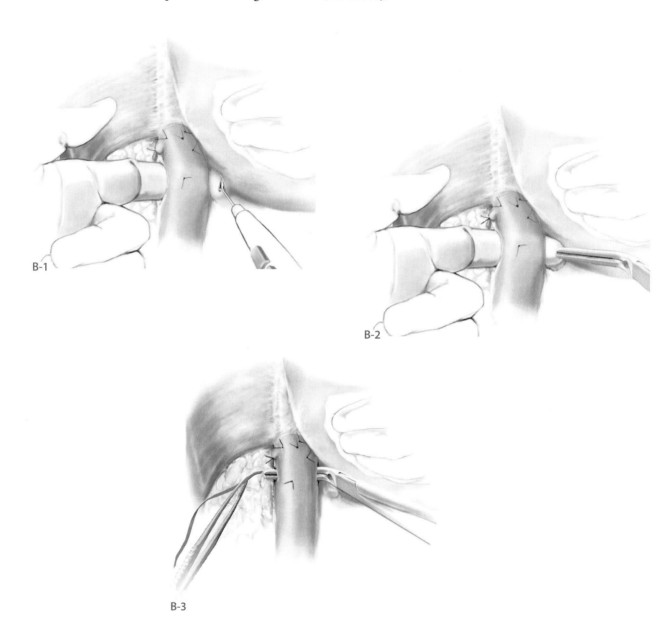

STEP 3

Mobilize the retrohepatic and suprahepatic vena cava up to the diaphragm. This is accomplished by passing a finger behind the vena cava and cauterizing the connective tissue. There are no venous branches in this area.

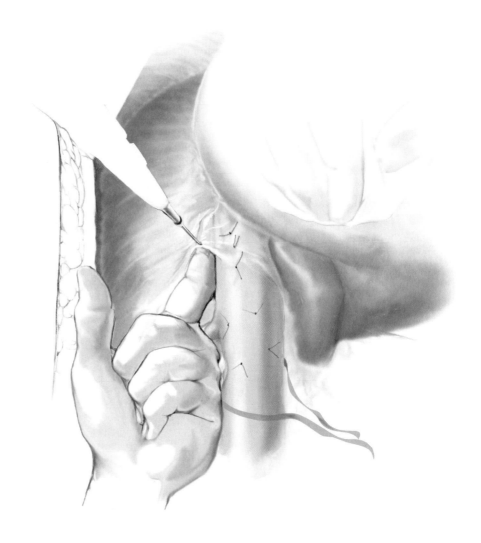

STEP 4

Occlude the infrahepatic cava with the corresponding tourniquet. If this is not tolerated, total vascular exclusion cannot be performed. If it is tolerated, lift up the left hepatic hemiliver and place a large curved vascular clamp from left to right on the suprahepatic cava as high as possible. Check if it can be closed, then occlude hepatic inflow by closing the tourniquet on the hepatoduodenal ligament. Clamp the suprahepatic vena cava including a little bit of diaphragm (if possible) (**A**). The liver is now in total vascular exclusion (**B**). We do not routinely use venovenous bypass in this setting (see section on venovenous bypass in the chapter "Orthotopic Liver Transplantation").

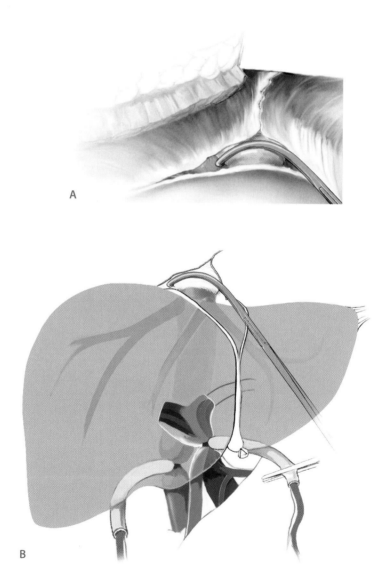

A

B

Reconstruction of Vena Cava

This technique is an alternative to associated cava reconstruction. It restores liver perfusion while working on the vena cava.

STEP 1

Open hepatic outflow by releasing the clamp on the suprahepatic vena cava.
Clamp the vena cava again below the hepatic veins.

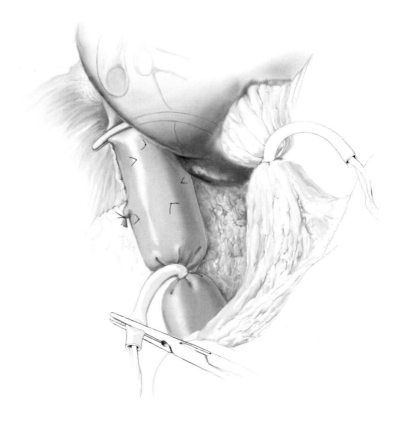

STEP 2

Open hepatic inflow by releasing the tourniquet on the hepatoduodenal ligament.
Now the retrohepatic cava is occluded while the liver is perfused.

STEP 3

The retrohepatic vena cava can now be resected. Reconstruction is accomplished with a Gore-tex interposition graft in an end-to-end fashion. Then release the cava clamp and the tourniquet on the lower cava.

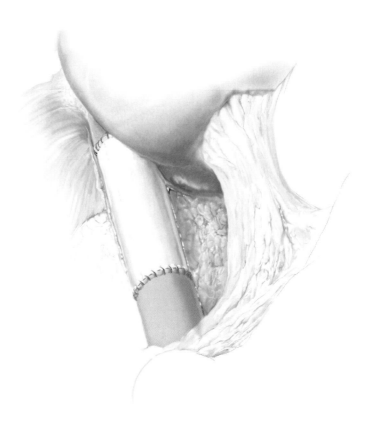

Tricks of the Senior Surgeon

- Always search for anatomical variants, especially an aberrant left hepatic artery. This has to be selectively clamped in addition to occlusion of the ligament.
- Best inflow occlusion is accomplished by pushing down the tourniquet, clamping the band right behind it to hold the tension and then pushing it down again with some force, before fixing it in position by clamping the tourniquet and the band. This can be repeated several times ("milking down technique"). When inflow occlusion is insufficient, especially in a very large hepatoduodenal ligament, a second tourniquet can be placed and occluded.
- When bleeding is encountered under total vascular exclusion the most likely reason is incomplete inflow occlusion. If an obvious reason cannot be identified, open outflow (but keep inflow occlusion and infrahepatic caval occlusion) and ask the anesthesiologist to lower the CVP.

Hanging Maneuver for Anatomic Hemihepatectomy (Including Living-Donor Liver Transplantation)

Jacques Belghiti, Olivier Scatton

In addition to the conventional approach described for liver resection in the chapters on conventional hepatectomies, the hanging maneuver has gained wide acceptance among liver surgeons. Depending on the situation, it can be used for resective liver surgery or for living related liver donation.

STEP 1

Suprahepatic preparation

After the hilar preparation, the anterior leaf of the coronary ligament and the anterior part of the right triangular ligament are dissected to expose the left side of the right hepatic vein. The space between the right and the median hepatic vein and the suprahepatic vena cava is freed by means of a vascular clamp.

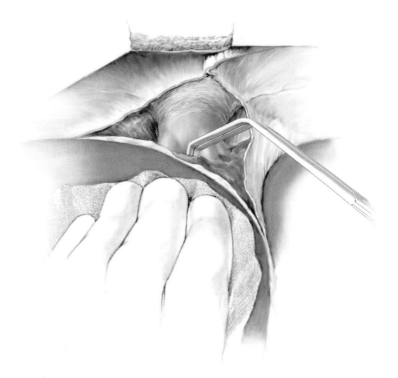

STEP 2   **Infrahepatic preparation of the vena cava**

Starting right above the origin of the right renal vein, the space between the vena cava
and the liver is freed. In order to prepare the tunnel where the tape will be passed, one or
two short veins to the caudate lobe need to be ligated. The tunnel is now prepared by
carefully opening the avascular plane between the liver and the anterior surface of the
vena cava with scissors. A tape is passed with an aortic clamp from the right side of the
median hepatic vein along the retrohepatic IVC to the inferior part of segment 1 (**A**),
which is divided to place the tape near the right portal pedicle (**B**).

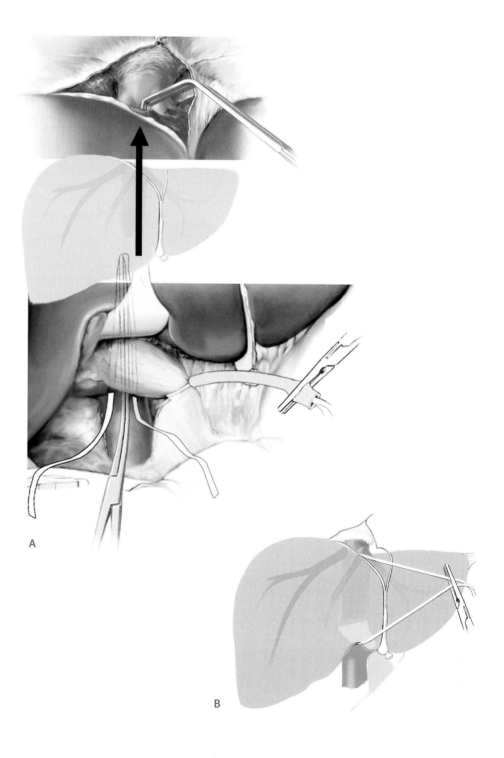

STEP 3   **Parenchymal transsection**

Slight traction on the tape leads to a separation of the right and the left hemiliver and allows easy identification of the right plane of parenchymal transsection. Depending on the situation, transsection is done with or without inflow occlusion and with the appropriate technique as described in the chapter on parenchymal transsection. Vessels with a diameter of less than 3 mm are coagulated while larger vessels are ligated using sutures or clips. At the end of the transsection, the two hemilivers are completely divided just joining together by hilar vessels and hepatic veins. The procedure is now continued depending on the situation (i.e., living related liver transplantation or liver resection for a tumor).

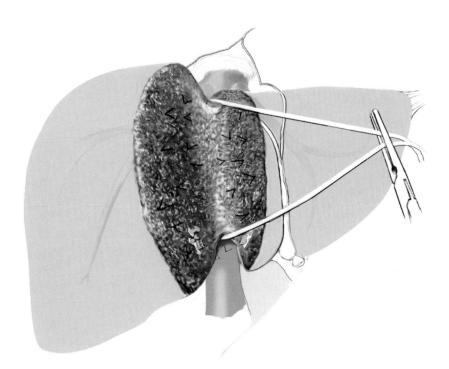

Modified Hanging Maneuver
for Middle Hepatic Vein Harvesting

For the harvest of the middle hepatic vein in a living donor procedure or for an oncologic extended resection, the hanging maneuver is adapted in order to facilitate the
transsection along the left side of the vein. First, the hepatotomy is started on the top,
near the median hepatic trunk, which allows identification of the left hepatic vein and
the median hepatic vein, respectively (**A**).

Once the median hepatic vein has been freed, the tape is switched to the left side of the
middle hepatic vein (**B**) and the procedure is continued as described in Step 3.

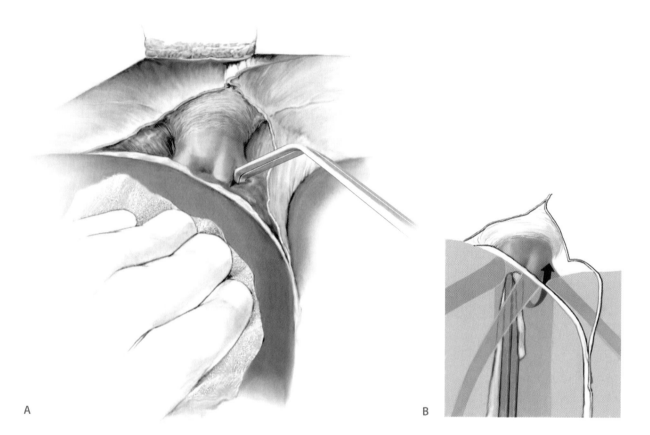

A   B

Tricks of the Senior Surgeon

- This maneuver should not be attempted in case of inflammatory adhesions
  (e.g., previous caval dissection, inflammatory process after multiple TACE)
  between the IVC and the liver capsule.
- The dissection on the upper part of the liver should be favoured since it
  facilitates the identification of the right plane in front of the IVC.

Liver Resections

Panco Georgiev, Pierre-Alain Clavien

Indications and Contraindications

Indications

- Primary and secondary malignancy (e.g., hepatocellular carcinoma, intrahepatic cholangiocarcinoma, colorectal metastases, neuroendocrine tumors)
- Benign neoplasia (e.g., adenoma, giant hemangioma)
- *Echinococcus multilocularis* (*alveolaris*)
- Abscesses refractory to conservative management
- Other benign diseases (e.g., Caroli syndrome)
- Living donor liver transplantation (modified technique; see chapter "Living Donor Liver Transplantation")
- Klatskin's tumor (modified approach to the bile duct; see Section 4
- Traumatic liver lesions

Contraindications

- Acute hepatitis (viral or alcoholic)
- Severe chronic hepatitis
- Poor liver reserve (e.g., Child-Pugh C cirrhosis)
- Severe portal hypertension (e.g., esophageal varices, ascites or hepatic venous pressure gradient >10 mmHg)
- Severe coagulopathy despite vitamin K administration
- Severe thrombopenia (platelet count <30,000/mm^3)

Preoperative Investigation and Preparation for the Procedure

History:	Alcohol, hepatitis and hepatotoxic medication, blood transfusions, tattoos, etc.
Clinical evaluation:	Encephalopathy, ascites, jaundice, nutritional status, signs of portal hypertension
Laboratory tests:	ALT, AST, bilirubin, alkaline phosphatase, albumin, coagulation parameters (PT, platelets), tumor markers and serologies (e.g., hepatitis, echinococcus) when indicated
CT scan or MRI	Assessment of liver volume (major resections) and resectability of the lesion
PET scan	Searching for extrahepatic lesions (e.g., colorectal metastases)

Postoperative Tests

- Postoperative surveillance in an intensive or intermediate care unit
- Coagulation parameters and hemoglobin for at least 48 h
- Check daily for clinical signs of liver failure such as jaundice and encephalopathy

Postoperative Complications

- Short term:
    - Pleural effusion
    - Ascites
    - Liver failure
    - Intra-abdominal bleeding
    - Bile leak
    - Subphrenic abscess
    - Portal vein thrombosis
- Long term:
    - Biloma
    - Biliary stricture
    - Bronchobiliary fistula

Right Hemihepatectomy

Panco Georgiev, Pierre-Alain Clavien

Procedure

STEP 1

Access, exposure and exploration

After a right subcostal incision, the round and falciform ligaments are divided, a retractor (e.g., Thompson) is installed and the abdomen is explored (**A-1**). Tumor size, number, and location in relation to vascular structures are evaluated by intraoperative ultrasound and a definitive decision regarding resectability of the lesion is made (**A-2**).

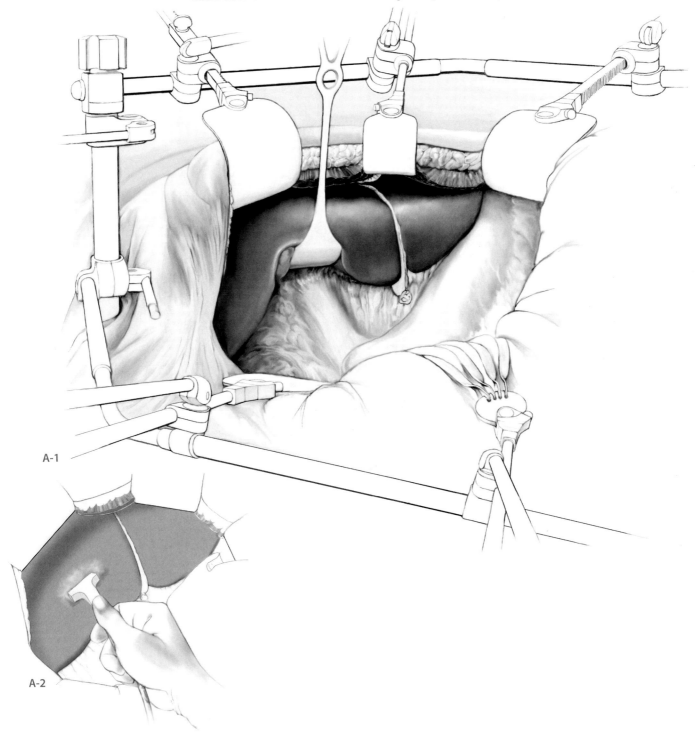

A-1

A-2

STEP 2   **Mobilization of the right lobe**

The right lobe is mobilized by dissection of the anterior leaf of the coronary ligament and the right triangular ligament. The assistant retracts the liver inferiorly and to the left using a gauze swab. The finger blade (Thompson) which is retracting the stomach and duodenum should be removed during this part of the procedure. Approaching the cava, the ligament can be exposed by means of a right angle or a Kelly clamp (**A-1**). Ligaments can be well presented by passing a finger between the diaphragm and the coronary ligament (**A-2**). Care must be taken to protect the phrenic vessels and secure hemostasis from phrenic collaterals.

Next, the Pringle maneuver is prepared as shown in the chapter "Techniques of Vascular Exclusion and Caval Resection." The falciform, round, and right coronary ligaments are divided and the gallbladder is removed as described in Sect. 4, chapter "Laparoscopic Cholecystectomy, Open Cholecystectomy and Cholecystostomy."

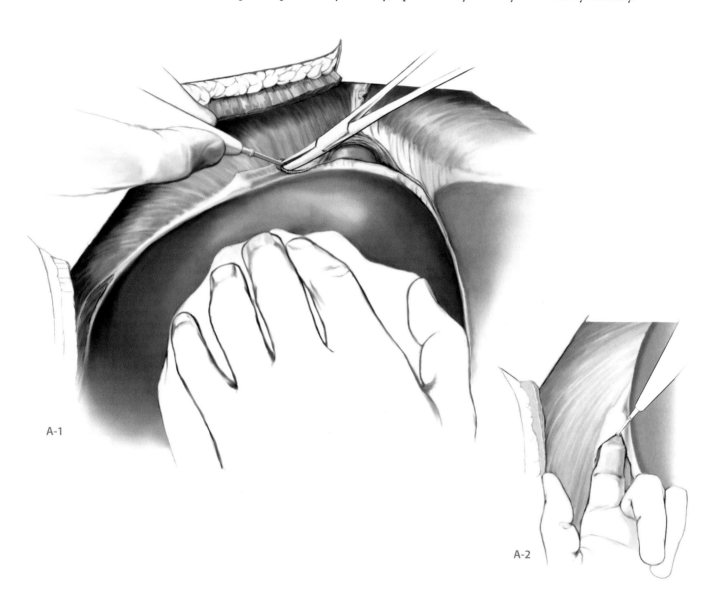

A-1

A-2

Mobilization of the right lobe

The suprahepatic vena cava and the right hepatic vein should be identified. Figure B depicts the mobilized liver as well as the structures which need to be identified during the next steps: hepatic artery, portal vein, and bile duct. An aberrant left hepatic artery (single asterisk in B) is found in about 20–25% of cases. It should be isolated for later possible inflow occlusion (**B**). An aberrant right hepatic artery (double asterisk in B) is present in 10-15% of cases.

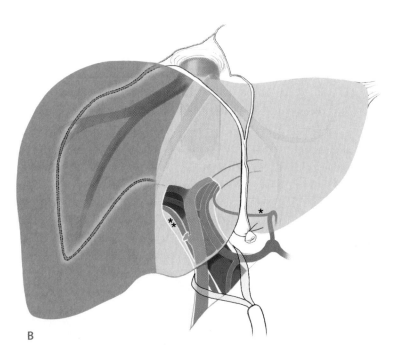

B

STEP 3

Preparation of the hilar structures and transsection of the right hepatic artery

The hepatoduodenal ligament is divided from the cystic duct to the left in order to identify the common hepatic duct and the right branch of the hepatic artery. No attempt is made to visualize or even secure the right hepatic duct (A).

To test the patency of the arterial blood supply to the left hemiliver, a "bulldog" is placed on the right branch of the hepatic artery. The patency of the left branch of the hepatic artery can now easily be assessed by palpating it through the hepatoduodenal ligament (B). Search for an aberrant right hepatic artery (10–15%, posterior and right to the portal vein, indicated by double asterisk in STEP 2 Figure B) from the superior mesenteric artery should be routinely performed prior to identification of the right portal vein.

Once the arterial anatomy is clearly identified, the right branch of the hepatic artery is divided between ties (C). In the presence of an aberrant right hepatic artery, the same maneuver should be applied.

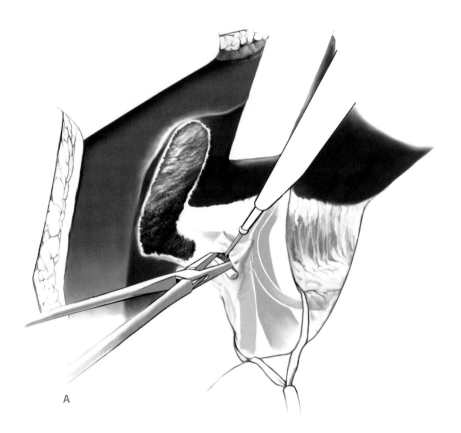

A

Preparation of the hilar structures and transsection of the right hepatic artery

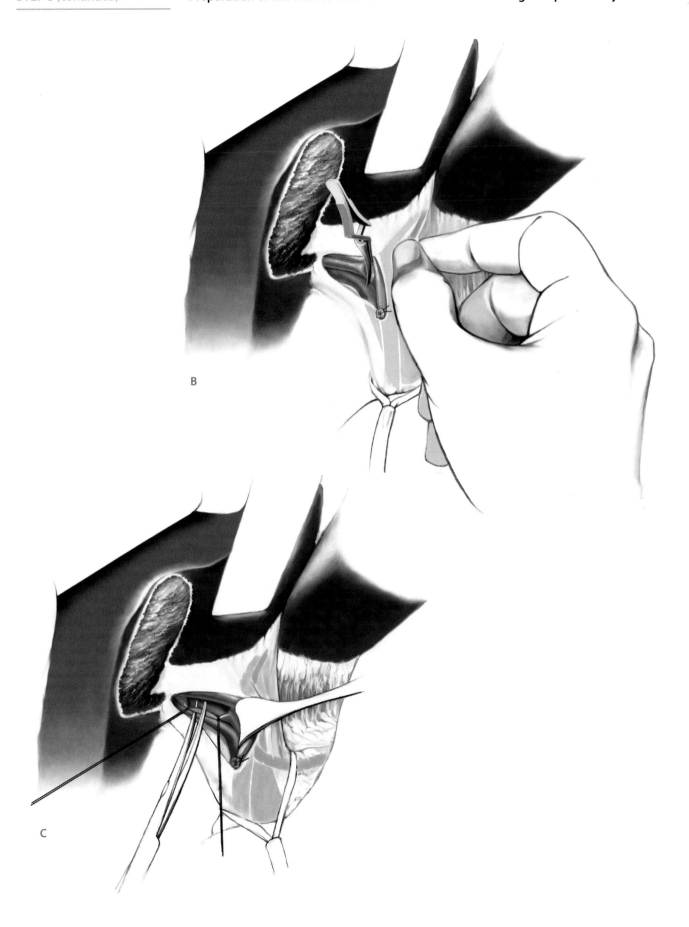

B

C

STEP 3 *(continued)*   **Preparation of the hilar structures and transsection of the right hepatic artery**

STEP 4

Transsection of the right portal vein

The bifurcation of the portal vein should be convincingly identified. A small branch to the caudate process is often present. By ligating it, about 2 cm of length along the right portal vein is obtained to facilitate safe ligation of the right portal vein (**A-1**).

Once the right branch of the portal vein is freed from the adventitial tissue, a right-angle clamp is passed around the vein (**A-2**).

A vascular clamp (e.g., small Satinsky clamp) is placed distally and the right portal vein is ligated with 1-0 silk. The distance to the bifurcation should be about 5 mm to avoid portal vein stenosis and subsequent thrombosis (**A-3**).

An alternative (e.g., in the case of a short right portal vein) is to use a small Satinsky clamp on the proximal right portal vein and a running Prolene 6-0 suture (**A-4**). As another alternative, a vascular stapler can be used in this position, but usually the small window in the porta hepatis through which this dissection is being performed lends itself more to a suture ligation than to a stapling. The portal vein on the liver side is controlled through suture ligature as a single ligature could slip away and cause bleeding. Now the demarcation line between the left and right hemiliver can be observed.

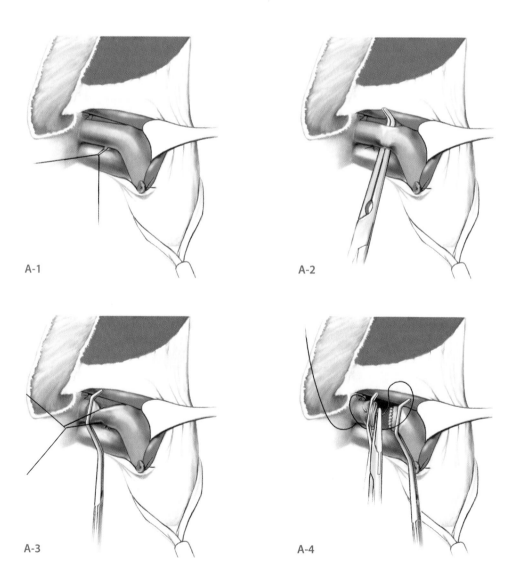

A-1

A-2

A-3

A-4

STEP 5

Transsection of short hepatic veins

The short hepatic veins on the right side are divided between ties. Clips should be avoided particularly on the caval side, as the clip can detach once the low CVP has been corrected postoperatively.

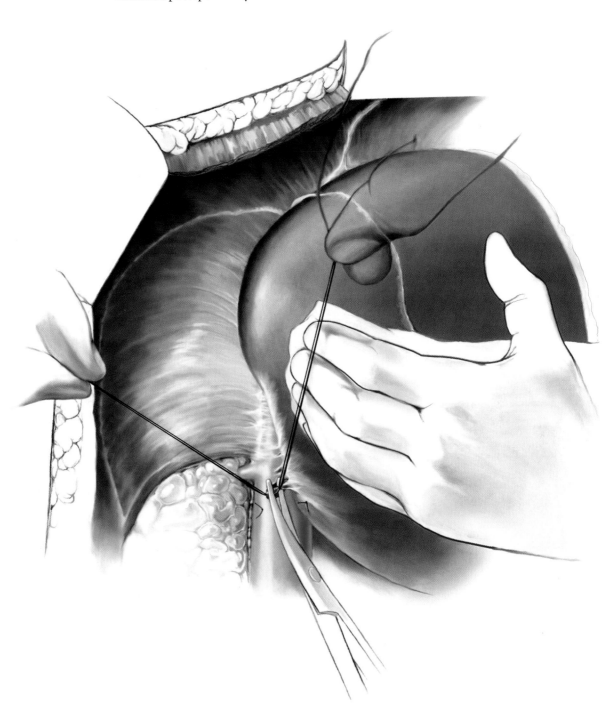

STEP 6   **Transsection of the right hepatic vein**

The right hepatic vein is prepared (separated from the mid and left hepatic vein) from the top and below on the cava by means of a Kelly clamp (**A-1**). A 1-0 silk or vessel loop is placed around the right hepatic vein. The transsection can be performed by means of a vascular stapler (**A-2**). An alternative technique is to occlude the right hepatic vein with a vascular spoon clamp and ligate the proximal hepatic side with a 1-0 silk ligature in combination with a large clip (**A-3**). Should bleeding occur despite the combined ligature and clip, it can easily be controlled by putting a finger on the transsected right hepatic vein. Just continue on the caval side, which is secured by a running 4-0 polypropylene suture. Once the caval side is secured, the bleeding on the transsected proximal hepatic vein can be controlled by a suture ligature.

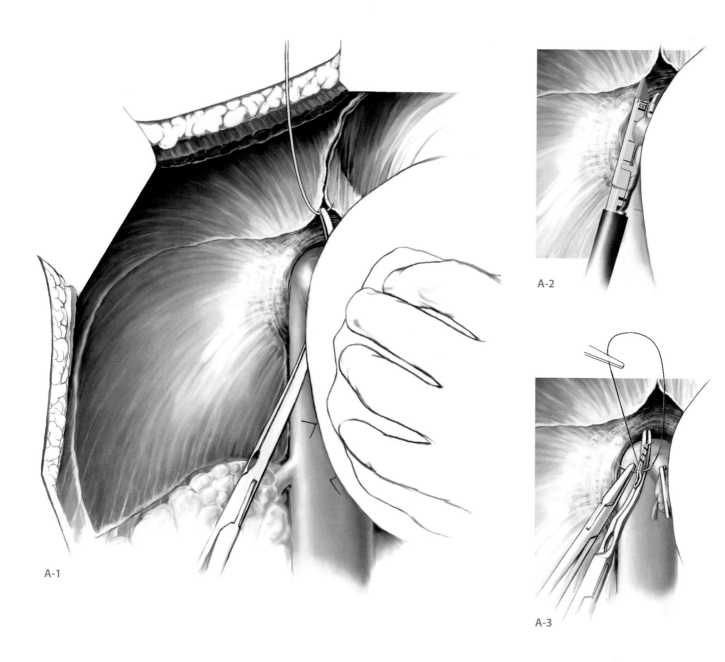

A-1

A-2

A-3

STEP 7

Transsection of the liver parenchyma

Two stay sutures (2-0 silk) are placed at the inferior margin of the liver, one on each side of the demarcation line. At this point, verify that CVP is low (below 3 mmHg). If the CVP is higher, ask the anesthesiologist to correct it and wait. The liver capsule is incised with diathermy a few millimeters on the ischemic side (A). Sometimes the resection line has to be extended to segment IV for oncological reasons.

The dissection of the parenchyma is started at the inferior margin between the stay sutures. The possible techniques for parenchyma dissection are described in the chapter "Techniques of Liver Parenchyma Dissection." The Pringle maneuver for continuous or intermittent inflow occlusion is used if needed. The dissection is continued posteriorly, then inferiorly, preserving the mid hepatic vein.

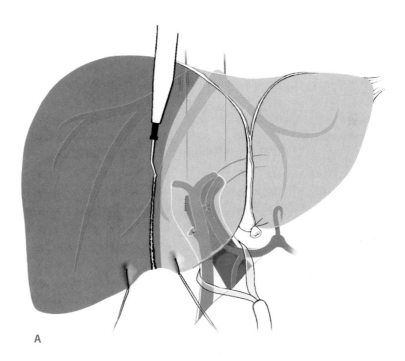

A

STEP 7 *(continued)*   **Transsection of the liver parenchyma**

The technique of bipolar forceps and Kelly clamp is shown (**B**). A band can be placed between the cava and the liver, which allows lifting and better exposure (see also the chapter "Hanging Maneuver for Right Hepatectomy"). As an alternative, the left hand of the surgeon can be placed between the liver and the cava. Each identified bile duct or vessel (>3 mm) is ligated on the left side and divided. In the hilum, the right bile duct is divided away from the main confluence above the caudate process.

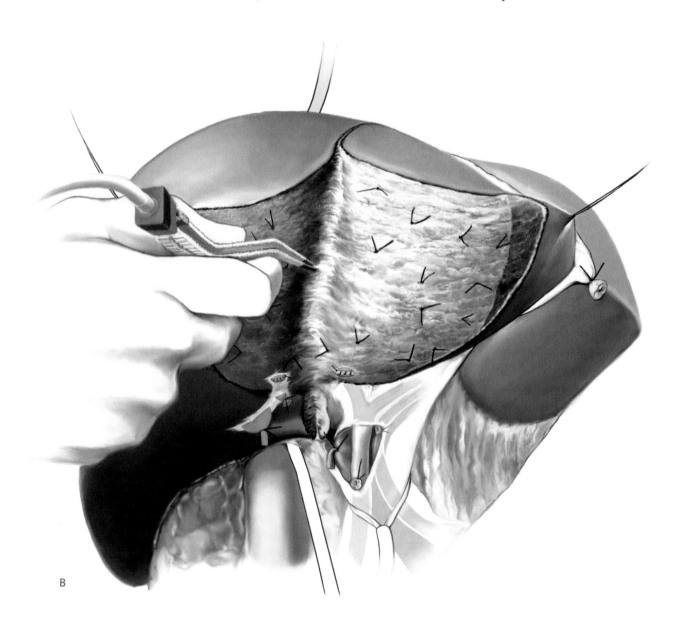

B

Transsection of the liver parenchyma

A gauze swab is placed on the resection surface and a slight compression is maintained for a few minutes or longer in case of diffuse bleeding. Each bleeding on the cut surface should be suture-ligated. At the end of the procedure, the gauze swab is removed and inspected carefully. Any bile leaks (yellow spots on the gauze swab) are oversewn by PDS 4-0 or 5-0. Some groups routinely inject methylene blue in the common bile duct to identify bile leaks. In order to prevent rotation of the left hemiliver, the falciform ligament needs to be reattached (C). The abdomen is closed without drainage.

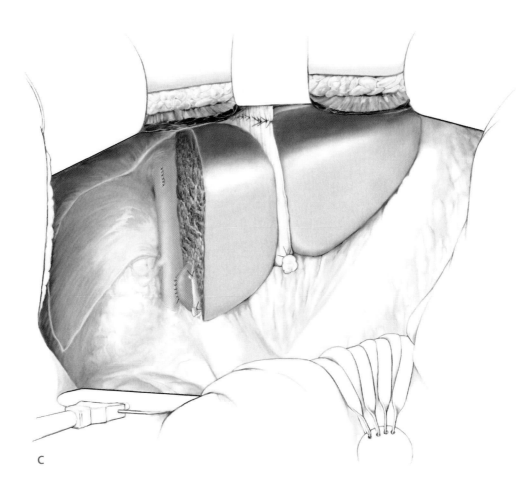

C

Tricks of the Senior Surgeon

- Ask the anesthesiologist early in the procedure for a low central venous pressure: this significantly reduces overall blood loss.
- If you use a ligature to secure the right hepatic vein on the liver side: add a large clip to the ligature – this prevents bleeding!
- If it bleeds despite the clip: do not panic! Compress the right hepatic vein with your finger and continue on the caval side.
- While you dissect the liver parenchyma, hold the right hemiliver with your left hand or a band for optimal exposure and protection of the cava.

Left Hemihepatectomy

Panco Georgiev, Pierre-Alain Clavien

Procedure

STEP 1 **Access and mobilization of the left hemiliver**

The abdomen is opened through a subcostal incision and the round and falciform ligaments are divided. The left hemiliver is mobilized by dividing the left triangular and
coronary ligament (A). Once the left hemiliver is mobilized, the liver can be evaluated by
ultrasound. After confirmation of the resectability, the Pringle maneuver is prepared for
by opening the hepatogastric ligament as shown in the chapter "Techniques of Vascular
Exclusion and Caval Resection." At this point an aberrant left hepatic artery can be
isolated for later clamping with a bulldog clamp.

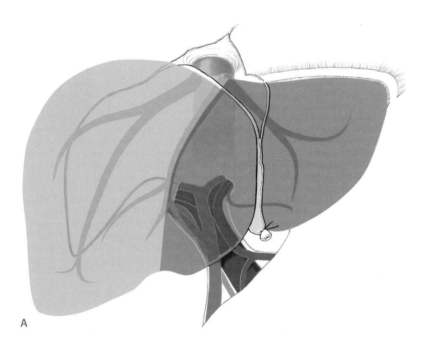

A

Access and mobilization of the left hemiliver

In contrast to the right side, the anterior and posterior leafs of the left coronary ligaments are attached to each other and separated close to the cava. The ligaments can be divided easily by electrocautery while the posterior structures (spleen, stomach, esophagus) are protected with a wet gauze swab (or a finger) placed behind the ligament (**B**). Alternatively, the ligament can be divided over a right-angle clamp.

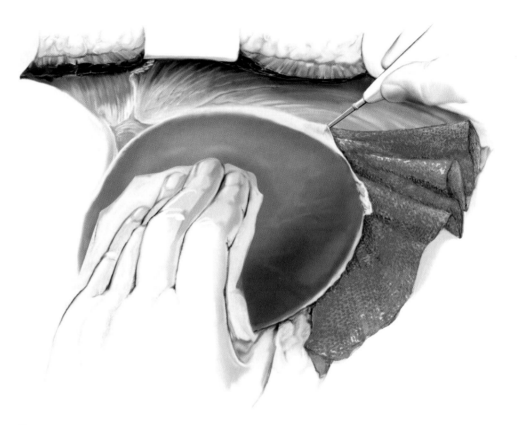

B

STEP 2   **Opening of the hepatoduodenal ligament**

A cholecystectomy is usually performed, although not necessary. Next, the hepatoduodenal ligament is opened from the left by means of a Kelly clamp and electocautery as illustrated. The common bile duct, the artery and the portal vein are visualized without any attempt to secure the left hepatic duct.

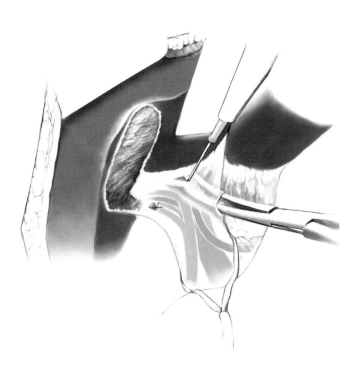

STEP 3

Identification and disconnection of the arterial blood supply to the left hemiliver

At this point the arterial anatomy has to be clarified. A possible aberrant left artery should be secured by means of a bulldog clamp. An aberrant right artery can be identified by palpation of the right border of the hepatoduodenal ligament. The left hepatic artery is identified left to the common and left bile duct and can then be isolated and clamped. The patency of the arterial blood supply to the right hemiliver can now easily be assessed by palpation of the right hepatic artery and/or an aberrant right artery. Once the arterial anatomy is clear, the left hepatic artery (and an aberrant artery to the left hemiliver if present) are divided between ties.

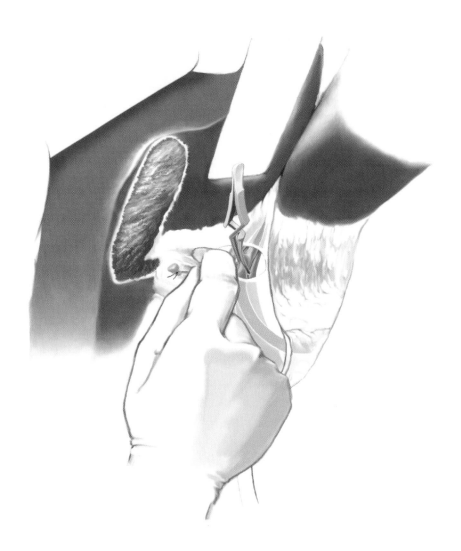

STEP 4 | **Preparation and ligation of the left portal vein**

As the left portal vein typically is situated behind the left branch of the hepatic artery it is easily identified. Following convincing identification of the bifurcation, the left portal vein should be freed from the adventitional tissue and the short branch to Sg1 on the back-left side is divided between ties. The vein can now be ligated with a 1-0 silk suture on both sides. The distance to the bifurcation should be at least 5 mm to avoid stenosis of the remaining right portal vein. Suture ligation with 5-0 Prolene or transsection by means of a vascular stapler are alternatives to a simple ligation (illustrated in the chapter "Right Hemihepatectomy").

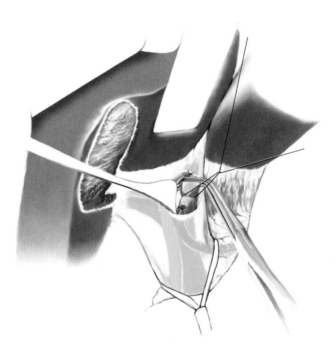

STEP 5   **Dissection of the Arantius' ligament and exposure of the left hepatic vein**

The anterior walls of the left and middle hepatic vein are usually exposed by extending
the dissection of the falciform and coronary ligament to the vena cava. In order to access
the posterior wall, the left hemiliver is lifted up and the lesser omentum is cut up to the
diaphragm. Next, the Arantius' ligament (ligamentum venosum) is identified between
the left hemiliver and Sg1. It runs from the left portal vein to the left hepatic vein or to
the junction between the left and the middle hepatic veins and is divided at its portal
origin between ties (a remnant of the ductus venosus might be present). The stump of
the ligament can now be grasped and dissected upward toward the inferior vena cava
until the ligament broadens into its attachment. By traction of the ligament cephalad
and to the left an avascular plane between the left hepatic vein and Sg1 can be seen and
developed. The left hepatic vein can be isolated by means of a right-angle or a Kelly
clamp. The left hepatic vein can be disconnected at this stage, but it is also possible to
divide it at the end of the parenchyma dissection as shown in Step 7.

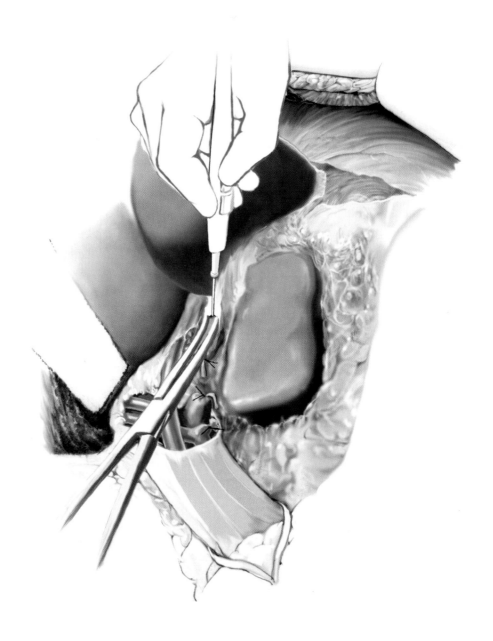

STEP 6   **Dissection of the liver parenchyma**

As the blood supply to the left hemiliver is now interrupted, a clear demarcation between the left and the right hemiliver is seen and identifies the line of resection along the main portal plane. Two stay sutures (2-0 silk) are placed at the inferior margin of the liver, one on each side of the demarcation line. At this point, verify that CVP is low (below 3 mmHg). The liver capsule is incised with diathermy a few millimeters on the ischemic side. The Pringle maneuver for intermittent or continued inflow occlusion is used as needed. The dissection starts on the inferior margin of the liver and is continued first on the caudate lobe, then right onto the surface of the vena cava. During the parenchyma dissection, care must be taken to protect the mid hepatic vein. The left bile duct is isolated and carefully ligated within the parenchyma.

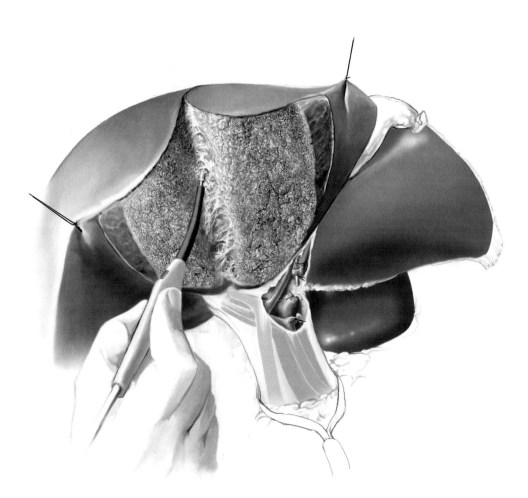

STEP 7   **Transsection of the left hepatic vein**

If the left hepatic vein has not been divided prior to the transsection of the parenchyma, care should be taken while approaching the top of the liver (2–3cm from the top). At this point a vascular stapler can be used to transsect the left hepatic vein. An alternative would be to use a spoon clamp. When a more accurate identification is necessary (e.g., a tumor in proximity), fine preparation of the vein can be achieved by palpation or devices such as the Cusa or Hydrojet (see chapter "Techniques of Liver Parenchyma Dissection").

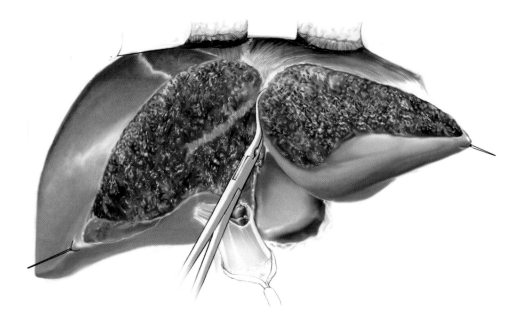

STEP 8

Situs at the end of the left hemihepatectomy with preservation of segment 1

A gauze swab is placed on the resection surface and a slight compression is maintained for a few minutes or longer in the case of diffuse bleeding. Each instance of bleeding on the cut surface should be suture-ligated. At the end of the procedure, the gauze swab is removed and inspected carefully. Any bile leaks (yellow spots on the gauze swab) are oversewn by PDS 4-0 or 5-0. Some groups routinely inject methylene blue into the common bile duct to identify bile leaks.

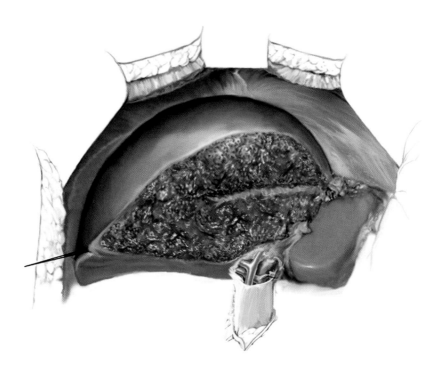

Tricks of the Senior Surgeon

- Ask the anesthesiologist early in the procedure for a low CVP: this significantly reduces overall blood loss
- Isolation and transsection of the LHV before the parenchyma dissection are not absolutely required. Forcing through the parenchyma or middle hepatic vein may cause severe bleeding. Thus, if difficulty is encountered in isolating the left hepatic vein, repetitive attempts should be avoided and the transsection performed at the end of the parenchyma dissection. The results in terms of blood loss are the same if a low CVP is maintained.

Extended Right Hemihepatectomy (Right Trisectionectomy)

The extended right hemihepatectomy (also called right trisectionectomy) includes resection of segments 4–8. For cholangiocarcinoma of the liver hilum (Klatskin's tumor) or carcinoma of the gallbladder, an en-bloc resection including segments 1 and 9 is usually performed. This procedure should only be performed if the remnant liver (segments 2 and 3) provides sufficient liver function. Therefore, preoperative assessment of liver function, a volumetric assessment of the expected remnant liver volume, and exclusion of liver fibrosis or cirrhosis are essential before extended resections.

Dependent on the vascular anatomy, two different approaches can be used for the anatomic resection of Sg4 in addition to segments 5–8. The classical anatomic resection of Sg4 is performed by selective ligation of the pedicle to Sg4 prior to tissue transsection. Alternatively, tissue transsection can be performed first with ligation of the pedicle to Sg4 during parenchymal transsection. Here, we describe the classical approach of resection.

STEPS 1–7 are the same as for a right hemihepatectomy.

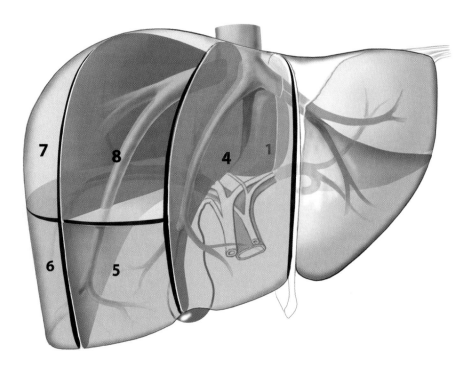

STEP 8   **Selective ligation of the pedicle to segment 4**

After mobilization of the right liver and ligation of the right branches of the hepatic artery and portal vein, careful blunt dissection along the left portal sheath is performed (A-1). The pedicle to segment 4 is then identified, carefully dissected and the vessels selectively ligated (A-2).

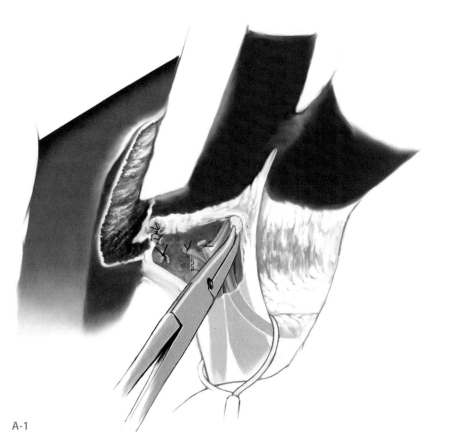

A-1

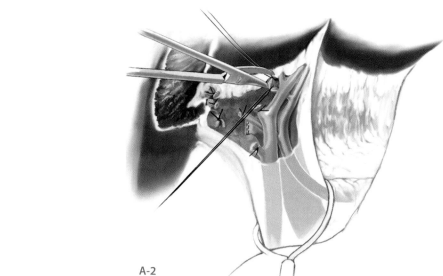

A-2

| STEP 9 | Exposure of the right hepatic vein and parenchymal transsection |

The right hepatic vein is isolated from below and marked with a rubber band as for a right hepatectomy. If the transection is going to be performed with a suspension technique, the right and middle hepatic veins can be isolated from the top as described in the chapter "Hanging Maneuver for Right Hepatectomy."

The resection margin for the extended right hepatectomy is the right side of the falciform ligament. Since the round ligament harbors the fetal connection of the umbilical cord with the left hepatic vein (Arantius' duct), it can be used as a guide. It is fixed with a Kelly clamp and retracted to the left, while a stay suture is placed to the right (A). Intraoperative ultrasound is routinely performed to define the exact extent of the lesion and to identify vascular anatomy.

Tissue transsection is started just to the right of the round ligament. All branches from the right side of the round ligament into the liver need to be ligated selectively (B). If not performed prior to the parenchymal transsection, the pedicle to segment 4 can now be selectively ligated (this approach can be advantageous in tumors involving the left portal sheath). The right bile duct and the bile duct to segment 4 can now be ligated safely.

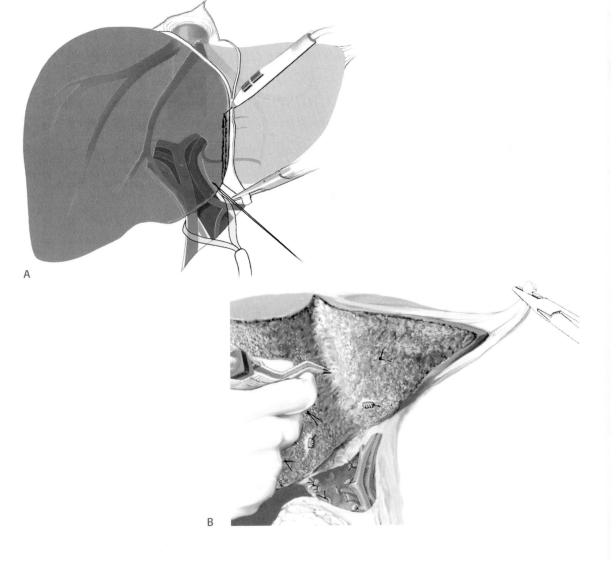

A

B

STEP 10   **Ligation of the right and middle hepatic veins**

Approaching the hepatic veins, the middle hepatic vein is now isolated. As the right
hepatic vein has been prepared before, both can be divided at the end of the
parenchymal dissection by means of a vascular stapler.

Of note, the middle and left hepatic veins usually share a common trunk. Make sure
that the left hepatic vein is preserved!

In addition to this extended right hemihepatectomy, the caudate lobe (segments 1, 9)
can be approached and resected en bloc, if needed (see Section 4).

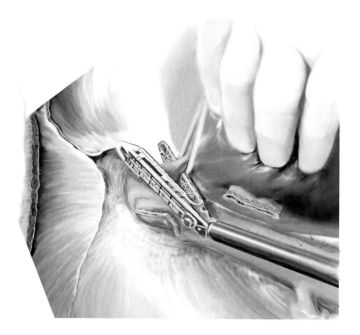

STEP 11

Reattachment of the falciform ligament

The falciform ligament must be reattached to prevent rotation of the remnant liver, since this can result in an acute Budd-Chiari syndrome (obstruction of the venous outflow of the liver), which is a fatal complication after extended right liver resections .

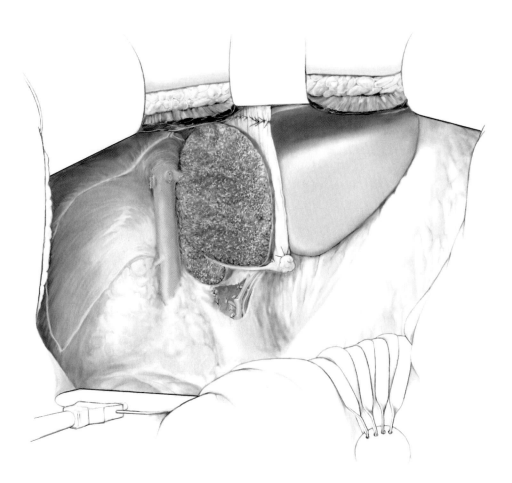

Extended Left Hemihepatectomy (Left Trisectionectomy)

The extended left hemihepatectomy includes resection of segments 2, 3, 4, 5 and 8.

This procedure should only be performed if the remnant liver (segments 1/9+6+7) provides sufficient liver function. Preoperative assessment of liver function, volumetric evaluation of the expected remnant liver volume and exclusion of liver fibrosis or even cirrhosis are essential.

Depending on the vascular anatomy, two different approaches can be used for the anatomic resection of segments 5 and 8 in addition to the left liver. The classical anatomic resection of segments 5 and 8 is performed by selective ligation of the pedicle to these segments prior to tissue transsection. Alternatively, tissue transsection can be performed with ligation of the pedicle to segments 5 and 8 during parenchymal transsection. Here, we describe the classical approach of resection.
STEPS 1–7 are the same as for a left hemihepatectomy.

To prepare an extended left hemihepatectomy, the right liver must be mobilized as for a formal right hemihepatectomy including the division of the short hepatic veins (see chapter "Right Hemihepatectomy").

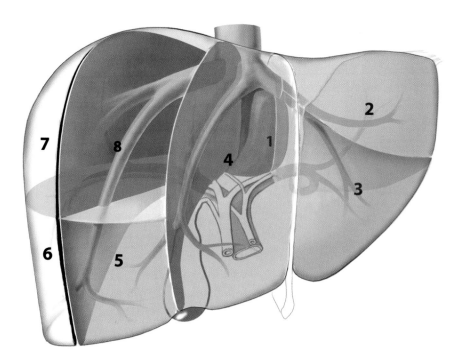

STEP 8   **Selective ligation of the pedicle to segments 5 and 8**

The pedicle to segments 5 and 8 (right anterior pedicle) is identified by careful blunt
dissection on the right portal sheath. The vessels are selectively ligated, while the right
posterior pedicle needs to be preserved. For tumors involving the right portal sheath,
the anterior pedicle should not be dissected in the hilum, but ligated during tissue
transsection. Intraoperative ultrasound is a helpful tool to define the exact extent of the
lesion and to identify vascular anatomy.

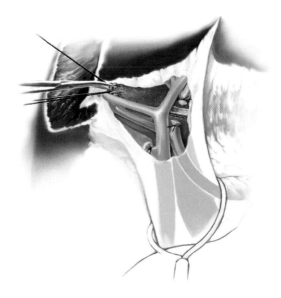

STEP 9   **Exposure of the left and middle hepatic vein**

The middle and left hepatic veins, which usually share a common trunk, are isolated
by careful dissection from above and marked with a rubber band for later dissection,
while the right hepatic vein is identified and preserved.

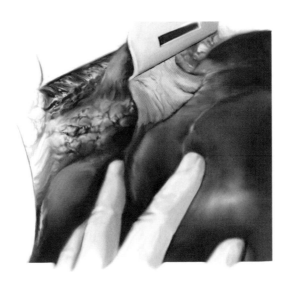

STEP 10   **Parenchymal transsection**

The resection is performed along the demarcation line, which can be seen after ligation of the pedicles to segments 5 and 8. Stay sutures allowing gentle traction are placed on each side of the demarcation. If the pedicle cannot be ligated first, the plane of trans-section is about 1 cm to the left of the right hepatic vein as defined by intraoperative ultrasound.

Particular attention must be paid to the right hepatic vein and its course needs to be known during the whole period of tissue transsection. The left bile duct and the bile duct to segments 5 and 8 can be safely ligated at the end of parenchyma dissection.

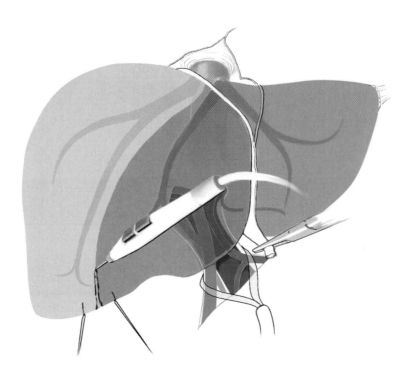

STEP 11

Ligation and transsection of the left and middle hepatic veins

At the end of tissue transsection, the left and middle hepatic veins are transsected by means of a vascular stapler and the resected part is removed, leaving segments 6 and 7 and the caudate lobe. In addition to this formal extended left hemihepatectomy, the caudate lobe can be approached and resected en bloc, if needed (see Section 4).

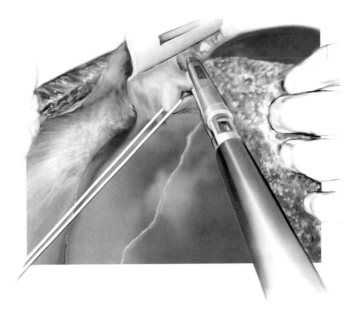

Tricks of the Senior Surgeon

- Extended hemihepatectomies are typically performed for large tumors partially invading segment 4 (extended right hemihepatectomy) or segments 5/8 (extended left hemihepatectomy) or hilar cholangiocarcinoma. In these cases, we do not selectively ligate the pedicles to segments 4 or 5 and 8, respectively, but rather perform a formal hemihepatectomy and extend the resection margin into the contralateral liver (extended wedge resection). This approach may spare liver parenchyma and operative time.
- In the case of tumor involvement of the hilum, dissection and selective ligation of segmental pedicles should be performed during tissue transsection.
- Similarly, in some situations preparation and transsection of the hepatic veins may prove difficult. Two strategies should be considered:
  - Transsection of the hepatic veins during parenchymal transsection without previous isolation.
  - Total vascular exclusion (TVE).
- Portal vein embolization with delayed hepatectomy (about 4 weeks) should be considered prior to resection, if the remnant liver is judged too small.

Segmentectomies, Sectionectomies and Wedge Resections

Norihiro Kokudo, Masatoshi Makuuchi

Introduction

Since hepatocellular carcinoma (HCC) and most metastatic diseases of the liver spread via intrahepatic portal branches, anatomical resection of a tumor bearing portal area, resection of a segment or a section, are basic procedures for treating liver tumors.

In this chapter, we feature anatomical resection of segment 8, segment 7, and right anterior sectionectomy as typical procedures, which contain most of basic techniques for anatomical liver resection. Other procedures including left lateral sectionectomy, left medial sectionectomy, central hepatectomy, and wedge resection are briefly presented.

Anatomical Resection of Segment 8

The standard three-dimensional anatomy of Sg8 is shown below.

The portal venous branches in Sg8 consist of two main branches, i.e., the dorsal branch (P8*dor*) and the ventral branch (P8*vent*), in 92% of patients. P8*vent* and one to three branches of Segment 5 (P5) form a trunk in 62% of patients. Between P8*vent* and P8*dor*, a thick branch of the middle hepatic vein (MHV) runs and drains Segment 8 (V8).

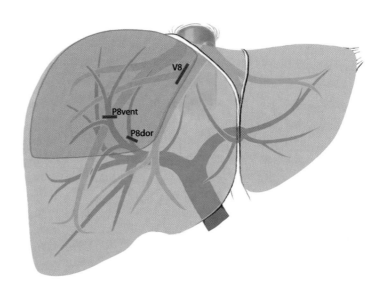

STEP 1	Access and identification of Sg8

A J-shaped thoracoabdominal incision is made entering via the 9th intercostal space. Using the operator's left hand, the right liver is easily lifted together with the diaphragm, and a wide surgical field for the right liver is obtained (**A**).

Under hepatic arterial occlusion with a soft jaw clamp, P8*vent* and P8*dor* are punctured with a 22G needle using intraoperative ultrasound. Approximately 5 ml of indigo carmine is slowly injected into each vessel (**B**). The liver surface of Sg8 is stained blue and the border is marked with electrocautery. Cholecystectomy and hilar dissection are performed when hemihepatic vascular occlusion is applied during hepatic parenchymal transection. No hilar dissection is needed when Pringle's maneuver is applied.

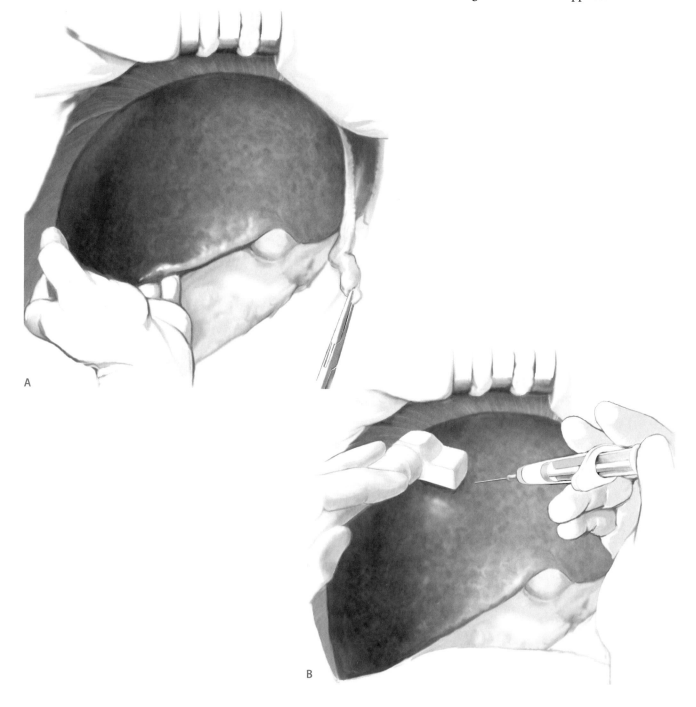

A

B

| STEP 2 | Hepatic parenchymal transection along the main portal fissure |

Using a curved forceps, hepatic parenchymal transection begins along the main portal fissure following the burned mark on the liver surface (A).

The trunk of the MHV is exposed and its tributaries draining Segment 8 are carefully ligated and divided (B).

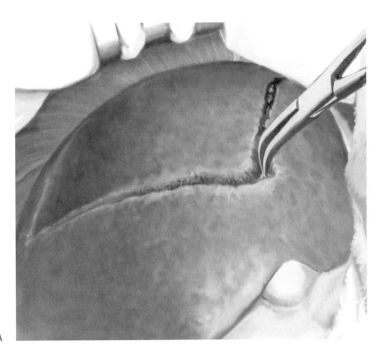

A

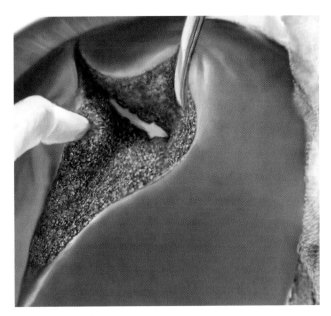

B

STEP 3   **Division of the portal pedicles for Segment 8**

The intersegmental plane between Sg8 and Sg5 is divided and the portal pedicle for the ventral part of Sg8 (P8*vent*) is isolated and divided. The dorsal portal pedicle (P8*dor*) is then ligated and divided. Hepatic parenchymal transection along the right portal fissure is done and the right hepatic vein (RHV) is exposed.

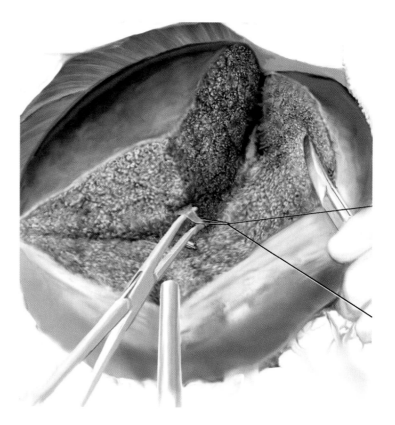

STEP 4   **Exposure of RHV trunk**

The root of the RHV is exposed and a thick venous tributary draining Sg8 is divided. The specimen can now be removed and the procedure is completed with careful hemostasis and suture-ligation of bile leaks. After removal of Segment 8, landmarks including MHV, RHV, and stumps of P8*vent* and P8*dor* are exposed.

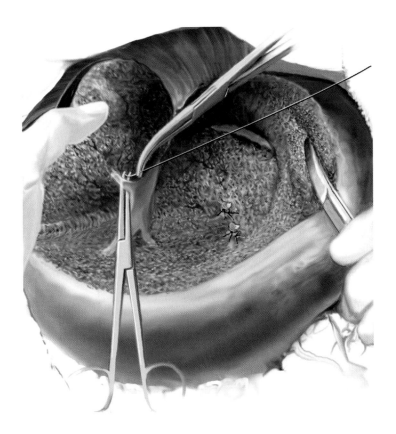

Anatomical Resection of Segment 7

Access to Sg7 is gained through a straight thoracoabdominal incision via the 8th intercostal space (left semilateral position), or through a right subcostal incision. An overview of the important anatomical structures is shown in the Figure.

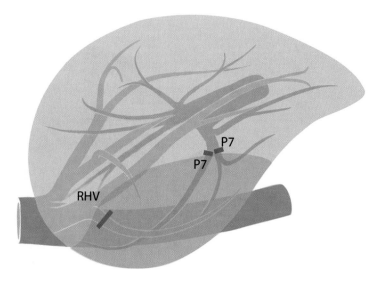

STEP 1   **Identification of the intersegmental plane and ligation
                                        of small hepatic vein branches**

The intersegmental plane between segments 7 and 6 is identified by injecting the die
into P6 (a counterstaining technique). A crushing method is applied using Pringle's
maneuver (**A**).

When a peripheral branch of the RHV is exposed, it is carefully traced proximally
and the trunk of the RHV is exposed. Tiny branches of the RHV are carefully ligated
with 4-0 silk (**B**).

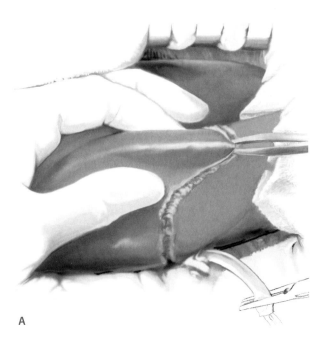

A

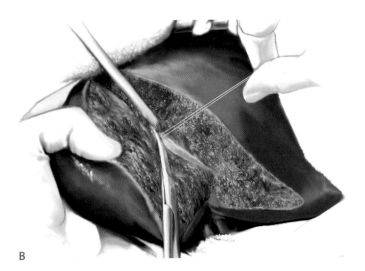

B

STEP 2   **Division of the portal pedicles for Segment 7 and exposure of the RHV**

The two major portal pedicles are exposed. Both are ligated and divided (**A**). The RHV is exposed and a thick drainage vein of Sg7 is ligated (**B**). After removal of Sg7, landmarks including RHV and stumps of P7 are exposed.

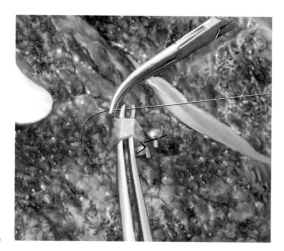

A

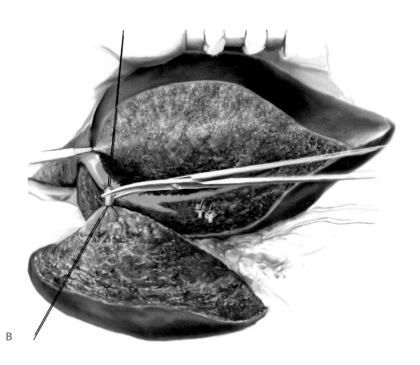

B

Right Anterior Sectionectomy (Right Paramedian Sectoriectomy, Anatomical Resection of Segments 5 and 8)

This procedure requires complete division of the main and right portal fissure, and thus the area of parenchymal transection of this procedure is the widest among all anatomical liver resections.

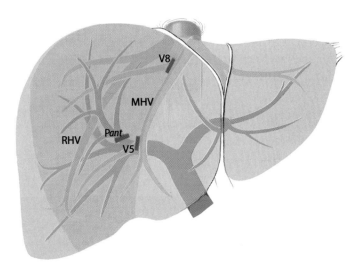

STEP 1

Hilar dissection and identification of the anterior section, transsection along the midplane of the liver

After cholecystectomy, the hepatic hilum is dissected and the right hepatic artery (RHA), the right portal vein (RPV), arterial and portal branches for the anterior and posterior section (Aant, Apost, Pant, Ppost), are isolated (for access to the hilum and preparation of right portal vein/right hepatic artery see also right hemihepatectomy and extended right hemihepatectomy) (A).

After clamping Aant and Pant, the liver surface of the anterior section is discolored and the demarcation lines are marked with electrocautery. This procedure confirms the secti-onal vascular anatomy and Aant and Pant can now be ligated and divided.

Next, under a selective vascular occlusion by soft vascular clamps of the left liver and anterior section, the hepatic parenchymal transection along the midplane of the liver is started (B). The MHV is exposed and tiny tributaries are carefully ligated and divided (C).

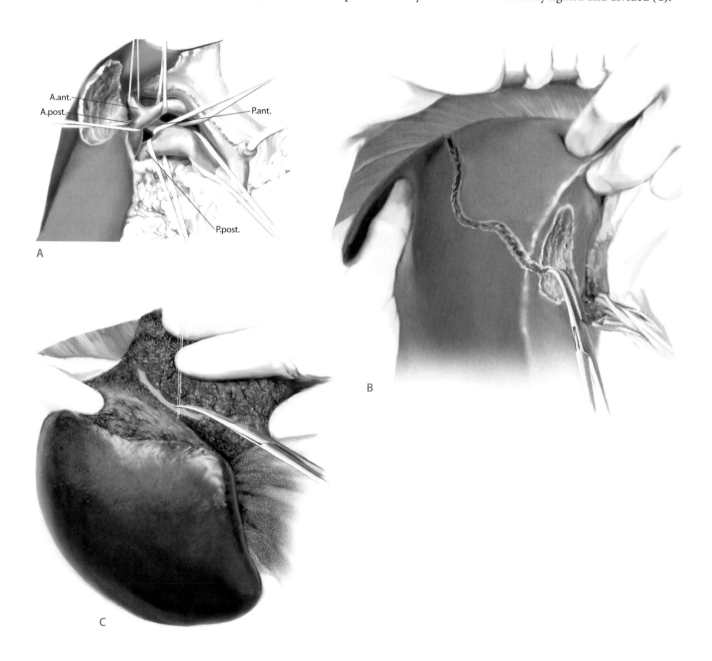

STEP 2

Hepatic parenchymal transection along the right intersectional plane

Under a right hemihepatic vascular occlusion, hepatic parenchymal transection along the right intersectional plane is started (A). The anterior section is lifted with the operator's left hand and the portal pedicle for the anterior section (P*ant*) is ligated and divided (B)

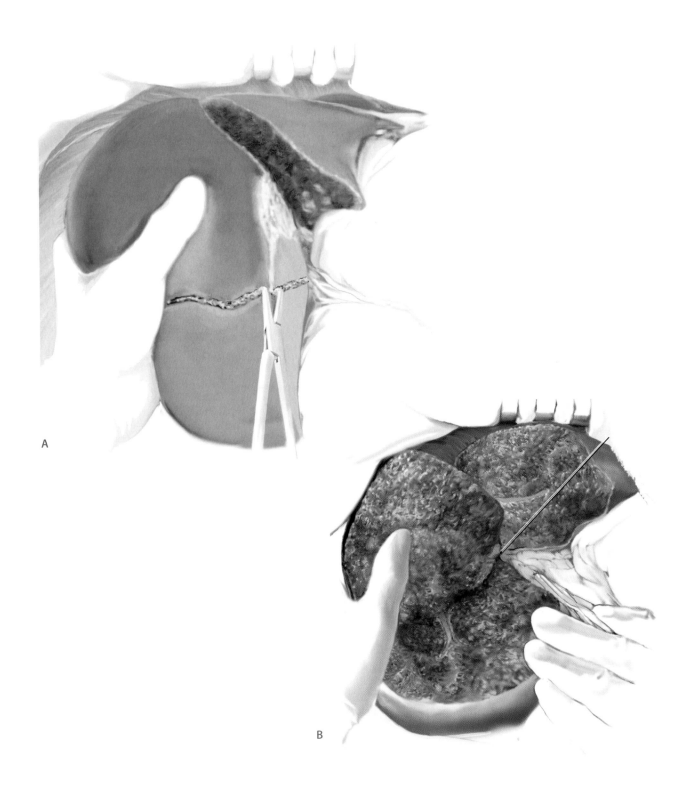

A

B

STEP 3   **Transsection of the RHV branch**

The RHV is exposed and a thick venous branch draining the anterior section is divided. After removal of the anterior section, landmarks including MHV, RHV, and the stump of P*ant* are exposed.

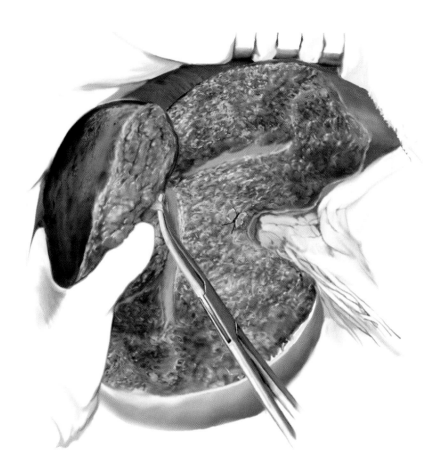

Left Lateral Sectionectomy
(Anatomical Resection of Segments 2 and 3)

The Figure depicts the important anatomical structures for this procedure.

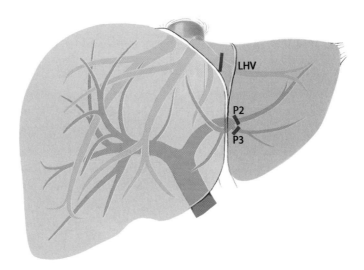

STEP 1	**Hepatic parenchymal transection along the left edge of the falciform ligament (the left intersectional plane)**

By pulling up the left liver via the round ligament, hepatic parenchymal transection is done along the left edge of the falciform ligament. The left wall of the portal pedicle for the umbilical portion of the portal vein is exposed, and all of the tributaries running into the lateral section are ligated and divided. When liver parenchyma of segment 3 and 4 is connected in the visceral side of the umbilical portion, the connecting part is divided during parenchymal transection.

STEP 2	**Division of portal pedicles for segment 2 and 3**

Along the left wall of the umbilical portion of the portal vein, there are a few thick portal pedicles for segment 3 (P3). All of them are ligated and divided. Portal pedicles for segment 2 (P2) are located in the cranial edge of the umbilical portion of the portal vein. They are usually thicker than P3s and only 2 or 3 cm caudal to the root of the left hepatic vein (LHV). They are ligated and divided.

STEP 3

Division of the left hepatic vein (LHV)

At the end of the hepatic parenchymal transection, the root of the left hepatic vein (LHV) is exposed and divided. The stump of LHV is ligated or is closed by running suture. The Figure shows the situation at the end of the procedure.

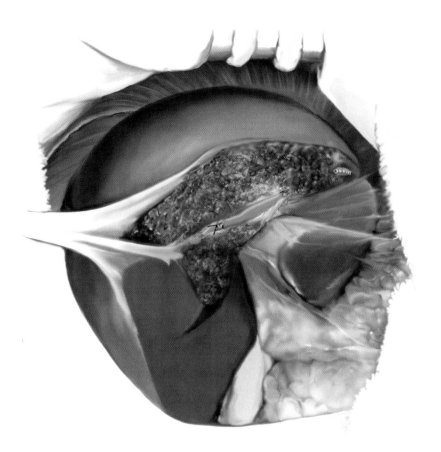

Left Medial Sectionectomy
(Anatomical Resection of Segment 4)

Figure A depicts the important anatomical structures for this procedure.

Hepatic parenchymal transection is done along the midplane of the liver and the right side of the umbilical portion of the portal vein (the left intersectional plane). After removal of the left lateral section, landmarks including MHV and stumps of P4s are exposed (B).

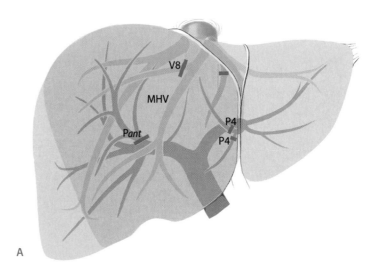

A

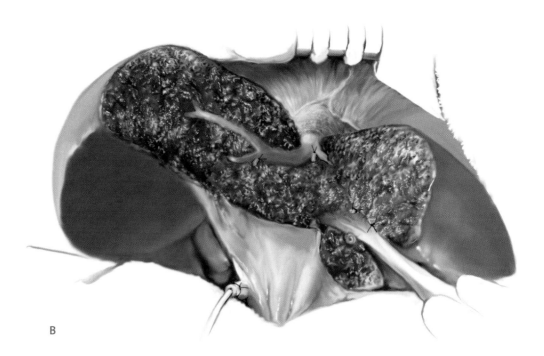

B

Central Hepatectomy
(Anatomical Resection of Segments 4, 5, and 8)

Figure A depicts the important anatomical structures for this resection.

Hepatic parenchymal transection is done along the right and left intersectional plane (i.e., the umbilical portion of the portal vein). The MHV is divided at its root. After removal of the left lateral section, landmarks including RHV and stumps of P*ant* and P4s are exposed (B).

For preparation of the right and anterior portal vein/right hepatic artery, and identification of the right intersectional plane, see also steps for anterior sectionectomy above.

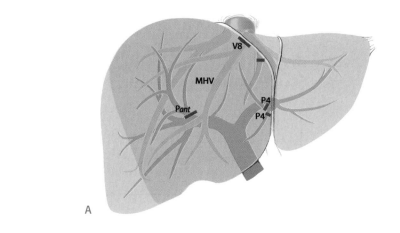

A

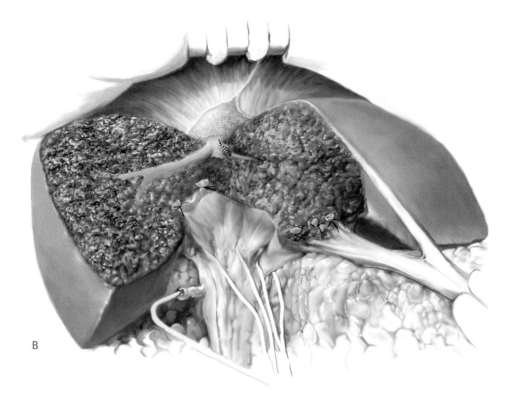

B

Wedge Resection (Limited Resection)

The aim of this procedure is a non-anatomical complete removal of the tumor with sufficient margin. A wide surgical margin (e.g., wider than 10 mm) is not necessary, but care should be taken not to expose the tumor on the cut surface.

Tricks of the Senior Surgeon

- Complete exposure of major hepatic veins, the landmarks for the intersegmental planes, is the key for successful segmentectomy and sectionectomy.
- Before starting hepatic parenchymal transection, branching patterns of the major hepatic veins in each patient should be examined thoroughly with intraoperative ultrasound.
- Major hepatic veins are first exposed at their root and distal edge in the cut surface. Then the middle part of the venous trunks is exposed from both ends.
- A tip of the Metzenbaum scissors is useful for dissecting hepatic veins, and all venous branches larger than 1 mm should be ligated.
- Very tiny branches can be pulled out from the parenchyma (not from the venous wall) with vascular pickups.
- CVP should be kept low (<3 mm Hg) to reduce blood loss during the parenchymal transection.

Laparoscopic Liver Resection

Daniel Cherqui, Elie Chouillard

Introduction

Unroofing of symptomatic simple liver cysts was the first laparoscopic liver procedure to be performed followed by resection of superficial, small-sized benign tumors. The first laparoscopic anatomical liver resection, a left lateral sectionectomy, was reported in 1996. More recently, larger hepatectomies and liver resections for malignant tumors have been described. Today, about 15–20 % of liver resections might be considered for a laparoscopic approach.

Indications and Contraindications

Indications

The indications for laparoscopic liver resections are the same as for open liver resections. Based on tumor size and location of the lesion, the following situations are most suitable for a laparoscopic approach:
- Non-pedunculated lesions less than 5 cm in diameter
- Lesions located in the anterior segments of the liver (segments 2–6; see Figure)
- Pedunculated lesions of any size

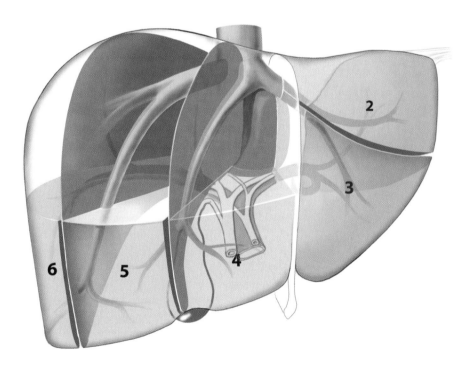

Contraindications

The contraindications are mainly anatomical and related to the size and location of the lesions.

- Large non-pedunculated tumors (>5 cm in diameter)
- Lesions of the hepatic dome (i.e., segments 7 and 8)
- Lesions located in the vicinity of major hepatic veins, the inferior vena cava and the hepatic hilum
- Severe portal hypertension (e.g. portal pressure >12 mm Hg)
- Severe coagulopathy (e.g. platelet count <30 000 ml)

Patient Position, Port Sites and Pneumoperitoneum

- For lesions in segments 2 through 5: Supine position with lower limbs apart and 5 ports are inserted (A). A gas-tight hand port placed in the right iliac fossa can be used for hand assistance. The same incision is then used for the specimen extraction (B)
- For limited resection of segment 6: A left lateral position may be used (C)
- We recommend the use of a 30° laparoscope. A low pressure CO_2 (12 mmHg) pneumoperitoneum is used

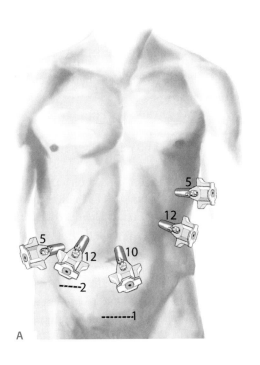

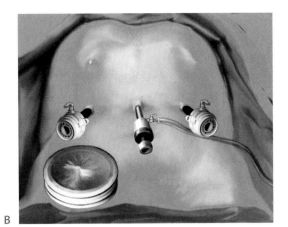

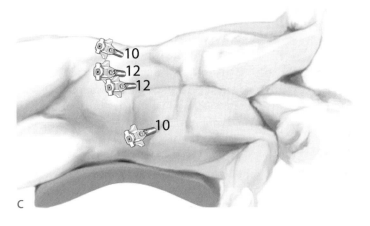

Procedures

Left Lateral Sectionectomy (bisegmentectomy 2, 3)

This is the most common anatomic liver resection performed laparoscopically.

STEP 1

Access, exploration, and mobilization of the left lateral section

After placement of the ports, the liver is explored by laparoscopic ultrasound to determine the size and location of the tumor, to detect additional lesions and to assess the quality of surrounding liver tissue as well as the feasibility of the laparoscopic resection. First, the round, the falciform, and the triangular ligament need to be divided and the lesser omentum is opened. The dissection of the falciform ligament is pursued to the inferior vena cava at the level of the insertion of the hepatic veins. The left triangular and coronary ligaments are divided.

STEP 2

Preparation for the Pringle maneuver and parenchymal transection

A tape is placed around the porta hepatis and passed through a 16-Fr rubber drain to be used as a tourniquet secured by a clip (A-1, A-2). The Pringle maneuver is not applied systematically but is used when required to reduce hemorrhage during transection. When present, an additional left hepatic artery originating from the left gastric artery should be either clamped or ligated and divided. Parenchymal transection follows the left margin of the round and falciform ligament from the anterior edge of the left lateral section up to the level of the origin of the left hepatic vein (B-1). The exposure during transection is maintained by traction of the round ligament towards the right and traction of an atraumatic forceps on the left lateral segment to the left. It is important that the line of transection remains on the left side of the ligaments to avoid injury to the pedicles of segment 4. Posteriorly, the line of transection follows the anterior margin of the Arantius' ligament. The technique of parenchymal transection includes division of the liver with step-by-step control and division of the encountered pedicles. In case of a parenchymal bridge covering the inferior aspect of the round ligament, it should be divided first. A harmonic scalpel is used for the superficial transection (the initial 2–3 cm of depth) for structures up to 3 mm in diameter. Its advantage lies in the ability to cut and coagulate simultaneously. However, it is a blind instrument which becomes more hazardous in the depth of the liver with a risk of injury to larger vessels.

Deeper vessels must be identified before division, and a CUSA with laparoscopic extended hand piece is the recommended device (B-2). Bipolar cautery is used for minor vessels while structures larger than 3 mm in diameter are clipped before division. We do not recommend the use of the argon beam coagulator during laparoscopy because severe gas embolisms due to sudden hyperpressure have been reported.

Portal pedicles to Segments 2 and 3 can be divided using a linear stapler. Stapler application must be performed on the left side of the round ligament (C).

STEP 2 *(continued)*   **Preparation for the Pringle maneuver and parenchymal transection**

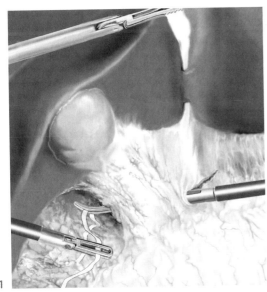

A-1

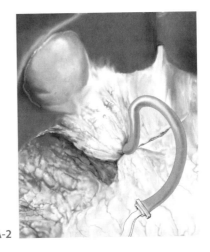

A-2

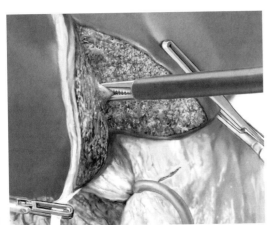

B-1

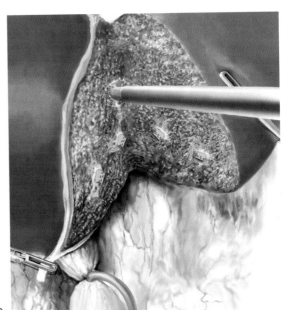

B-2

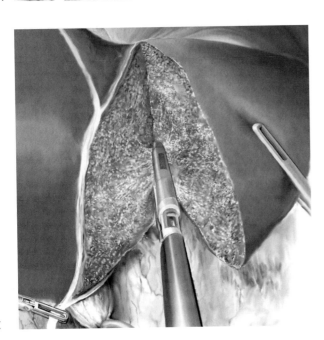

C

STEP 3   **Transection of the left hepatic vein and extraction of the specimen**

Once the portal pedicles have been divided, an ultrasonic dissection can progress cephalad to identify the left hepatic vein, which can then be divided using the same linear stapler, finishing the transection (A).

Additional hemostasis or biliostasis of the transected surface can be achieved by cautery, further clipping or suturing.

A 5-cm incision is usually sufficient for a left lateral section specimen. The incision can be a previous appendectomy incision or a suprapubic incision. At the chosen location, skin and subcutaneous incisions are made without incising the fascia to maintain the pneumoperitoneum. A 15-mm trocar is inserted under internal visual control for the insertion of a large specimen bag (B). The specimen is placed in the bag, which is then extracted with the 15-mm trocar. CO_2 insufflation is stopped and the fascia is incised to allow externalization of the bag. After reinsufflation, hemostasis is checked again and completed if necessary. CO_2 pneumoperitoneum is vented as completely as possible to reduce postoperative pain and the fascia of port sites >5 mm is carefully closed with absorbable suture material.

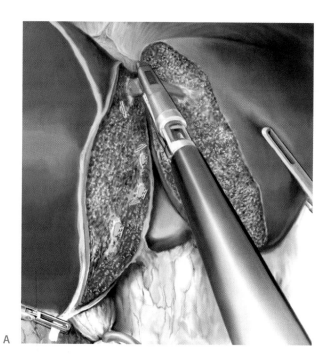

A

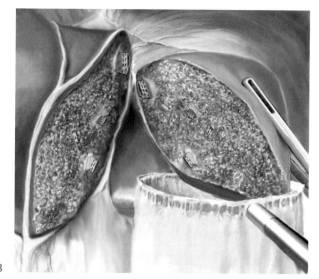

B

Non-anatomical or Wedge Resection for a Peripheral Lesion

These resections are for small lesions located on the edge of the anterolateral segments of the liver (i.e., Segments 3–6).

The liver is exposed and explored as for a left lateral sectionectomy. Although a Pringle maneuver is rarely necessary for these types of resections, it is a safety measure to prepare for the possibility of clamping in case of bleeding. The preparation is the same as for the left lateral sectionectomy.

Resection limits are marked on the liver surface with electrocautery. No wide margins are required in case of benign lesion, while a 10-mm margin is recommended for malignant tumors of the liver.

Parenchymal transection follows the margins marked on the liver surface by cautery.

Since this is a peripheral resection, the harmonic scalpel (Ethicon EndoSurgery) is usually very convenient and sufficient. Additional hemostasis is achieved by bipolar cautery and according to the size of the encountered pedicles. Staplers are usually unnecessary except for pedunculated lesions, whose pedicles can be divided by stapler applications.

The specimen is extracted as shown for the left lateral sectionectomy. While the size of the incision should be adapted to the specimen, port sites >5 mm need to be sutured.

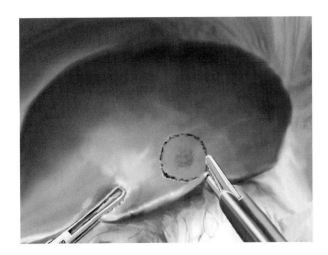

Laparoscopic Living Donor Left Lateral Sectionectomy for Liver Transplantation in Children

This procedure consists of a laparoscopic left lateral sectionectomy without vascular clamping or division in order to minimize parenchymal ischemia. General principles of patient installation and instrumentation are the same as for the left lateral sectionectomy. The mobilization is the same as for a conventional left lateral sectionectomy. For open living donor left lateral sectionectomy see chapter by Tanaka and Egawa.

STEP 1	Preparation of the left portal pedicle

The left arterial and portal branches are dissected, encircled, and marked with a vascular band in the hepatoduodenal ligament (**A**). Arterial and portal branches to segment 1 are divided between clips (**B**).

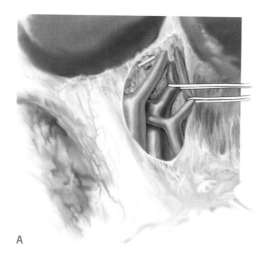

A

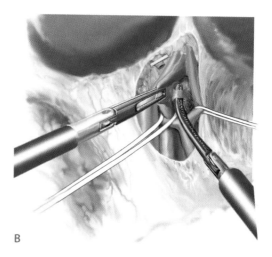

B

STEP 2	**Parenchymal transection**

In contrast to the conventional resection of the left lateral section, the parenchymal transection for living donation needs to be performed along the right aspect of the falciform ligament. The harmonic scalpel is used for the superficial part of the transection and the CUSA for deeper transection. Bleeding is controlled only by using bipolar cautery and clips without any vascular clamping. Segment 4 portal pedicles are divided inside the liver parenchyma with a linear stapler or clips depending on their size.

STEP 3	**Left bile duct division**

Once parenchymal transection has reached the hilar plate and the left hepatic duct becomes visible, the left bile duct is divided using sharp scissors. Its proximal stump is sutured using absorbable running sutures (PDS 5-0).

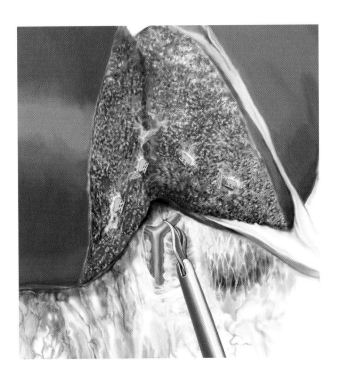

STEP 4

End of transection and isolation of the left hepatic vein

After bile duct division, transection progresses cephalad with section of Arantius' line and progressive dissection of the left hepatic vein. At that stage, the graft is only attached by its vessels.

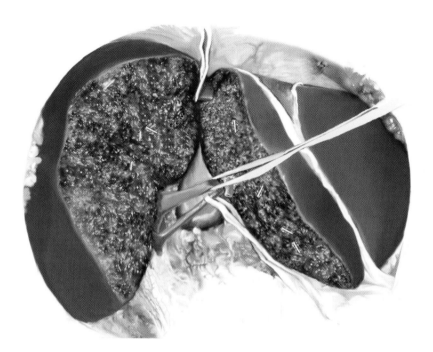

STEP 5

Graft harvesting

An 8–10 cm suprapubic, transverse incision is performed in order to extract the left lobe to be transplanted. Only the skin and subutaneous tissue are opened and a 15-mm trocar is inserted to fit the extraction bag. The left lobar arterial branch is clipped and divided. The left portal branch is then divided initiating warm ischemia. In order to preserve an adequate length of the left portal vein, an Endo-TA stapler (endoTA, Tyco, USA) with one-sided stapling on the remaining donor liver side is used. In addition, a bulldog is placed on the side of the graft in order to prevent bleeding. Finally, the left hepatic vein is stapled with the same one-sided stapling device.

The graft is placed in the bag and extracted through a suprapubic incision after incision of the fascia as for a conventional left lateral sectionectomy.

The graft is handed to another team for perfusion with the preservation solution. Warm ischemic time is usually less than 10 min.

Final hemostasis and biliostasis remain the same as for the conventional left lateral resection.

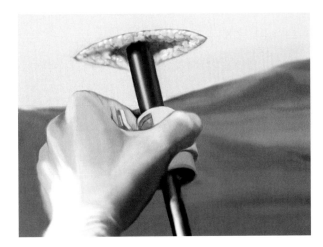

Tricks of the Senior Surgeon

- Laparoscopic hepatectomy is a difficult procedure requiring expertise in both hepatic and laparoscopic surgery. This may require the association of two surgeons.
- In cases of technical difficulty such as persistent bleeding, insufficient exposure or vision, the risk of tumor rupture or insecurity with respect to the tumor margin, one should convert to an open procedure. A conversion, in contrast to a less than optimal outcome, is not a failure of the procedure.
- Abdominal pressure of less than 12 might reduce the risk of gas embolism.
- Before new tools become available, a combination of harmonic scalpel and ultrasonic aspirator is the recommended combination for laparoscopic parenchymal transection.

Cryosurgery

Koroush S. Haghighi, David L. Morris

The goal of hepatic cryosurgery is complete destruction of tumors for curative or palliative reasons as an alternative to resection where resection is not feasible.

Indications and Contraindications

Indications

Malignant liver tumors in the case of:
- Cirrhosis – if risk of resection is excessive
- Bilobar disease where resection would not leave enough hepatic parenchyma
- Debulking of neuroendocrine tumors
- As an adjunct to resection (i.e., resect one side and cryoablate the other side)
- Edge cryotherapy when resection margins are less than 1 cm

Contraindications

- Non-resectable extrahepatic disease (except neuroendocrine tumors)
- High number of lesions (i.e., > nine lesions; other centers may consider > five lesions as a contraindication)
- Tumors >5 cm
- Synchronous bowel resection and hepatic cryoablation (increased risk of liver abscess)

Preoperative Investigation and Preparation for the Procedure

In addition to the preoperative investigations before liver resections:
- In the case of neuroendocrine tumors: H1 and H2 blockers and somatostatin (double existing dose or 100 μg twice daily if not on it) 48 h preoperatively
- Bowel preparation (facultative)
- Make sure there is liquid N_2 in the machine

Procedure

STEP 1	Evaluation of the tumor

In order to exclude extrahepatic disease, the procedure is started with a diagnostic laparoscopy or a mini-laparotomy. The liver is examined bimanually and the tumors are investigated by ultrasound with respect to number, size and distance of bile ducts and vascular structures. Next, the lesser sac is opened and suspicious lymph nodes are sent for histological examination. Heated bed blankets should be used to prevent hypothermia.

STEP 2	Insertion of the probe and applying cryotherapy

Access to the liver is gained by a bilateral subcostal or triradiate incision. For safety reasons, the probes need to be checked for leaks under water with liquid N_2 running. Using ultrasound guidance (A-1), the probes (3–10mm in diameter) can be inserted at the center of the tumor (A-2).

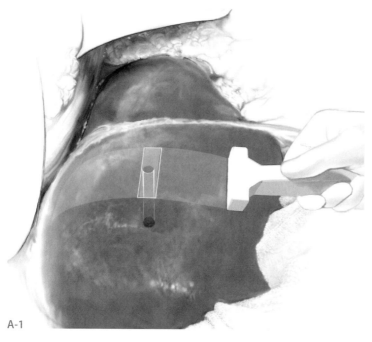

A-1

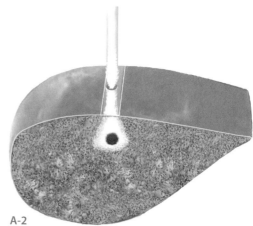

A-2

Insertion of the probe and applying cryotherapy

For larger tumors multiple probes in a predetermined relationship are used (**B**). Cryosurgery can also be combined with a partial hepatectomy. In such cases an edge probe is used to destroy the remnant tumor at the resection surface. This probe does not need to be inserted into the liver (**C**).

The iceball made by cryoablation should extend ≥1 cm beyond the tumor margin. This should be demonstrated with ultrasound guidance. Since it is not possible to see through the ice, the posterior margin is visualized by ultrasound from behind the liver.

After demonstration of a 1-cm margin, we thaw passively and wait for 1 cm to thaw out and then refreeze. Twin freeze-thaw cryotherapy lowers local recurrence rate.

A single cryoablation cycle takes approximately 7–10 min, depending on the size of the lesion.

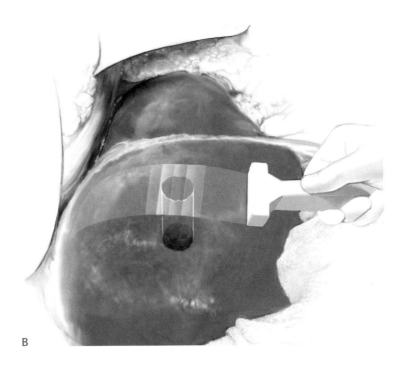

B

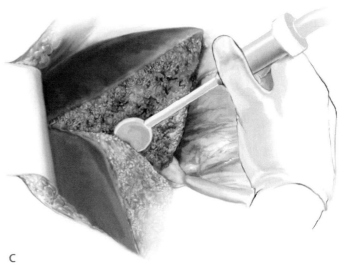

C

STEP 3

Removing the probes

Before the probe can be taken out, it has to be rewarmed with warmed nitrogen gas. Then, the probe can gently be pulled out of the liver, and the tract can be filled with surgical or alternate hemostatic foams.

STEP 4

Cracks

The changes in temperature can cause fractures in the liver which can cause bleeding. These "cracks" need to be managed by liver sutures and packs.

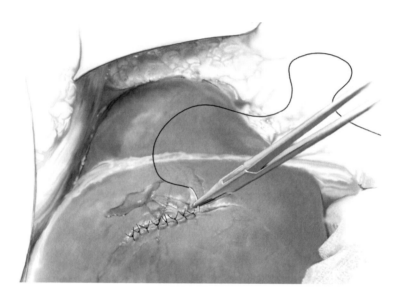

Postoperative Tests

Prediction of Cryoshock

- Full blood count (FBC), looking for thrombocytopenia particularly on day 3
- Liver function test (LFT), especially aspartate aminotransferase (AST), highest rise day 1
- Kidney function tests

Postoperative Complications

Cryoshock

Cryoshock is a syndrome of multiorgan failure including renal impairment, pulmonary edema, coagulopathy, and disseminated intravascular coagulation. The incidence of cryoshock is around 1% and is only seen with large volume distraction and especially with the complete twin freeze-thaw technique.

Hepatic Abscess

Very rare, except with synchronous bowel resection and cryoablation.

Pleural Effusion

Common, especially during right-sided hepatic ablation.

Biloma or Biliary Leak

Biliary Strictures

Biliary strictures can occur but are very rare within the liver. The main risk is for large lesions in segment IV lying at the bifurcation of the PVS.

Tricks of the Senior Surgeon

- Do not wash the lesion or the abdominal cavity with warm saline to speed thawing, as this can result in dramatic cracking.
- Make sure there is liquid N_2 in the machine before you start the procedure.
- Use multiple probes for multiple lesions simultaneously to increase the speed of procedure. However, single lesions are better treated by one large probe than several small probes due to the risk of cracking between small probes.
- Large lesions need more than one probe.
- Before closing the abdomen, make sure the iceball has thawed completely and there is no bleeding from any cracks.
- Aim for a high urine output (intra- and postoperatively) to prevent kidney failure.

Radiofrequency Ablation of Liver Tumors

Michael M. Awad, Michael A. Choti

Indications and Contraindications

Indications

- Unresectable malignant tumors of the liver (e.g., hepatocellular carcinoma, colorectal metastases, neuroendocrine tumors, selected other types of metastases)
- Tumors <5 cm in size (most effective for lesions <3 cm)
- Palliative treatment of symptomatic tumors (e.g., neuroendocrine metastases)
- Bridge to liver transplantation (hepatocellular carcinoma)
- Access:
  - Open:
    - In combination with resection
    - When resection is planned, but unresectability is found at time of laparotomy
    - In difficult locations or selected cases when multiple ablations are required
    - percutaneus: not discussed in this atlas
  - Laparoscopic:
    - Patient fulfills basic requirements to undergo surgery
    - Lesion(s) amenable to laparoscopic approach
    - percutaneus: not discussed in this atlas

Contraindications

- Extrahepatic disease (unless extrahepatic sites are resectable or when there is palliative indication)
- Perihilar tumor location
- Significant coagulopathy or thrombocytopenia
- Ascites
- Previous bilio-enteric anastomosis (relative contraindication due to the increased risk of hepatic abscess following radiofrequency ablation, RFA)

Preoperative Investigation and Preparation for the Procedure

CT or MRI:	Assessment to rule out resectability and determine if lesions are ablatable
PET:	Evaluation for presence of extrahepatic disease (e.g., colorectal metastases)
In operating room:	Grounding pads (varies depending on RFA manufacturer)
	– Place greater than 50 cm from electrode
	– Orient pads with long axis perpendicular to body axis
	– Use multiple pads when indicated

Guidance Imaging Modality

Imaging is used for lesion localization, probe guidance, and ablation monitoring. The following features of each imaging modality must be considered.

- Ultrasound
  - Most common method used
  - Inexpensive and real time feedback
  - Sometimes difficult to visualize lesion adequately
  - Increased echogenicity from microbubbles
  - Microbubbles are not a true representation of zone of coagulation necrosis
  - Echogenicity may obscure further needle positioning
- Alternatives: CT or MRI
  - Transaxial needle track required
  - CT fluoroscopy is a useful adjunct
  - For MRI, a compatible RFA needle is required

Probe Selection

A number of different probes are commercially available for performing RFA (A-1, A-2, A3). Probes are typically 14–17.5 gauge, 15–25 cm long, insulated cannulas containing one to three straight needle electrodes (ValleyLab) or five to ten individual hook-shaped electrode arms or tines (RITA Medical, Boston Scientific). Some of the newer probes have a cooled-tip system utilizing circulating saline (ValleyLab, Berchtold), or local saline infusion (RTA Medical).

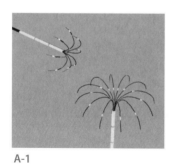

A-1

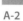

A-2

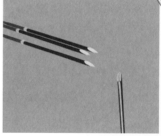

A-3

Procedures

Open Technique

STEP 1

Access and assessment of tumors

Incision, evaluation, palpation and mobilization of the liver are performed as for a liver resection. The abdomen is explored for the presence of extrahepatic disease and the evaluation is completed by intraoperative ultrasound (IOUS) to identify/confirm the location and the size of the lesions (A). The feasibility of the ablation is determined and the number of needed ablations is calculated.

STEP 2

Placement of the probe and ablation of tumors

The probe is aligned so that its trajectory lies in the plane of the ultrasound image and does not intersect vital structures such as blood vessels and bile ducts. It is advanced under image guidance until the tip is either close to the proximal edge of the tumor or near the distal edge, depending on the probe type (B-1). The deployed probe is visualized in perpendicular view to confirm adequate tip position and deployment (A). The probe tines are deployed and radiofrequency energy is applied according to the manufacturer's directions (B-2, B-3).

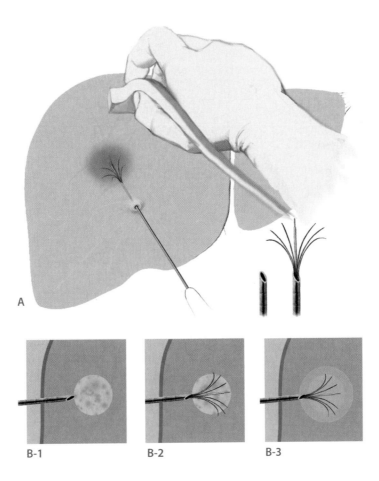

A

B-1   B-2   B-3

STEP 3   **Ablation of large or irregularly shaped lesions and tract ablation**

For large or irregularly shaped lesions, multiple ablations may be needed (Step 2 is repeated as necessary). A pattern of overlapping spheres or cylinders is used to cover the lesion while maintaining adequate margins.

With some devices, tract ablation is performed to cauterize the tract and to minimize seeding. The probe is withdrawn 1 cm at a time in tract ablation mode on the radio-frequency generator, allowing temperature to reach >70 °C at each step. This is continued until the probe is completely removed.

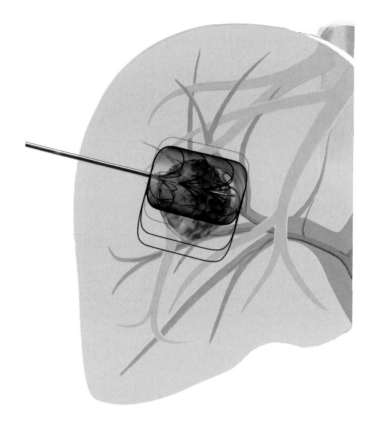

Laparoscopic Approach

Positioning of the patient and access

Depending on the location of the tumor(s), the patient is placed in the supine or left lateral decubitus position. A minimum of two laparoscopic trocars are placed: a 12-mm periumbilical camera port and a 12-mm laparoscopic ultrasound port in the right flank. The radiofrequency probe can be placed percutaneously, through a sheath, or through a 5-mm right subcostal port. More ports may be required if additional procedures are to be performed (e.g., liver mobilization, partial resection) (A-1).

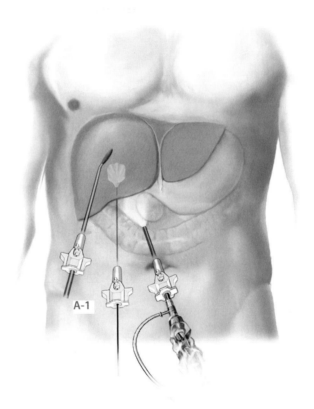

STEP 2   **Assessment of tumors and ablation**

Laparoscopic intra-abdominal ultrasound (IOUS) is performed by either rigid or
flexible IOUS probes to identify/confirm the location and the size of the lesions.
The abdomen is explored for the presence of extrahepatic disease. As described
for the open technique, the RFA probe is oriented parallel with the IOUS crystal to
facilitate probe guidance (A-2). Limited mobility can make this more difficult than
with the open technique. The ablation process and monitoring is otherwise performed
as described with the open approach.

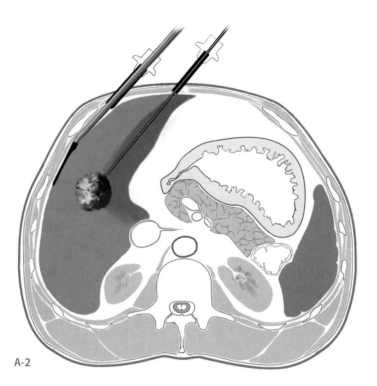

A-2

Postoperative Testing

Follow-up postablation imaging (CT or MRI) is performed 3–7 days after procedure to assess completeness of ablation.

Postoperative Complications

- Short term:
  - Pleural effusion
  - Regional hemorrhage into needle track or into RFA lesion
  - Fever
  - Hepatic abscess (more common with enterobiliary anastomosis)
  - Biliary stricture secondary to ablation near major bile duct
  - Grounding pad burns
- Long term:
  - Biloma
  - Biliary fistula
  - Ascites
  - Hepatic insufficiency
  - Arteriovenous fistula

Tricks of the Senior Surgeon

- When the lesion lies near a major blood vessel, thermal energy from the probe may be drawn away from the ablation zone, limiting ablation efficacy. This is known as the "heat-sink" effect. This can be limited using in-flow occlusion techniques (e.g., Pringle maneuver) or repositioning the array closer to the vascular structure.
- Stabilization of the radiofrequency probe at the skin or liver surface should be done during deployment to avoid "push back."
- Depending on the device, monitoring of the impedance pattern and tine deployment shape by ultrasound can confirm success of the ablation in real time.
- With some devices, temperature profiles can also be helpful at confirming successful ablation, including consistent tine temperatures and adequately slow cool-down temperatures.

Selective Hepatic Intra-arterial Chemotherapy

Christopher D. Anderson, Ravi S. Chari

Hepatic intra-arterial infusion pump (HAIP) placement provides hepatic specific continuous infusion of chemotherapeutic agents. The chemotherapeutic agents selected for use with HAIP should exhibit a high degree of first pass kinetics in order to minimize systemic toxicity. Agents used include cisplatin, fluodeoxyuridine (FUDR), mitomycin C, and Adriamycin.

Indications and Contraindications

Indications	■ Unresectable hepatic metastatic colorectal carcinoma
	■ Liver specific adjuvant chemotherapy following resection of colorectal metastases
	■ Use in hepatocellular carcinoma and other metastatic carcinomas can be considered under certain circumstances
Contraindications	■ Portal hypertension (portal pressure >12 mm Hg)
	■ Known extrahepatic malignancy
	■ Poor liver reserve (e.g., Child B or C cirrhosis)
	■ Severe coagulopathy (e.g. platelets <30 000 ml)
	■ Active hepatitis

Preoperative Studies

History:	Specific for hepatic function (e.g., alcohol use, hepatitis)
Clinical evaluation:	To rule out obvious extrahepatic malignancy (lymph node exam) and underlying liver dysfunction (ascites, nutrition status, signs of portal hypertension)
Triple phase CT, CT angiogram (CTA) or MRI of abdomen:	For definition of tumor and arterial anatomy
Chest CT:	To rule out pulmonary metastases, except in the case of colorectal carcinoma
FDG-PET:	In cases of metastatic colorectal carcinoma
Hepatic arteriogram:	Not mandatory if HAIP is to be placed via laparotomy, but it may decrease operative time. Mandatory if HAIP to be placed laparoscopically, and CTA or MRA not performed

Procedure

STEP 1   **Incision and exposure**

A right subcostal approach is used. The falciform ligament is divided and the porta hepatis is exposed further by gentle superior retraction of the liver. Cholecystectomy is performed to eliminate the postoperative complication of chemical cholecystitis induced by infusional chemotherapy. The gastrohepatic ligament is divided with care to avoid injury to a replaced left hepatic artery (if present). All duodenal and antral vessels must be ligated to eliminate the possibility of reflux of chemotherapy into these regions as this may lead to chemical duodenitis or gastritis. The common hepatic, gastroduodenal, and proper hepatic arteries are identified by dissection of the hepatoduodenal ligament and marked with vessel loops.

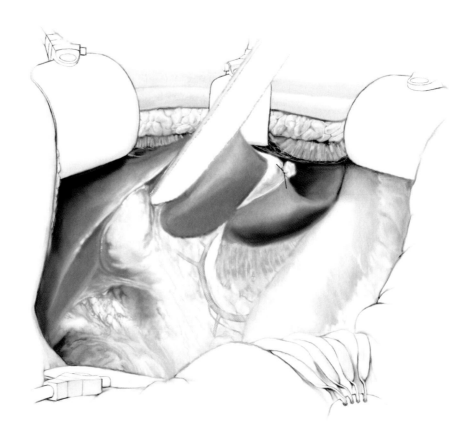

| STEP 2 | Determination of arterial anatomy |

At this point it is imperative to accurately determine the hepatic arterial anatomy if no preoperative arteriogram was performed. The more common variants in hepatic arterial anatomy are shown in the figure: (**A-1**) the common hepatic artery may originate from the celiac trunk (typical). (**A-2**) A replaced right hepatic artery (RRHA) may arise directly from the superior mesenteric artery. (**A-3**) A replaced left hepatic artery (RLHA) may arise directly from the left gastric artery. (**A-4**) Common origin of the right hepatic artery, left hepatic artery and gastroduodenal artery. This is commonly referred to as the "trifurcation anatomy."

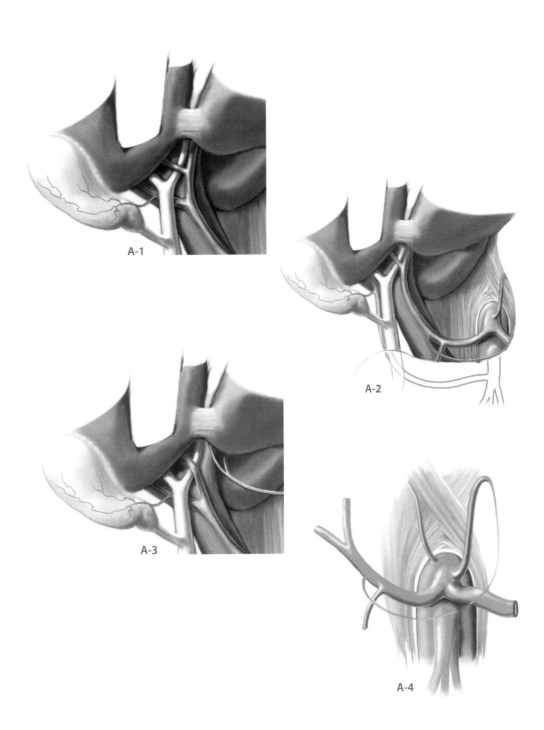

A-1

A-2

A-3

A-4

STEP 3   **Placement of the infusion pump in subcutaneous pocket**

The pump pocket is created in the right lower quadrant by making a transverse incision at the level of the umbilicus and dissecting to the anterior rectus sheath and the external oblique fascia. The pocket is extended laterally to near the iliac crest and inferiorly to just above the inguinal ligament. Some surgeons prefer that the pocket be developed through the initial subcostal incision, while others prefer it not to communicate with the laparotomy incision. The pump is primed with heparinized saline and proper pump function should be established before anchoring it to the fascia with 2-0 nonabsorbable braided suture. The arterial catheter is passed into the pocket by direct puncture.

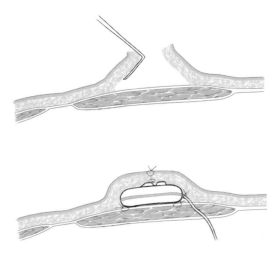

STEP 4	Placement of the arterial catheter

Cannulation typically should be performed with a single catheter placed in the gastro-duodenal artery (GDA). The origin of the GDA from the common hepatic artery is identified, and the proper hepatic artery from the GDA to the liver is skeletonized. Any branches leading to intestinal viscera are individually ligated and divided. This step prevents visceral misperfusion injuries. The GDA is further skeletonized for approximately 2 cm distal to its origin and then ligated near the pancreas. A noncrushing vascular clamp is used to occlude the GDA at its origin. A transverse arteriotomy is made in the GDA approximately 1.5 cm from its origin. The beaded infusion catheter is cut such that its port does not enter the common hepatic artery, but that at least one bead is in the GDA. The catheter tip should not enter the common hepatic artery to lessen the risk of catheter associated common hepatic artery thrombosis. The GDA is secured around the catheter using 4-0 nonabsorbable suture both proximally and distally to the catheter bead. This prevents advancement or retraction of the catheter.

To insure proper hepatic perfusion, 1–5 cc of fluorescence is bolused into the catheter, and the liver is observed under a Woods lamp. Alternatively, 1–5 cc of methylene blue will also visually confirm adequate perfusion; this is a useful method when placing HAIP laparoscopically.

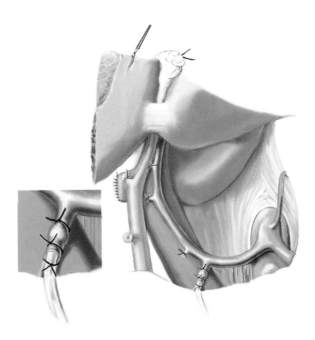

STEP 5

Dealing with atypical arterial anatomy

Following a hepatic resection, management of aberrant arterial anatomy is contingent upon the arterial supply of the remnant hepatic parenchyma. However, without a liver resection, the most common arterial variant encountered is the trifurcation anatomy. This may be approached by ligation of the GDA and directly cannulating the common hepatic artery well proximal to the bifurcation of the right and left hepatic arteries. The common hepatic artery is skeletonized and occluded proximally and distally with noncrushing vascular clamps. A longitudinal arteriotomy is performed and the catheter is inserted with the bead remaining outside the arteriotomy (A-1). A pursestring suture (6-0 nonabsorbable) is used to close the arteriotomy around the catheter and secure the catheter in place (A-2).

Replaced hepatic arteries may undergo isolation and clamping. If clamping is tolerated, the replaced vessel may be ligated and the liver can be perfused via the typical catheter placement. If clamping is not tolerated, a replaced right hepatic artery may be approached by placing one catheter in the GDA to perfuse the left hepatic and a second catheter directly into the replaced right hepatic artery as described for the trifurcation anatomy. A similar approach may be used for a replaced left hepatic artery. If two catheters are placed, it is important not to connect them to a single pump via a Y connector because of differential resistance in each vessel.

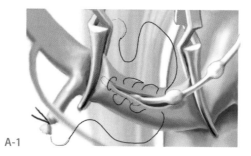

A-1

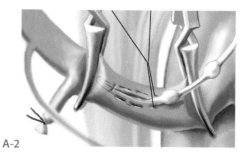

A-2

Postoperative Studies

Some centers routinely perform a nuclear medicine study of the HAIP on postoperative day 3–5 to rule out extrahepatic perfusion. This consists of a sulfur colloid outline of the liver and then bolus injection of technetium micro-albumin aggregate (MAA) via the pump bolus port. The two images are superimposed to insure adequate hepatic perfusion and to rule out extrahepatic visceral perfusion.

Complications

- Early:
  - Visceral misperfusion
  - Arterial injury and postoperative bleeding
  - Hematoma or seroma of the pump pocket
- Late:
  - Biliary stricture
  - Hepatic artery thrombosis
  - Occlusion or displacement of the catheter
  - Pseudoaneurysm
  - Pump pocket infection

Tricks of the Senior Surgeon

- Prime the pump and test its function early in the case. Be familiar with the specifics of the various pumps and the needles used to bolus/prime and fill the pump.
- When accessory vessels are known to exist or are discovered at the time of laparotomy, determination of their contribution to hepatic perfusion can be gauged by clamping and observing the parenchyma for color change: this should be performed early in the case so there is adequate time to determine the consequences of ligation versus the need for a second pump system.
- A postoperative MAA perfusion study is not essential and may be omitted if clear intraoperative studies indicate uniform hepatic perfusion with lack of reflux into the duodenum or stomach. In cases where accessory vessels are ligated, and a single catheter and pump are placed, an MAA study 1 month after placement should be performed to demonstrate uniform perfusion of the hepatic parenchyma.

Unroofing and Resection for Benign Non-Parasitic Liver Cysts

Juan M. Sarmiento, David M. Nagorney

Hepatic cysts are classified according to the presence or absence of a parasitic etiology. They seldom lead to hepatic dysfunction and are mostly asymptomatic. The treatment is always individualized according to the origin and presence of symptoms. The choice between unroofing versus resection is dictated by site, number of cysts, malignant potential (cystadenoma/cystadenocarcinoma), and parasitic infection (see next chapter). Malignant potential is rare and is not a primary concern.

Indications and Contraindications

Indications	■ Pain significantly affecting lifestyle
	■ Jaundice
	■ Infection
	■ Hemorrhage
	■ Portal hypertension
	■ Abdominal fullness or mass
Contraindications	■ Asymptomatic patients
	■ Patients amenable to percutaneous cyst aspiration and/or alcohol sclerosis under US or CT guidance (simple cysts lacking or with minimal capsular extension or cysts in segments 7 and 8)

Preoperative Investigation and Preparation for Procedure

History:	Polycystic disease of the kidney
Clinical evaluation:	Abdominal pain, jaundice, signs of portal hypertension
Laboratory tests:	AST, ALT, alkaline phosphatase, bilirubin, tumor markers (CEA, CA 19–9) and serologies (hydatid)
CT scan:	Location, accessibility to laparoscopic versus open approach, amount of remaining healthy parenchyma
US:	Location, compression of main vessels (especially hepatic veins), biliary dilatation
MRI:	Polycystic liver disease or complicated cases

Procedures

Laparoscopic Unroofing of a Simple Cyst

STEP 1   **Access and exploration**

Usually three ports are used: camera, grasper for the cyst wall, and cutting instrument (cautery, harmonic scalpel, or scissors). Placement varies according to the anatomic location of the cyst . One of the working ports should be 10 mm for clip application.

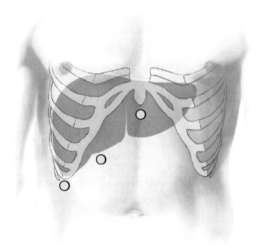

STEP 2 | **Unroofing**

The dome of the cyst is elevated with a grasper. Incising the cyst and draining its contents makes the cyst wall flaccid and easier to handle (**A, B**). The wall of the cyst is resected with electrocautery. Excision should be as close as possible to the interface between the cyst and the remnant liver. It is very important to resect the maximal amount of the wall of the cyst to enhance retraction of the remnant edge of the cyst, thus preventing reapproximation of the rim by contraction with subsequent recurrence. Cytology of the aspirate is performed if indicated and if the cyst is complex with mural nodules. Effaced ducts or vessels at the cyst-liver interface should be stapled or clipped. After removal, the cyst wall is assessed histologically.

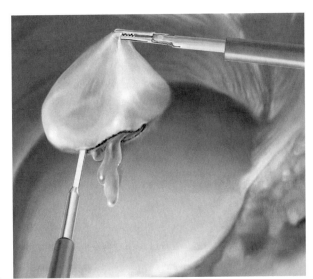

A

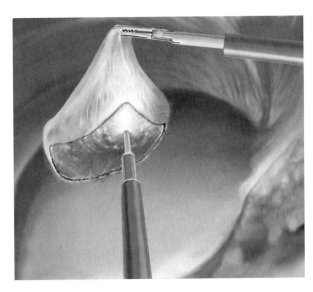

B

STEP 3

Inspection of the cyst

After unroofing, the residual cyst wall is inspected carefully. Irregularities within the concavity of the cyst are biopsied. When less than 50 % of the cyst has been removed, ablation of the remnant cyst lining directly by cautery, argon beam coagulation, or topical sclerosant may reduce the incidence of recurrence. Omentum can be placed within the cyst remnant to prevent recurrence in this circumstance.

Open Unroofing of a Simple Cyst

STEP 1

Access and approach

Cysts located superiorly in segments 7 and 8 are usually unroofed in an open fashion. A right subcostal incision is indicated in these cases; the triangular and a portion of the coronary ligaments are divided to rotate the liver (see chapter "Right Hemihepatectomy"). Using the nondominant hand, the surgeon pulls the liver toward the midline to complete the exposure of the cyst. The same principles dictated for the laparoscopic approach are followed and the cyst is unroofed. Alternatively, the cyst can be enucleated en toto.

STEP 2	Inspection of the cyst

There is no cyst wall left above the level of the hepatic parenchyma. Occasionally, blood vessels or bile ducts can be seen on the cavity. No drains are necessary after cyst excision.

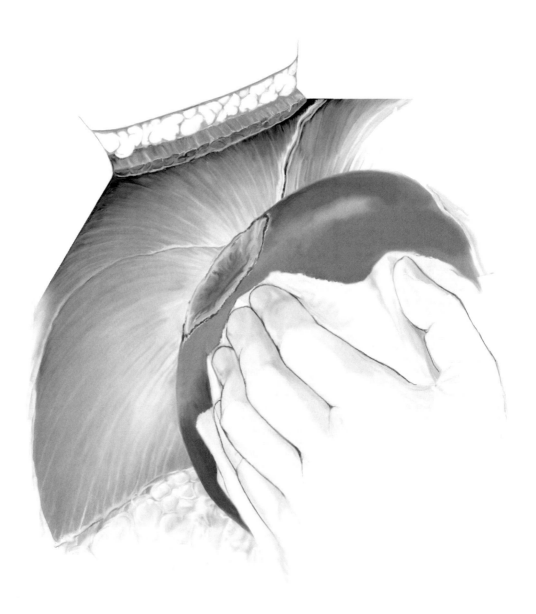

Enucleation of Biliary Cystadenoma

STEP 1

Enucleation of the cyst (A)

After mobilization of the liver, countertraction is maintained by the nondominant hand of the surgeon (B). The interface between the cyst and the hepatic parenchyma is identified and developed; the wall of the cyst is usually thick and rarely ruptures. With deeper dissection, compressed vessels and bile ducts become evident and should be preserved. The dissection is completed circumferentially and the cystadenoma is enucleated and sent for histologic analysis to exclude occult cystadenocarcinoma.

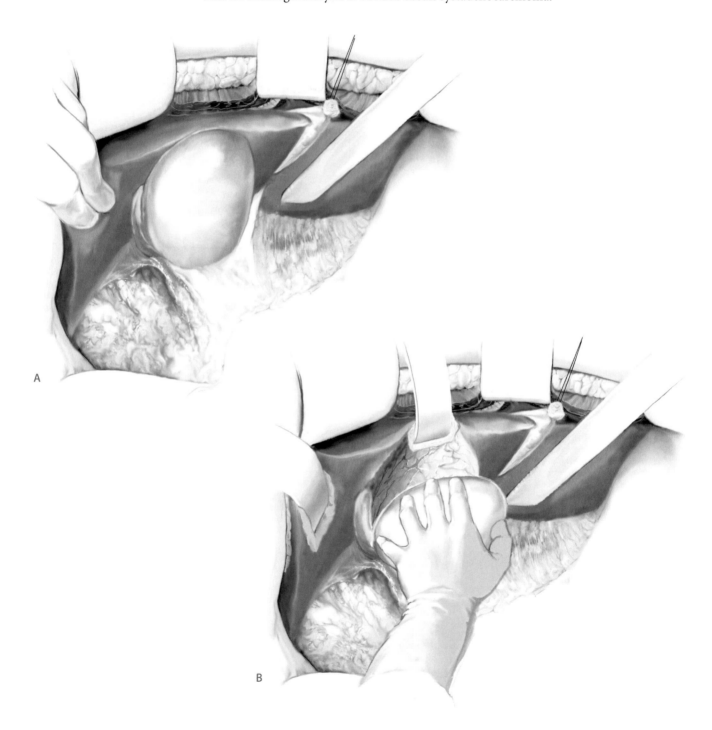

A

B

STEP 2   **Repair of vasculobiliary injuries**

When inadvertent injury of the bile ducts occurs, a fine (4-0 or 5-0 absorbable) interrupted suture is used for repair. Abdominal drainage is optional. Importantly, complete excision of the cystadenoma eliminates risk of recurrence.

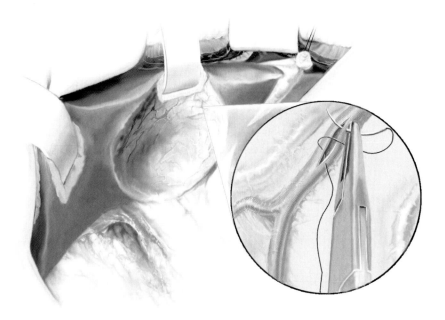

Laparoscopic Resection of Cysts

STEP 1

Access, approach and parenchymal transection

Laparoscopic resection is used to treat peripheral cysts, especially those in the left lateral sector (Sg2 and 3) or in the anterior segments (Sg4B, 5, and 6). The CT scan and the picture illustrate a simple cyst in Sg3. The approach described previously is undertaken. Three ports are usually used, and their placement depends on the site of the cyst.

The most common instruments used for this purpose are the Harmonic Scalpel, Tissuelink, CUSA, and surgical staplers. The surgeon needs to determine the most direct route for positioning the instrument to achieve a complete cyst resection with sparing of healthy parenchyma. Since these lesions are usually peripheral and the parenchyma is thin, at times the stapler has the capability of securing tightly both the superior and the inferior edges of the line of transection and results in a nearly bloodless margin. Identification of individual vasculobiliary structures in this situation is not necessary (A). When the tissue is too thick for stapling devices, the initial transection can be done with ultrasonic shears (B) or any other method of vascular sealing, and the pedicle taken with the staplers. The Pringle maneuver is usually not required for this type of transection.

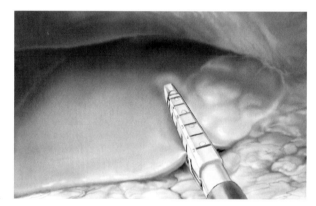

A

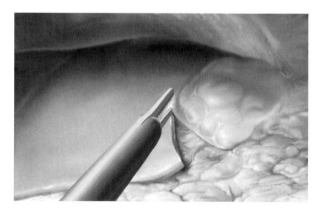

B

STEP 2

Resection of the specimen

After the transection of the hepatic parenchyma is completed, hemostasis must be confirmed by direct inspection. Sometimes it is useful to "feel" or abrade the transection line to exclude a vessel that has stopped bleeding temporarily but may act as a site of remnant bleeding once the pneumoperitoneum is evacuated and normal intra-abdominal pressure returns. If identified, hemostasis is secured by electrocautery, surgical clips, and hemostatic agents or devices when still available.

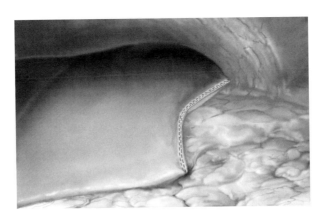

Postoperative Tests

- Routine postoperative surveillance for most patients
- Intermediate care or intensive care units for complicated cases of polycystic disease of the liver

Postoperative Complications

See chapter "Right Hepatectomy."

Tricks of the Senior Surgeon

- Although unroofing is simple, enucleation carries risk of hemorrhage. Make certain the hepatic duct and ligament is accessible for a Pringle maneuver if needed.
- Look for small biliary radicals after enucleation; drainage is not a good alternative to repair or suture ligation.
- During laparoscopic resection of hepatic cysts, be aware that major pedicles may not be amenable to sealing devices. Surgical staplers are still the best mechanism to secure structures.
- Like in any laparoscopic procedure with potential bleeding, do not hesitate to open up the patient in the presence of significant bleeding. Safety is still better than pride!

Pericystectomy for Hydatid Liver Cyst

Lucas McCormack

Patients with hydatid cysts in the liver used to present a therapeutic challenge. Although surgical techniques have improved, considerable controversy still exists regarding the most effective operative technique. The main principle of the surgery is to eradicate the parasite and prevent intraoperative spillage of cyst contents avoiding peritoneal spread. Pericystectomy provides a radical treatment removing the whole cyst "en bloc" including the adventitia without resection of healthy liver tissue.

Preoperative Treatment

Albendazol orally 10–14 mg/kg/day in two doses administered 2–4 weeks before and after surgery.

Indications and Contraindications

Indication	■ Peripheral hydatid cyst of the liver
Contraindications	■ Intrahepatic major vascular invasion ■ Invasion of right or left hepatic duct ■ Deep cyst within the liver parenchyma (>2–3 cm from liver surface) ■ General contraindication of liver resections

Procedure

| STEP 1 | Incision, exposure, and staging |

Access is performed as shown in the chapters on liver resection. Careful exploration of the abdominal cavity is done to exclude extrahepatic disease. The liver should be completely mobilized as for a major liver resection. Since accidental opening of the cyst may occur during mobilization, always have a cup with povidone-iodine (or hypertonic saline solution) ready to use in case of intraoperative spillage of cyst contents.

Inspection and manual exploration of both lobes of the liver need to be done with caution. Intraoperative ultrasound using a 5-MHz T-shaped probe is used to assess the number and location of the cysts. Particular attention is directed toward the relationship of the cysts with the portal veins, major hepatic veins, and the vena cava. In addition, meticulous examination of the cyst and the adjacent liver parenchyma can sometimes demonstrate a biliary communication.

| STEP 2 | Definition of the surgical approach |

Most of the cysts located in the right liver are easy to dissect away from the diaphragm. If not safely feasible, a partial resection of the diaphragm must be performed.

In case of major vascular involvement or with invasion of the left or right hepatic duct, an anatomical liver resection is indicated.

In case of a cyst located deep within the liver, liver resection is also recommended. However, when depth from the liver surface is less than 2–3 cm, a hepatotomy allows the cyst to be reached and a standard pericystectomy can be performed.

For cysts located close to the vena cava in segments 6 or 7, the liver needs to be mobilized as for a right hepatectomy.

STEP 3   **Preparation prior to pericystectomy**

The central venous pressure should be below 3 mmHg before starting the liver transection. A tourniquet is placed around the porta hepatis for inflow occlusion in case of bleeding. To prevent accidental spillage of the cyst contents, the whole space around the liver is packed using gauze swabs. A pack placed behind the right liver usually offers better exposure. The contents of the cyst should never be evacuated before resection. Stay sutures should not be placed in the cyst wall. However, stay sutures with silk 2-0 are placed in the liver parenchyma around the emerging part of the cyst to enable traction and better exposure during resection.

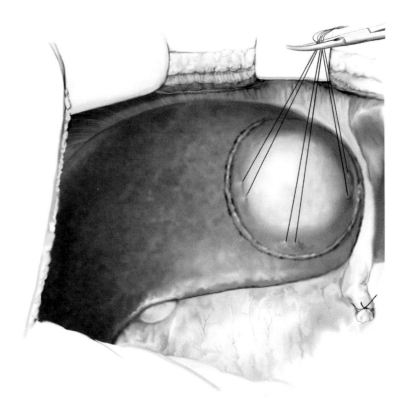

STEP 4

Resection of the cyst

The liver capsule is incised with diathermy. Careful identification of the correct plane of cleavage is crucial to avoid bleeding or spillage of the cyst contents (A). Intrahepatic vessels are coagulated selectively with bipolar forceps or ligated with metallic clips, ties or suture-ligatures depending on the diameter. Although several possible techniques for liver parenchyma dissection can be used (see chapter "Techniques of Liver Parenchyma Dissection"), we prefer the water jet, which enables a selective and safe separation of the cyst wall from the liver parenchyma (B). Small bile ducts should be carefully identified and tied. Hemostasia of the exposed raw surface of the liver can be improved with argon beam coagulator or topical fibrin derivates.

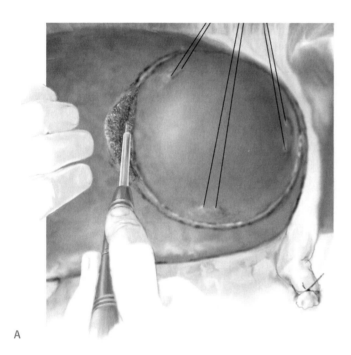

A

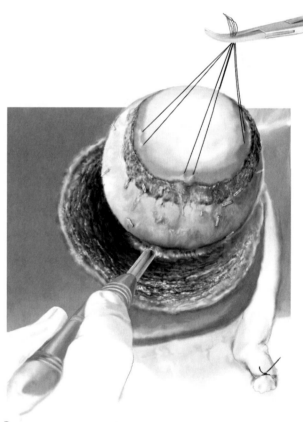

B

Postoperative Complications

■ Same complications as in liver resections
■ Biliary fistula is less common than in partial resection

Tricks of the Senior Surgeon

■ Use magnification loops to control bile leaks after pericystectomy. Careful repair should be done with suture-ligatures with Prolene 4-0 to 5-0.
■ At least two drains with powerful suction should be available in case of rupture of the cyst to avoid peritoneal spread of the contents.
■ Always have a cup with povidone-iodine (or hypertonic saline solution) ready to use in case of intraoperative spillage of cyst contents into the peritoneal cavity.
■ In case of intraoperative bleeding and technical difficulties during surgery, remember that adequate conservative surgery (e.g., partial resection of the cyst) can also achieve excellent results. The strategy can be changed anytime!

Special Maneuvers in Liver Trauma

Denis Castaing, Olivier Scatton, Marius Keel

Introduction

Liver injuries most often (>90% of all cases) are associated with other injuries such as ipsilateral rib fractures, lung contusions, other intra-abdominal lesions, or injuries of the extremities, the pelvis and the head. Hepatic injuries are graded according to the Organ Injury Scale of the American Association for the Surgery of Trauma (AAST-OIS) (Table 1).

Because clinical examination of the abdomen is unreliable in trauma patients with an altered level or loss of consciousness, a Focused Assessment with Sonography for Trauma (FAST) should be undertaken as an adjunct to the primary survey. In hemodynamically unstable patients with free fluid in FAST, a diagnostic laparotomy without further investigation is indicated. In stable patients, CT scanning of the abdomen represents the gold standard with evaluation of hemoperitoneum, parenchymal fractures, as well as vascular mapping including a three-phase study (arterial, portal and venous) as a preparation for a possible arterial embolization. The decision for operative or non-operative management of blunt hepatic trauma after CT scan is made according to the grade of liver injury and diagnosed or suspected other abdominal injuries, whereas for penetrating abdominal injuries an operative exploration of the abdomen is still standard.

Table 1. Grading of hepatic injuries according to the Organ Injury Scale of the American Association for the Surgery of Trauma (AAST-OIS)

Grade	Injury description	Incidence	Mortality
I	Subcapsular hematoma, <10% surface area Capsular tear, <1 cm in depth	20%	0%
II	Subcapsular hematoma, 10–50% surface area Intraparenchymal hematoma, <10 cm in diameter Laceration, 1–3 cm in depth, <10 cm in length	55%	<10%
III	Subcapsular hematoma, >50% surface area expanding or ruptured with bleeding Intraparenchymal hematoma, >10 cm in diameter or expanding Laceration, >3 cm in depth	15%	25%
IV	Parenchymal disruption involving 25–75% of lobe or one to three segments	7%	45%
V	Parenchymal disruption of >75% of lobe or more than three segments Juxtahepatic venous injury	3%	>80%
VI	Hepatic avulsion	<1%	Near 100%

Non-operative Management

Liver injuries grade I–III should be treated non-operatively. In case of active bleeding (diagnosed by CT scan), an angiographic embolization should be performed in patients with injuries grade I–IV. However, the following conditions should be fulfilled:

- Patient without altered level or loss of consciousness
- Hemodynamic stability or rapid stabilization after initial fluid resuscitation
- Exclusion of hypothermia, acidosis or severe coagulopathy
- No doubt about another abdominal lesion
- Intensive care unit available with continuous pulse and arterial blood pressure monitoring, repeated measurements of Hb, Hct and coagulation parameters, and careful follow-up clinical examination and sonography
- Availability of a surgical team
- Arteriography and experienced radiologist available

Indications and Contraindications

Indications for Laparotomy

- Hemodynamic instability
- Peritonitis on physical examination
- Other abdominal injuries in diagnostic studies
- Failed non-operative treatment

Procedure

Incision and abdominal exploration

A midline incision and, depending on the type of injury, an extension into the chest by median sternotomy or left or right thoracotomy is performed. The initial step in a trauma laparotomy is to pack all four quadrants of the abdomen in order to control hemorrhage as quickly as possible. The next step is to determine the site(s) of bleeding and injuries by exploration of the whole abdomen with special attention to the pancreas and the right retroperitoneal area. Packs are removed from one quadrant at a time, starting in the non-injured area and ending in the most seriously injured area. Injuries of the small or large bowel and of the biliary tree are repaired.

In addition, a rapid transfusion device with warmed crystalloids and blood is essential. After exclusion of hollow organ injuries, blood should be collected in the peritoneal cavity for autotransfusion (cell saver). Dilutional coagulopathy may follow massive blood transfusions, prompting the need for transfusion of platelets, fresh frozen plasma and/or activated factor VII.

In general, three situations can be found after laparotomy:

1. Diffuse severe active bleeding or cardiac arrest at the opening:
   The control of massive exsanguinating hemorrhage requires clamping of the aorta and/or inferior vena cava (IVC). Aortic control can be approached through a sternotomy or left thoracotomy allowing supradiaphragmatic, intrathoracic aorta cross-clamping and open cardiac massage in situations with cardiac arrest. This is predictable if an external cardiac massage on a "dying person with a tense abdomen" is performed. Furthermore, the suprarenal abdominal aorta can be approached through the gastrohepatic ligament or after medial rotation of the splenic flexure of the colon (Mattox maneuver). The infradiaphragmatic IVC can be controlled by direct digital pressure or clamping after an extended Kocher maneuver or right side to medial visceral rotation (Cattel Braasch maneuver).
2. No active bleeding from the liver:
   Simple hepatic injuries such as grades I, II or III without active bleeding do not require further operative investigation or treatment.
3. Active bleeding from the liver:
   Proceed with Step 2.

STEP 2   **Manual compression of the liver**

In case of active hemorrhage from the liver, the surgeon or ideally the assistant performs initial tamponade by manual compression for at least 10 min.

Then, two situations can be found:

1. When the hemorrhage can be controlled by manual compression, a competent team is available for appropriate assessment, and the patient is hemodynamically stable without hypothermia or acidosis, a one-step intervention leading to definitive surgical repair can be decided (see step 3).

2. When the hemorrhage is not controllable and hemodynamic instability, hypothermia, acidosis and coagulopathy occur, a liver packing (see step 9) with or without vascular control (see step 10) needs to be performed.

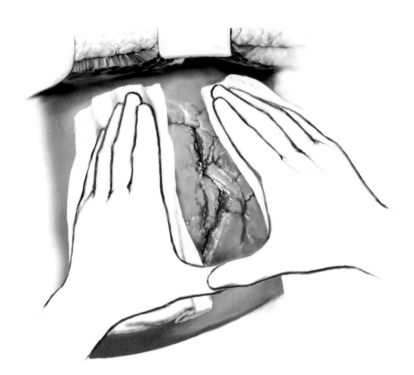

STEP 3

Mobilization of the liver

The liver can be fully mobilized to facilitate the examination and exploration of the posterior surface and the retrohepatic vena cava. It must be carefully done to avoid hepatic vein damage. After dissection of the falciform ligament, the right triangular, the coronary and the left triangular ligaments are divided while the assistant is taking care of the fracture by manual compression.

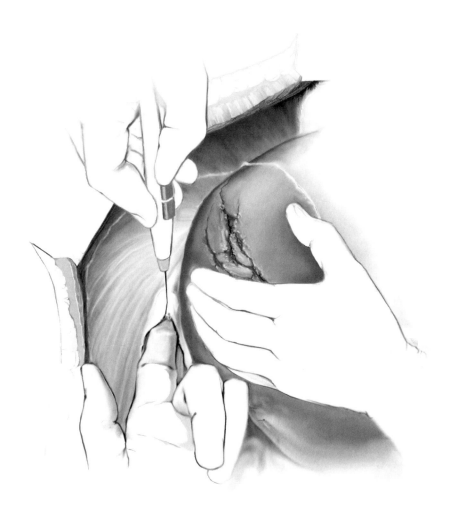

STEP 4   **Risk of hepatic vein damage during liver mobilization**

When liver packing is needed (step 9), hepatic mobilization is not recommended since this maneuver increases the risk of hepatic vein damage and aggravates the initial liver injury.

Major hepatic lesions are usually caused by a deceleration trauma leading to a liver fracture at the level of the right triangular ligament along the right hepatic vein. This location is often difficult to access. To stop the bleeding, the fracture should be closed by placing the assistant's hand beyond the fracture, while traction should be avoided.

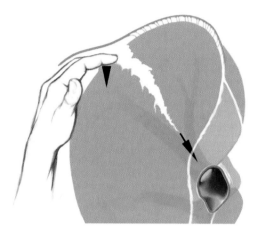

STEP 5   **Vascular ligation**

The wound may require enlargement to visualize the source of bleeding by utilizing finger-fracture technique and retractors (hepatotomy). Bleeding vessels can be controlled using sutures, surgical clips, and electrocautery. However, deep stitches, which could lead to ischemic areas, should be avoided.

While a Pringle maneuver might be required, prolonged pedicle clamping must be avoided whenever possible as it may aggravate ischemic injury caused by hypotension. If pedicle clamping longer than 30 min is needed, intermittent clamping is recommended (15 min of clamping and 5 min of reperfusion).

Hepatic defects can be filled by vascularized omentum (omentoplasty). This helps to eliminate dead space, tamponades venous oozing and may reduce the risk of a significant bile leakage.

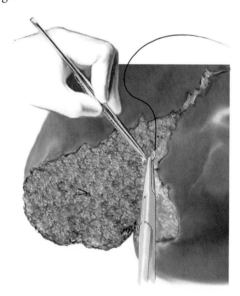

| STEP 6 | Resectional débridement |

Devitalized hepatic tissue needs to be removed because of the risk of abscess. The hepatic parenchyma is divided along the line of fracture in the plane between devascularized liver and the remaining parenchyma using the back of the scalpel handle. When resistance is encountered, this indicates the elastic tissue of vessels or biliary ducts, which are doubly clamped, divided and suture ligated. In most instances, a non-anatomical resection rather than a standard anatomical hepatectomy is preferred. A major hepatectomy is rarely indicated in the presence of extended injuries.

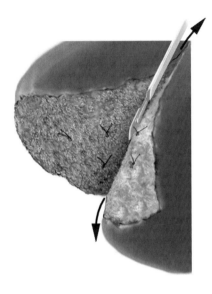

| STEP 7 | Ruptured subcapsular hematoma |

In case of a ruptured subcapsular hematoma, hemostasis is performed using an argon beam coagulator and the capsula is glued onto the bleeding parenchyma. The glue can be injected between the parenchyma and the glissonian capsule. Alternatively, the dissecting sealer (Tissue Link) can be used.

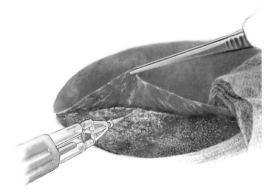

STEP 8   **Methylene blue test and cholangiography**

After complete hemostasis, the integrity of the biliary tract is evaluated by a methylene blue test. The test can be performed through a gallbladder puncture combined with a manual choledochal compression. Biliary leaks are repaired by selective ligations.
The opening of the gallbladder wall must be closed carefully (cholecytorrhaphy). In case of limited liver trauma, a cholecystectomy is referred, allowing cholangiography through the cystic duct to detect biliary leaks into the fracture line.

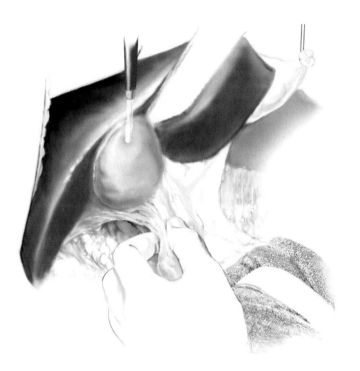

STEP 9

Packing

Packing is the mainstay of damage control. The principle is to perform a compression of the liver against the diaphragm (upper and posterior direction), which works very well for venous bleeding. Gauze swabs are placed around the liver – not inside the lesion – in order to compress the fracture and keep the compression against the diaphragm. However, no pack should be placed between the liver and the diaphragm to avoid a compression of portal veins and vena cava compromising venous return and resulting in decreased cardiac inflow and a portal venous thrombosis. However, the elevation of the diaphragm leads to a high peak airway pressure with hypoventilation which needs to be taken into account in the postoperative care.

The abdomen is closed under tension without drainage to maintain pressure on the packs. The increased intra-abdominal pressure represents a major risk for an abdominal compartment syndrome and therefore needs to be checked regularly.

If the hemorrhage is not controlled, manual compression is performed again and the liver is packed one more time. If this does not lead to control of the bleeding, partial or total vascular exclusion of the liver needs to be performed (Step 10).

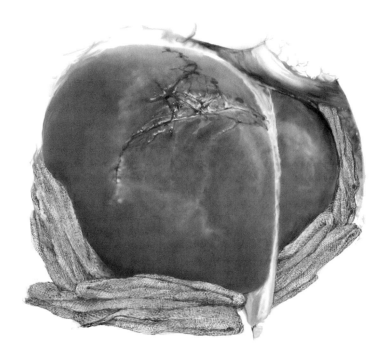

STEP 10   **Vascular control**

If packing fails to control hemorrhage in complex liver injuries, the Pringle maneuver allows hemorrhage control from the hepatic artery and portal venous system. The technique also helps to rule out other sources of bleeding such as retrohepatic veins and the vena cava. If this does not lead to control of the bleeding (grade VI lesions), total vascular exclusion of the liver is performed by clamping the supradiaphragmatic IVC after sternotomy and the infradiaphragmatic IVC (see chapter "Techniques of Vascular Exclusion and Caval Resection"). The appropriate and early use of vascular control allows for accurate identification of the injury and the control of hemorrhage.

STEP 11   **Hepatic venous exclusion**

In case of a retrohepatic caval injury, an atrial-caval shunt to the superior vena cava or a hepatic venovenous bypass should be employed additionally to the Pringle maneuver early in the operation to preserve venous return while repairing the retrohepatic caval injury. An atrial-caval shunt can be performed with a large chest tube through the right atrial appendage placed and advanced into the IVC distal to the renal veins. Additional side holes are cut in the tube at the atrial level. Tourniquets are tightened around the vena cava at the level of the supradiaphragmatic and suprarenal cava levels and the atrial appendage.

STEP 12   **Intrahepatic balloon tamponade**

Hemorrhage control for through-and-through penetrating liver injuries can be
achieved by an intrahepatic balloon, avoiding an extensive hepatotomy (tractotomy).
The intrahepatic balloon is created from a Penrose drain that acts as a balloon and
hollow catheter. Inflation of the balloon causes a tamponade within the liver
parenchyma. Alternatively a simple Foley catheter can be taken. The tamponade is
maintained for 48h.

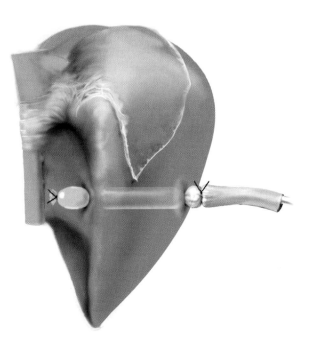

Postoperative Management

- Postoperative care on the intensive care unit requires a correction of hypovolemia and the "triad of death": hypothermia, acidosis, and coagulopathy.
- Frequent intra-adominal pressure measurements by means of a Foley catheter in the bladder should be made after primary closure of the abdomen to detect the development of an abdominal compartment syndrome.
- If packing is decided upon, a planned reintervention (second look) with removal of the packs, as well as repacking, definitive hemostasis and definitive abdominal closure or abdominal vacuum assisted closure, is necessary after the resuscitation period. The time point of the second look depends on rewarming, correction of acidosis and coagulopathy, which usually takes 24–48h.

Postoperative Complications

- Short term:
  - Hemorrhage
  - Abdominal compartment syndrome
  - Bile leaks
  - Liver failure
  - Acidosis, coagulopathy and hypothermia with multiple organ failure
- Long term:
  - Biloma
  - Biliary fistula
  - Biliary stricture
  - Abscess and hematoma infection

Tricks of the Senior Surgeon

- Do not hesitate to call for help (HPB surgeon).
- Request experienced anesthesiologists.
- Ask regularly for temperature and quantity of transfusions.
- Do not mobilize the liver until volume replacement has been achieved.
- Alert the anesthesiologist prior to clamping of major vessels, as a sudden decrease in venous return is tolerated poorly by hypovolemic patients.
- A decision to use packing is usually the best in a complex situation.

Technique of Multi-Organ Procurement (Liver, Pancreas, and Intestine)

Jan Lerut, Michel Mourad

Introduction

The growing success of liver transplantation led to the development of a flexible procedure for multiple cadaveric organ procurement as introduced by Starzl in 1984. The subsequent development of pancreas, multivisceral and intestinal transplantation has required modification and improvement of the initially described technique.

Different procedures, varying from isolated procurement of the different abdominal organs to total abdominal evisceration, were described during the 1990s.

The aim of every multiple organ cadaveric procurement should be the maximal use of organs, the minimal dissection of their cardinal structures as well as an adequate repartition of their vascular axes.

A technique combining minimal in situ dissection, rapidity, safe repartition of organs and easy acquisition of technical skills should become standard in today's organ transplantation practice.

Procedures

En Bloc Pancreas-Liver Procurement

STEP 1   **Access to the abdominal vessels**

A midline xyphopubic incision is performed. After exploration of the abdominal organs for previously undiagnosed pathologies, the white line of Toldt is incised, the right colon is mobilized to the left, duodenum and bowel are extensively kocherized, and the peritoneal root of the mesentery is divided from the right iliac fossa to the ligament of Treitz.

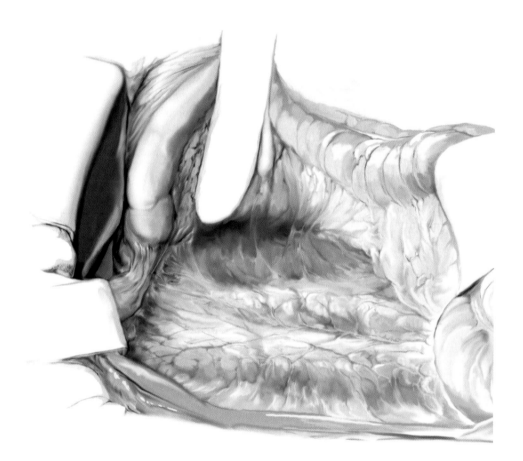

STEP 2   **Preparation of the major abdominal vessels**

The distal abdominal aorta and the inferior vena cava (IVC) are freed from their bifurcation to the level of the left renal vein. Slight traction on the distal duodenum by the assistant allows the procurement surgeon to identify the superior mesenteric artery, located just above the left renal vein. The periarterial solar plexus is incised longitudinally on its left side in order to visualize the first 2–3 cm of the superior mesenteric artery. This maneuver allows aberrant liver vascularization to be individualized (e.g., a right hepatic artery originating from the superior mesenteric artery) (A).

Next, the hepatoduodenal and hepatogastric ligaments are inspected for anatomic variants (e.g., a left hepatic artery originating from the left gastric artery).

The supraceliac part of the aorta is prepared for later occlusion by encircling it at the supra- or infradiaphragmatic level by means of a vessel loop (B).

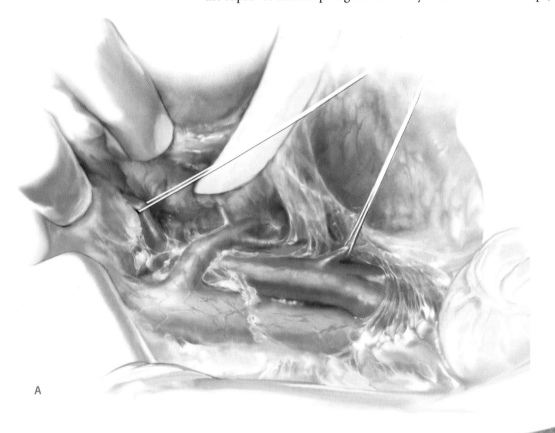

A

B

STEP 3   **Access to the pancreas**

The stomach is gently separated from the transverse colon by dividing the gastrocolic
ligament. This allows the whole pancreas to be visualized. The splenic artery can be
encircled and marked close to its origin from the celiac trunk; this mark can be helpful
during later ex-situ division of the pancreas – liver bloc.

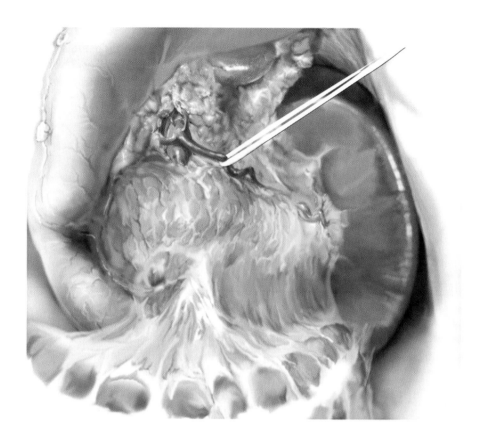

STEP 4 | Preparation and perfusion of the abdominal organs

The gallbladder fundus is opened with the electric cautery and gallbladder and bile ducts are flushed out with saline. Manual compression of the distal bile duct allows a better proximal duct cleansing, which should be completed through a small catheter once the bile duct is transected (A).

When the thoracic team is ready for procurement, heparin is given (500 units/kg body weight) and the aortic canula is inserted right above the aortic bifurcation. If the thoracic team prefers to clamp the suprahepatic IVC during the procurement, the IVC can be canulated at the same level as the aorta in order to obtain better decompression and clean exsanguination. For both the aorta and the IVC, chest drains can be used (B).

The portal vein does not need to be perfused in situ, but only during the back-table preparation.

The supraceliac aorta is clamped or ligated at the beginning of aortic perfusion with the preservation solution (e.g., 60 ml of UW solution/kg body weight) and the intravascular cooling of the abdominal organs is completed by abundant topical irrigation using cold saline.

The bile duct is transected just above the duodenal arch and needs to be rinsed once more with saline through a small catheter.

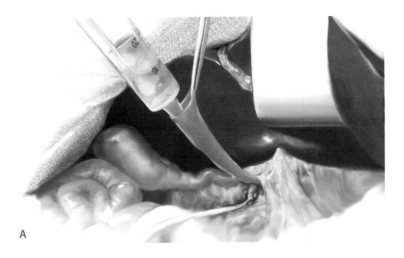

A

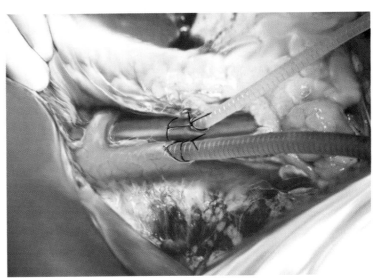

B

STEP 5

Preparation and procurement of the arterial axis

Once the abdominal organs are discolored and the thoracic procurement is completed, the en-bloc liver-pancreas procurement can start. The dissection of the superior mesenteric artery trunk is completed at the anterior side of the abdominal aorta. Retroperitoneal tissue and solar plexus located between IVC and aorta are transected from the left renal vein towards Winslow's foramen in order to fully expose the right side of the aorta and the superior mesenteric artery. Next, the anterior side of the aorta is incised just distally to the origin of the superior mesenteric artery. After visualization of the orifices of the renal arteries, an arterial aortic Carrel patch encompassing the origin of both superior mesenteric artery and celiac trunk is created. The simultaneous excision of the vascular roots of the tissue bloc is an important step of the en-bloc liver-pancreas procurement.

Afterwards, colon and intestine are repositioned in the abdomen. All branches of the left gastric artery are transected closed to the stomach, allowing the preservation of a possible left hepatic artery (LHA) originating from the left gastric artery.

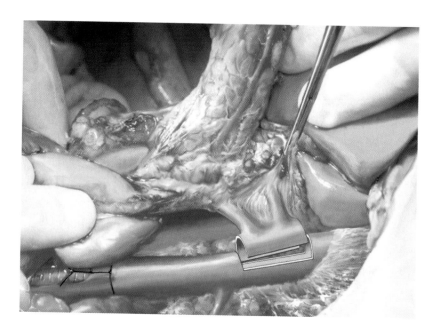

STEP 6	Preparation of the duodenum and the pancreas

After instillation of a betadine solution through a gastric tube, the duodenum and the jejunum are stapled distal to the pylorus and the ligament of Treitz, respectively. The mesenteric root is transected distally of the pancreas using the GIA stapling device. The splenocolic ligament is taken down and the spleen and the pancreas are freed retroperitoneally. Finally, the IVC is transected at the level of the right adrenal gland, the liver is mobilized by transection of the falciform ligament and the liver-pancreas bloc is removed containing a large diaphragmatic patch.

The *ex-vivo separation* of liver and pancreas is done on the back-table after identification of the vascular anatomy (see back-table work).

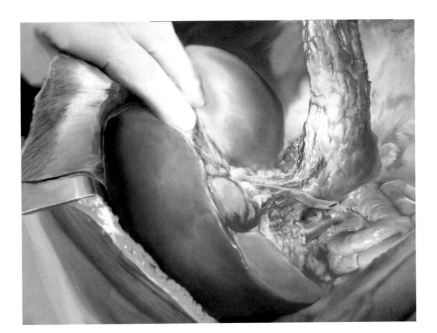

Modifications of the En-Bloc Liver Pancreas Procurement

Pancreas Removal for Islet Transplantation
For islet procurement, the pancreas is removed together with the liver and the duodenum is simply removed from the pancreatic head.

Procurement of Intestine for Transplantation
After initial preparation of the superior mesenteric artery and the celiac trunk, the intestine is repositioned adequately in the abdominal cavity. The first jejunal loop is transected about 10 cm distal to the ligament of Treitz using a GIA stapler . The transected jejunal loop is pulled up by the assistant in order to better individualize the mesenteric root. A second assistant maintains the intestine in place to avoid traction on the superior and inferior mesenteric veins, as malpositioning causes reduced splanchnic perfusion.

Several small branches of the jejunal mesentery are transected close to the serosa (as is usually done in a duodenopancreatectomy). The proximal part of the mesenteric vessels are freed for about 2 cm, so the small pancreatic veins joining the right part of the SMV are ligated, as well as those branches of the SMV draining the pancreatic isthmus. Once the SMV is freed, the abdominal organ perfusion can be started.

As soon as the perfusion is completed, the liver-pancreas-small bowel bloc can be retrieved. In case of an isolated intestinal transplant it can be necessary to extend the superior mesenteric vein and artery using free iliac venous and arterial grafts.

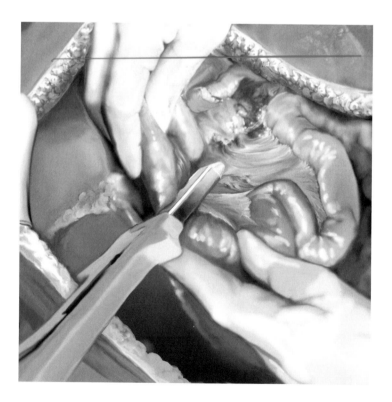

Back-table Work

First, the gallbladder and the bile ducts need to be flushed again to avoid mucosal damage by precipitating bile salts. Next, ex-vivo portal flushing is done through a canula introduced in the SMV. The tip of the portal vein catheter is positioned with slight finger compression.

The liver-pancreas bloc is positioned as in the abdominal cavity; the aorta patch, containing the celiac trunk and the superior mesenteric artery, is dissected free. Splenic, celiac, hepatic and left gastric artery should all be individualized; one should look as well for the RHA and the LHA. Bile duct and the portal vein and splenomesenteric venous confluence also need to be dissected. The final repartition of all vascular axes is dictated by their anatomical variability.

A. In the presence of standard arterial anatomy, the celiac trunk should be kept with the whole pancreas transplant. By doing so, a reconstruction with a Y-graft can be avoided as the superior mesenteric artery can be directly connected to the ostium of the common hepatic artery (for illustration see chapter "Orthotopic Liver Transplantation"). The repartition of the venous vessels is usually unproblematic if the *recipient* portal vein is transected close to the liver parenchyma.

B. If the liver-pancreas bloc contains an LHA originating from the left gastric artery, the celiac trunk should go to the liver graft. In this case, a vascular reconstruction between splenic artery and superior mesenteric artery is necessary using a free iliac arterial graft (see Sect. 6, chapter "Pancreas Transplantation").

C. In the presence of an aberrant RHA with a complete *extrapancreatic* course, one can decide to divide the superior mesenteric artery between the head of the pancreas and the origin of the aberrant right hepatic artery (see Figure). This allows for three different types of reconstruction (for illustrations see chapter "Orthotopic Liver Transplantation"):

   - Anastomosing the stump of the superior mesenteric artery on the ostium of the splenic artery
   - Anastomosing the celiac trunk or the common hepatic artery on the proximal ostium of the superior mesenteric artery
   - Anastomosing the aberrant right hepatic artery to the gastroduodenal artery

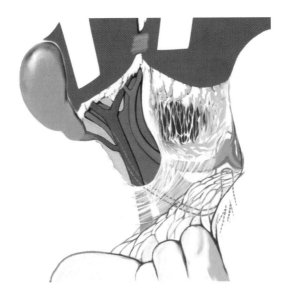

In the case of an *intrapancreatic* RHA, division of this artery should only be performed after discussion with the pancreas and liver teams. If this artery is transected proximal to the pancreatic head, it must be possible for the liver surgeon to implant the RHA into the ostium of the gastroduodenal or the splenic artery.

Both recipient teams must finally decide if both organs should be implanted because of technical difficulties.

The only anatomical absolute contraindication to simultaneous whole pancreas and liver transplantation is the presence of an important pancreatico-duodenal artery originating from an aberrant RHA. In this case, vascularization of the pancreatic head can be compromised, as the gastroduodenal artery and thus the superior pancreatico-duodenal artery are kept to retain the common hepatic artery for the liver allograft.

Tricks of the Senior Surgeon

- The correct procurement of iliac, superior mesenteric, carotid and jugular vessels is crucial as complex vascular reconstructions might be required during the implantation. Therefore, the whole iliac axis down to the inguinal ligament must be taken.
- The bile duct should be routinely rinsed by means of a small feeding tube through the cut end, as remaining bile salts precipitate and may damage the biliary epithelium. Flushing the biliary tree through the gallbladder cleans only the distal bile duct and thus is not enough!
- Correct back-table bath temperature must be guaranteed. Warming up of the solution and direct contact with the ice can both be harmful and can easily be avoided by separating the allograft from the crushed ice through a cold saline buffer.

Orthotopic Liver Transplantation

Robert J. Porte, Jan Lerut

Since its introduction into clinical practice in 1963 by Starzl et al., the technique of orthotopic liver transplantation has been refined progressively. The original technique included resection of the recipient inferior vena cava (IVC) and the use of extracorporeal venovenous bypass. More confidence with the technique and the more frequent use of technical variants in pediatric liver transplantation have led to the development of recipient cava-preserving hepatectomy techniques without use of venovenous bypass and with or without use of a temporary portocaval shunt, independently of anatomical and general status of the recipient. Regardless of the exact technique, orthotopic liver transplantation is characterized by three stages: the pre-anhepatic, the anhepatic and the post-anhepatic stage. The technique of orthotopic liver transplantation, either with or without preservation of the recipient IVC, will be described following these three stages.

Indications and Contraindications

Indications

a) Chronic liver failure (cirrhosis) due to:
 – Chronic hepatitis B, B and D (coinfection), and C
 – Alcoholic liver disease
 – Autoimmune hepatitis
 – Cryptogenic cirrhosis
 – Congenital liver fibrosis
 – Primary and secondary biliary cirrhosis
 – Primary sclerosing cholangitis
 – Biliary atresia
 Metabolic liver diseases:
 – Wilson's disease
 – Alpha$_1$-antitrypsin deficiency
 – Hemochromatosis
 – Protoporphyria
 Vascular diseases
 – Budd-Chiari syndrome
b) Acute liver failure
 – Viral [hepatitis A, B, D (coinfection), E]
 – Intoxications (e.g., acetaminophen, Amanita phalloides)
 – Acutely decompensated chronic liver disease (e.g., Wilson's disease)
 – Extensive liver trauma
 – Budd-Chiari syndrome
c) Metabolic disorders (e.g., tyrosinemia, familial amyloid polyneuropathy, primary hyperoxaluria)
d) Liver tumors
 – Hepatocellular carcinoma: single tumors <5 cm, or up to three tumors <3 cm (Milan criteria, extended criteria center dependent)
 – Metastases of neuroendocrine tumors
 – Benign (polycystic liver disease, giant hemangioma, Caroli's disease)

Contraindications
- Untreated systemic infections or sepsis
- Extrahepatic malignant disease
- Irreversible multiorgan failure

Preoperative Investigation and Preparation for the Procedure

History and physical examination:

Laboratory tests:	Liver tests, coagulation studies, kidney function, electrolytes, hepatitis and HIV serology
Doppler ultrasound:	Check for patency and flow of liver vessels (portal vein, hepatic artery, and hepatic veins)
CT scan or MRI:	Check for tumors, vascular collaterals, aneurysms of the splenic artery or splanchnic thrombosis
MRCP or ERCP:	May be indicated in primary sclerosing cholangitis
Angiography:	In case of portal vein thrombosis, planned retransplantation, and in case of hepatocellular carcinoma for TACE (trans-arterial chemo-embolization)
Classification:	According to the Child-Pugh criteria (bilirubin, albumin, prothrombin time/INR, ascites, encephalopathy) and/or according to the Model for End-Stage Liver Disease (MELD) score (serum creatinine, bilirubin, international normalized ratio, INR)
Histological examination:	Graft biopsy in case of suspected steatosis

Procedures

Orthotopic Liver Transplantation: The Pre-anhepatic Stage

STEP 1   **Access, exposure, exploration, and dissection of the hepatoduodenal ligament**

After a bisubcostal incision, the round and falciform ligaments are divided. Care must be taken to avoid injury of large collaterals or a repermeabilized umbilical vein, which may be present in the umbilical ligament due to portal hypertension. A retractor (e.g., Thompson) is installed followed by a careful mobilization of the left and right hemiliver. The left and right triangular and coronary ligaments are divided as for a left and right hemihepatectomy and the hepatogastric ligament is transsected by cautery or after step-wise suture ligation. A possible aberrant or accessory left hepatic artery needs to be identified and ligated. All these steps have to be performed with a particularly careful technique, as portal hypertension and consecutive dilation of the vascular bed leads to more fragile vessels which are prone to bleeding.

Next, the hepatoduodenal ligament needs to be palpated and checked for aberrant arterial anatomy, i.e., an aberrant or accessory right hepatic artery from the superior mesenteric artery, running behind the common bile duct. The peritoneum is opened on the ventral aspect of the ligament and the proper hepatic artery is identified.

A. Dissect the proper hepatic artery towards the liver. Ligate and divide the left and right hepatic artery distal from the bifurcation (A-1).

B. Encircle the common bile duct as high as possible (usually at the level of the cystic duct or above) in the porta hepatis, preserving an adequate amount of tissue surrounding it to avoid devascularization. Again, check for a possible aberrant right hepatic artery. Divide the common bile duct and ligate and divide the aberrant right hepatic artery, if present (A-2).

C. Dissect the portal vein completely free from its surroundings along the length of the hepatoduodenal ligament.

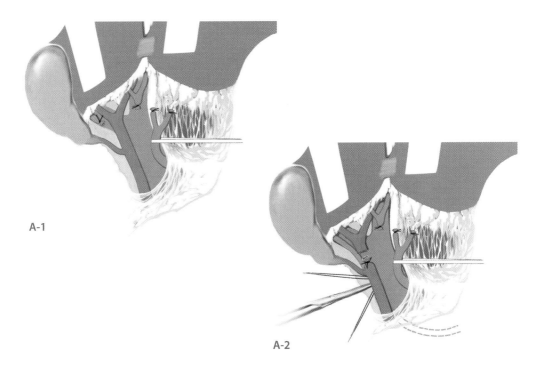

A-1

A-2

STEP 2   **Mobilization of the infrahepatic inferior vena cava**

At this stage of the operation, the planes of dissection are different for the classical (with resection of the IVC) and the cava-sparing (or piggyback) technique. The latter technique is more demanding but has the advantage of avoiding interruption of the caval venous return and of a shorter warm ischemia time during implantation, because only one instead of two IVC anastomoses have to be performed.

The two techniques will be described separately.

The Classical Technique with Resection of the IVC
The liver is turned to the left and the infrahepatic inferior vena cava is exposed. The right adrenal vein is identified and ligated between ties. The inferior vena cava is mobilized circumferentially by opening the peritoneal reflection along the right side of the cava with cautery. Care must be taken not to injure the right hepatic vein. The same technique is applied on the left side of the cava.

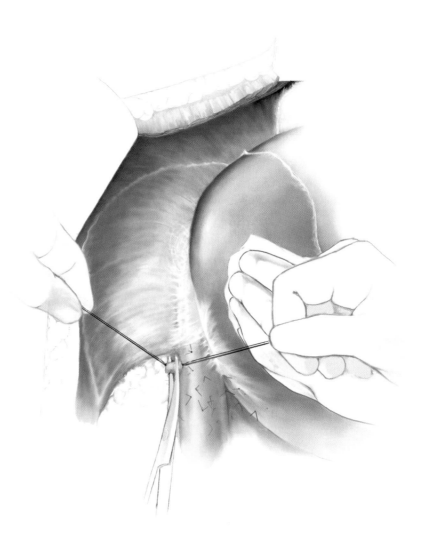

Mobilization of the infrahepatic inferior vena cava

The Cava-Sparing (or Piggyback) Technique

For this technique the right liver is rotated to the left upper quadrant in order to expose adequately the right and anterior sides of the retrohepatic IVC. The tissue between the retrohepatic IVC and the posterior surface of the liver is divided. All smaller Spigelian veins draining the caudate lobe and the right accessory veins when present are selectively ligated and divided from below upwards. In this way, the hepatic veins are approached. The right hepatic vein is encircled and transected using a vascular endostapler. Precise stapler application close to the liver parenchyma permits safe and tight transsection of the right hepatic vein without narrowing the retrohepatic IVC. The transsection of the right hepatic vein allows the retrohepatic-IVC to be turned away from to a further extent and makes the safe isolation of the middle and left hepatic veins much easier.

Some surgeons construct a temporarily end-to-side portal-caval shunt to reduce splanchnic pressure and bleeding and to facilitate mobilization of the liver (not shown).

In the case of a retransplant following a previous classical liver transplant with IVC replacement, the previous allograft's IVC is preserved. The plane between the parenchyma and the previous donor IVC will have remained intact. In case of a retransplant after previous cava-sparing transplant, the graft can be removed without interfering with IVC flow.

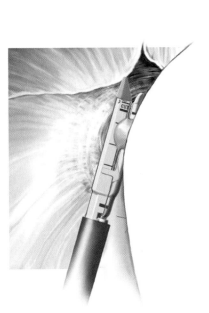
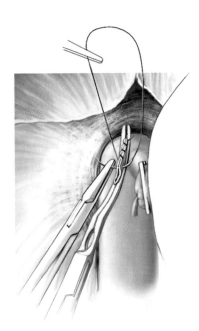

The Anhepatic Stage

STEP 3   **Removal of the native liver**

Before completion of the recipient hepatectomy, hemostasis of the retroperitoneal bare
areas is performed using an argon beam coagulator. The bare areas are not routinely
oversewn in order to keep the available space for the allograft to the maximum.

The Classical Technique with Resection of the IVC
Ligate and divide the portal vein as high up into the hilum as possible (A-1). Place
vascular clamps on the suprahepatic and infrahepatic IVC and transsect it (A-2).

The Cava-Sparing (or Piggyback) Technique
After clamping and division of the portal vein high up in the liver hilum, the middle and
left hepatic veins are clamped and transected and the native liver is removed.

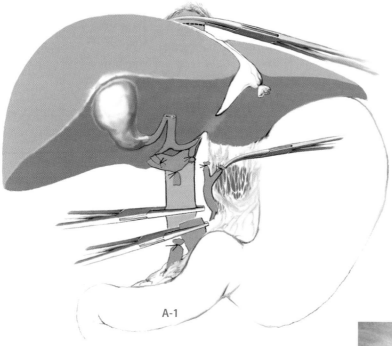

A-1

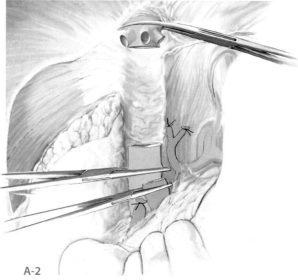

A-2

| STEP 4 | Anastomosis of the IVC |

The Classical Technique with Resection of the IVC

The suprahepatic vena cava of the recipient is sutured to the suprahepatic cava of the donor liver in an end-to-end fashion, using running polypropylene 3-0. During each step, the vessel wall is everted to obtain nice endothelium to endothelium apposition.

Identical procedure for the infrahepatic vena cava. A sterile suction catheter can be positioned in the retrohepatic cava transanastomotically for venting upon. Do not tie the infrahepatic anastomosis yet (A-1).

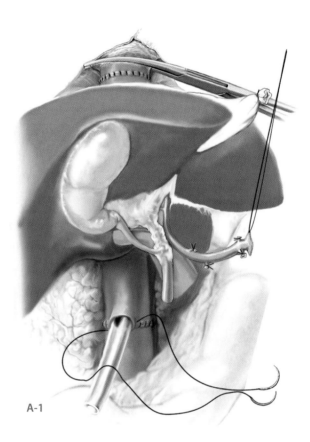

A-1

Anastomosis of the IVC

The Cava-Sparing (or Piggyback) Technique
The retrohepatic IVC of the allograft needs careful preparation on the back-table. The upper cava cuff is shortened flush to the hepatic veins. The lower cava cuff of the allograft is shortened up to the level of the first major vein draining segment 1 and subsequently oversewn with a running polypropylene 4-0 or 5-0 suture. A suctioning catheter can be positioned through this suture to facilitate flushing of the liver upon reperfusion (see below).

From here on, three different methods can be used to anastomose the donor and recipient IVC:

a) *End-to-end anastomosis.* The ostia of the three hepatic veins are interconnected to create a wide opening for the suprahepatic caval anastomosis (A-2) and an end-to-end anastomosis is performed with the suprahepatic IVC of the donor liver (A-3). This technique
    is becoming less popular because of the risk of (partial) venous outflow obstruction due to kinking of this relatively narrow anastomosis.

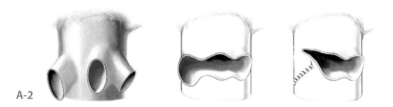

A-2

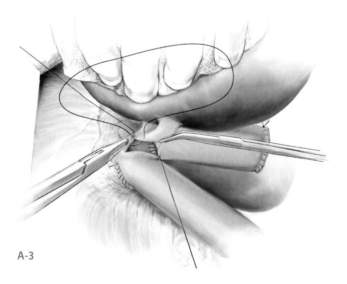

A-3

STEP 4 (continued) **Anastomosis of the IVC**

b) *Side-to-side cavo-cavostomy.* The donor suprahepatic IVC is closed as well with running polypropylene 4-0 suture, and a 6-cm-long cavotomy is made on the left posterior side of the donor IVC. This cavotomy should encompass the orifices of the major hepatic veins in order to obtain optimal venous allograft drainage and to permit later procedures such as transjugular biopsy or TIPS placement (A-4). A *large* anastomosis is made between the left posterior wall of the donor IVC and the anterior wall of the recipient IVC using partial clamping of recipient IVC (A-4). The anastomosis is performed from the right (or the left) side by using two running sutures of polypropylene 4-0. This anastomosis is rendered easier using a specially designed caval clamp.

c) *End-to-side cavo-cavostomy.* The suprahepatic end of the donor IVC is spatulated on the dorsal side over 4 cm, allowing a wide anastomosis. The anterior wall of the recipient IVC is partially clamped as described above. A wide (>6 cm) anastomosis is subsequently made between the spatulated suprahepatic IVC of the allograft and the recipient IVC in an oblique end-to-side fashion, using two running sutures of polypropylene 4-0 (A-5). An advantage of this technique is that the anastomosis can be made as wide as possible and that the blood flow from the hepatic veins follows a more direct course into the IVC, compared to the side-to-side technique.

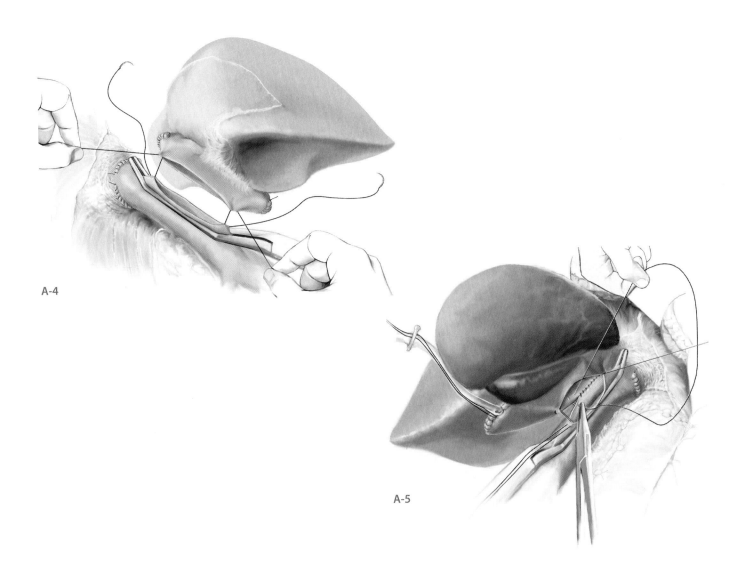

A-4

A-5

STEP 5   **Anastomosis of the portal vein**

From here on, the procedure is essentially the same for both the classical and the IVC-sparing techniques.

After cutting the donor portal vein to adequate length, the portal vein is anastomosed end-to-end, using running polypropylene 5-0 or 6-0. Avoid kinking or rotation and flush the recipient portal vein briefly to remove any clots. Ensure an adequate growth factor of about 3/4 the diameter of the vessel (A-1).

When the recipient portal vein is not suitable for anastomosis (i.e., after longstanding thrombosis), or when the two portal vein stumps are too short, a segment of common iliac vein from the donor can be used to extend the donor portal vein or as a jump graft to the superior mesenteric vein (A-2, A-3). In case of portal vein thrombosis, cannalization can usually be obtained using the eversion thrombectomy technique.

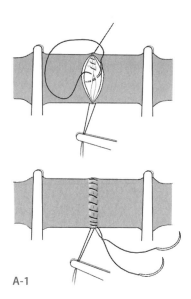

A-1

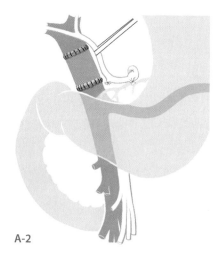

A-2

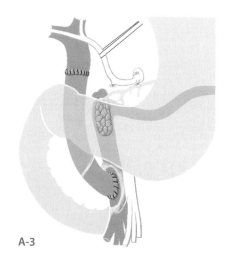

A-3

The Post-anhepatic Stage

STEP 6   **Reperfusion of the donor liver**

Reperfusion can be done in different ways.

- Remove the vascular clamp from the portal vein and reperfuse the liver, flushing 300–400 ml of blood via the catheter in the infrahepatic IVC to remove air, preservation solution and potassium from the graft. Remove the catheter in the inferior vena cava and tie the suture at the infrahepatic cava. Subsequently, slowly remove the vascular clamp at the suprahepatic and infrahepatic vena cava (in case of a classical procedure) or the clamp at the anterior aspect of the IVC (in case of a cava-sparing technique).
- When anastomosing the portal vein, the allograft can also be flushed retrogradely via the IVC. Advantage of this technique is complete restoration of the caval venous return to the heart before reperfusion of the graft.
- Once the liver is reperfused, topical irrigation of the liver with warm saline facilitates rewarming.
- Some centers flush the liver with albumin solution prior to reperfusion.

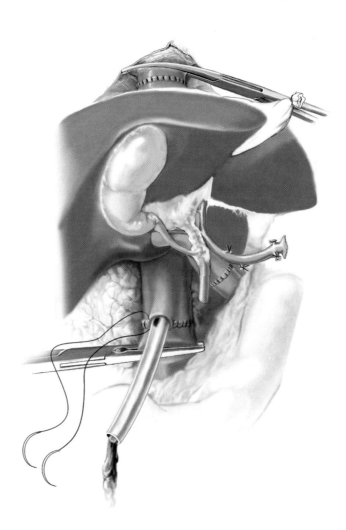

STEP 7   **Arterial anastomosis**

There are several options for the arterial anastomosis. In most cases, an end-to-end anastomosis is made between the common hepatic artery or celiac trunk of the donor and the common hepatic artery or the bifurcation of the left and right hepatic arteries of the recipient, using running or interrupted polypropylene 6-0 or 7-0 (A-1). Depending on the length and diameter of the vessels, alternative sites for anastomosis are possible. The recipient artery should be adequately flushed to remove clots, before completing the anastomosis.

Accessory or aberrant donor arteries should be revascularized by either making a direct anastomosis to the recipient artery or by anastomosing it to the stump of the gastroduodenal artery or splenic artery of the graft (A-2.1, A-2.2, A-2.3).

When the recipient artery is not suitable for grafting (i.e., hepatic artery thrombosis or severe stenosis of the celiac trunk), a segment of iliac artery from the donor should be used as a conduit to make a direct anastomosis with the supratruncal or infrarenal abdominal aorta. In some cases, the donor artery is long enough to make a direct anastomosis between the donor celiac trunk and recipient supratruncal aorta (A-3). When an iliac conduit is used, it can either be anastomosed in an end-to-side fashion to the supratruncal aorta after removal of the native liver (A-4), or to the infrarenal aorta, when the anastomosis is delayed until after reperfusion of the liver via the portal vein (A-5). In the latter situation, clamping of the aorta during construction of the anastomosis will not interfere with the portal perfusion of the graft.

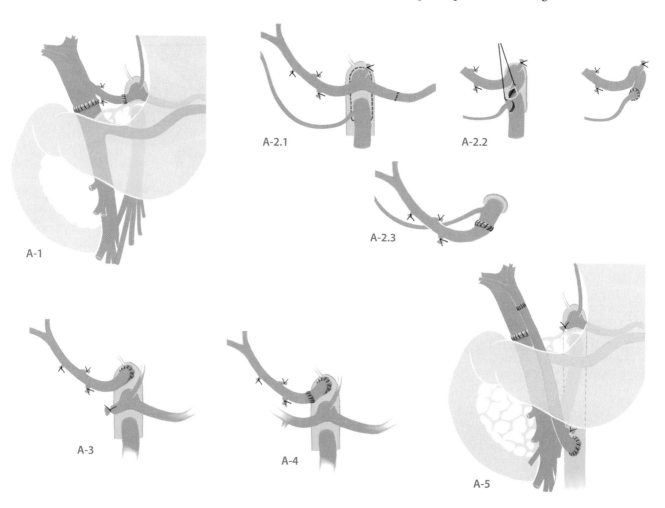

A-2.1

A-2.2

A-2.3

A-1

A-3

A-4

A-5

STEP 8   **Bile duct reconstruction**

The bile duct is shortened on both the donor and the recipient side, until adequate bleeding is obtained from both ends. The bile duct anastomosis can be made in an end-to-end fashion, using interrupted PDS 5-0 to 7-0. An alternative is a side-to-side anastomosis (as shown in the chapter on biliary anastomoses). A biliary catheter can be introduced via the recipient common bile duct and placed transanastomotically using a T-tube. In patients with primary disease of the bile ducts, such as primary sclerosing cholangitis, the bile duct usually should be reconstructed by a Roux-Y hepatico-jejunostomy. However, some surgeons would perform a direct duct-to-duct anastomosis when extrahepatic strictures and inflammation have been excluded.

Before closure, three abdominal vacuum drains are placed (Redon or Jackson Pratt drain): two subdiaphragmatic drains (one on the left and one on the right side) and an infrahepatic drain behind the anastomosis.

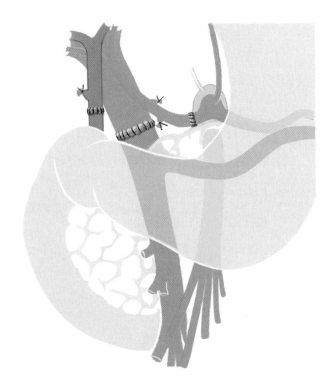

Venovenous Bypass (Optional)

Depending on the center, a venovenous bypass will be used systematically, occasionally, or never. When venovenous bypass is used during the anhepatic stage, this usually includes drainage of (a) the portal vein and (b) the lower part of the body via the left greater saphenous vein into the left axilliary, brachial or internal jugular vein. An alternative for direct cannulation of the portal vein stump is cannulation of the inferior mesenteric vein. The centripetal Biopump with heparin-coated, armed cannulas is the most widely used one. Before use, the cannulas are primed with normal saline or an equivalent solution.

A 6-cm longitudinal incision is made in the left groin, just below Poupart's ligament, and the proximal end of the greater saphenous vein is isolated and encircled with sutures. After ligation of the distal side, the cannula of the venovenous bypass is inserted via a small venotomy in the proximal side of the greater saphenous vein and advanced into the femoral vein. The portal vein can be cannulated either directly by inserting and securing the cannula into the stump of the recipient portal vein or by cannulation of the inferior mesenteric vein. The axillary vein is cannulated following an identical procedure as for the saphenous vein, via a small longitudinal incision in the left axilla. It is also possible to insert a large bore catheter transcutaneously into the internal jugular vein.

Some centers perform a temporary portosystemic shunt, which will not be covered in this chapter.

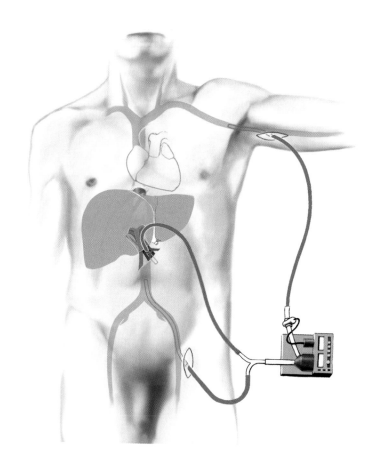

Postoperative Tests

- Laboratory tests: liver tests, coagulation studies, kidney function, monitoring of levels of immunosuppressive drugs
- Doppler ultrasound: check for patency of the liver vessels
- Liver biopsy when rejection is clinically suspected

Postoperative Complications

- Early (<14 days):
  - Hepatic artery thrombosis or stenosis
  - Primary non-function (death of patient without retransplantation)
  - Initial poor function (definition center dependent)
  - Acute rejection
  - Massive ascites
  - Budd-Chiari syndrome
  - Portal vein thrombosis
  - Biliary leakage
  - Bleeding
- Intermediate/late (>14 days):
  - Acute or chronic rejection
  - Abdominal infections
    - Intra-abdominal abscess
    - Infected ascites
  - Systemic infections
    - Viral [e.g., cytomegalovirus (CMV) or Epstein-Barr virus (EBV)]
    - Fungal
    - Bacterial
  - Biliary complications
    Intra- and/or extrahepatic stenosis and/or sludge formation
  - Vascular complications
    - Hepatic artery thrombosis
    - Portal vein thrombosis
    - Venous outflow tract obstruction
  - Recurrent disease
    - Malignancies
    - Post-transplant lymphoproliferative disorders
    - Skin cancer

Management of the Most Common Complications

- Primary non-function (<5%): early retransplantation
- Rejection: increased immunosuppression
- Hepatic artery thrombosis: immediate surgical thrombectomy with or without intra-hepatic thrombolysis. If severe ischemic biliary strictures or hepatic necrosis develop, retransplantation should be considered
- Infectious complications should be treated as usual (e.g., surgical or percutaneous drainage and appropriate anti-infectious chemotherapy)
- Ascites/edema: Avoid fluid overload in the first week after transplantation, diuretics if necessary

Tricks of the Senior Surgeon

- For both the classical approach and the cava-sparing technique, the central venous pressure should be kept as low as possible. Otherwise the dissection of the liver from the retrohepatic IVC and the dissection of the Spigelian veins is rendered more difficult, which leads to increased blood loss.
- A short period of hypotension is usually seen upon reperfusion of the graft. This can be due to bleeding or metabolic changes (i.e., "post-reperfusion syndrome"). When venous bleeding occurs from the (retrohepatic) inferior vena cava or dorsal side of the liver, provide temporary packing for the retrohepatic space and wait for hemodynamic stabilization before attempting to place any sutures.
- In case of preexisting portal vein thrombosis, adapt donor and recipient operations to reduce ischemic time. Be assured, before starting the allograft implantation, of the method of portal revascularization. First make the arterial anastomosis and revascularize the liver via the artery. This will provide more time to remove clots and perform the anastomosis of the portal vein, without extending the cold or warm ischemia time.

Partial Cadaveric Liver Transplantation: Donor Procedure and Implantation

Massimo Del Gaudio, Xavier Rogiers, Daniel Azoulay

In 1989 Pichlmayr et al. were the first to report a case of splitting a cadaveric liver for two recipients, an adult and a child. In the same year, Bismuth et al. performed the first transplantation of a single liver into two adult recipients with fulminant hepatitis. Today, donor livers are split for an adult and a pediatric recipient or, less frequently, for two adults.

Indications and Contraindications

General Donor Criteria

- Age <55 years
- Weight >70 kg
- Hemodynamic stability
- Normal liver function tests
- No macroscopic aspect of liver steatosis
- Graft-to-recipient body weight ratio >1 %

Donor Procedure: *Ex-Situ* Versus *In-Situ* Splitting

In general, the liver graft can be split either during the procurement procedure (i.e., in situ) or on the back-table after a conventional donor procedure (*ex situ*).

For *ex-situ* splitting of the liver, the whole organ is retrieved as described in the chapter "Technique of Multi-Organ Procurement." Grafts are then prepared in the recipient transplant center. An alternative is the *in-situ* splitting technique, which is closely related to the techniques established for living related donor procurement.

Although the *ex-situ* split is the most widely used method to transplant two patients with one liver, extended cold ischemic time and some rewarming due to the longer back-table procedure as compared to conventional liver transplantation increase the risk of graft dysfunction in the recipient. While *in-situ* splitting potentially eliminates this problem, its application is limited due to a more time-consuming and technically more demanding explantation procedure.

Back-Table Procedure for *Ex-Situ* Splitting

During back-table splitting, attention should be paid to keep the liver cold. After standard procurement of the liver graft, the presence of a portal bifurcation is checked by inserting a blunt metallic probe into the portal trunk. The anatomy of the hepatic artery and the bile duct is identified by dissection, probing or back-table X-ray with contrast medium.

The ultimate dissection of the portal vein, the hepatic artery, the biliary tree and the suprahepatic veins is performed on the back-table.

Procedures

In-Situ Split Liver Donor Procedure for an Adult and a Pediatric Recipient

The goal of this procedure is to obtain the following grafts:

- Graft for adult recipient: Segments 4–8
- Graft for pediatric recipient: Segments 2 and 3

STEP 1

Mobilization and transection of the left lateral segments

Segments 2 and 3 are mobilized and prepared in an identical manner as for a living donor procedure. The left hepatic artery and the left portal vein are isolated. Particular attention is paid to preserve the arterial branch to segment 4 whenever possible. The left hepatic vein is identified and controlled by placing a vessel loop around it to allow vessel-loop guided parenchymal transection (see the chapter "Hanging Maneuver for Right Hepatectomy").

Optionally a cholangiography can be performed as shown in the chapters on living donor procedures.

Parenchymal transection is performed along the falciform ligament (resection line 1 in A-2). The hepatic veins are separated, the left hepatic vein remaining with the left graft, whereas the right and the middle hepatic veins remain with the right graft in continuity with the inferior vena cava.

Once the division of the parenchyma reaches the hilar plate it is cut straight with a scalpel slightly toward the left side, thus cutting the left hepatic duct blindly. This avoids unnecessary dissection of the bile duct which would compromise the biliary arterial blood supply.

Segment 1 is partially resected, with ligation of portal branches originating from the posterior aspect of the portal bifurcation and the hepatic veins draining into the inferior vena cava.

This will help the implantation of the right graft on the recipient's inferior vena cava.

The resection encompasses the left part of segment 1 and extends to the right side of the IVC. Although the resection of the left part of segment 1 is not mandatory, it is recommended as it permits better exposure of the left hepatic vein during the implantation procedure.

In case of a too large right graft or when the perfusion of segment 4 is not optimal, segment 4 can be resected after implantation (resection line 2 in A-2).

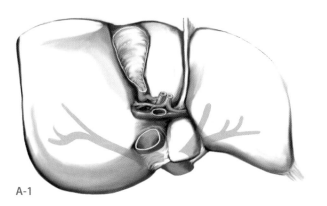

A-1

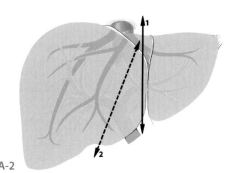

A-2

STEP 2   **Procurement of the grafts**

Now the graft is prepared for procurement. Flushing of the organs is performed as in a
standard multiorgan procurement. The left or right portal vein is cut at its origin and
the orifice is closed with a 7-0 monofilament running suture. If the portal vein is to be
cut at the origin of the left branch, the branches from the first centimeters of the left
branch of the portal vein to segment 1 are secured between ligatures and divided in
order to gain length and to allow for coaxial anastomosis to the recipient's portal vein.
In a standard situation, the artery is divided at the origin of the right hepatic artery,
leaving the celiac trunk with the left graft. The left hepatic vein is divided and the left
graft is removed and stored. Then the right graft is removed.

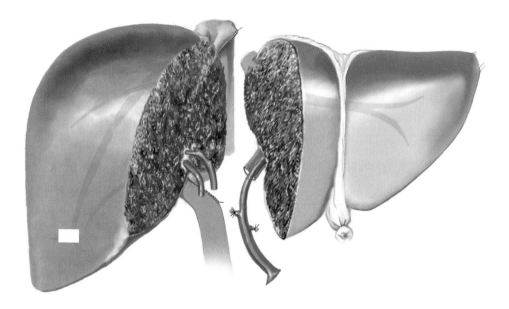

In-Situ Splitting for Two Adult Recipients

The goal of this procedure is to obtain the following grafts:

- Right graft: Segments 5–8
- Left graft: Segments 2–4

The hepatic dissection starts with complete mobilization of the right liver including isolation of the right hepatic vein, which is prepared for vessel loop guided parenchymal transection. Short accessory hepatic veins draining the right liver are preserved if they are larger than 5 mm as they need to be anastomosed during implantation of the right graft.

The portal vein and the hepatic artery are prepared as described in the section on adult and pediatric split liver procedure. In a standard situation, the celiac axis remains with the left graft. Regarding portal bifurcation, the portal vein trunk is kept in continuity with the left graft. In case of portal trifurcation, the portal trunk is kept with the right graft. The plane of transection is to the right of the middle hepatic vein, so the whole of segment 4 is included in the left graft. This procedure yields two grafts as shown in **A-1**, **A-2**. In contrast to the split liver procedure for an adult and a pediatric recipient, in this situation the cava remains with the left graft.

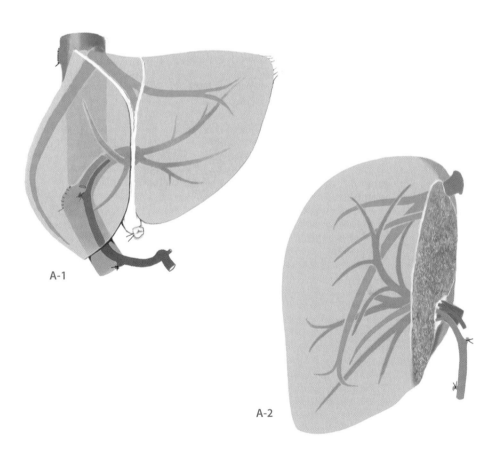

A-1

A-2

Implantation

Implantation of the Right Graft When the Liver is Split for an Adult and a Pediatric Recipient

STEP 1	Preparation of the graft

As in this situation the cava remains with the right graft, side-to-side cavocavostomy is possible and yields optimal allograft outflow. The preparation of the graft consists of resection of the upper and lower inferior vena cava cuffs at a level beneath the first major hepatic veins draining the residual part of Sg1. A 6-cm-long cavotomy at the right posterior side of the inferior vena cava encompasses the orifices of the major hepatic veins (A-1, A-2).

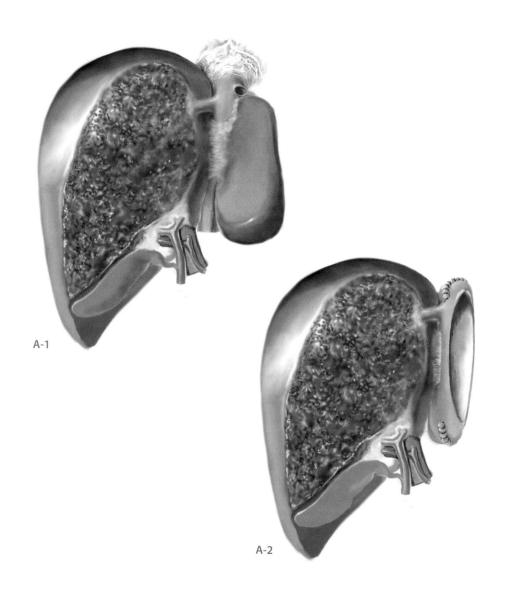

A-1

A-2

STEP 2

Side-to-side cavocavostomy

A side-to-side cavocavostomy using partial clamping of the recipient inferior vena cava is performed (see also chapter "Orthotopic Liver Transplantation"). Resection of the retrocaval and left part of Sg1 during back-table procedure improves exposure and thereby easy anastomosis between the two caval veins. The same technique can be applied for the left graft in a procedure for two adult recipients, as in this situation the cava remains with the left liver.

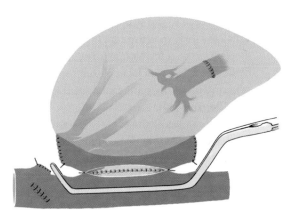

STEP 3

Portal vein, hepatic artery and bile duct anastomoses

An end-to-end portal vein anastomosis is performed between the right branch of the portal vein of the graft and the common trunk of portal vein of the recipient. If long enough, the right hepatic artery is anastomosed to the hepatic artery of the recipient at the level of the bifurcation with the gastroduodenal artery. Otherwise it is anastomosed to the right or common hepatic artery. Finally, the right hepatic duct is connected to the common bile duct of the recipient applying the same technique as in orthotopic liver transplantation.

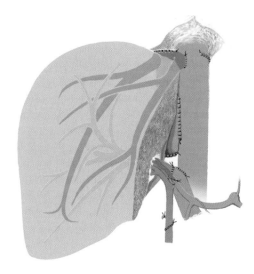

**Implantation of the Right Graft After Splitting for Two Adult Grafts
or After Right Living Donor Procurement**

Implantation of the left graft when the liver is split for two adult recipients is described in the chapter on left living donor transplantation.

In the situation of living donor procurement or split liver procedure for two adult recipients, the cava remains in the donor or with the left graft, respectively. Therefore, the venous outflow is reconstructed by anastomosing the donor's hepatic veins to the recipient's vena cava. The hepatectomy in the recipient is performed as for an orthotopic liver transplantation with preservation of the inferior vena cava. The orifices of the middle and left hepatic veins are oversewn or stapled; the right hepatic vein is directly anastomosed to the stump of the right hepatic vein or to a wider orifice in the recipient's vena cava. Any inferior hepatic veins more than 5 mm in diameter are also anastomosed directly to the inferior vena cava. A significant hepatic vein from segment 5 or 8 needs to be drained. This can be achieved by constructing a jump graft by means of a saphenous vein or, depending on the anatomic situation, by creating a common orifice with the right hepatic vein.

Anastomoses of the portal vein and the hepatic artery are performed as for the split graft for adult and pediatric recipients and the biliary continuity can be restored by biliodigestive anastomosis as shown in the Figure or by the direct connection between right hepatic duct of the right graft and common bile duct of the recipient.

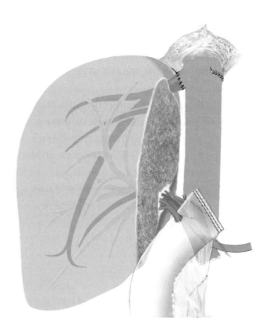

Implantation of the Left Graft in a Pediatric Recipient (Sg2 and 3)

As in this situation the cava stays with the right graft, the left hepatic vein is anastomosed directly on the inferior vena cava of the recipient. It is fundamental to keep the hepatic vein short as too long a vein can lead to kinking of the caval anastomosis. End-to-end anastomosis of the portal vein between the donor's left portal vein and the recipient common trunk is performed. Finally, the celiac axis of the left graft is anastomosed to the hepatic artery of the recipient at the level of the gastroduodenal artery and biliary continuity is reconstituted by a Roux-en-Y biliodigestive anastomosis.

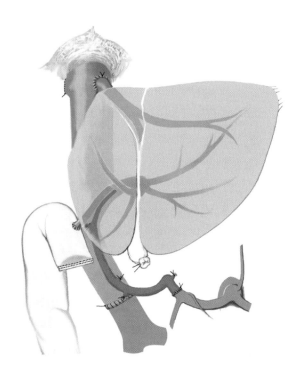

Alternative Management of the Hepatic Venous Outflow in Split Liver Transplantation for Two Adults

In split liver transplantation for two adults, the maintenance of an optimal venous outflow is of great importance to safeguard a maximal parenchymal integrity. In principle the same venous reconstructions and anastomoses are made as in right liver donation, including reanastomosis of segment 6 veins and reconstruction of larger segment 5 or 8 veins as shown. Additionally two techniques, not usable in living donation, can be applied to make the implantation easier while maintaining optimal venous outflow.

Splitting of the Inferior Vena Cava

This technique can be used in the *in-situ* as well as in the *ex-situ* technique. The front- and backwall of the vena cava are cut longitudinally, thus obtaining a caval patch on both grafts containing the respective hepatic veins as well as a possible segment 6 vein on the right side and Sg1 veins on the left side. At implantation the caval patches are sewn into the front wall of the preserved recipient vena cava.

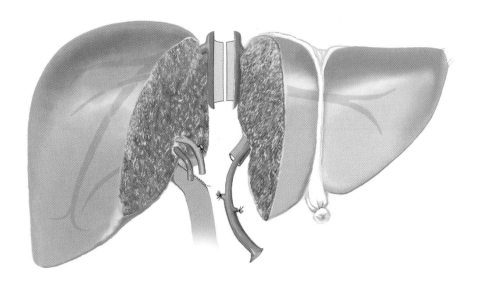

Splitting of the Middle Hepatic Vein

This technique can only be performed in *ex-situ* splitting. During parenchymal transection the middle hepatic vein is cut through the middle, in continuity with its orifice in the vena cava (A). On both sides it is reconstructed using donor iliac vein patches. In this way larger segment 5 or 8 veins are drained without the need for any further reconstructions or anastomoses (B-1, B-2).

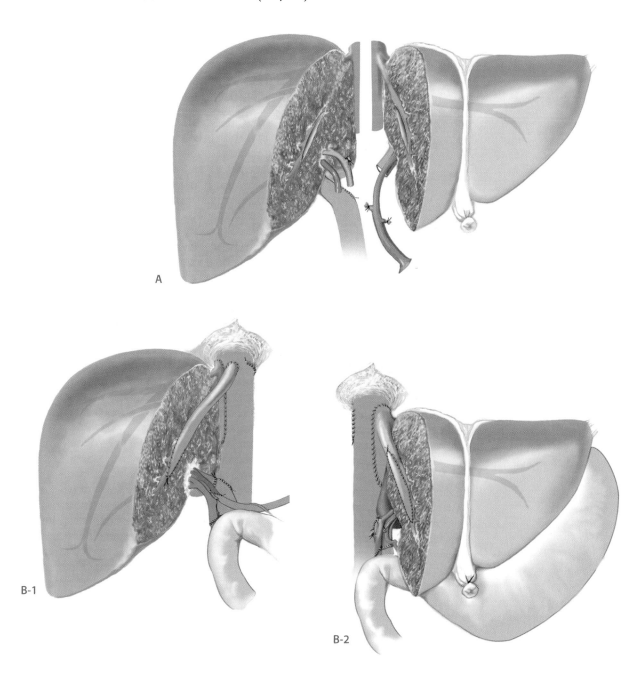

Routine Postoperative Tests

- Doppler ultrasound examination daily in the intensive care unit, then weekly until discharge
- Laboratory parameters as for orthotopic liver transplantation

Postoperative Complications

- Biliary leaks from the raw surface, which usually resolve with percutaneous drainage
- Other complications are the same as for orthotopic liver transplantation or living donor transplantations and should be treated accordingly

Tricks of the Senior Surgeon

- Sharp transection of the parenchyma is preferred as it leaves a flat surface allowing for most efficient hemostasis.
- Clips have a propensity to drop off during the implantation procedure. Therefore, every individual vessel seen on the cut surface is closed with stitches. During this step, care is taken to avoid liver rewarming by applying cold towels, leaving only the cut surface exposed.

Right Living Donor Hemihepatectomy

Zakiyah Kadry, Pierre-Alain Clavien

Indications and Contraindications

General Donor Criteria	■ Age 18 and 60 years ■ ABO compatibility between donor and recipient ■ No major medical problems ■ Significant long-term emotional relationship to the potential recipient ■ Donor competent to give informed consent
Donor Contraindications	■ Donor age <18 years or >60 years ■ ABO blood group incompatibility ■ Significant co-morbid condition (e.g., morbid obesity, coronary artery disease) ■ Multiple previous upper abdominal operations ■ Hepatic steatosis >30% (cut off center dependent) ■ Donor remnant liver volume <5% of the total liver volume ■ Significant celiac artery stenosis ■ Anatomic variations (center dependent) ■ Body mass index >28 (if a liver biopsy is not performed)

Right Lobe Living Donor Workup

■ Psychological evaluation and clinical examination
■ Laboratory tests for undiagnosed liver disease
■ Non-invasive tests for the assessment of liver volume and anatomy:
  – CT scan or MRI for volumetry and vascular reconstruction
  – Magnetic resonance cholangiopancreatography (MRCP) or CT cholangiography for biliary anatomy (center dependent)
■ Invasive tests:
  – Liver biopsy (center dependent)
  – ERCP (center dependent)

Procedure

STEP 1	Access and intraoperative evaluation

After a bilateral subcostal incision an appropriate retractor (e.g., Thompson retractor) is placed as for a conventional right hemihepatectomy. The division of the round and falciform ligaments is followed by a careful exploration of the abdominal cavity. The falciform ligament should be cut at a distance from the liver as it will be sutured to the diaphragm at the end of the procedure. The left triangular ligament is also preserved to fix the remnant left liver. Guided by intraoperative ultrasound (A-1), the position of the middle hepatic vein is marked by electrocautery (A-2) and any intrahepatic lesions missed on the preoperative workup are excluded.

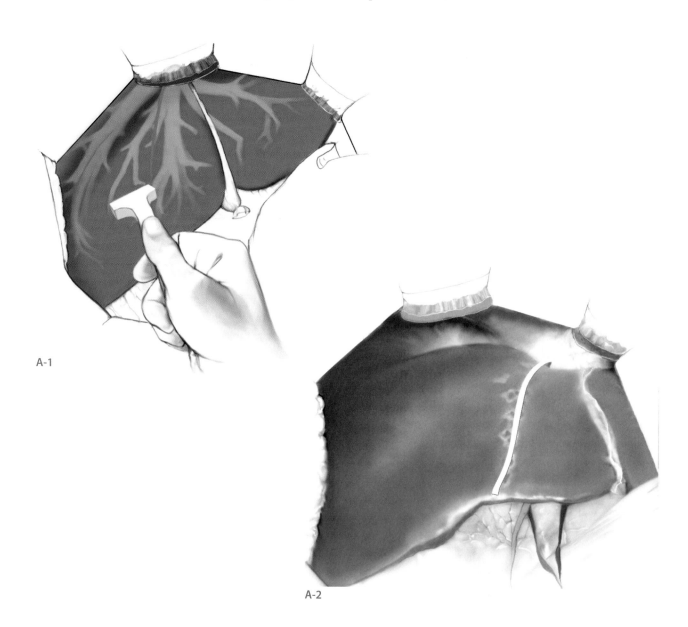

A-1

A-2

STEP 2

Hilar dissection

A cholecystectomy is performed and an intraoperative cholangiogram is obtained with a radiopaque marker such as a metallic clip or a small metal bulldog clamp placed near the point where the right hepatic duct is thought to lie. At completion of the cholangiogram and once no contraindications to living donation are identified on exploration, the recipient is brought to the operating room.

Next, the hepatic hilum is exposed and the posterior right aspect is palpated to check for a right hepatic artery arising from the superior mesenteric artery (SMA). The peritoneum and lymphatic tissue are divided on the right lateral aspect of the hepatic hilum avoiding skeletonization of the common bile duct as this could lead to strictures. After identification of the right hepatic artery on the posterior aspect of the bile duct it is followed both to its bifurcation distally and to its origin proximally without traction. The proximal point may occasionally be just distal to the point of origin of the segment 4 branch (which should be preserved to avoid vascular compromise of segment 4), the gastroduodenal artery or the origin of the left hepatic artery. An adequate length of right hepatic artery is required and the point of proximal transection is variable depending on the donor anatomy.

The right portal vein branch is identified posterior to the bile duct in the right hilum. When isolating the right portal vein, care must be taken to identify clearly the confluence of the right and left portal veins as well as the main portal vein trunk. The posterior branch arising from the right portal to the caudate process should be identified and divided between ligatures to avoid accidental tearing and hemorrhage. A vessel loop can be placed around the right portal vein.

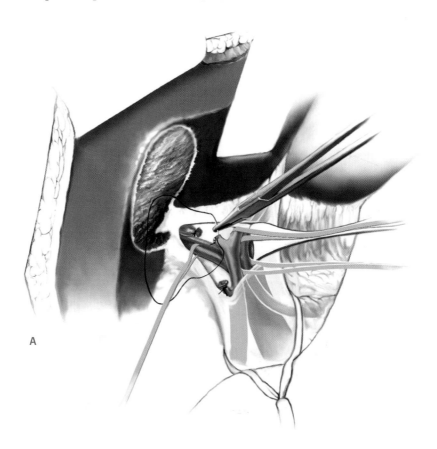

A

Hilar dissection

If a portal vein trifurcation is present, the anterior and posterior branches should be individually identified and separately encircled.

The point of transection of the right hepatic duct as decided by intraoperative cholangiography is marked either with a metallic clip or a fine suture. The division of the right hepatic duct is started on its anterior wall at 2–3 mm from the confluence with the left hepatic duct. Then, the posterior wall of the right hepatic duct is divided, leaving an adequate cuff to close the remaining donor side using a continuous suture of 5-0 or 6-0 resorbable PDS or Maxon without causing a stricture of either the common or left hepatic ducts. If there are an additional one or two bile ducts draining segments of the right liver into the left hepatic duct, they are identified and divided during the parenchymal dissection.

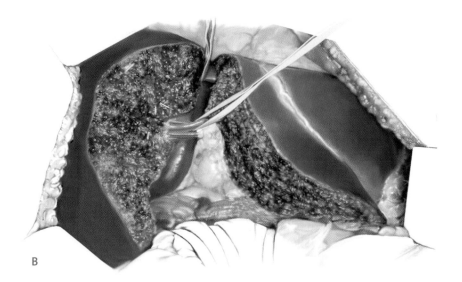

B

STEP 3	Mobilization of the right lobe and preparation of the right hepatic vein

The right liver is mobilized basically as for a conventional right hemihepatectomy with the important difference being that short accessory hepatic veins greater than 5 mm in diameter should be preserved for venous reconstruction in the recipient.

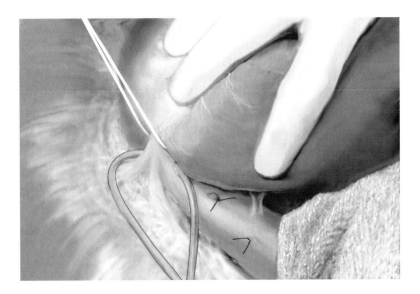

STEP 4

Hepatic parenchymal transection

The line of hepatic transection should be approximately 1 cm to the right of the middle hepatic vein, identified and demarcated at the start of the procedure by intraoperative ultrasound. The line of demarcation can also be checked by placing a vascular or bulldog clamp on the right hepatic artery and right portal vein.

Alternatively, a partial Pringle maneuver involving the left hemiliver by temporarily occluding the left hepatic artery and portal vein using an umbilical tape is also possible. This allows demarcation of the line of transection, which can be marked using electrocautery. Next, two stay sutures (2-0 silk) are placed on either side of the line of demarcation on the inferior border of the liver as for a conventional right hemihepatectomy.

The anesthesiologist is asked to maintain a low central venous pressure below 3 mmHg. In case the hanging maneuver (see chapter "Hanging Maneuver for Right Hepatectomy") is used, it is prepared at this stage. Although different techniques for liver dissection can be used, Hydrojet or CUSA without inflow occlusion is preferred in most centers.

In a standard right donor hepatectomy, the middle hepatic vein is conserved and remains with the donor left liver. When V5 and/or V8 are significant and have to be preserved, they are carefully identified during the dissection and divided between a vascular metal clip on the right side and a ligature of 2-0 silk on the left side close to the middle hepatic vein. This preserves the V5 and V8 veins for venous drainage reconstruction in the recipient.

On completion of the parenchymal transection, time is taken to re-check for hemostasis and any potential bile leakage on both the graft and donor side.

STEP 5   **Right graft explantation**

When the parenchymal transection is complete, the right graft is separated and only remains attached to the donor by the right hepatic artery, right portal vein, right hepatic vein and possibly accessory veins to the cava. The right hepatic duct is usually divided either just prior to or at the end of the parenchymal division.

There are two methods of right liver graft removal: either an "in situ" perfusion with cold preservation solution, or graft removal after placement of vascular clamps and "ex situ" back-table perfusion. In some centers an intravenous bolus of heparin is administered to the donor 5 min prior to graft explantation.

Ex situ perfusion technique: the right hepatic artery is proximally tied and divided. A vascular clamp is placed on the right portal and hepatic veins, which are also divided respectively. The graft is removed and flushed on the back-table with a cold preservation solution. As for a cadaveric liver transplantation, the bile duct needs to be flushed separately.

In situ perfusion technique: cannulation of the right portal is started by placing a vascular clamp closed to the portal vein bifurcation without obstructing the left portal vein. A catheter is introduced into the right portal vein and is fixed with a 2-0 silk ligature just distal to the clamp. The right hepatic vein is divided followed by the right hepatic artery while the perfusion of the right hemiliver through the catheter is started. The right graft is then removed and subsequently further perfused with cold preservation solution on the back-table.

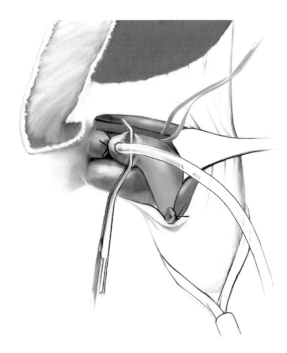

STEP 6   **Closure of donor vessels and hepatic duct**

Both the right portal vein and right hepatic vein should be cut at the time of graft explantation with an adequate cuff on the remaining donor vessel. This is especially important in the case of the portal vein, where iatrogenic stricture and twisting should be avoided at all costs. In the case of a portal vein trifurcation, the right anterior and right posterior portal vein branches should be divided separately without attempting to obtain a common cuff to avoid causing a stricture of the remaining donor portal vein. The hepatic vein stump is closed with a continuous 4-0 Prolene suture, and the portal vein stump is oversewn with a continuous 5-0 or 6-0 Prolene suture.

The transected border of the left liver is again checked for hemostasis. Potential bile leaks may be identified by placing a wet gauze sponge on the cut surface for 5–10 min. Any areas of bile leakage are oversewn with a 5-0 PDS suture and re-checked. The remnant liver is fixed by suturing the attached falciform ligament to the diaphragm. This prevents potential rotation of the left liver and an iatrogenic Budd-Chiari syndrome in the postoperative period. The abdomen is closed without placement of a drain.

Complications

These are the same as for right hemihepatectomy, the most common being:
- Biliary fistula
- Sustained hepatic dysfunction
- Biliary strictures

Tricks of the Senior Surgeon

- In performing the hilar dissection, start on the right lateral aspect when identifying the right portal vein and hepatic artery. This avoids excessive dissection and skeletonization of the right hepatic duct and bile duct.
- Identification of the biliary anatomy by intraoperative cholangiography should be performed early in the operation. A radiopaque metal clip or small bulldog should be used to mark the area of the right hepatic duct during the cholangiogram. An atraumatic bulldog can be placed on the distal bile duct to avoid passage of contrast into the lower bile duct.
- Marking the pathway of the middle hepatic vein by intraoperative ultrasound helps decide the parenchymal transection line, which should be 1 cm to the right of the middle hepatic vein.
- Central venous pressure should be maintained low by anesthesia as it helps to reduce blood loss.
- The hanging maneuver makes the parenchymal dissection easier, particularly in the last part.

Living Donor Transplantation:
Left Hemiliver Donor Procedure and Implantation

Koichi Tanaka, Hiroto Egawa

For laparoscopic left hemiliver donor procedure see chapter by D. Cherqui.

Open Donor Procedure for Left Living Donor Liver Grafts

STEP 1 | **Access and mobilization**

Access is gained through a bilateral subcostal incision with cranial extension. The falciform ligament is divided leaving enough length on the liver side as it needs to be fixed in the recipient. Finally a retractor (e.g., Takasago retractor) is installed (**A**).

The lateral segment is lifted up and a towel is placed in front of the spleen for its protection. A sponge is placed behind the left triangular ligament and the lateral segment is placed back. The left liver is pulled downward and the left coronary ligament and the left triangular ligament are divided by a cautery knife (**B**).

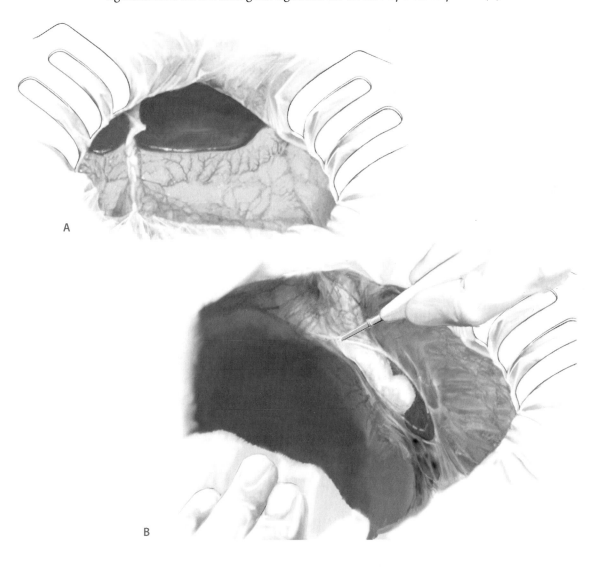

A

B

STEP 2   Approach to the left hepatic vein and the left side of the cava

The lateral segment is rotated to the right, and the ligamentum venosum is encircled, ligated and divided near the inferior vena cava (A). The connective tissue is detached from the superior aspect of the Spigelius lobe to expose the left side of the inferior vena cava as well as the posterior surface of the left hepatic vein (B).

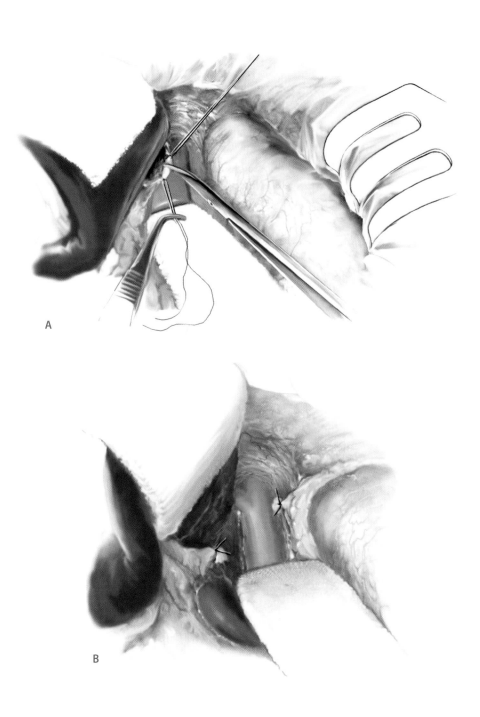

A

B

STEP 3 · · · Dissection of the hepatoduodenal ligament

The serous membrane on the ventral aspect of the hepatoduodenal ligament is detached at the level of the cystic duct and the hepatic arteries are identified. The left and middle hepatic arteries are dissected out at the hepatic hilum up to the bifurcation of the right and left hepatic artery (A). The middle hepatic artery can be cut off when it is clearly smaller than the left hepatic artery.

When the anterior aspect of the hepatoduodenal ligament is separated, the common bile duct can be identified. After the left hepatic duct is identified a small vascular clip is placed to the predetermined cut line on the bile duct. A 24-G puncture needle with a trocar is inserted into the common bile duct and cholangiography is obtained (B).

In some cases, the left hepatic duct may be located inside the hepatic parenchyma and it is difficult to be identified. In such cases, it can be identified during the dissection of the parenchyma.

The cholangiography provides information of the biliary anatomy and allows to determine the dissection line of the left hepatic duct (C). After the cholangiography, the catheter is removed and the puncture site is closed by a 6-0 Prolene stitch. The left hepatic duct can now be encircled at the point of predetermined cut line (D).

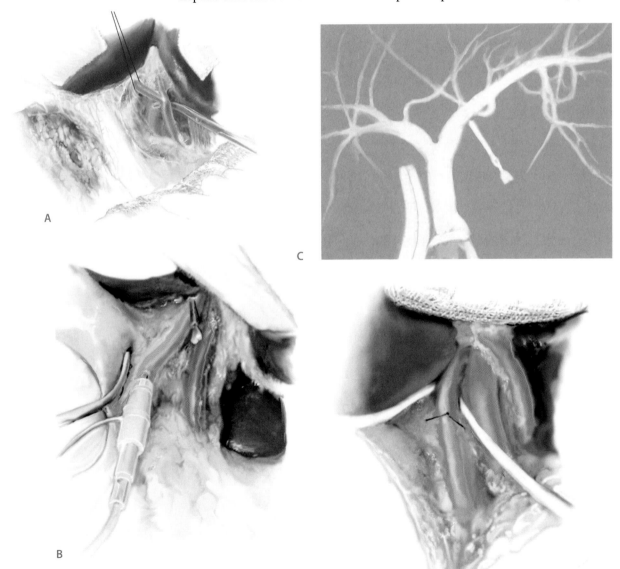

A

B

C

D

STEP 4   **Parenchymal dissection**

For a Left Lateral Segment Graft (Sg2 and 3)

A cutting line is marked on the surface with a cautery knife approximately 1 cm to the right of the falciform ligament (**A**). Without any vascular obstruction during parenchymal dissection, the liver surface is incised with a cautery knife and the parenchyma is dissected with a Cavitron Ultrasonic Surgical Aspirator (CUSA) in combination with a bipolar cautery with irrigation system for hemostasis.

Small vessels are dissected with the cautery knife while thicker vessels (i.e., diameter >3 mm) are ligated or clipped. Large vessels are clamped, dissected and suture-ligated by 5-0 or 6-0 Prolene stitches.

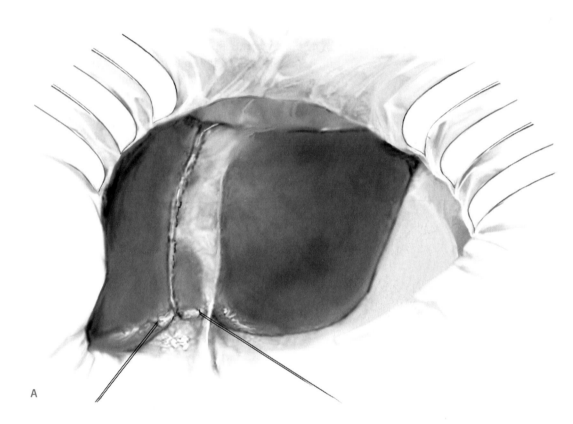

A

STEP 4 *(continued)*   **Parenchymal dissection**

For a Left Lateral Segment Graft (Sg2 and 3)

The left hepatic duct can be found where the parenchymal dissection line meets the hepatic hilus region (right side of the left portal branch) (B). The left hepatic duct is cut at the previously determined site. The hilar plate and the stiff fibrous tissue are dissected with a cautery knife. The left hepatic duct is closed with 6-0 Prolene suture on the donor side.

In the left lateral segment graft, reconstruction of the Sg4 hepatic duct is not necessary and it can be closed after confirming the direction. The Sg4 duct can be closed on the donor side too.

It is crucial to free the left portal vein branch completely through ligation and isolation of the caudate branches. They extend from the horizontal part of the origin of the branch.

For the parenchymal dissection, curved DeBakey forceps are used as a guide. The tip of the forceps is inserted between the caudate lobe and the lateral segment from the head direction of the portal vein. The forceps are lifted and fixed. The cutting line of the parenchyma is made between the marked incision of the surface and the tip of the forceps (C).

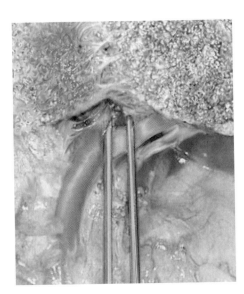

B

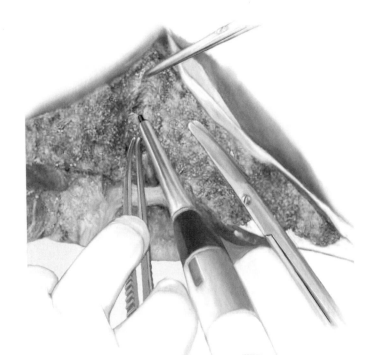

C

STEP 4 *(continued)*   **Parenchymal dissection**

For a Full Left Hemiliver Graft without caudate lobe (Sg2–4)

The cutting line for left hemiliver graft is marked on the surface with electrocautery starting from the right side of the middle hepatic vein to the liver bed of the gallbladder. The location of the middle hepatic vein is confirmed with ultrasonography before parenchymal dissection. The cutting line on the posterior side starts from the liver bed and reaches to the right side of the predetermined cutting point of the left hepatic duct.

The parenchymal dissection follows the sagittal plane from the top surface until the level of the middle hepatic vein (line 1). When the entire middle hepatic vein is included in the graft side, the direction of the dissection is changed in an oblique plane (line 2). To prevent injury of the middle hepatic vein and its small venous branches, some parenchymal tissue should be left on the middle hepatic vein. After dissection of the left hepatic duct, the direction is changed toward the space between the lateral segment and the caudate lobe (line 3). The curved DeBarkey forceps are useful as a guide as in left lateral segmentectomy.

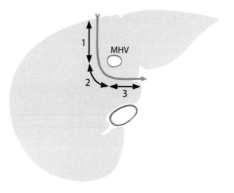

STEP 5   **Preparation of the hepatic veins**

The tissue around the hepatic veins is separated and the confluence of the left hepatic vein and the middle hepatic vein is exposed using the CUSA. Small branches around the confluence should be stitched with 6-0 Prolene suture and divided. Do not use hemostatic clips as they might interfere with the vascular clamp.

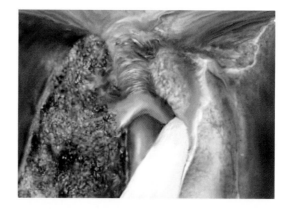

STEP 6

Perfusion and removal of the graft

After accomplishing the parenchymal dissection, the donor is systemically administered 1,000 units of heparin. The left hepatic artery is clamped with two clips and divided. The anterior wall of the left portal vein is opened and the tip of the catheter for perfusion is inserted into the lumen. Subsequently the left portal vein is divided (A-1). The left hepatic veins is clamped with a spoon clamp and divided. Immediately after dividing the left hepatic vein (A-2), the graft is perfused with preservation solution [histidine-tryptophan-ketoglutarate (HTK) or University of Wisconsin [UW] solution] (A-3). The artery is not rinsed. The hepatic duct is washed with the solution.

The donor hepatic vein is closed with 5-0 Prolene, the donor portal vein with 6-0 Prolene and the donor hepatic artery is closed with 6-0 Prolene suture or 3-0 silk double ligation.

If the left hepatic vein has a septum close to the orifice, it is cut sharply with scissors and sutured to make a single orifice with enough length of the cuff (B).

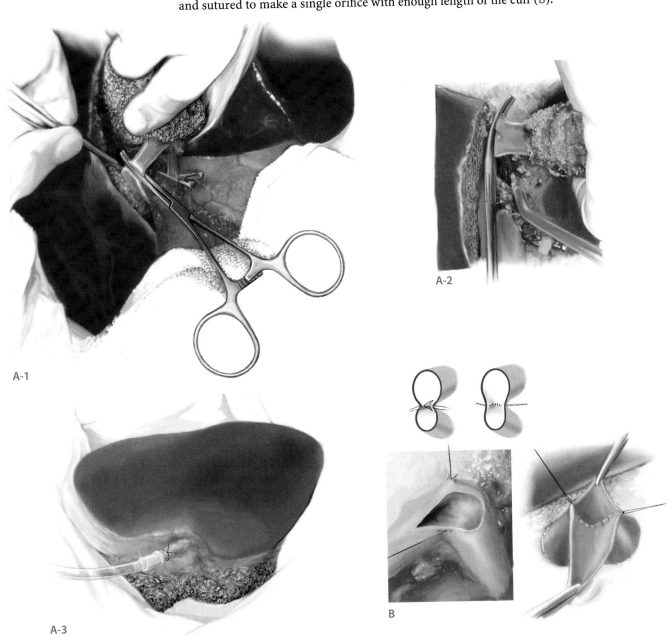

A-1

A-2

A-3

B

Implantation Procedure for Left Living Donor Liver Grafts

STEP 1   **Access and hilar dissection**

A bilateral subcostal incision with an upper midline extension to the xiphoid is the preferred access. The most important point to consider during the hilar dissection in living donor liver transplantation is to leave the pedicle of the vessels and bile duct with the greatest possible length, because they are much shorter than those in a cadaveric liver graft. The hepatic arteries are dissected carefully and transected close to the liver to provide adequate length and enough options for arterial reconstruction. In children suffering from biliary atresia the hepatic artery frequently has a larger size than expected. In this particular situation, dissection of the hepatic artery inside the liver of the recipient is required to adjust the size of hepatic artery between the graft and the recipient. Double ties on the proximal side of the hepatic arteries are recommended to prevent injury to the intima. The first ligation is done loosely just to occlude the lumen with 4-0 silk. The second tie is placed tightly just distal to the first.

The portal pedicle is elongated by dissecting the tissue around the portal vein up to the confluence of the superior mesenteric and splenic vein. Removal of the lymph nodes around the portal vein is helpful as it provides the desired smooth curve of the portal vein. The portal flow should be confirmed by unclamping the portal vein. The left gastric vein is divided routinely to increase portal flow.

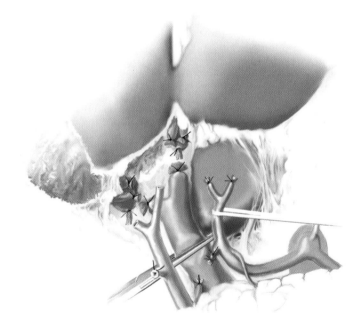

STEP 2	Reconstruction of the hepatic vein

We have three standard procedures for hepatic vein reconstruction in left-sided graft implantation: (a) one orifice using all of the hepatic veins, (b) the left and middle hepatic vein orifices and an additional incision of the IVC, and (c) the right hepatic vein and an additional incision of the IVC (A).

Preparation of a single orifice by using all of the hepatic veins is shown in the following figures: The inferior vena cava is entirely clamped to include all hepatic venous stumps (B-1). All septa are opened to create a single hole (B-2) and the size is measured (B-3). If the hole is too large for the hepatic vein of the graft, the diameter is adjusted by 5-0 Prolene suture at the left corner of the hole. Stitches with double armed 5-0 Prolene or PDS are placed on the right and left corners (B-4). The posterior anastomosis is made by the intraluminal method. After accomplishing the anastomosis, another small vascular clamp is placed just proximal to the anastomosis and the large one is removed to resume blood flow of the inferior vena cava.

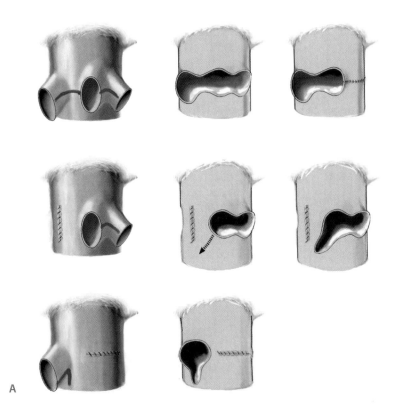

A

STEP 2 *(continued)*

Reconstruction of the hepatic vein

Preparation of a single orifice by using all of the hepatic veins is shown in the following figures: The inferior vena cava is entirely clamped to include all hepatic venous stumps (B-1). All septa are opened to create a single hole (B-2) and the size is measured (B-3). If the hole is too large for the hepatic vein of the graft, the diameter is adjusted by 5-0 Prolene suture at the left corner of the hole. Stitches with double armed 5-0 Prolene or PDS are placed on the right and left corners (B-4). The posterior anastomosis is made by the intraluminal method. After accomplishing the anastomosis, another small vascular clamp is placed just proximal to the anastomosis and the large one is removed to resume blood flow of the inferior vena cava.

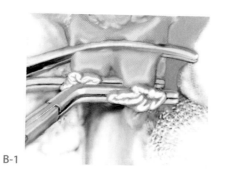

B-1

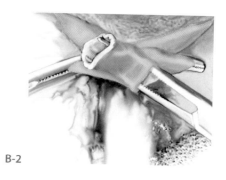

B-2

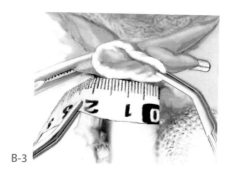

B-3

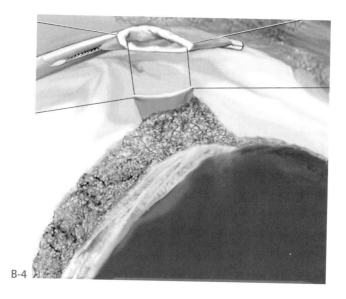

B-4

STEP 3   **Portal vein anastomosis**

Different techniques can be used for portal vein preparation (A), including: (a) with a branch patch, (b) with an oblique incision, (c) graft interposition, and (d) a patch graft. The first two are the simplest and most frequently used to adjust the graft size of the portal vein. If the portal vein wall is damaged or narrow, it should be changed with a venous graft. When the available venous graft is too small for interposition, the patch graft technique using a patch made from a small venous graft which is longitudinally opened is recommended.

Before the portal anastomosis is started, the portal vein should be briefly unclamped and washed with heparinized saline to check the flow and to remove possible coagula. The anastomosis is started by placing two double armed 6-0 Prolene or PDS sutures at the right and left corner of the graft portal vein. Anastomosis of the posterior wall is first carried out from the inside, in a running suture fashion. During the anastomosis, the suturing stitch should be kept loose to prevent anastomotic stricture (B). When this technique is used, creation of a growth factor is not required.

This continuous suture is our standard technique in most cases. However, interrupted sutures are used for the anterior wall subsequent to a running suture for the posterior wall in cases of a size mismatch or a small diameter using 7-0 Prolene or PDS.

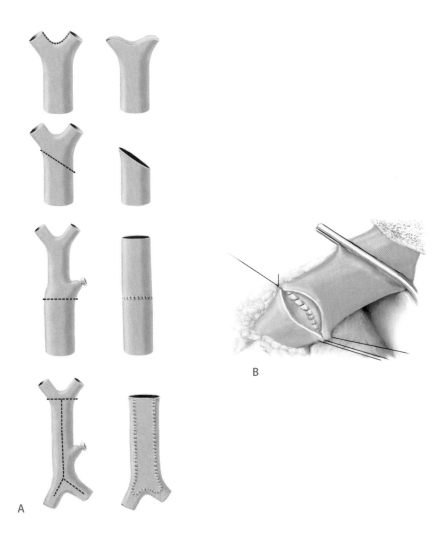

A

B

STEP 4   **Arterial anastomosis**

A surgical microscope and magnifying glasses should be used to perform the arterial anastomosis. First, excellent front flow of the recipient artery needs to be confirmed. Both arteries are clamped with fine vascular clips and are freed from the surrounding connective tissue with microscissors until the smooth adventitial surface is reached. The anastomosis is carried out with an interrupted 8-0 Prolene suture.

Size mismatch between the graft and recipient artery is frequently encountered. In most cases it can be managed by simple mechanical dilatation of the smaller artery using fine forceps. When the mismatch is significant, several techniques for adaptation can be used. In cases of multiple arteries, a larger one is chosen for the first anastomosis. When excellent arterial backflow is observed from the second artery after the first anastomosis, the second artery can be ligated.

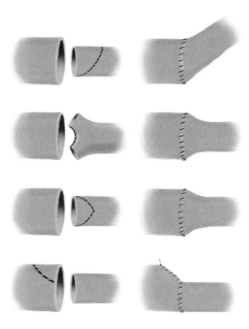

STEP 5

Biliary anastomosis

In patients with biliary atresia, pediatric patients with small-diameter bile ducts, or in patients with primary sclerosing cholangitis and a sclerotic common bile duct, a hepatico-jejunostomy should be performed. In other cases, a duct to duct anastomosis can be performed in a similar way as for orthotopic or right living donor liver transplantation.

A small hole is made in the Roux-en-Y limb close to the proximal end. A 4-Fr polyvinyl alcohol tube is inserted through the hole into the intestinal lumen as an external stent and is led out of the intestinal wall again. Two double-armed 6-0 PDS sutures are placed on the right and left corner of the graft hepatic duct. The stitch of the right corner is pulled with a small clamp to open the hepatic duct. Anastomosis of the posterior wall is made first with a running suture using the stitch of the left corner (A). After completion of the posterior wall, the inside needle of the stitch of the right corner of the graft is passed through the corner of the jejunum from inside to outside. After insertion of the tip of the stent into the duct lumen, anastomosis of the anterior wall is made using another needle of the left corner in running fashion (B). When the diameter of the hepatic duct is small, an incision on the anterior wall along the axis can be used to enlarge it.

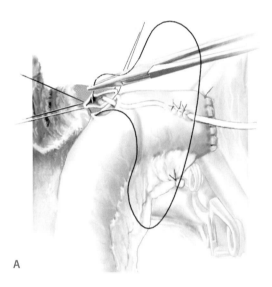

A

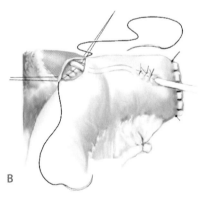

B

Tricks of the Senior Surgeon

- Preparation of the hepatic artery for a left lateral segment liver graft:
  In case a small middle hepatic artery disturbs the hilar dissection, it can be cut after confirmation of a sufficiently large left hepatic artery. By contrast, the left hepatic artery should be kept even if it seems to be too small for anastomosis until the anatomy of the left and middle hepatic artery is clarified.
- Preparation of the hepatic duct for a left lateral segment liver graft:
  When the left hepatic duct is cut above the B 4 bifurcation to preserve it for the donor, this is likely to result in two separate bile ducts (B2 and B3), which would complicate the biliary anastomosis. Therefore, we recommend the preparation of a single biliary orifice even if B4 needs to be sacrificed for this purpose. Since the inflow to Sg4 is usually limited it usually shrinks which leads to a compensatory enlargement of the remnant liver. Hence, the occlusion of B4 will not be a problem for the recipient.
- "Monosegment grafts":
  In cases where the lateral segment is too large, the graft can be reduced by cutting the lateral half or two thirds. If this reduced graft is still too large, the caudal 1/3 can be removed.
- To prevent twisting of the hepatic vein secondary to dislocation of the graft into the right subphrenic space, the falciform ligament should be reattached before the abdomen is closed.

Auxiliary Liver Transplantation

Karim Boudjema, Philippe Compagnon, Jean-Pierre Campion

The principle of auxiliary liver transplantation is the implantation of a right or left hemiliver into the abdominal cavity to restore normal liver function temporarily, while the native liver recuperates. Once the native liver has recovered, the graft can be removed or left in place without immunosuppression leading to atrophy.

Indications and Contraindications

Indications

- Fulminant and subfulminant liver failure (approximately 10% of all liver transplant indications) as defined by the King's College or the Clichy criteria
- Fulminant rather than subfulminant form of acute liver failure (interval jaundice/encephalopathy <2 weeks)
- Preferentially acute liver failure due to viral hepatitis (A and B), mushroom intoxication or drugs that are known to induce reversible acute liver failure

Exclusion Criteria

- General contraindications to transplantation
- Presence of fibrosis (or cirrhosis) on a frozen section biopsy performed during the procedure

Special Considerations

- Since there is not enough space in the abdominal cavity to harbor two entire livers, the graft has to be reduced.
- The reduced liver graft can be implanted heterotopically, i.e., below the native liver, but this technique may lead to a portal steal syndrome and compromise graft vascularization.
- Orthotopic implantation of the graft is more physiologic and is widely accepted as the standard technique. It implies resection of a native hemiliver. Consequently, two types of auxiliary partial orthotopic liver transplantation (APOLT) can be performed depending on the type of graft that is used:
    - Right APOLT (A-1): right hemihepatectomy of the native liver and implantation of a right liver graft (Sg5, 6, 7 and 8 and right part of the dorsal sector)
    - Left APOLT (A-2): left hemihepatectomy of the native liver and implantation of either a left lateral section (Sg2 and 3) or a left hemiliver (Sg2, 3 and 4)
- The liver graft can be harvested from a living donor or a cadaveric donor. When harvested from a cadaveric donor, the liver can be split in situ or ex situ.
- Two teams are mandatory and work simultaneously:
    - A donor team which procures and splits the graft
    - A recipient team which fits up the recipient abdominal cavity and performs the transplantation

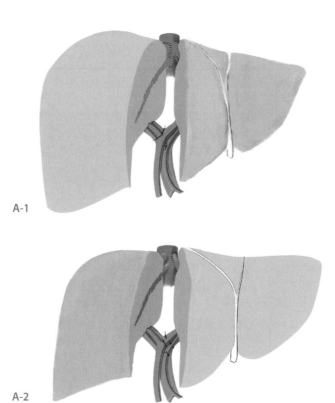

A-1

A-2

Specific Postoperative Complications

- Primary non-function of the liver graft
- Bleeding from the cut surfaces of both native and auxiliary livers
- Stricture of the portal vein anastomosis and subsequent portal steal syndrome and graft non-function
- Hepatic artery thrombosis and subsequent biliary tract necrosis of an atrophic graft

Procedures

Right Auxiliary Partial Orthotopic Liver Transplantation

Right APOLT is recommended for adult patients in order to raise the graft weight/patient weight ratio above 1%.

This part of the procedure mimics removal of a right living donor procedure except that it can be performed under selective occlusion of the right portal triad.

STEP 1   **Exploration, mobilization and resection of the native right hemiliver**

After visual and manual exploration of the liver and the entire abdominal cavity, the vascular structures (median hepatic vein and its branches from segments V and VIII) are evaluated by ultrasound with a special emphasis on anatomical variations that may complicate the procedure (i.e., absence of right portal trunk). Next, a wedge biopsy is performed for the evaluation of fibrosis, as the presence of fibrosis or cirrhosis is a contraindication for auxiliary liver transplantation. Parenchymal necrosis is common and its intensity does not necessarily predict the likelihood of recovery.

After cholecystectomy, the right hemiliver is mobilized. Of note, the distal end of the right hepatic vein can be encircled from below using a lace but should not be transsected at this stage.

The lateroposterior peritoneal sheath of the right part of the hepatoduodenal ligament is opened and the right hepatic artery is gently dissected from behind the common hepatic duct up to its bifurcation and marked with a vessel loop. The right branch of the portal vein is cautiously freed from the hilar plate. This maneuver cannot be performed safely without having controlled and cut one or two small branches to the caudate process. The vein is also marked with a vessel loop.

The right hepatic artery and the right portal vein are temporarily occluded with vascular clamps in order to reveal the demarcation line between left and right hemiliver. Then both vessels are divided between ligatures, as distally as possible.

The right hepatic duct should not be isolated extrahepatically. It can easily be transsected during the parenchymal dissection.

The liver parenchyma is transected 1 cm to the right of the main portal fissure, preserving the median hepatic vein. Transection is conducted posteriorly to the retrohepatic vena cava and the right hepatic duct is divided through the liver parenchyma at the confluence of its anterior and posterior branches. The bile duct from segment one is carefully preserved. Then, the right hepatic vein is transected by means of a vascular stapler (or another technique; see chapter "Right Hemihepatectomy"). At the end the retrohepatic segment of the inferior vena cava is widely exposed, ready to receive the right hepatic graft.

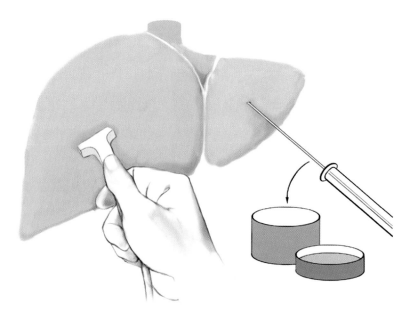

STEP 2

Preparation of the right liver graft

A right cadaveric graft is ideally split in situ. If performed ex situ the median hepatic vein should be preserved on the graft side in order to avoid congestion and bleeding of the graft cut surface at the time of revascularization. The graft includes (A):

- Segments 5–8
- The right branch of the hepatic artery
- The right branch of the portal vein
- The right hepatic duct(s) along with the confluence and the common hepatic duct
- The right and median hepatic vein both attached to the retrohepatic inferior vena cava. Since the left hepatic vein has been divided by retaining a narrow patch from the common trunk, the defect has to be closed by transverse suture

In a right living donor graft (see also chapter on living donor liver transplantation), the retrohepatic vena cava, median hepatic vein, and extrahepatic biliary tract must stay on the donor side. Consequently, the graft includes (B):

- Segments 5–8
- The right branch(es) of the hepatic artery
- The right branch(es) of the portal vein
- The right hepatic duct(s)
- The right hepatic vein

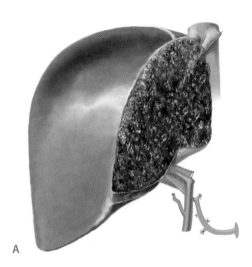

A

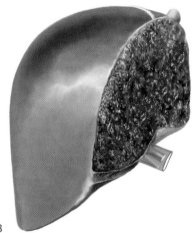

B

Implantation of a Right Liver Graft from a Cadaveric Donor

STEP 3   Caval anastomosis

In a cadaveric graft, a caval implantation is performed. The native IVC is clamped laterally and opened for about 5 cm including the ostium of the right hepatic vein. The left
side of the graft IVC is widely opened and a side-to-side cavocavostomy with a continuous 4-0 Prolene suture is performed. While the posterior layer is stitched, the graft is
flushed with Ringer's or 4% albumin solution.

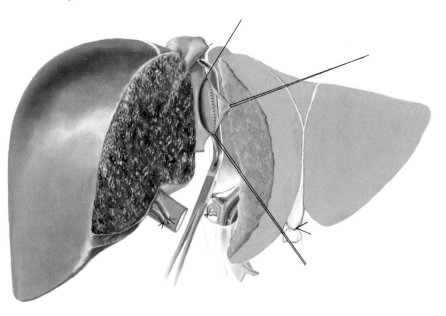

STEP 4   Portal vein and arterial anastomosis

The native right portal branch stump is clamped at its origin, and it is widely opened.
The length of the graft portal vein is accurately adjusted in order to avoid tearing or
kinking. An end-to-end anastomosis is performed between the donor and recipient right
portal branch with a 5-0 or 6-0 Prolene running suture, leaving a growth factor of about
5 mm. The graft is then revascularized and careful hemostasis performed.

    The standard artery reconstruction is an end-to-end anastomosis between the
donor and recipient right hepatic artery, using separate stitches of 8-0 Prolene. Donor
saphenous vein interposition may be necessary to implant the graft artery more
proximally on the recipient celiac axis.

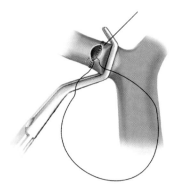

| STEP 5 | Reconstruction of the biliary tract |

After careful hemosthasis, a standard direct duct-to-duct anastomosis with separate PDS 6-0 stitches is performed and a T-drain is inserted. If a standard choledocho-choledochostomy cannot be performed, a Roux-en-Y hepaticojejunostomy would be performed.

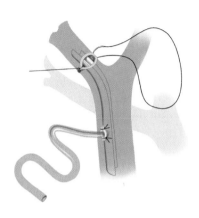

Note: Implantation of a Right Liver Graft from a Living Donor
The right liver graft from a living donor differs from the cadaveric graft implantation at step 1 only. Since the IVC has been left to the donor, the graft's right hepatic vein is implanted in an end-to-side fashion to the recipient IVC

Left Auxiliary Partial Orthotopic Liver Transplantation

Left APOLT is recommended for children since an adult right liver graft may be too large. An adult left lobe or left hemiliver graft is sufficient to provide a graft weight/patient weigh ratio above 1%.

Removal of the native left hemiliver and preparation of the graft

The resection of the native left hemiliver can be performed under selective occlusion of the left portal triad (see chapter "Segmentectomies, Sectionectomies and Wedge Resections") and includes resection of segment 1 with preservation of the median hepatic vein in the right hemiliver. The left side of the retrohepatic segment of the inferior vena cava is widely exposed to facilitate the left hepatic graft implantation.

For the preparation of the graft, resection of Sg1 is recommended, regardless of the type of graft (Sg2 and 3 or left hemiliver) or the type of donor (cadaveric or living).

The left grafts include:

- The left branch of the hepatic artery (living donor) or the entire hepatic artery including the celiac trunk (cadaveric donor)
- The left branch of the portal vein
- The left hepatic duct
- The retrohepatic IVC is never left attached to the left graft
- Either segments 2 and 3, drained through the left hepatic vein (left lateral section)
- Segments 2, 3 and 4, drained through the left and the median hepatic vein (left hemiliver graft) (A-1, A-2)

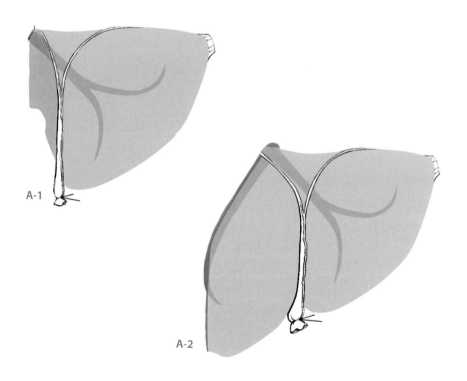

A-1

A-2

STEP 2

Implantation of left liver grafts

The native IVC is clamped anterolaterally, using the remaining stump of the left hepatic vein to expose the vessel. Then, the native IVC is opened vertically on 2 cm, beginning at the ostium of the left hepatic vein. An end-to-side anastomosis is performed using a continuous 4-0 Prolene suture between the recipient vena cava and the graft left hepatic vein or common median-left stem. The portal vein is adjusted and implanted with a growth factor as for the right side. The standard artery reconstruction is an end-to-side anastomosis between the graft celiac axis and the recipient common hepatic artery or splenic artery. End-to-end anastomosis between the donor and recipient left hepatic artery is used in case of a living donor graft.

The standard technique for biliary tract reconstruction is a direct duct-to-duct anastomosis, with separate PDS 6-0 or 7-0 stitches, and with insertion of a T-drain. A Roux-en-Y hepaticojejunostomy is performed in case a direct anastomosis cannot be performed

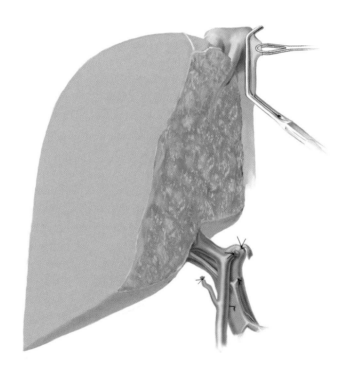

Tricks of the Senior Surgeon

- Never start the recipient procedure before the split procedure has been shown to be anatomically feasible.
- Two teams need to work simultaneously, headed by two experienced liver surgeons.
- Never start before a biopsy of the recipient liver has been performed. Fibrosis or cirrhosis would lead to perform orthotopic rather than auxiliary liver transplantation.

Biliary Tract and Gallbladder

Yuman Fong

Introduction

Yuman Fong

Diseases of the biliary tract represent some of the most challenging problems for the surgeon. Gallstone disease is a common ailment, for which surgical treatment has been recorded since ancient times. In the following chapters, authorities in the field will describe the often performed procedures of cholecystectomy and common bile duct exploration. Versions of these procedures performed as open surgery will be presented as well as the laparoscopic versions, which are arguably one of the major advances in general surgery in the past two decades. Surgery to fix the most feared complication from treatment of gallstone disease, namely bile duct injury, will also be presented.

We will then proceed to discussions of treatments for diseases that are much rarer: congenital malformations of the biliary tree and malignancies of the proximal/mid bile duct and gallbladder. Resections of these conditions are extremely challenging from a technical perspective. The principles, operative conduct, and "tricks of the senior surgeon" are presented by accepted masters of this trade. Distal bile duct problems will be presented in the chapters on pancreatic resection.

Finally, palliative bypasses for obstructions of the biliary tree will be presented. These chapters will describe the general approach to performing a facile biliary-enteric anastamosis, as well as methods of specific bypass procedures such as a choledochoduodenostomy or a hepaticojejunostomy. Even though biliary stent placement by endoscopic or percutaneous routes is widely used for patients who have clearly unresectable malignancies, for patients with benign disease or with disease found unresectable at surgery, such bypasses offer durable palliation with little added morbidity over the surgical exploration.

Laparoscopic Cholecystectomy, Open Cholecystectomy and Cholecystostomy

George A. Fielding

Laparoscopic Cholecystectomy

Mouret performed the first laparoscopic cholecystectomy in Lyon in 1988, and the first written report was by Dubois in 1989. Reddick popularized the procedure in the United States in 1990.

Indications and Contraindications

Indications

- Same as for open procedure
- One of the most important indications is that the surgeon be adequately trained to perform the procedure
- All manifestations of symptomatic gallstones – biliary colic, history of jaundice, chronic cholecystitis and acute cholecystitis
- Gallstone pancreatitis
- Acalculous cholecystitis
- Large gallbladder polyps

Contraindications

- There are no absolute contraindications to laparoscopic cholecystectomy
- Relative contraindications include cirrhosis and portal hypertension, bleeding diathesis, pregnancy
- Technical modifications can be made to suit these three problems

Preoperative Investigation and Preparation for the Procedure

Preoperative investigations include liver function tests and typically an ultrasound examination. If the laparoscopic cholecystectomy is being performed for acalculous cholecystitis, patients may have had nuclear studies to assess gallbladder function. If there is the suspicion of gallbladder cancer or big polyps, a CT scan is required.

There is no place for routine preoperative endoscopic retrograde cholangio-pancreatography (ERCP) in laparoscopic cholecystectomy.

The patient should have prophylactic antibiotics on induction and appropriate anti-thromboembolic measures.

Procedure

STEP 1

Access

The procedure should be performed on a table allowing operative cholangiography. There is no routine need for a nasogastric tube or Foley catheter.

Typically there is no requirement for invasive anesthetic monitoring.

Patients are placed supine, legs together with a slight reverse Trendelenburg position. There is little to gain by using a steep reverse Trendelenburg position.

Safe access:

Open insertion of a Hasson cannula through a transumbilical incision. Eversion of the umbilicus creates access via the gap in the linea alba at the base of the umbilicus.

The Hasson cannula can be sat directly in the peritoneal cavity. There is no need for stay sutures nor to suture the port in place. A 30° telescope is used; insufflation pressures are set at 15 mmHg. Placement of other access parts is as shown in the figure.

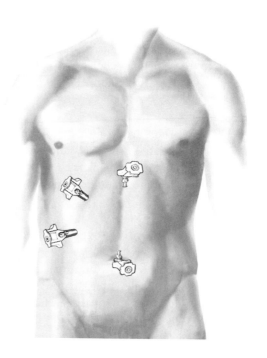

<table>
<tr><td>STEP 2</td><td>Retraction and dissection of Calot's triangle</td></tr>
</table>

STEP 2

Retraction and dissection of Calot's triangle

Once caudad retraction of the fundus is established, the crucial maneuver is lateral retraction of Hartmann's pouch by the upper lateral 5-mm port. This places Calot's triangle on the stretch and will greatly reduce the chance of injury of the common bile duct.

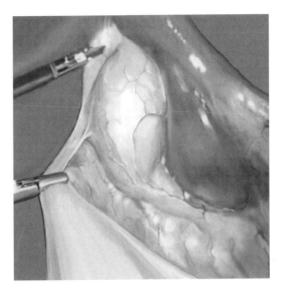

STEP 3

Then incise the posterior peritoneal attachment behind Hartmann's pouch to separate Hartmann's pouch from the liver to further stretch out Calot's triangle.

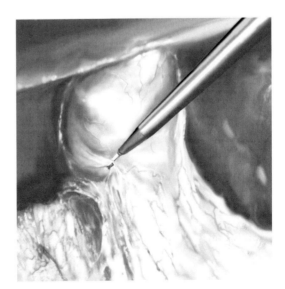

STEP 4

Once these two maneuvers are instituted, hook dissection can be performed, staying close to the gallbladder to incise the anterior sheet of peritoneum over Calot's triangle. This will expose one or two cystic arteries and the cystic duct . Windows should be developed between all these structures before anything is divided.

Once the anatomy is determined (see anatomical variations and tricks), the cystic arteries are divided between clips and a clip is placed below Hartmann's pouch to the proximal end of the cystic duct.

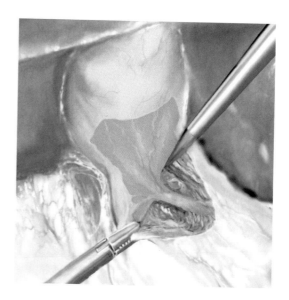

STEP 5   **Cholangiography**

Lateral retraction of Hartmann's pouch is maintained by a grasper, this time coming from the subxiphoid port.

The cystic duct is incised through the right (A). The cystic valve can occasionally make this difficult.

A No. 4 ureteric catheter with an end hole is inserted through the Olsen-Reddick cholangiogram clamp into the cystic duct and the clamp closed around the duct (B).

Operative cholangiography is then performed with aid of C-arm fluoroscopy. Cholangiography confirms the biliary anatomy and reveals the common duct stones, allowing laparoscopic duct exploration.

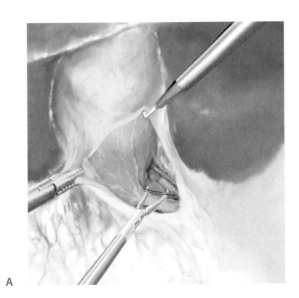

A

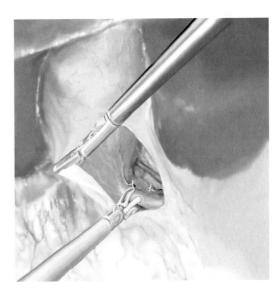

B

STEP 6   **Removal of gallbladder**

Once cholangiography is completed, the ureteric catheter is removed and the cystic duct is clamped. The gallbladder is then removed from the liver bed using hook diathermy. This is done through a combination of elevating the peritoneum, burning with the hook and pushing so that the gallbladder is removed toward the fundus and finally separated from the liver at the fundus. There is very little place for fundus-first laparoscopic cholecystectomy.

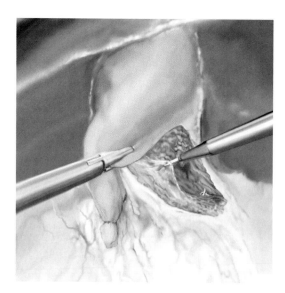

Anatomical Variations

- The major anatomical variations are involved with the common bile duct and the right hepatic artery.
- A very small common bile duct can be mistaken for the cystic duct and completely excised. Even more worrisome is the variant of a low junction of the left and right hepatic ducts (A) or a low junction of the right anterior and right posterior hepatic ducts (B). In these situations the cystic duct can enter the right hepatic duct or the right posterior hepatic duct. The right or right posterior ducts can therefore be mistaken for the cystic duct and divided.
- More rarely, but even more difficult, particularly in the setting of acute cholecystitis, is when there is no cystic duct and Hartmann's pouch opens directly underneath the right hepatic duct or the common duct.

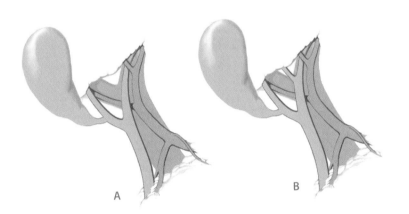

Complications

Bleeding

The major intraoperative complication is bleeding. This is typically from a very short cystic artery or from the right hepatic artery itself. Bleeding from the portal vein is very rare, but in contrast to hepatic and cystic artery bleeding, it is always torrential and the patient must be opened.

Failure to Progress

The second major complication is failure to progress. If the surgeon is not making any progress, the patient should be converted to an open cholecystectomy.

Bile Duct Injury

Proper retraction, careful dissection, steady control of hemorrhage and recognition of an appropriate time to convert to open cholecystectomy should minimize the chance of the most feared intraoperative complication – bile duct injury or bile duct resection.

If a duct injury is recognized the surgeon should just stop, collect his or her thoughts, and ring a hepatobiliary colleague immediately.

Postoperative Complications

- Most bile leaks are low volume and will settle spontaneously.
- A high volume bile leak is suggestive that the clip has come off the cystic duct or there is a major unrecognized duct injury. ERCP will determine this, allowing appropriate management.
- Subphrenic collection may require percutaneous drainage.
- Pneumonia – best treated with physiotherapy and antibiotics.
- Jaundice suggests major duct obstruction or excision – ERCP or referral to a hepatobiliary specialist.

Tricks of the Senior Surgeon

- In cases with portal hypertension and cirrhosis, patients should be considered for a partial cholecystectomy, where the back wall of the gallbladder is left on the liver bed. Failure to do so can result in life-threatening hemorrhage. Furthermore, with laparoscopic surgery, you simply will not be able to see the operative field due to the blood.
- In severe acute cholecystitis, the first step is to decompress the gallbladder by inserting the trocar directly into the gallbladder and aspirating the contents. This will convert a tense, unmanageable gallbladder to a collapsed thick-walled gallbladder that can be grasped and maneuvered.
- If there is a stone impacted in Hartmann's pouch, it should be pushed back into the gallbladder to allow safe manipulation of Calot's triangle.

Open Cholecystectomy

Until 1989 open cholecystectomy was the procedure of choice for all the complications of symptomatic gallstones. It has largely been supplanted by laparoscopic cholecystectomy as a freestanding elective procedure. The principle of open cholecystectomy is removal of the gallbladder and its contents with preservation of the biliary tree.

Indications and Contraindications

Indications

- Failed laparoscopic cholecystectomy
- Whipple resection or bile duct resection as part of hepatectomy
- Patient choice
- Suspected malignant gallbladder polyp

Contraindications

- There are no absolute contraindications to cholecystectomy
- A severely ill patient where a cholecystostomy may be the best option

Open cholecystectomy is now performed most frequently as part of other major procedures as listed above. If it is in the setting of a failed laparoscopic procedure it is often a very difficult cholecystectomy and it is vital in this situation to make an adequate incision.

Preoperative Investigation and Preparation for the Procedure

- Liver function tests
- Ultrasound
- Planning of associated major procedure
- Clinical preparation and prophylactic antibiotics
- Anti–deep vein thrombosis therapy of choice

Procedure

STEP 1

Positioning and incision

Operative table allowing C-arm fluoroscopy. If done for patient choice, and there are no other contraindications, a 5-cm transverse incision is centered over the lateral border of the rectus sheath made.

STEP 2

After conversion from laparoscopic cholecystectomy, it is essential to make an adequate incision, as the main reason for conversion is an anatomical difficulty usually in the setting of an inflamed gallbladder. A long right subcostal incision is made a finger's width below the costal margin. The rectus sheath is divided in the line of the incision and this is taken down to the peritoneum using diathermy coagulation.

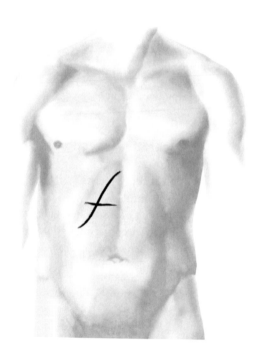

STEP 3

The peritoneal cavity is elevated with the fingers and the wound incised along its full length. Three packs are inserted – one behind the liver, one on the colon and one over the gastroduodenal area and retractors are placed over the gastroduodenal area and one over the liver to place Calot's triangle on the stretch.

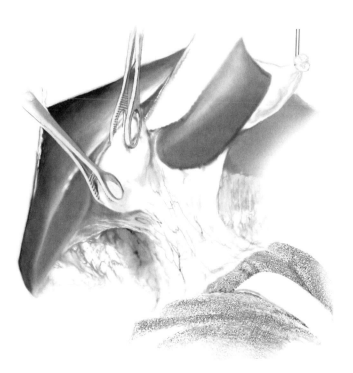

The key step in open cholecystectomy is division of the cystic artery, which allows Hartmann's pouch to swing out and allow clear definition of the biliary anatomy. The cystic duct is clipped and the gallbladder is retracted inferiorly and dissected free of the liver.

Cholangiography is typically performed through the cystic duct using the same equipment as for laparoscopic cholecystectomy.

Once the anatomy has been determined and cleared, the gallbladder is removed. This is typically done starting from Hartmann's pouch, but in the case of severe inflammation it may be better done with the fundus first dissection, carefully dividing in the plane between the liver and the gallbladder (A-1, A-2).

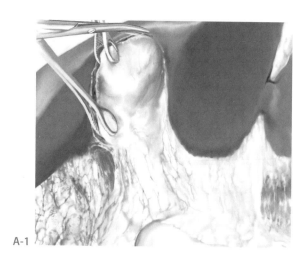

A-1

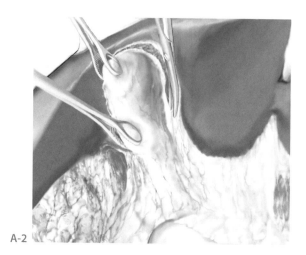

A-2

Complications

These complications are the same as those for laparoscopic cholecystectomy.

Cholecystostomy

Indications and Contraindications

Indications

- Percutaneous cholecystostomy is used most commonly in the setting of a severely ill patient with underlying gallbladder sepsis.
- Operative severe inflammation of Calot's triangle at surgery where the safest option is to decompress the gallbladder.

Procedure

Cholecystostomy may be performed open but this is much more typically found at laparoscopic cholecystectomy.

STEP 1

The 5-mm lateral trocar is inserted directly into the gallbladder and the gallbladder aspirated. The gallbladder will collapse, typically showing a large stone in Hartmann's pouch; if this can be milked back and removed it should be done.

STEP 2

A Foley catheter is inserted via the lateral port directly into the gallbladder. Cholangiography can be completed via this if indicated.

STEP 3

The trocar is removed from the gallbladder, leaving the Foley catheter in place, which is then insufflated. The gallbladder is sutured 2nd request around the Foley catheter.

The Foley catheter is then left on free drainage and should be left in place at least 6 weeks to allow the gallbladder to settle prior to returning to complete the laparoscopic cholecystectomy.

The Foley catheter should be irrigated twice daily with 20 ml of saline.

Resection of Gallbladder Cancer, Including Surgical Staging

Rebecca Taylor, Yuman Fong

Introduction

Gallbladder cancer was first described in 1777. The average age at diagnosis is 65 years, with women being three times more affected than men. In gallbladder cancer, 90 % of the cancers are adenocarcinomas. Gallstones and chronic inflammation of the gallbladder are associated with malignant disease. It is estimated that 1 % of patients undergoing cholecystectomy for gallstones are found to have cancer. Twenty percent to 60 % of gallbladders with calcifications (porcelain gallbladder) will develop cancer.

Natural History

- Patients with incompletely resected gallbladder cancer have a 5-year survival rate of less than 5 %
- Completely resected patients have a 5-year survival rate of 17–90 % depending on stage of disease

Indications and Contraindications for Resectional Procedures

Indications
- Gallbladder cancer with T1–4, N0/1 and M0

Relative Contraindications
- Lymph node metastases to N2 compartment

Contraindications
- Peritoneal carcinomatosis or other distant metastases (M1)

Presentation

- Mass in segment 4/5 associated with gallbladder
- During surgery for presumed cholelithiasis or as pathologic finding after cholecystectomy for presumed gallstone disease
- One-third of patients will present with jaundice

Preoperative Investigations and Preparation for the Procedure

History: Biliary colic, jaundice, itching, weight loss, previous gallbladder
                            or biliary surgery
Physical examination: Right upper quadrant mass

Imaging

- Ultrasound
- Contrast-enhanced CT scan (CT angiogram is preferred)
- Magnetic resonance cholangiopancreatography (MRCP)
- Cholangiography [if invasive cholangiography is necessary, percutaneous cholan-
  giography (PTC) is preferred over endoscopic retrograde cholangiopancreatography
  (ERCP)]
- Direct arteriography (rarely needed)
- Important anatomic details: porcelain gallbladder, mass, enlarged/necrotic lymph
  nodes, arterial involvement, portal venous involvement, adjacent organ (colon,
  duodenum) involvement, peritoneal metastasis
- Gallbladder polyp [solitary, sessile, large (>1 cm) polyps are worrisome for cancer]
- Look at anomalous pancreaticobiliary duct junction, choledochal cyst, and of course
  hepatic arteries

Extent of Resection According to Stage

Patients presenting with gallbladder mass on imaging or operative exploration:
- *T2/3, N0/1, M0:* radical cholecystectomy and lymph node dissection
- *Unilateral vascular involvement:* extended lobectomy and lymph node dissection
- *T4, N0/1, M0:* extended lobectomy and lymph node dissection, possible adjacent
  organ resection
- *N2 or M1:* no curative surgery, possible palliation by biliary or gastric bypass

Patients with cancer discovered as an incidental finding after cholecystectomy for
presumed cholelithiasis:
- *T1 with negative liver and cystic duct margin:* no further therapy
- *T1 with positive cystic duct margin:* re-resection of cystic duct or common bile duct
  to negative margins
- *T2/3/4, M0:* extended lobectomy, common bile duct resection, lymph node dissection,
  and resection of laparoscopic port sites
- *N2 or M1:* no curative surgery (palliation)

Procedure

A radical cholecystectomy (including segments 4b and 5) resection will be described. If an extended lobectomy is necessary because of the bulk of the tumor or because of vascular invasion, the dissection of the porta hepatis and hilar areas is performed as described below. With gallbladder cancer, when an extended resection is necessary, it is usually an extended right lobectomy. The liver resection is then performed as described in Sect. 3, "Liver," after the vasculature to the left side is dissected free and protected and the left hepatic duct has been divided.

Incision

- *No previous surgery:* A low right subcostal (hockey stick) incision is favored (see Sect. 1, chapter "Positioning and Accesses" for descriptions of incisions and division of falciform)
- *Previous cholecystectomy:* Subcostal incision to incorporate excision of previous open or laparoscopic port incisions plus separate excision of umbilical port

---

STEP 1

Surgical exploration

Exposure and exploration: installation of the retractor (see Sect. 1, chapter "Retractors and Principles of Exposure") and inspection of possible port site and peritoneal metastasis

Ultrasound to evaluate location of the primary tumor in relation to vascular structures (portal vein, hepatic artery, hepatic vein) and to rule out discontiguous liver metastases

Careful inspection of vascular variation

STEP 2

Area resected by radical cholecystectomy, and regional lymph node and connective tissue dissection

The two segments (4b and 5) contiguous with the gallbladder bed are resected.

N1 lymph nodes (blue): those in the hepatoduodenal ligament (No. 12) and common hepatic (No. 8) and celiac arteries (No. 9) are resected. Positive N2 nodes (red), retropancreatic nodes (No. 13), perigastric nodes or aortocaval nodes indicate incurable disease.

Nerve plexuses around the hepatic artery should be dissected.

Full kocherization allows inspection of these nodal stations and facilitates subsequent dissection.

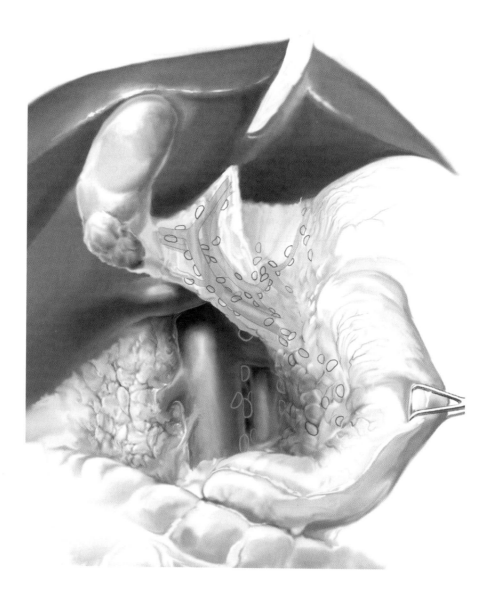

STEP 3   **Excision of the highest peripancreatic lymph node**

After kocherization, the highest peripancreatic lymph node is excised. This node is sent for frozen section histologic analysis. After excision of this node, retraction of the bile duct anteriorly allows visualization of the portal vein and facilitates safe dissection of nodal and connective tissues. Frozen section staging using this node also guides the operative procedure. If this node is positive and the patient is at high medical risk, then the radical resection is usually abandoned. A radical resection performed in the setting of a positive node should include a retropancreatic nodal dissection and aortocaval nodal dissection, with or without a pancreaticoduodenectomy.

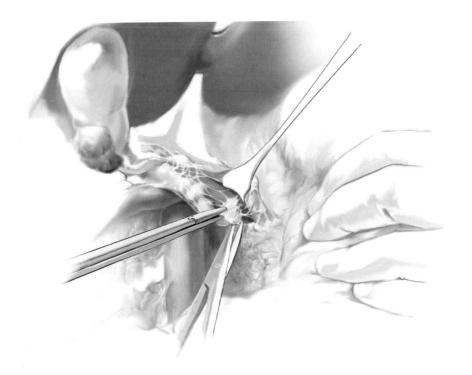

STEP 4

Common bile duct resection

Except in the very thin patient, it is very difficult to adequately excise the nodal tissue in the porta hepatis without resecting the common bile duct. This is particularly true if the patient has recently had a cholecystectomy, so that the scars from such surgery further complicate identification of nodal tissue and tumor. Resecting the common bile duct also allows the most certainty of resection of the cystic duct–common duct junction. Furthermore, resecting the common duct allows the safest dissection and inspection of the portal vein and hepatic arteries behind the tumor and in the hilar area.

The bridge of liver tissue between segments 4b and 3, overlying the base of the falciform, is divided (**A**) to allow access to the left portal pedicle. The common bile duct is divided immediately above the pancreas and reflected upward (**B**). The resection margin must be examined by frozen section. All nodal and connective tissues, including the celiac, hepatoduodenal, and portal-caval nodes, are dissected with the common duct, leaving behind only the skeletonized portal vein and hepatic artery.

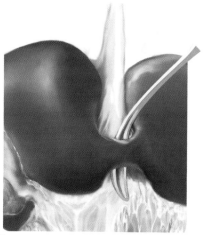

A

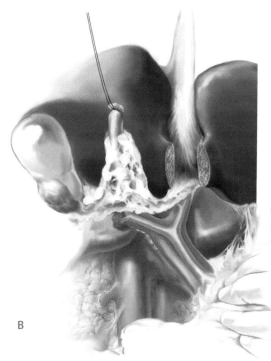

B

| STEP 5 | Assessment of the portal vein and hepatic artery |

With the common duct and portal nodal tissue reflected upward, the main, left, and right portal veins and arteries are dissected. If the main portal vein is involved, a portal vein resection and reconstruction may be necessary (see below). If the right hepatic artery and/or right portal vein are involved, an extended right liver resection is warranted. Once the arterial anatomy and possible arterial variations are clearly identified, the right or left hepatic artery is skeletonized distally to the right and left extremes of the hilar plate. In doing so, the left and right hepatic ducts are dissected free.

| STEP 6 | Transection of the left and right hepatic ducts |

The left hepatic duct is then identified and transected at the base of the umbilical fissure. Unlike the dissection for a hilar cholangiocarcinoma, the junction of the left and right hepatic ducts can usually be freed from the liver. Retraction of the left hepatic duct stump upward then allows a good look at the right hepatic duct from the posterior-inferior aspects. A stay suture is then placed on this duct before transection.

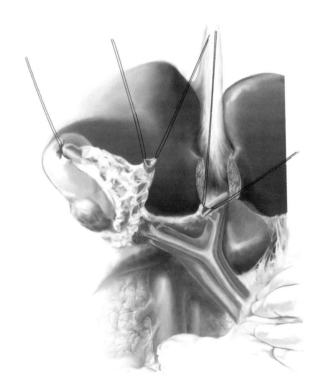

STEP 7   **Liver resection**

After transection of the right hepatic duct, tissue from both the left and right ductal margins is sent for frozen section analysis. The entire gallbladder bed including segments 4b and 5 is then resected along the dotted lines shown. The portal veins and hepatic arteries are protected under direct vision. Liver parenchymal transaction is as described in Sect. 3, chapters "Liver Resections" and "Left Hemihepatectomy," usually with inflow occlusion by the Pringle maneuver, and with central venous pressure (CVP) maintained below 3 cm H_2O (see Sect. 3, chapter "Extended Hemihepatectomies").

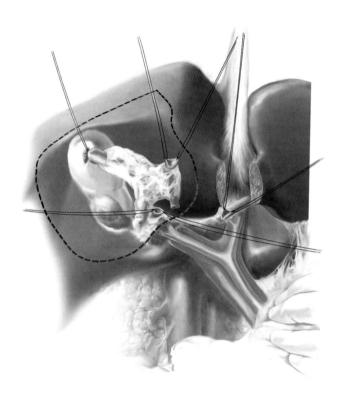

STEP 8

Biliary reconstructions

Before bilioenteric anastomosis, the left and right hepatic ducts can be joined by interrupted, absorbable sutures (4-0 or 5-0 Vicryl or PDS) to minimize the number of the anastomosis. Alternatively, the two ducts can be anastomosed separately. A 70-cm Roux-en-Y jejunal loop is lifted through the shortest route that allows for no tension on the anastomosis: retrocolic or retrogastric. For details on the biliary anastomosis, please see this section, chapters "Intrahepatic Biliodigestive Anastomosis Without Indwelling Stent" and "Reconstruction of Bile Duct Injuries." If a plastic biliary stent has been placed before surgery, it is removed and not replaced. If a metal stent has been placed, it is usually safest to cut across the metal stent at a site believed to be free of cancer. The jejunal loop is then sewn to the duct and the stent.

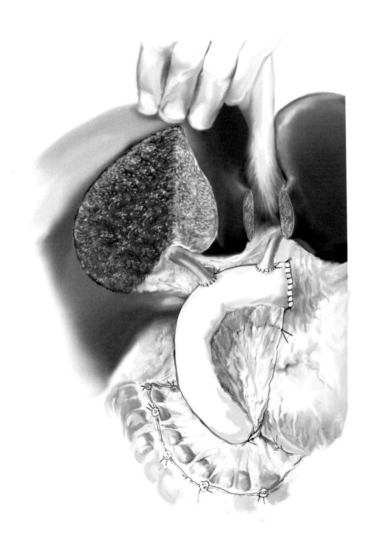

STEP 9

Portal vein reconstruction

Tumors that occupy the neck of the gallbladder or the cystic duct often invade into the right portal vein or the main portal vein. Patients presenting with jaundice are at particularly high risk for portal invasion. If the left portal vein and artery are free of tumor, these vascularly invasive tumors may often be resectable by combined extended lobectomy, portal lymphadenectomy, and portal vein resection and reconstruction.

Splitting the liver along the umbilical fissure, on the line of the extended lobectomy, provides access to the hilar area and allows for easier control of the portal vein and safer reconstruction. After cutting the left hepatic duct, this duct is reflected to the patient's left. The right hepatic artery is then transected to allow for unobstructed access to the portal vein. Vascular clamps are then placed on the main portal vein and the left portal vein (A-1). After transection, anastomosis of the main and left portal vein is accomplished with a running, nonabsorbable suture (e.g., 5-0 Proline) (A-2).

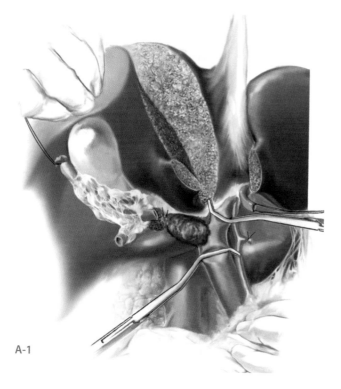

A-1

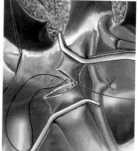

A-2

| STEP 10 | Liver resection and biliary reconstruction |

An extended right hepatic resection is then performed as described in Sect. 3, chapter "Extended Hemihepatectomies." The figure illustrates the subsequent reconstruction utilizing a retrocolic Roux-en-Y hepaticojejunostomy.

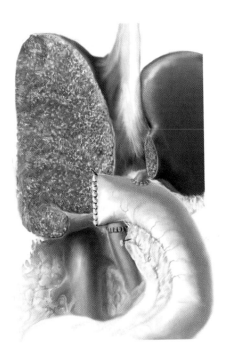

| STEP 11 | Drainage after reconstruction |

After completing hemostasis in the surgical field, closed drains are placed in the right upper quadrant near the biliary anastomosis. If a percutaneous transhepatic stent has been removed, a drain should also be placed near the site of the stent entry site on the liver surface. We do not usually use stents for the anastomosis. Nasogastric tube decompression of the gastrointestinal tract is usually continued until return of bowel function. This is particularly important if the bile duct used for anastomosis is small. Nasogastric decompression prevents swelling of the Roux-en-Y limb and possible disruption of the anastomosis.

Postoperative Tests

- Postoperative surveillance in an intensive or intermediate care unit (for extended procedures)
- Coagulation parameters and hemoglobin for at least 48 hours
- Liver function test and electrolytes (including phosphorus) for at least 48 hours

Postoperative Complications

- General:
  - Pleural effusion
  - Pneumonia
  - Deep vein thrombosis
  - Pulmonary embolism
- Abdominal:
  - Intra-abdominal bleeding
  - Infected collection/abscess
  - Liver failure (extended procedures)
  - Bile leak with biloma formation
  - Leakage of biliodigestive anastomosis (procedures with common bile duct resection)
  - Portal vein thrombosis

Tricks of the Senior Surgeon

- If the patient presents with a radiologic T3 or T4 gallbladder cancer, laparoscopic staging is warranted because of the high incidence of peritoneal metastases.
- For surgical planning, any patient with a tumor in the neck of the gallbladder or in the cystic duct, or presenting with jaundice, should be scrutinized on preoperative scans for signs of right hepatic arterial involvement. If the right artery is encased, a minimum of an extended lobectomy is necessary for resection.
- Accessory or replaced left hepatic arteries do not reside in the porta hepatis, but rather pass across the lesser omentum and enter the base of the umbilical fissure. Patients with these anomalous vessels can therefore often be resected even when extensive involvement of the porta exists.
- Stay sutures should be placed before dividing the intrahepatic bile duct; otherwise the small segmental duct can slip away and retract within the liver parenchyma.
- The lymphatic vessels throughout this dissection should be tied to prevent postoperative lymphorrhea.

Exploration of the Common Bile Duct: The Laparoscopic Approach

Jean-François Gigot

Introduction

Stone migration is a common situation encountered during the management of gallstones. Common bile duct (CBD) exploration (CBDE) thus remains the cornerstone of complete surgical treatment of gallbladder and common bile duct stones (CBDs). The first laparoscopic choledochotomy was reported in 1991 by Petelin.

Indications and Contraindications

Indications

- CBD stone disease
- Failed endoscopic removal of stones

Choice of Route
- The choice of optimal strategy for laparoscopic CBDE (LCBDE) will be guided by the features of intraoperative cholangiography (IOC), according to the characteristics of the stone and to the biliary anatomy.

The transcystic (TC) route is chosen when there is:
- A patent cystic duct
- A limited number of stones
- Small stone size (stone size ≤ cystic duct size)
- Stones located below the cystic duct (CD)–CBD junction
- Adequate biliary anatomy of the CD–CBD junction (the ideal case is a perpendicular angle of insertion of CD into the CBD)

Choledochotomy is chosen when there is:
- Dilated CBD ≥7–8 mm
- Accessible porta hepatis (no acute inflammation)

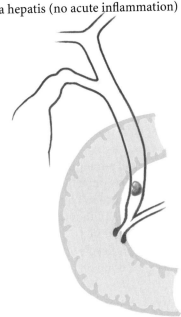

Contraindications

General

- High risk patients (ASA III or IV) for whom an endoscopic approach is preferred
- Dense peritoneal adhesions due to previous upper abdominal surgery (a limitation for the laparoscopic approach)
- Liver cirrhosis with portal hypertension/severe coagulation disorders

Transcystic

- Presence of obstructive cystic valves (associated with a risk of instrumental CD or CBD injury)
- Stones too large for TC stone extraction
- Stones located in the common hepatic duct or in intrahepatic bile ducts
- Inadequate biliary anatomy of the CD (tortuous, etc.) and the CD–CBD junction (parapapillary insertion, acute angle of insertion of CD into CBD, etc.)

Choledochotomy

- Thin CBD (risk of stricture after suturing)
- The presence of severe inflammation (gangrenous cholecystitis, acute necrotizing pancreatitis, etc.) at the porta hepatis, precluding a safe identification of CBD

Preoperative Investigations

History and evaluation:	Previous and actual clinical history of biliary symptoms Pain, jaundice, fever, chills, signs of pancreatitis
Laboratory tests:	White blood cell (WBC) count, CRP, bilirubin, ALT, AST, alkaline phosphatase, amylase, lipase, coagulation parameters
Preoperative radiologic assessment:	Ultrasound, MR cholangiography, endoscopic ultrasonography

Conditions for LCBDE

- Adequate experience in open biliary surgery *and* in laparoscopic advanced procedures, in suturing techniques and in endoscopic techniques
- Routine practice of Intraoperative cholangiography (IOC)
- Adequate technical environment (instrumentation, fluoroscopy, flexible scopes, etc.)

Instrumentation/Material

LCBDE is a technically demanding operation requiring:
- High volume insufflator
- High energy light source
- Fluoroscopic intraoperative cholangiographic equipment
- Dormia basket or balloon extraction baskets
- Flexible endoscope 3.5 mm (fine, fragile and expansive)
- Contact or laser lithotripsy device (optional)
- Laparoscopic knife
- Laparoscopic needle holder
- Transcystic drain or T-tube

Procedure

Incision

- Same four-trocar technique as for laparoscopic cholecystectomy.
- An additional atraumatic soft fifth trocar is placed below the right costal margin, serving as the port for the introduction of the scope.

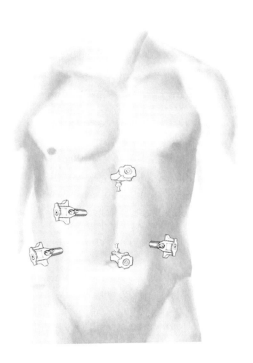

Exposure

- LCBDE is performed during cholecystectomy after completion of IOC, when the dissection of Calot's triangle is completed, the gallbladder remaining in place
- The hepatoduodenal ligament is stretched by pulling up on the quadrate lobe. The patient is placed in an anti-Trendelenburg position to allow gravity to pull down on the duodenum.

Laparoscopic Transcystic CBDE

STEP 1

Introduction of instruments

The cystic duct incision done for performing IOC is used for transcystic CBDE (TCBDE). Care is taken to avoid a cystic duct incision too close to the CBD, in order to reduce the risk of instrumental CBD injury. The incision must also not be too far from the CBD, because the presence of obstructive cystic valves may preclude instrumental TCBDE. If the caliber of the sufficiently large CD is not dilated enough, it can be carefully dilated using a soft, flexible dilator, with care taken to avoid instrumental CBD injury.

STEP 2

Instrumental stone extraction

Stone extraction through TCBDE can be performed using a three-wire soft Dormia basket with three different approaches:
- By blunt introduction of the instrument into the CBD through the CD.
- Under fluoroscopic guidance (safer for ensuring stone capture and avoiding instrumental CBD injury).
- Under visual cholangioscopic guidance (for small stones).

A balloon catheter is not used during TCBDE, in order to avoid stone migration in the upper part of the CBD. In the case of huge, impacted, obstructive stones not amenable to extraction by using standard instrumental or endoscopic methods, the stone can be fragmented by using an endoluminal electrohydraulic or laser lithotripsy probe under endoscopic visual control.

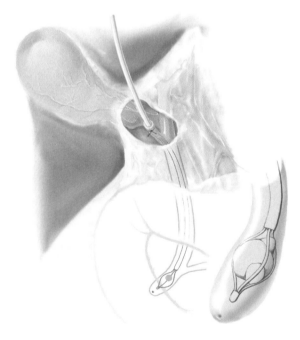

STEP 3

Stone clearance assessment

The assessment of complete stone clearance is performed in two different ways:

- By control cholangiography.
- By using flexible choledochoscopy (A-1, A-2): the scope is introduced under fluoroscopic or visual guidance into the CBD to assess the presence of residual CBDs. When used through a TC approach, choledochoscopic stone clearance assessment is usually only possible in the lower part of the CBD, except in the case of a wide angle of insertion of the CD into the CBD. In this case (15–20% of cases), the scope can be guided into the upper part of the biliary tract.

In case of residual CBDS, an additional endoscopic attempt at stone extraction can be performed by introducing a Dormia basket through the operative channel of the scope, and also by guiding stone capture under visual control. When the number of stones is limited and when stone clearance is complete, the CD can be primarily clipped.

When doubt exists about the completeness of stone clearance, the CBD can be drained by using a transcystic duct drain, carefully secured with an endoloop or an extracorporeal suturing technique.

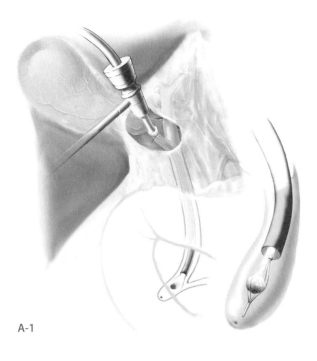

A-1

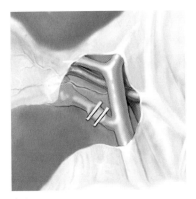

A-2

STEP 4

Routine subhepatic drainage is used.

Laparoscopic Choledochotomy

STEP 1

The anterior wall of the CBD is additionally dissected within the porta hepatis, by using blunt or instrumental dissection (avoiding the use of electrocautery close to the CBD).

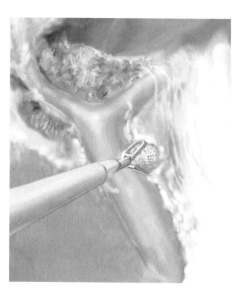

STEP 2

A longitudinal incision is made with a laparoscopic knife into the CBD after having blown up the CBD with saline solution through the transcystic cholangiographic catheter. The size of the incision is dependent on the size of the largest CBDS to be extracted from the CBD.

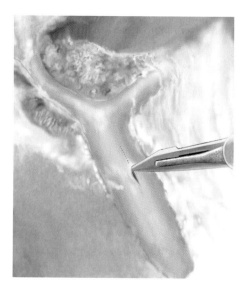

STEP 3	Stone extraction

- By blunt introduction of a Dormia basket or a balloon catheter through the choledo-cholithotomy (A-1, A-2).
- Under endoscopic visual control by introducing a Dormia basket or a balloon catheter through the operative channel of the flexible scope.
- If a large, obstructive stone is encountered, an endoscopic electrohydraulic or laser lithotripsy technique can also be used.

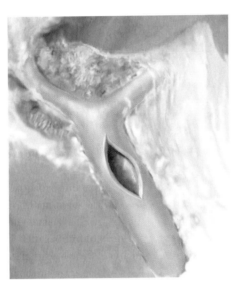

A-1

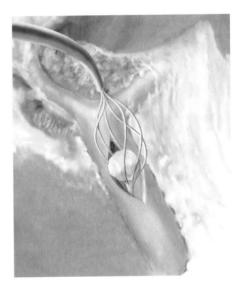

A-2

STEP 4

Stone clearance assessment

- Is performed only by the use of a flexible choledochoscope through the choledochotomy. In this setting, a complete assessment of the lower and upper biliary tract is easily possible, up to the intrahepatic bile ducts (A-1, A-2).
- In case of residual CBDs, endoscopic stone extraction can be performed under visual control.

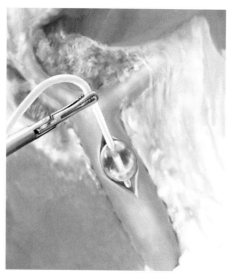

A-1

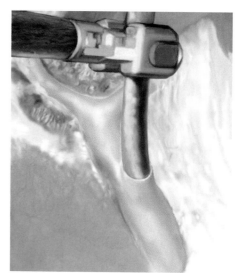

A-2

| STEP 5 | Suture of the choledochotomy |

- Closure of the choledochotomy is performed by using interrupted or continuous suture with resorbable 4-0 or 5-0 stitches.
- The use of resorbable or nonresorbable clips to block a continuous suture of the choledochotomy is contraindicated, to avoid further intraductal clip migration.
- At the end of the suturing, a water-tightness test is employed by blowing the CBD through the TC cholangiographic catheter, before clipping the CD or through the T-tube.

| STEP 6 | CBD drainage |

Several options can be used, including primary closure of the CBD (see Step 5), external biliary drainage (by a TC drain or a T-tube) or internal drainage (using an endoprosthesis).

- *Primary CBD closure:* is used when there is no doubt about the complete CBD vacuity, in the absence of severe cholangitis and when papillary obstruction is absent (permeable sphincter of Oddi, absence of edema due to transpapillary instrumental maneuvers, etc.).
- *External biliary drainage:* by using a transcystic drain (see TCBDE) or a T-tube. In case of T-tube placement, the tube is fenestrated and then inserted into the CBD through the choledochotomy. The CBD suture is started after having pushed the tube at the upper corner of the choledochotomy (A). Then the T-tube is exteriorized through the site of the fifth trocar.
- *Internal biliary drainage using an endoprosthesis:*
  - *Indication:* When the number of CBDs is limited, the stone clearance is accurate and in the absence of pancreatitis or Oddi dysfunction.
  - *Technique:* The endoprosthesis is pushed under fluoroscopic guidance on a guidewire into the CBD and through the papilla into the duodenum. Adequate transpapillary positioning is assessed by transcystic cholangiography at the end of the procedure (B).
    - The endoprosthesis is removed 3 weeks later by a standard duodenoscopy.

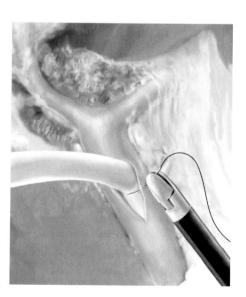

A

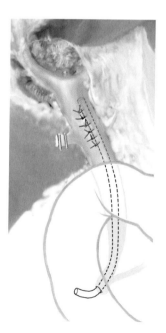

B

STEP 7

Perform control cholangiography at the end of the procedure to detect biliary leak or transcystic drain or T-tube misplacement.

STEP 8

Routine peritoneal drainage is used.

Postoperative Tests

- Clinical assessment
- Check biliary drains
- Laboratory tests: liver function tests, pancreatic enzymes
- Control cholangiography at postoperative days 2–3 (before hospital discharge) if a TC or a T-tube drain is in place, to exclude a residual CBDS or a biliary leak

Postoperative Complications

Local Complications
- Residual CBDS
- Bile leak
- Hemorrhage
- Subhepatic abscess
- Late biliary stricture

Due to External Biliary Drain
- Patient discomfort
- Electrolyte abnormalities
- Postradiologic cholangitis
- Tube obstruction
- Accidental tube removal
- Wound infection
- Bile peritonitis at extraction

Tricks of the Senior Surgeon

- Look carefully at pictures of IOC to decide the optimal strategy for CBDE; this will save operative time and decrease possible instrumental complications.
- Use soft, atraumatic instruments in the CBD and perform instrumental TCBDE under fluoroscopic guidance, to avoid CBD injury.
- When the suture of choledochotomy is completed, use a water-tightness test by blowing up the CBD with saline solution or methylene blue through a transcystic cholangiographic catheter or drain or through the T-tube.
- In case of failure of CBDE, postoperative endoscopic sphincterotomy can be planned. In these circumstances, placement of a transcystic biliary drain will optimize the success rate of the further endoscopic procedure.

Exploration of the Common Bile Duct: The Open Approach

Introduction

The first choledochotomy through laparotomy was reported by Kehr in 1896 and was the surgical treatment of choice for many years. However, since the 1990s, the open approach has been increasingly abandoned in favor of the laparoscopic procedure for CBDE.

Indications and Contraindications

Indications

- After conversion to open cholecystectomy
- When laparoscopic and endoscopic expertise is not available

Contraindications, Preoperative Investigations, Postoperative Tests and Postoperative Complications

These are similar to those for LCBDE.

Procedure

Incision and Exposure

Right subcostal or upper middle-line incision. The hepatoduodenal ligament is more easily stretched than for LCBDE, by pulling up the quadrate lobe using a retractor and pulling down the pancreatic head by using the assisting surgeon's hand.

Choledochotomy

Indications and techniques, including methods of stone extraction and stone clearance assessment, are similar to those for laparoscopic CBDE. However, external biliary drainage is classically used during open CBDE (OCBDE), by using either a TC drain or more often a T-tube. However, primary closure of the CBD might be indicated under the same conditions as for LCBDE. Internal biliary drainage is usually not reported during OCBDE.

- Stay sutures are placed on the CBD on either side of the planned choledochotomy, and the CBD is openedless (A).
- The common duct stone is then extracted either by choledochoscopy (B-1) or by use of stone forceps (B-2).
- The CBD is then closed over a T-tube (C).

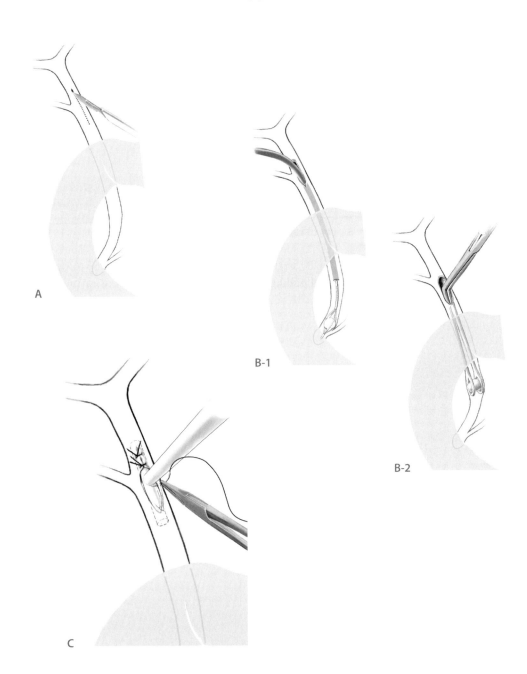

A

B-1

B-2

C

Bile Duct Resection

Yuji Nimura

Introduction

Resection of tumors at the bifurcation of the left and right hepatic duct requires one of the most difficult operations. The surgical procedure requires not only a portal lymphadenectomy and bile duct resection, but almost always a liver resection. The goals of this operation are: (1) resection of the primary tumor, (2) resection of the lymphatic drainage of the liver and (3) reestablishment of biliary continuity.

Indications and Contraindications

Indications
- Primary malignancies (e.g., intrahepatic cholangiocarcinoma involving the hepatic hilus, hilar cholangiocarcinoma, gallbladder carcinoma involving the hepatic hilus, diffuse carcinoma of the extrahepatic bile duct)
- Benign diseases (e.g., primary sclerosing cholangitis, inflammatory pseudotumor)
- Traumatic lesion at the hepatic hilus

Absolute Contraindications
- Biliary carcinoma with distant organ metastasis (liver, lung, bone, peritoneum)
- Uncontrollable severe cholangitis with or without sepsis
- Poor liver reserve with prolonged cholestasis
- Severe coagulopathy despite vitamin K administration

Relative Contraindication
- Locally advanced cholangiocarcinoma with bilateral hepatic arterial encasement

Preoperative Investigation and Preparation for the Procedure

History:	Biliary surgery
Clinical evaluation:	Jaundice, cholangitis, nutritional status
Laboratory tests:	Bilirubin, alkaline phosphatase, ALT, AST, albumin, coagulation parameters (prothrombin time, platelets), indocyanin green test, tumor markers carbohydrate antigen 19–9 (CA19–9) and carcinoembryonic antigen (CEA)
Radiology:	Ultrasonography, cholangiography (PTC, ERCP, MRCP), 3D CT (angiography), CT volumetry
Endoscopy:	Peroral cholangioscopy, percutaneous transhepatic cholangioscopy. The above procedures should be performed to make a differential diagnosis or to define the intraductal spread of cancer by taking a biopsy.

What we should not do

A metallic stent should not be used in resectable biliary carcinoma.

Preparation Prior to Surgery

- Antibiotics sensitive to bile culture
- Percutaneous transhepatic biliary drainage (endoscopic biliary drainage is not advisable)
- Portal vein embolization for major hepatectomy
- Internal biliary drainage or bile replacement through a nasogastric tube for patients with external biliary drainage

Procedure

Access

Incision, division of round and falciform ligament (see Sect. 1, chapters "Positioning and Accesses" and "Retractors and Principles of Exposure").

STEP 1

Exposure and exploration: installation of the retractor (see Sect. 1, chapter "Retractors and Principles of Exposure") and inspection of possible peritoneal metastasis.

Percutaneous transhepatic biliary drainage (PTBD) catheters are moved to the operative field to maintain intraoperative biliary drainage.

Ultrasound to evaluate location of the tumor in relation to vascular structures (portal vein, hepatic artery, hepatic vein).

Careful inspection of vascular variation.

STEP 2

Regional lymph node and connective tissue dissection

Lymph nodes in the hepatoduodenal ligament (No. 12), along the common hepatic (No. 8) and celiac arteries (No. 9) and retropancreatic nodes (No. 13), should be dissected (A) while placing a vessel loop around the common, proper, right, middle and left hepatic arteries and common bile duct (B).

Nerve plexuses around the hepatic artery should be dissected.

Confirmation of vascular variation.

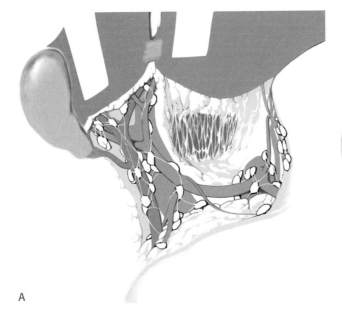

A

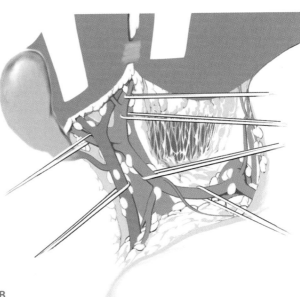

B

STEP 3   **Distal bile duct resection**

The Kocher maneuver is performed to mobilize the duodenum and allow dissection of the distal bile duct. The distal bile duct is dissected down to the head of the pancreas and divided above the pancreas. The resection margin must be examined by frozen section.

In some cases this procedure should be advanced more distally to detach the bile duct from the pancreatic tissue and resect the duct in the pancreas with a free margin.

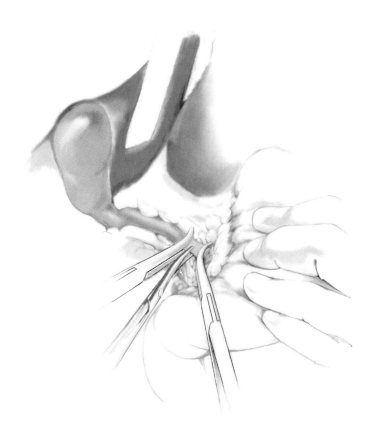

STEP 4

Skeletonization of the upper part of the hepatoduodenal ligament

The transected distal bile duct is pulled up and the distal portion of the hepatic artery and portal bifurcation exposed (A). After dividing the caudate lobe branches of the portal vein (A), the right and left portal veins are encircled by a vessel loop (B).

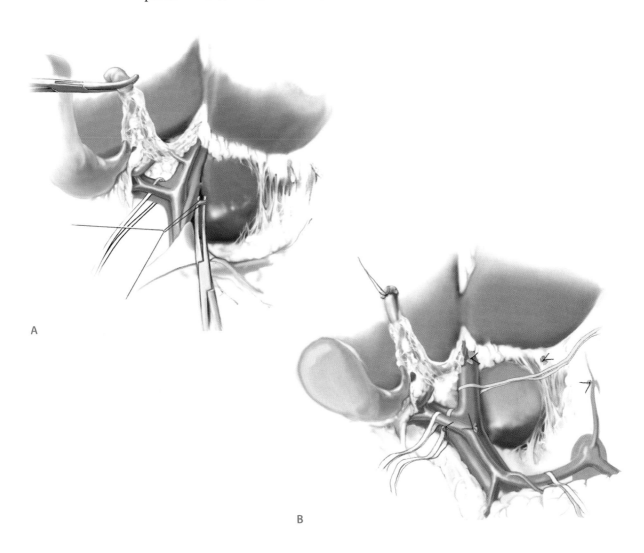

A

B

Left Hepatic Resection

STEP 5

Dividing the hepatic artery

Once the arterial anatomy and possible arterial variation are clearly identified, the left and middle hepatic arteries (and cystic artery) or right hepatic artery are divided at the origin (see Figure B of STEP 4). The remaining left hepatic artery is skeletonized more distally to encircle the right anterior and posterior branches at the right extremity of the hilar plate or the middle and left hepatic artery at Rex's recess.

STEP 6

Transection of the left portal vein

The left portal vein is divided and ligated distally to the bifurcation. An alternative is to use a small vascular clamp on the proximal side and oversew the venous stump with a running suture of 5-0 Prolene.

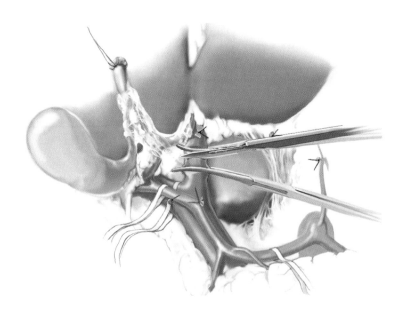

STEP 7 — Mobilization of the caudate lobe with division of the short hepatic veins

In case of left side hepatectomy, the short hepatic veins are divided in the same manner from the left caudal side to the right cranial side. Finally the distal end of the canal of Arantius is ligated and divided at the confluence of the left hepatic vein or the vena cava.

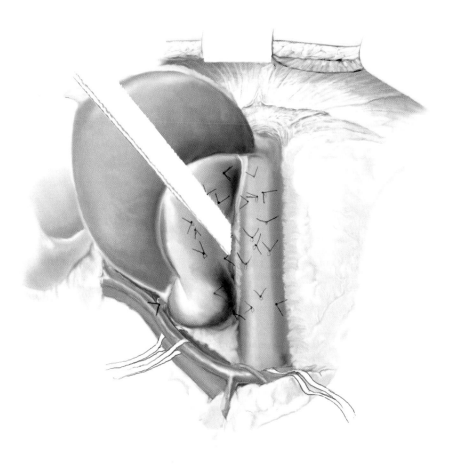

STEP 8 — Exposure and transection of the left hepatic vein

In case of a left hepatectomy, the left hepatic vein is not transected before liver dissection. A vessel loop is placed around the common trunk of the left and middle hepatic vein. In case of a left trisectionectomy, the common trunk of the left and middle hepatic veins is transected before the liver.

STEP 9

Demarcation and incision of the liver capsule

In case of a left hepatectomy with caudate lobe resection, dorsal demarcation appears between the caudate process and segment 7 after complete devascularization of the caudate lobe.

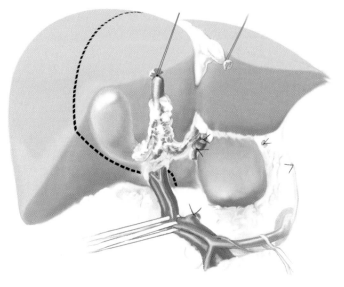

STEP 10

Division of the draining veins of the pericaval segment

In case of a total caudate lobe resection, draining veins of the pericaval segment (segment 9) are identified behind the middle hepatic vein and carefully divided. Liver transection is continued until the left hepatic vein is reached, divided and closed at its confluence of the middle hepatic vein. The right intrahepatic bile duct is identified behind the middle hepatic vein, and the posterior wall is carefully detached from the right anterior branch of the hepatic artery, which runs in the connective tissues between the bile duct and the portal vein. Two stay sutures are placed caudally and cranially and the bile duct is incised from the caudal edge where the anterior branch or the bile duct of segment 5 is opened.

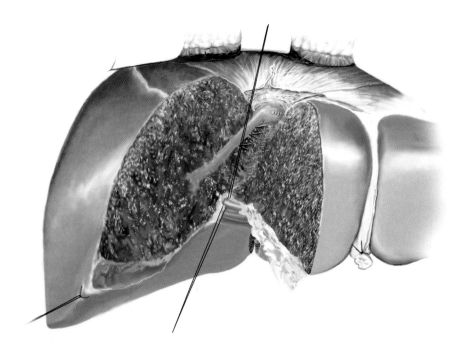

STEP 11

Intrahepatic bile duct resection

Further extension of the incision opens the segmental or subsegmental bile ducts of segment 8 (B8, B8a, B8bc) and the right posterior duct. The surgical field after removal of the left lobe and caudate lobe is shown.

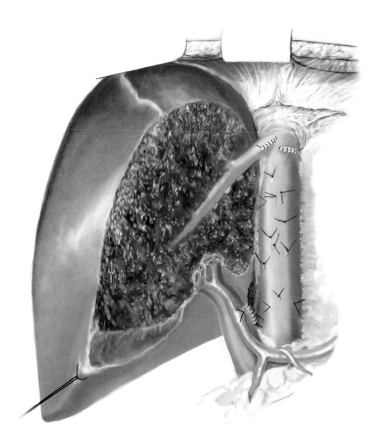

STEP 12   **Extended lymph node dissection**

After removing the hemiliver and the caudate lobe, para-aortic node dissection is
carried out from the level of the ligamentum crus to the origin of the inferior mesenteric
artery. The lymph nodes behind the left renal vein are carefully dissected by taping the
left renal vein and the right renal artery. Right celiac ganglionectomy is also performed
during this procedure.

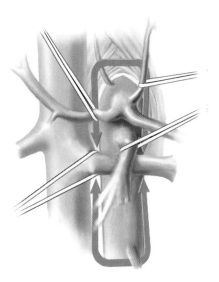

STEP 13

Biliary reconstructions

Before bilioenteric anastomosis, hepaticoplasty should be performed with 5-0 PDS sutures to minimize the number of anastomoses (A).

A Roux-en-Y jejunal loop is lifted through the shortest route: the retrocolic and retrogastric route. A jejunostomy tube is also introduced from the proximal edge of the jejunal limb before hepaticojejunostomy (B).

The posterior wall is first anastomosed with 4-0 PDS sutures and a biliary drainage tube is placed in each anastomosis. Finally the anterior wall is anastomosed. See chapter on biliary anastomosis.

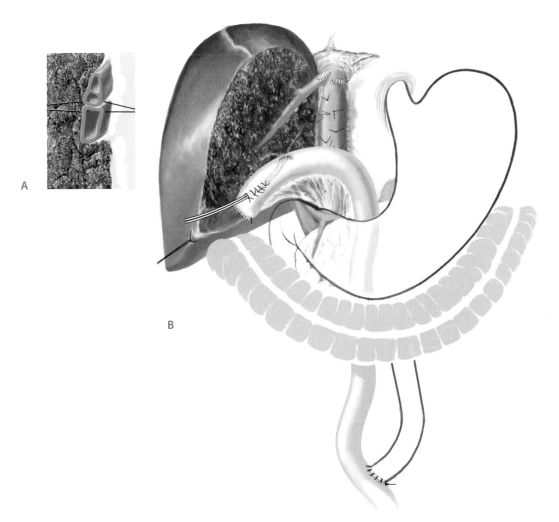

STEP 14

Drainage after reconstruction

After completing hemostasis in the surgical field, closed drains are placed in the foramen of Winslow, the pericaval space along the aorta and along the cut surface of the liver. Biliary drainage catheters and a jejunostomy tube are fixed on the skin, and the abdomen is closed. Although some groups do not use biliary stents, externally drained bile is mixed with elemental diet and ingested through the jejunostomy tube from the second postoperative day.

Right Hepatic Resection

Dividing the hepatic artery and portal vein

Once the arterial anatomy and possible arterial variations are clearly identified, the right
hepatic artery is divided at its origin. The remaining right hepatic artery is skeletonized
more distally to encircle the right anterior and posterior branches at the right extremity
of the hilar plate or the middle and left hepatic artery at Rex's recess. The figure
demonstrates a right predominant lesion and ligation of the right portal vein and
segment 4 veins that is necessary. Also illustrated is the ligated right hepatic artery.

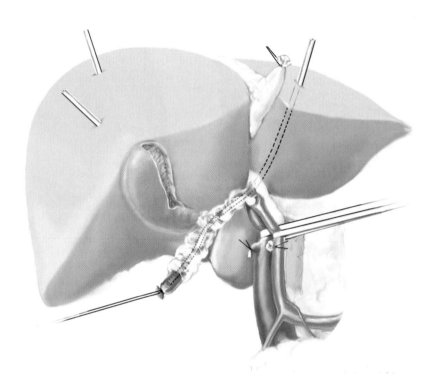

STEP 6

Mobilization of the right hepatic lobe and caudate lobe with division of the short hepatic veins

The right liver is mobilized and the entire short hepatic veins are divided between ties on the caval side and clips on the liver side from the right caudal side to the left cranial side.

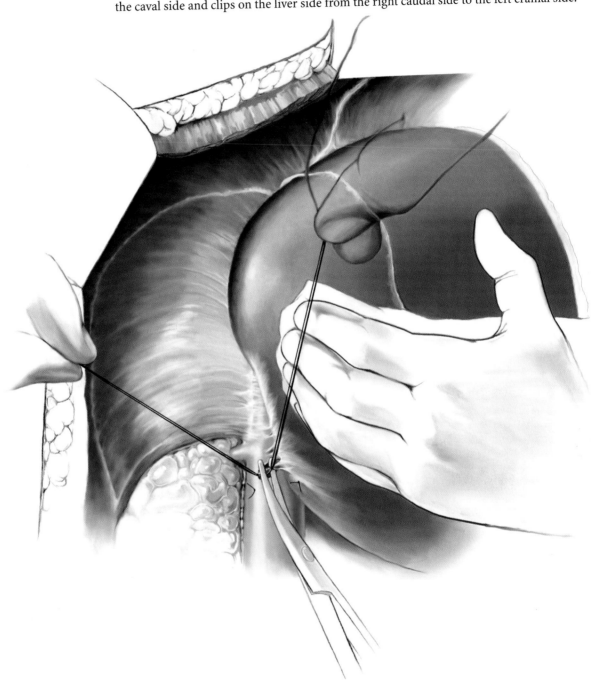

STEP 7

Exposure and transection of the right hepatic vein

A vessel loop is placed around the right hepatic vein, and vascular clamps are placed on the caval side and the liver side. The transection can be performed between the clamps. The caval side is secured by a running 4-0 Prolene suture and the other side with a 3-0 silk suture. An alternative technique is to transect the right hepatic vein with a vascular stapler (see the chapter on right hemihepatectomy).

STEP 8

Demarcation and marking of the liver capsule

A stay suture is placed at the inferior margin of the ischemic side of the liver, and the liver capsule is incised with monopolar diathermy or bipolar scissors along the demarcation. At this point, central venous pressure (CVP) should be maintained below 3 cm H_2O.

In case of a right hepatectomy with caudate lobectomy, a transection line on the visceral surface of the liver is turned transversely from the Cantlie line about 1 cm above the hilar plate to maintain a surgical margin and reach to the right edge of Rex's recess.

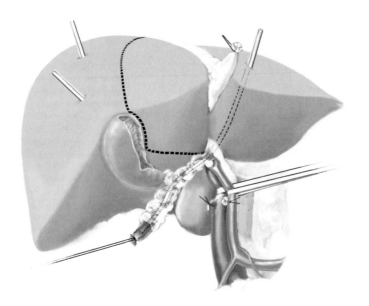

STEP 9

Transection of the liver

The liver dissection is started from the inferior margin under intermittent occlusion of the hepatic artery and the portal vein. The dissection is continued cranially and posteriorly, preserving the middle hepatic vein.

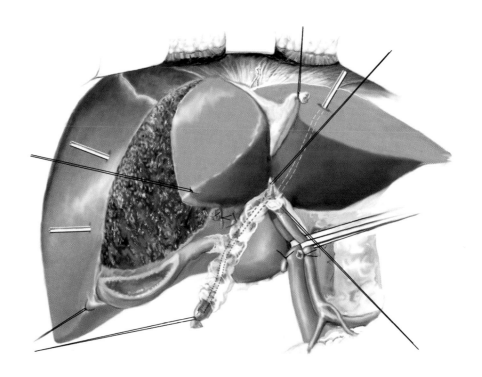

STEP 10   **Intrahepatic bile duct resection**

The left intrahepatic bile duct is identified at the right edge of Rex's recess. Two stay sutures are placed ventrally and dorsally (**A**), the left hepatic duct is transected perpendicularly, and the right liver, caudate lobe and extrahepatic bile duct are removed (**B**). At the ventral edge of the resected margin of the left hepatic duct, the bile duct of segment 4 is opened followed by the segments 2 and 3 dorsally.

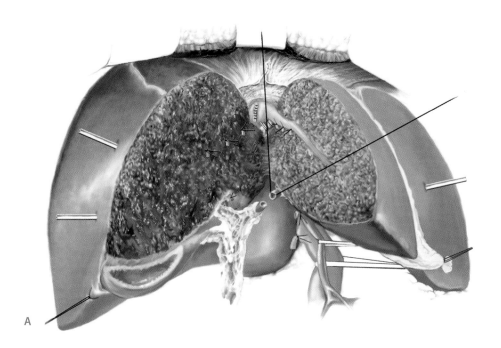

A

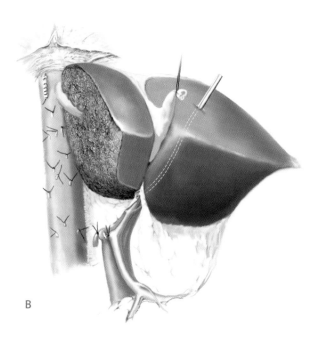

B

STEP 11

Extended lymph node dissection is performed as above.

STEP 12

Biliary reconstructions

A Roux-en-Y jejunal loop is lifted through the shortest route: the retrocolic route. A jejunostomy tube is also introduced from the proximal edge of the jejunal limb before hepaticojejunostomy.

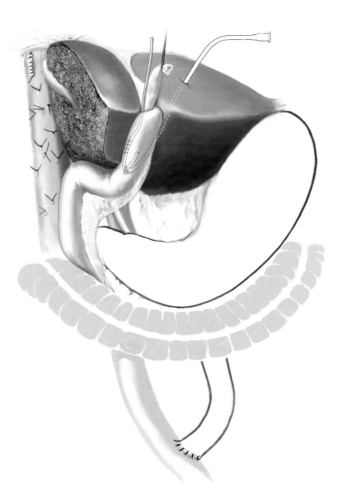

Postoperative Tests

- Postoperative surveillance in an intensive or intermediate care unit
- Liver function test (bilirubin, ALT, AST, albumin), coagulation parameters, hemoglobin, red blood cell (RBC), withe blood cell (WBC), CRP
- Color Doppler ultrasound to estimate the blood flow of the portal vein and hepatic artery

Local Postoperative Complications

- Short term:
  - (Pleural effusion)
  - Wound infection
  - Bile leak from hepaticojejunostomy or raw surface of the liver
  - Subphrenic or subhepatic abscess
  - Intra-abdominal bleeding
  - Liver failure
  - Portal vein thrombosis
- Long term:
  - Cholangitis
  - Anastomotic stricture
  - Chronic liver failure

Tricks of the Senior Surgeon

- Check the intraoperative external biliary drainage to prevent unexpected biliary congestion from which septic complications may develop.
- Suture the large short hepatic veins or caudate lobe veins in detaching the caudate lobe from the vena cava.
- Check the CVP in the monitor before liver transection. If the CVP is higher than $3\,cm\,H_2O$, do not start to transect the liver.
- The hepatic vein on the liver side should be closed by a running suture to prevent bleeding during the handling of the liver.
- Stay sutures should be placed before dividing the intrahepatic bile duct, otherwise the small segmental duct will slip away and be hidden by the liver parenchyma.
- The lymphatic vessels should be tied in a para-aortic lymph node dissection to prevent postoperative massive lymphorrhea.

Editor's Comments

- Tissue diagnosis is not a prerequisite for surgical resection of suspected cholangio-carcinoma – clinical presentation and radiographic appearance is enough.
- ERCP and peroral cholangioscopy are avoided for high bile duct obstruction since these are unlikely to define the problems or palliate obstruction, and can lead to cholangitis.
- Percutaneous drainage is not always necessary prior to surgery. The patients who will benefit from preoperative drainage are those who (1) have cholangitis, (2) have renal dysfunction, (3) have possible vascular invasion on the side that will be the remnant liver after resection or (4) should undergo portal vein embolization.
- In mobilizing the candidate lobe for a patient who will be subjected to a left lobectomy and caudate resection, it is usually safest to mobilize the caudate from the right to the left. Only in the thinnest patients is it safe to perform the mobilization from the left.
- Some surgeons believe that caudate resection is an essential part of every resection for hilar cholangiocarcinoma, while others believe that resecting this portion of the liver is indicated only when the caudate lobe is directly involved by tumor.

Resection of the Mid Common Bile Duct

Chandrajit P. Raut, Jean-Nicolas Vauthey

Introduction

True mid bile duct tumors are very rare. Most patients with mid bile duct obstruction should be considered to have gallbladder cancer until proven otherwise. Mid bile duct resections are usually performed for the rare mid duct cholangiocarcinomas or for patients with early gallbladder cancer and tumor at the cystic duct margin.

Indications and Contraindications

Indications

- Diagnosis of biliary strictures without confirmed malignancy
- Diagnosis of suspected benign disease
- Confirmed malignant disease confined to mid common bile duct (CBD) in patients unfit for more extensive resection (pancreaticoduodenectomy or liver resection)

Contraindications

- Malignant disease involving biliary confluence (hilar cholangiocarcinoma)
- Vascular invasion involving the main trunk of the portal vein or the proper hepatic artery
- Bilateral vascular involvement of hepatic arterial and/or portal venous branches

Preoperative Investigation and Preparation for the Procedure

History:	Alcohol intake, cholelithiasis, choledocholithiasis, primary sclerosing cholangitis/ulcerative colitis, choledochal cysts, Caroli's disease, recurrent pyogenic cholangiohepatitis, biliary parasites, exposure to chemical carcinogens
Clinical evaluation:	Jaundice (90–98% of patients), weight loss (51%), abdominal pain (45%), fever (20%)
Laboratory tests:	Alkaline phosphatase, γ-glutamyl transpeptidase, ALT, AST, coagulation parameters
	Assess intra- and extrahepatic biliary obstruction, presence of gallstones, tumor extension, vascular involvement
CT scan, CT angiography or MRI:	Identify metastases, define relationship between tumor mass (if detectable) and liver, assess lobar atrophy or compensatory hypertrophy, hepatic arterial anatomy
PTC/ERCP/MRCP:	Delineate proximal extent of tumor, number of tumors (10% of cases will have multiple tumors)
Cytology:	Percutaneous catheter drainage (positive in 47% of cases), fine needle aspiration (sensitivity 77%), endoscopic transpapillary biopsy, ERCP brushing

Procedure

STEP 1   **Exposure and exploration**

The abdomen is explored through a bilateral subcostal incision. Retraction is maintained with broad blade retractors from a fixed support, elevating the costal margin. A soft retractor blade (malleable) may be inserted from above to retract segment 4. The ligamentum teres is divided, and the falciform ligament is separated from the anterior abdominal wall. Cephalad traction on the ligamentum teres provides additional exposure of the undersurface of the liver. If present, the bridge of liver parenchyma between segment 4 and the left lateral bisegment is divided with electrocautery; bleeding is easily controlled as this tissue rarely contains large vessels. This maneuver exposes the umbilical fissure for a later step.

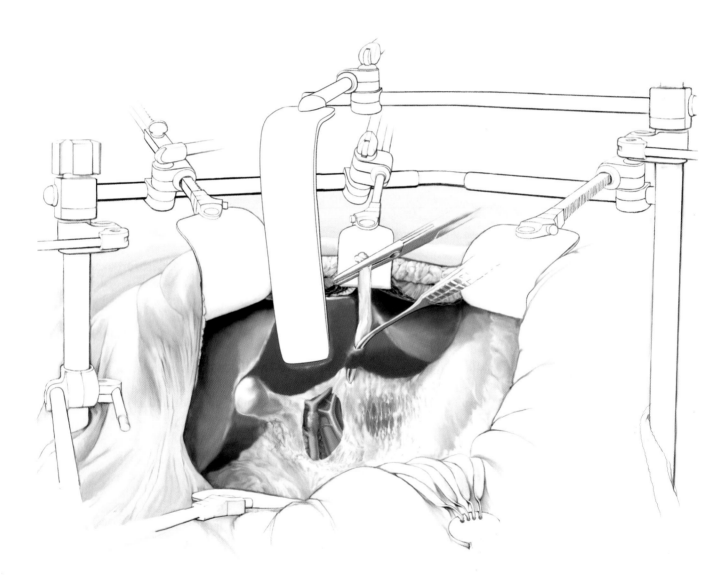

STEP 2	**Division of the distal CBD**

The gallbladder, if present, is dissected free from its liver bed. The proximal CBD and the right and left hepatic ducts are dilated proximal to the stricture, unless stenting across the stricture has drained the obstruction. The distal CBD is isolated and divided early in the dissection above the superior edge of the pancreas and a frozen section analysis of the margin is obtained. The distal CBD stump is ligated in a figure-of-eight fashion with 4-0 PDS suture on an SH needle.

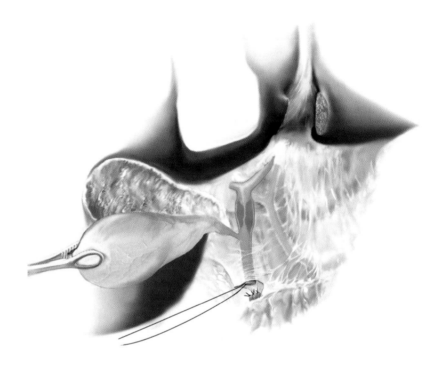

STEP 3   **Division of the proximal CBD**

The CBD, gallbladder and hepatoduodenal lymph nodes are reflected superiorly en bloc, exposing the hilar vessels and confirming resectability. Dissection is continued between the tumor anteriorly and the hepatic artery posteriorly. The hilar plate is lowered by dividing the peritoneal reflection at the base of segment 4 and the umbilical fissure is opened to expose the extrahepatic left bile duct (A). As this exposure is extended to the left, a branch of the portal vein or hepatic artery to segment 4 may be encountered and should be preserved. This exposure allows the base of segment 4 to be elevated; the malleable blade retracting the quadrate lobe may be repositioned. The proximal duct is transected at the confluence of the right and left hepatic ducts, and the specimen is marked for orientation. Additional duct margins are submitted for intraoperative microscopic frozen section examination. The opening in the proximal duct at the site of transection can be extended into the extrahepatic left bile duct sharply using Pott's scissors (B).

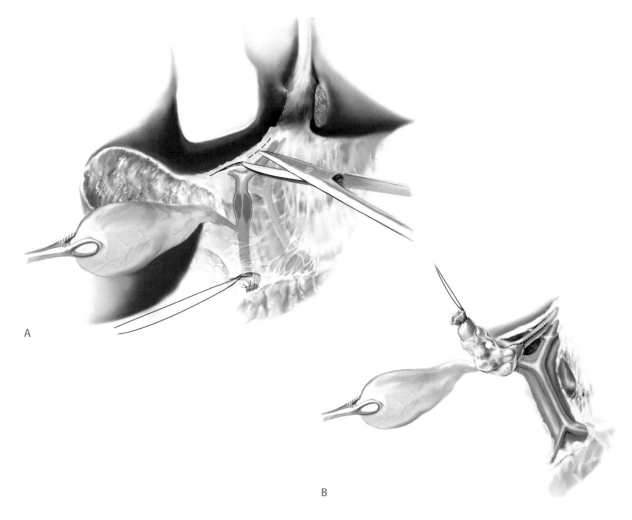

A

B

If the proximal bile duct is dilated, there may be no need to lower the hilar plate or extend the incision to the left hepatic duct – Y.F.

STEP 4

Hepp-Couinaud reconstruction

The biliary-enteric continuity is restored with a side-to-side retrocolic Roux-en-Y hepaticojejunostomy with a single layer of interrupted, absorbable sutures (5-0 PDS vs. an shRVI needle as preferred by the authors). This technique incorporates the extrahepatic portion of the left duct in the anastomosis, as first described by Hepp and Couinaud, thus creating a wide side-to-side hepaticojejunostomy. A 70-cm jejunal Roux-en-Y limb is prepared and brought through the transverse mesocolon to the right of the middle colic artery; the stapled end does not need to be oversewn. Both the left duct and the jejunum are incised longitudinally for a 2-cm-wide anastomosis. The anterior row of No. 5-0 absorbable sutures is brought through the bile duct wall and the needles are left intact (A). A Gabbay-Fisher suture guide (Genzyme Co., Fall River, MA) facilitates the management of these free sutures by organizing them; each guide holds up to 16 sutures. Gentle retraction on these sutures superiorly allows exposure of the posterior edge of the ductal incision. Precise mucosa-to-mucosa anastomosis is established with interrupted No. 5-0 absorbable sutures between the posterior edge of the ductal incision and the posterior edge of the jejunal incision. The posterior sutures are tied with the knots on the inside (B). The anterior stay sutures are then placed through the jejunum to complete the anterior row of sutures. These are tied such that the knots are exterior (C). Internal stenting is not required. A drain on bulb suction is left near the anastomosis and brought through the abdominal wall in the right upper quadrant.

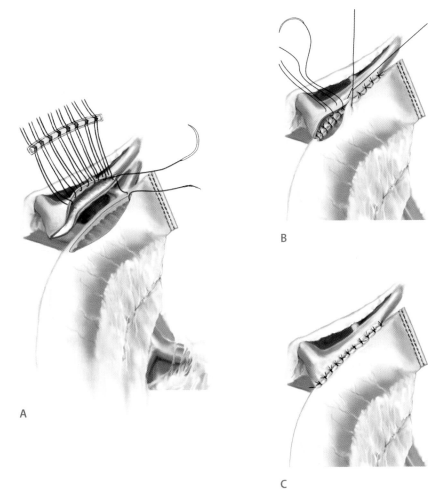

A

B

C

Local Postoperative Complications

- Short term:
  - Bile leak
- Long term:
  - Cholangitis (rare)

Tricks of the Senior Surgeon

- Preoperative biliary drainage with a transtumoral catheter may be of technical assistance for the hilar dissection and biliary enteric anastomosis, but does not reduce perioperative morbidity or duration of hospitalization. Drainage is only indicated in patients with sepsis and cholangitis.
- If present, the bridge of liver parenchyma between segment 4 and the left lateral bisegment is divided by electrocautery.
- Duct margins should be submitted for intraoperative frozen section analysis.
- A Gabbay-Fisher suture guide facilitates the management of these free sutures by organizing them to minimize entanglement; each guide holds up to 16 sutures.
- Internal stenting is not required.
- Resection and reconstruction utilizing the Hepp-Couinaud approach, which employs a wide mucosa-to-mucosa anastomosis extended to the left hepatic duct, has the advantage over an end-to-side anastomosis of having a lower rate of stricturing.

Intrahepatic Biliodigestive Anastomosis Without Indwelling Stent

William R. Jarnagin

Introduction

The technique for reestablishing continuity of the extrahepatic bile ducts to the intestinal tract is described. Multiple biliary lumen may be encountered even with minor dissection into the hepatic parenchyma. All lumens should either be anastomosed or ligated with permanent sutures.

Indications and Contraindications

Indications

- Reconstitution of biliary-enteric continuity after bile duct resection or combined hepatic and biliary resection for malignancy involving the proximal bile duct – typically hilar cholangiocarcinoma or gallbladder cancer
- Palliative biliary drainage for proximal biliary obstruction due to locally advanced malignancy
- Provision of durable biliary drainage in the setting of a benign stricture/injury of the proximal bile duct – often associated with multiple prior attempts at repair

Contraindications

- Elective, palliative intrahepatic biliary-enteric bypass for malignancy is best avoided in the face of widespread metastatic disease, extensive intrahepatic disease or portal vein obstruction.
- Portal hypertension in patients with benign strictures is a lethal combination and should rarely be attempted.

Procedures

General (End to Side)

The general technique for intrahepatic (and proximal extrahepatic) biliodigestive anastomoses is shown. This technique is quite useful in all cases where access to the bile duct is limited by space. In such situations, approaches that might be appropriate for a straightforward distal bile duct anastomosis usually cannot be used. For example, one may be tempted to complete the posterior row as the first step, as one would in a distal bile duct anastomosis, only to find that completion of the anterior row is now extremely difficult, if not impossible, due to steric hindrance from the bowel. The technique described allows precise placement of sutures under direct vision, before apposition of the bowel and bile duct hinders access. In all cases, anastomosis is performed to a 70-cm retrocolic Roux-en-Y jejunal loop. Absorbable suture material (3-0 or 4-0 Vicryl or PDS) should be used.

STEP 1	Identification of transected bile ducts

After adequate exposure of the duct has been obtained, a tension-free jejunal loop is brought through the transverse mesocolon. It is imperative that the surgeon identify all exposed ductal orifices for inclusion in the anastomosis (see below). Failure to provide adequate drainage of all ducts often leads to serious postoperative complications, such as persistent bile leak or subhepatic abscess, biliary fistulation, lobar atrophy, cholangitis or hepatic abscess.

The jejunal limb is temporarily anchored with a stay suture at some distance from the bile duct to allow precise placement of the sutures.

STEP 2	**Placement of anterior stitches**

Working from left to right, the anterior row of sutures is placed on the bile duct (inside to out) (A).

The sutures are sequentially clamped and the needles are retained. It is important to keep the sutures in order so that they can be easily retrieved (B).

STEP 3	**Placement of posterior stitches**

Once the anterior row has been placed on the bile duct, the posterior row is placed.

Working from left to right, full-thickness sutures are placed from the jejunal limb (inside to out) to the back wall of the bile duct (outside to in) (B).

The sutures are not tied but are sequentially clamped with the needles removed. Again, it is important to keep the sutures in order.

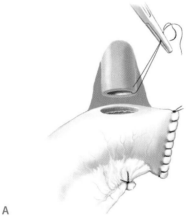

A

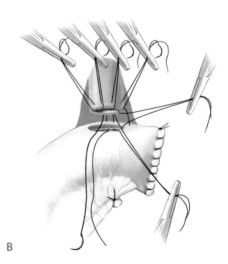

B

STEP 4   **Approximating the posterior anastomosis**

The jejunal loop is then slid upward along the posterior row of sutures until the back
wall of the bowel and the bile ducts are apposed.
  The posterior sutures are then tied and the sutures are cut.

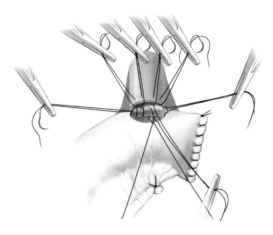

STEP 5   **Completing the anterior anastomosis**

The previously placed sutures on the anterior wall of the bile duct are now used to
complete the anastomosis.
  Working from right to left, the needles are passed sequentially through the anterior
jejunal wall (outside to in).
  The sutures are not tied at this point but are sequentially clamped with the needles
removed.

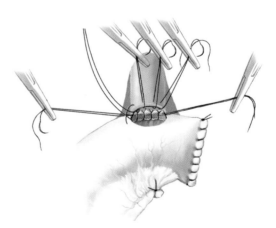

| STEP 6 | Tying the anterior stitches |

The anterior layer is then completed by securing the sutures, tying from left to right (A).

The completed anastomosis is shown (B).

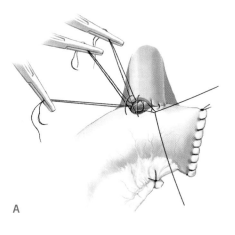

A

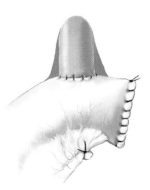

B

Anastomosis to Multiple Ducts (End to Side)

Resection of the biliary tree above the confluence often results in multiple disconnected ducts, all of which must be included in the anastomosis. Failure to do so often results in life-threatening complications, as described above. If possible, two or more disconnected duct orifices should be approximated with sutures and treated as a single duct for the purposes of the anastomosis. When this is not possible, the same general technique can be used to perform multiple simultaneous anastomoses. By placing the entire anterior row of sutures on all exposed ducts followed by the posterior row, as described above, the separated orifices are treated as if single. Interference from the jejunal limb usually precludes creation of a second anastomosis after the first has been completed.

Single Anastomosis to Multiple Exposed Ducts

STEP 1   **Identification of all lumens**

All exposed ducts are identified.

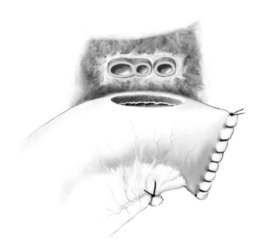

STEP 2   **Anastomosis to a single jejunal opening**

Ducts that are not connected by a septum are brought into apposition by placing two or three interrupted sutures. The complex of exposed ducts can be treated as a single ductal orifice, and the anastomosis is created to a single jejunal opening. The anastomosis is carried out using the general technique described in "Procedures", "General (End to Side)".

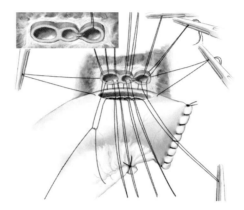

Multiple Simultaneous Anastomoses to Separated Ducts

If the surgeon determines that the ductal orifices are too widely separated to create a single anastomosis, multiple simultaneous anastomoses will be required, using the same general approach as described in "Procedures", "General (End to Side)". Working from left to right, the anterior row of sutures is placed on all exposed bile ducts (inside to out). The sutures are sequentially clamped and the needles are retained, keeping the sutures in order so that they can be easily retrieved (A).

The jejunal loop is then slid upward along the posterior row of sutures until the back wall of the bowel and the bile ducts are apposed, making sure that the jejunal openings are properly aligned to the respective ductal orifices. The posterior sutures are then tied and the sutures are cut (B).

The previously placed sutures on the anterior wall of the bile duct are now used to complete the anastomosis, as in "Procedures", "General (End to Side)", making certain that the ductal sutures are correctly placed to the corresponding jejunal opening (C).

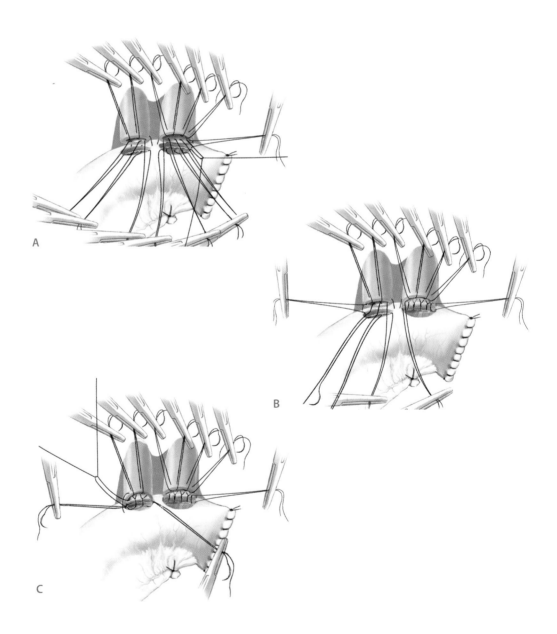

Side-to-Side Intrahepatic Anastomosis

Side to side intrahepatic biliary-enteric anastomoses are generally undertaken for palliative biliary drainage in patients with unresectable cancer, most commonly hilar cholangiocarcinoma or gallbladder cancer; they are much less frequently used in cases of benign strictures/bile duct injuries. The most common approaches are to use the segment 3 duct or the right anterior sectoral duct. Techniques have been described for exposing the segment 5 duct at the base of the gallbladder fossa, although this is difficult and rarely used. The anastomotic technique used is identical to that described in "Procedures", "General (End to Side)" above. There are several general points worth emphasizing regarding these approaches:

- In patients with advanced cancer, the right and left ductal systems are often isolated. Decompression of the right or left side alone will result in normalization of the serum bilirubin if at least 30 % of the functional hepatic parenchyma is adequately drained.
- A bypass created to a lobe with ipsilateral portal vein occlusion or gross atrophy is doomed to failure and should be avoided.
- If the right and left ductal systems are isolated, the contralateral side will not be adequately drained. In patients with advanced malignancy, this is acceptable, provided that the contralateral biliary tree has not been contaminated (i.e., prior instrumentation). If this is the case, interventional radiologists may be able to place an internal wall stent from left to right (or right to left), allowing decompression of the contralateral system through the bypass; if not, the patient will require a permanent external biliary drain.
- For benign strictures, unlike palliative bypass for malignancy, intrahepatic bypass approaches require continuity at the hilus so that complete biliary decompression is achieved.

Tricks of the Senior Surgeon

- When multiple ducts are encountered, it is particularly important to find the open caudate ducts. If these are left without anastomoses to the intestinal tract, a chronic fistula may occur.
- If a small open duct is encountered that is too small for anastomosis, ligation with a non absorbable suture is the most expedient solution.

The Ligamentum Teres Approach and Other Approaches to the Intrahepatic Ducts for Palliative Bypass

Michael D'Angelica

Introduction

When the hilus of the liver is not accessible for decompression of obstructive jaundice, use of intrahepatic ducts for surgical bypass is a safe and effective technique as originally described by Bismuth and Corlette in 1975 and later by Blumgart and Kelly in 1984. The general principle is to identify intrahepatic healthy bile duct mucosa proximal to a point of biliary obstruction and to create a mucosa-to-mucosa anastomosis to a long Roux-en-y loop of jejunum. Anastomosis should provide biliary drainage and relief of symptoms such as jaundice and pruritis.

Indications and Contraindications

Indications

- Malignant obstruction (most commonly gallbladder carcinoma and hilar cholangiocarcinoma) of the biliary confluence when access to the common hepatic duct is not possible
- Life expectancy greater than 6 months
- Extensive benign stricture involving the biliary confluence when access to the common hepatic duct is not possible
- Complete obliteration of the biliary confluence and consequent disconnection of the right from the left liver is *not* a contraindication

Exclusion Criteria

- Lack of safe access to healthy bile duct mucosa for an adequate anastomosis
- Bypass to a portion of liver that is atrophied or fibrotic

Investigation/Preparation

Clinical:	Signs and symptoms of cholangitis, cirrhosis and portal hypertension
Laboratory:	Liver function tests, nutritional parameters, clotting parameters, renal function
Radiology:	Duplex ultrasound, magnetic resonance cholangiopancreatography (MRCP); consider direct cholangiography (percutaneous transhepatic) with or without preoperative stenting
Preparation:	Bowel preparation, perioperative broad-spectrum antibiotics, adequate treatment of cholangitis with drainage and antibiotics

Procedure

Access and General Principles

- The incision must provide adequate access to the hilum of the liver as well as provide the ability to completely mobilize the liver if necessary.
- Potential incisions: right subcostal incision with a midline vertical extension (hockey stick), bilateral subcostal incision with or without midline vertical extension (chevron, rooftop).
- In the special case of right lobe atrophy, extension of the incision to a thoraco-abdominal approach from the midpoint of the right subcostal portion up through the 7th intercostal space can be invaluable.
- Retraction with a Goligher retractor with wide blades pulling the ribs in an anterior and cephalad direction.
- Intraoperative ultrasound to determine the relationship of tumor/stricture and adequately dilated bile ducts.
- Intraperitoneal drain is placed and left for gravity drainage postoperatively.

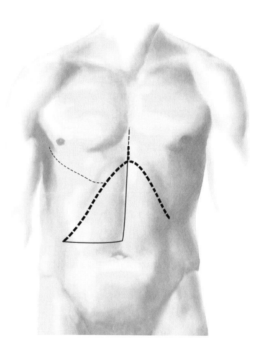

Approach to the Left Hepatic Duct

STEP 1   **Dividing the bridge between segments 3 and 4**

The ligamentum teres is divided and the falciform ligament is freed from the abdominal wall and diaphragm. A tie is left in place on the hepatic side of the ligamentum teres, which serves as a retractor to help elevate the liver. The bridge of liver tissue between the quadrate lobe (segment 4b) and the left lateral segment is divided. There are never major vessels in this tissue and it can be divided easily with electrocautery. This maneuver exposes the umbilical fissure completely and makes dissection at the base of segment 4 easier.

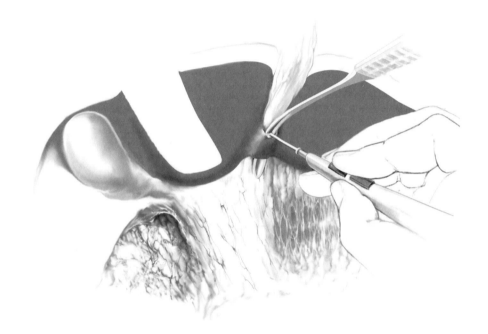

STEP 2   **Exposing the duct**

Segment 4 is elevated superiorly, exposing its base. Sharp dissection is used to dissect
the plane between Glisson's capsule and the left portal triad, thus lowering the hilar
plate (A). The left hepatic duct is exposed and dissected throughout its transverse extrahepatic course at the base of segment 4 before it enters the umbilical fissure. Dissection
to the right side can expose the biliary confluence and the right hepatic duct origin as
well (B). Minor bleeding can occur in this area and is almost always controllable with
light pressure. A thin curved retractor placed at the base of segment 4 from above can
help with exposure. A large tumor in this area may make exposure difficult, mandating
local excision or abandonment of this approach.

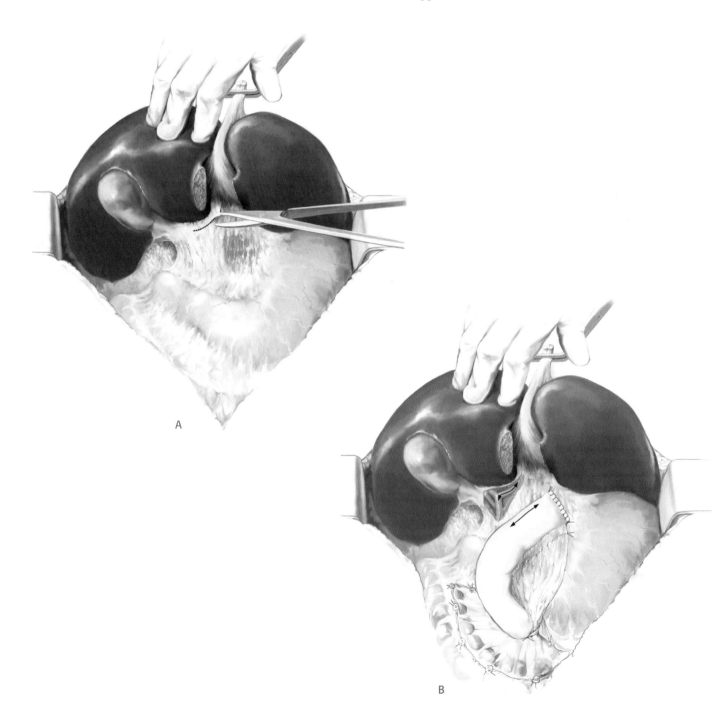

A

B

STEP 3   **Biliary-enteric amastomosis**

A 70-cm Roux-en-y loop of jejunum is brought up to the hilum in a retrocolic fashion and a side-to-side anastomosis is performed.

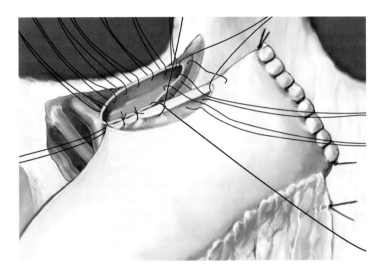

Ligamentum Teres (Round Ligament) Approach
(See also chapter "Intrahepatic Biliodigestive Anastomosis Without Indwelling Stent")

STEP 1   Controlling the round ligament

The ligamentum teres is divided and the falciform ligament freed from the abdominal wall and diaphragm. The bridge of liver tissue between segment 4 and the left lateral segment is divided.

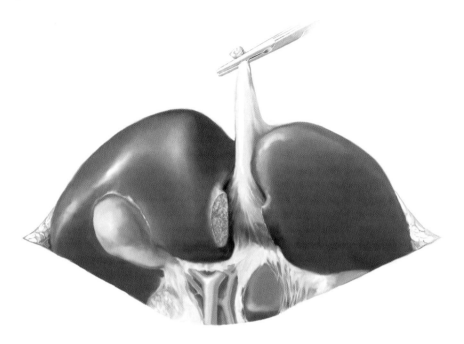

STEP 2   Mobilizing and positioning the round ligament

While holding the liver upward, the ligamentum teres is then pulled downward and its attachments to the liver are released, exposing its base.

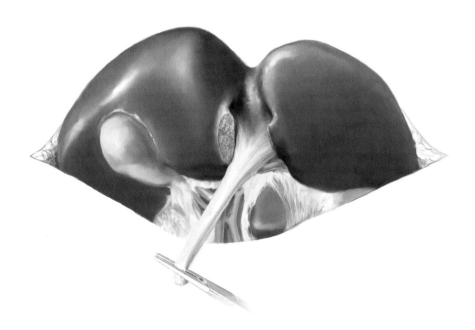

STEP 3

Dissection is then carried out to the left of the upper surface of the base of the ligamentum teres. A number of small vascular branches to the left lateral segment will be encountered and sometimes must be ligated and divided. The main portal pedicle to segment 3 can usually be preserved. This dissection can be tedious and must be done carefully because bleeding in this area can be difficult to control. A small aneurysm needle can be helpful in isolating and encircling these small branches.

STEP 4

Exposing the segment 3 duct

The segment 3 duct is exposed in its position above and behind the portal vein branch. The duct is opened longitudinally just beyond the branching of the segment 2 and 3 ducts. A side-to-side hepaticojejunostomy to a 70-cm retrocolic Roux-en-Y jejunal loop is carried out.

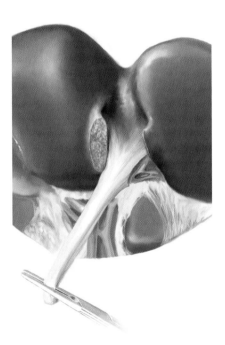

STEP 5

Partial hepatectomy to facilitate exposure

An alternative approach or a helpful adjuvant technique to expose the segment 3 duct is to split the liver just to the left of the falciform ligament superiorly (**A**) and to divide the tissue until the duct is reached from above (**B**). This can assist identification of the duct or be the primary means of approach. The added benefit of this approach is the lack of devascularization to segment 3 that is usually necessary for the dissection in the umbilical fissure.

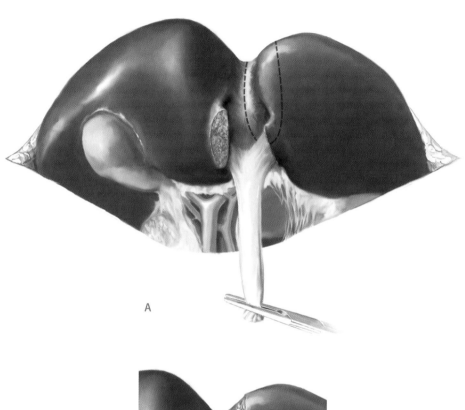

A

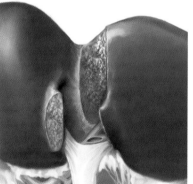

B

Approach to Proximal Right Sectoral Ducts

STEP 1

The ligamentum teres is divided and the falciform ligament is freed from the abdominal wall and diaphragm. A tie is left in place on the hepatic side of the ligamentum teres, which serves as a retractor to help elevate the liver.

STEP 2	Identification of the right portal pedicle

Hepatotomies are made at the base of the gallbladder and at the caudate process and the main right portal pedicle is identified. The tissue in front of the main right portal pedicle is divided by blunt dissection and ligation and excised.

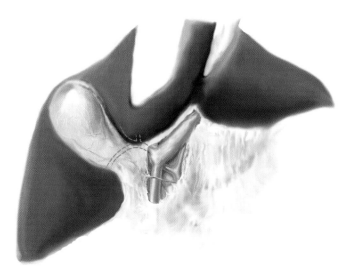

STEP 3	Exposing the right hepatic ducts

With the main right portal pedicle exposed, intrahepatic dissection is continued along either the anterior (more commonly) or the posterior pedicle until a satisfactory length is demonstrated. The bile duct is then dissected and exposed longitudinally. A longitudinal incision is then made in the bile duct.

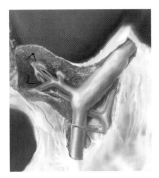

STEP 4

A side-to-side hepaticojejunostomy to a retrocolic 70-cm Roux-en-Y loop of jejunum is performed.

Postoperative Tests

- Coagulation parameters and hematocrit in the first 48 hours
- Daily liver function tests
- Daily assessment of renal function
- Daily assessment of drain output for bile leakage

Postoperative Complications

- Short term:
    - Bile leakage
    - Biloma
    - Abscess
    - Liver dysfunction/liver failure
    - Intra-abdominal bleeding
    - Early stricture of anastomosis
- Long term:
    - Recurrent benign biliary stricture
    - Recurrent malignant biliary stricture
    - Cholangitis

Tricks of the Senior Surgeon

- In the round ligament approach, a small branch of the portal vein passing to segment 3 usually lies immediately anterior to the segment 3 duct. This branch usually needs to be divided for adequate ductal exposure.
- Even if the malignant obstruction has isolated the left biliary tree from the right, drainage of only the left liver most often will suffice to relieve jaundice. This is particularly true if the tumor occupies predominantly the right liver and has produced right hepatic atrophy.
- Because of technical difficulties, right-sided bypasses have largely been abandoned in favor of percutaneous drainage.

Choledochojejunostomy and Cholecystojejunostomy

Henricus B.A.C. Stockmann, Johannes J. Jeekel

Introduction

For any patient with a life expectancy of greater than 6 months, surgical biliary bypass can provide durable palliation for jaundice. The preferred surgical method for palliative treatment of biliary obstruction is a side-to-side anastomosis, because it allows the possibility of making a large anastomosis, and of draining the intrahepatic bile duct as well as the part of the bile duct distal to the anastomosis. If local anatomy does not allow a side-to-side anastomosis, an end-to-side anastomosis should be made taking into account the possibility of stasis of pancreatic juice in the pancreatic part of the bile duct.

Indications and Contraindications

Indications	■ Inoperable or M1 malignant tumors of the head of the pancreas or the papilla Vateri ■ Primary (inoperable) duodenal malignancy (adenocarcinoma, neuroendocrine tumors, lymphoma, sarcoma) ■ Secondary (inoperable) malignancy in the ligamental area (carcinoma, melanoma, lymphoma, leukemia, sarcoma)
Absolute and Relative Contraindications	■ Life expectancy less than 6 months (preferred method of treatment: transmural percutaneous or endoscopic stent placement) ■ Severe coagulation disorders due to the biliary obstruction (preoperative correction through vitamin K administration) ■ Local infectious disease: cholangitis, abscesses ■ Quality of biliary, ligamental or intestinal surgical anatomy (e.g., portal hypertension, sclerosing cholangitis, short bowel syndrome) ■ Comorbidity (e.g., Child-Pugh C liver cirrhosis)
Indications for Choledochojejunostomy	■ High insertion of cystic duct into the common bile duct (CBD) in patients with low obstruction

Investigation and Preparation

Clinical
- Pain in the right upper abdomen
- Weight loss/catabolic state
- Icterus
- Pruritus
- Coagulopathy
- Hepatorenal dysfunction
- Cholangitis

Laboratory Tests

Liver-specific function:	Lactate dehydrogenase (LDH), ALT, AST, γ–glutamyl transpeptidase (GGT), and alkaline phosphatase, bilirubin
Prothrombin time:	Coagulation test in case of an interrupted enterohepatic circle

Radiology

Ultrasound:	Origin, location and type of the obstruction, width of the intra- and extrahepatic bile ducts and the possibility of relieving the bile ducts by percutaneous transhepatic drainage
Three-phase CT scan:	Extent of the obstructive lesion, local resectability and relation to the surrounding structures (the portal vein and the common hepatic artery)

What We Should Not Do

Preoperatively, one should consider whether the morbidity and mortality of the surgical procedure outweigh the life expectancy of the patient. Often one is confronted with inoperability during exploration. In such situations, biliary bypass can be performed as a palliative measure. However, postoperative stent placement is preferred if life expectancy is short.

If preoperative drainage of the obstruction is required, plastic endoprotheses are the equipment of choice, because they are easier to remove during surgery. The placement of wall stents should be avoided in obstructive bile duct disease.

Preparation Prior to Surgery
- Correction of the coagulopathy through administration of vitamin K
- Preoperative drainage may lead to increased morbidity because of biliary infections. However, preoperative drainage is done in the majority of cases for logistic reasons
- Antibiotic prophylaxis

Procedure

Access

Either a subcostal incision, with the possibility of extending this incision to the left side of the abdomen, or a midline incision may be chosen. If percutaneous transhepatic cholangiography (PTC) is in place, the incision should be chosen to avoid having to remove the PTC perioperatively.

STEP 1

Exposure

In first-access operations it is usually not necessary to mobilize the flexura hepatica of the colon and to mobilize the duodenum by means of a Kocher procedure; however, this may facilitate exposure. In redo operations the preferred method is to carefully perform adhesiolysis and mobilize the liver from the abdominal wall starting at the right subhepatic area. Then by gentle preparation one should follow the edge of the liver dorsally and cranially in order to reach the hilus of the liver. Stay close to the liver! After careful mobilization, a retractor (e.g., Thompson) is installed (A, B).

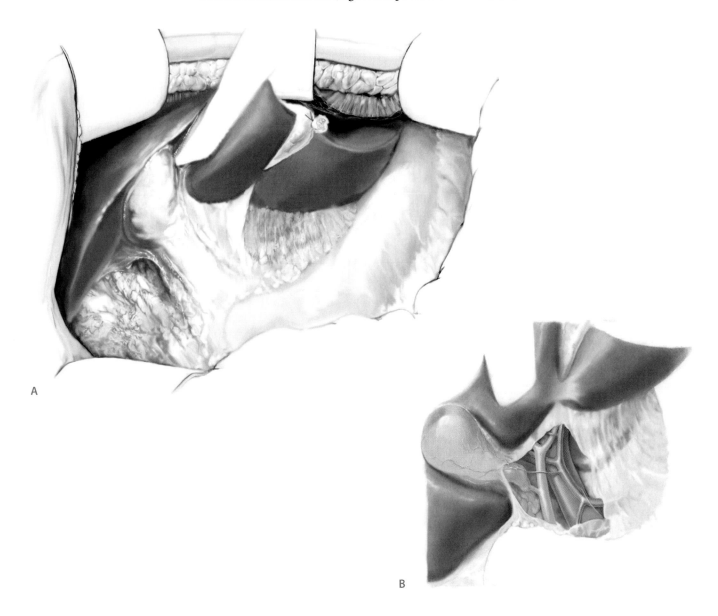

A

B

STEP 2

Opening of the hepatoduodenal ligament

Cholecystectomy is performed as described in the chapter "Laparoscopic Cholecystectomy, Open Cholecystectomy and Cholecystostomy."

The hepatoduodenal ligament is divided following the cystic duct medially until its
entrance in the common hepatic duct. Next is the preparation of a segment of the
jejunum, 40 cm distal to Treitz's ligament, where it is divided with the TLC (Ethicon), and
again 40 cm distal to this point an end-to-side anastomosis is made. The blind end of the
jejunum is secured with a suture and brought to the common hepatic duct through a
hole made in the mesocolon. Because of the multiplicity of anatomic variations and the
consequences of inadvertent injury to vascular structures, it is imperative to identify
definitely the exact location of the hepatic duct and common bile duct within the hepatoduodenal ligament before any clamping or incising is done. The purpose of the procedure is to identify healthy bile duct mucosa proximal to the site of obstruction, to
prepare a segment of the gastrointestinal tract, usually a Roux-en-Y loop of the jejunum,
and to direct mucosa-to-mucosa anastomosis between the bile duct and the gut. A small
hole (about 1–1.5 cm) is made in the jejunum (usually a puncture with the diathermia is
enough) and a stay suture is placed on the left lateral side.

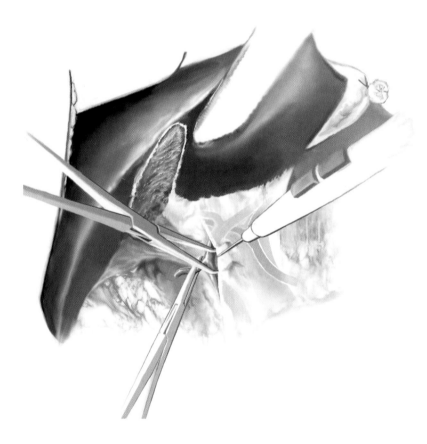

Side-to-Side Anastomosis

STEP 3

Opening of the jejunum and the choledochal duct, placement of stay sutures

The common hepatic duct is opened and a stay suture is placed on the median side in order to provide a good view of both sides of the anastomosis. Then, the anastomosis is started using a long 3-0 or 4-0 PDS suture, with needles on both ends, inside-out in the common hepatic duct and outside-in through the jejunal wall. Both ends should be of equal length and a clamp should be put on one side, and the started suture used to continue suturing the dorsal part of the anastomosis. The first two to three stitches may be placed without traction (as a "parachute"), after which the jejunum is firmly pulled against the ductal wall. The suture should be guided by the assistant operator.

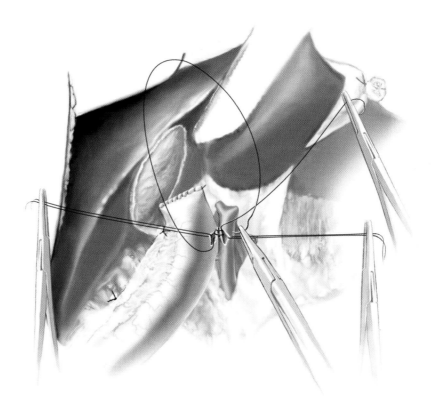

STEP 4

Continuous running suture of the dorsal part of the anastomosis

A continuous running suture of the dorsal side is performed using full thickness bites of both the duct and the jejunum. With every stitch, mucosa-to-mucosa contact should be ensured using a forceps while bringing the suture to tension. Intraoperative bile leakage is not a problem. Spill from the intestines should be avoided or removed to reduce the possibility of postoperative infection, possibly leading to dehiscence of the anastomosis.

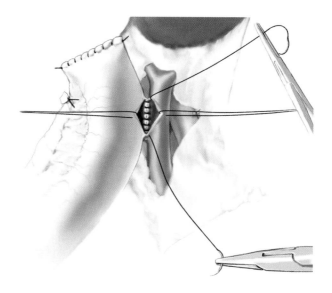

STEP 5

Continuous running suture of the ventral part of the anastomosis

One or two sutures are made around the corner at the duodenal side of the anastomosis, after which this side of the suture is put on a clamp and the other end is used to continue the suture for the ventral part of the anastomosis from the top. At this point the stay-sutures may be removed .

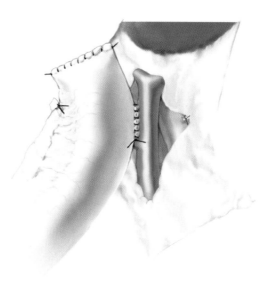

STEP 6   **Final situation, side-to-side choledochojejunostomy**

After the anastomosis is finished, a drain is left in situ behind the anastomosis to indicate postoperative blood loss and/or bile leakage. No suction on the drain is needed.

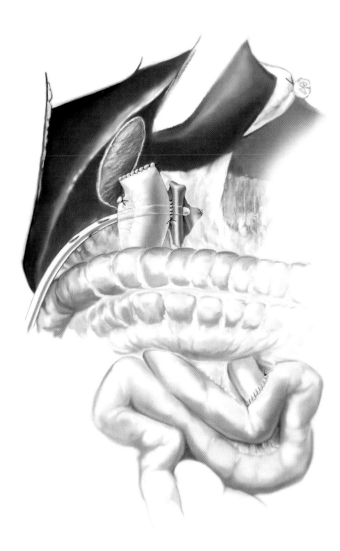

End-to-Side Choledochojejunostomy

STEP 7

Opening of the jejunum and division of the choledochal duct, closure of the duodenal part; placement of stay-sutures

After exploration of the hepatoduodenal ligament (Steps 1 and 2, see above), the chole-dochal duct is cut and the duodenal side is closed using a continuous slowly resorbable monofilament suture. This is usually done in the supraduodenal part, which is about 3.5 cm long; however, the middle or retroduodenal and distal or pancreatic parts of the choledochal duct are at least 2–3 cm long. Stasis of pancreatic juice in this part is possible and could lead to rupture into the abdomen. If this is anticipated, the distal part should be anastomized separately during the operation or stented peri- or postopera-tively. Damage to pancreatic tissue should be left untreated perioperatively; however, in order to protect the hepaticojejunostomy a drain should be left in place. To facilitate the making of the anastomosis, stay-sutures are placed in the ventral side of the choledochal duct as well as in the opening of the jejunal loop. The anastomosis is started using a long 3-0 PDS suture, with needles on both ends, inside-out in the jejunum and outside-in in the hepatic duct on the median side (suturing toward oneself). Both ends should be of equal length and a clamp is placed on one side and the other suture used to continue the closure of the dorsal part of the anastomosis. Again the "parachute" technique may be used (see Step 3).

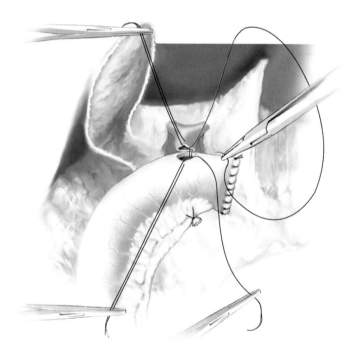

STEP 8 — Continuous running suture of the dorsal part of the anastomosis

Full thickness bites of both the duct and the jejunum should be taken while suturing. Mucosa-to-mucosa contact should be ensured with every stitch using a forceps while bringing the suture to tension. Tearing of the diseased ductus requires anastomosis on a level closer to the hilus of the liver.

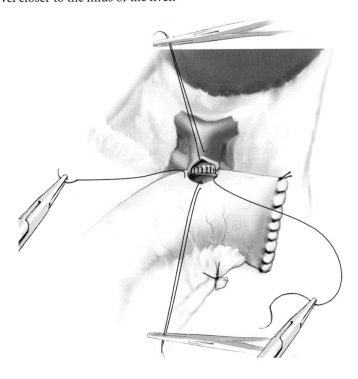

STEP 9 — Running suture of the ventral part of the anastomosis

One or two sutures are made around the corner on the lateral side of the anastomosis, after which this side of the suture is put on a clamp and the other end used to continue the suture for the ventral part of the anastomosis.

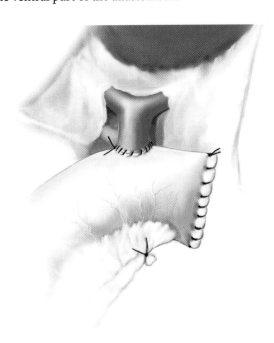

Cholecystojejunostomy
Facile bypass for those with distal common duct obstruction and high resection of cystic duct.

STEP 10   **Preparation and dorsal running suture**

If obstruction in the hepatoduodenal ligament and in the distal biliary tree is such that the bile duct cannot be reached, a cholecystojejunostomy is performed. However, before this procedure is started, one should be certain that the cystic duct and the proximal part of the bile duct are not obstructed. Since the anatomic structures are more on the surface, this solution is an option when minimally invasive or endoscopic surgery is desirable. The gallbladder is left in situ and opened for at least 2–3 cm. A jejunal loop is created as described previously and an opening of the same size is made. One should clearly identify the gallbladder and the jejunal wall, and free it from omental adhesions, in order to perform adequate through-wall stitches. A continuous running 3-0 PDS is used to anastomose the gallbladder onto the jejunum, starting on the medial side (A).

While suturing, one should take care to take full thickness bites of both the gallbladder wall and the jejunum. With every stitch, mucosa-to-mucosa contact should be ensured using a forceps while bringing the suture to tension. The size of the opening in the gallbladder as well as in the jejunum may be adjusted while making the anastomosis in order to create a perfect fit and thereby avoid postoperative leakage (B).

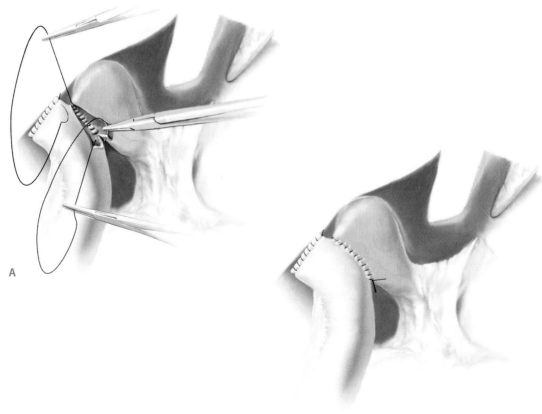

A

B

STEP 11   Completed cholecystojejunostomy

A drain is left in situ after finishing the anastomosis, to indicate postoperative bleeding or bile leakage. If a drain is really indicated, drainage is set up as shown in Sect. 1, chapter "Principles of Drainage"

Postoperative Tests

- Check daily for clinical signs of biliary obstruction (fever, icterus and pain). However, bile obstruction may be considered normal for the first few days postoperatively due to edema of the operative area.
- If an enterohepatic drain is in place, a cholangiography through the outside drain on day 5 will reveal possible leakage of the anastomosis (in case of leakage, the drain should not be removed at day 5 but should be left in place for at least another 6 weeks).

Postoperative Complications

- Bleeding usually occurs within 24 hours and may require immediate reexploration and control of the bleeding after full exposure of the cause.
- If a bile leakage from the anastomosis is recognized within 24 hours, a reexploration is indicated and usually can be easily restored. If bile leakage happens later, drainage is usually the treatment of choice, which may be helped by the placement of a stent in the hepaticojejunostomy with endoscopic retrograde cholangiopancreatography (ERCP). At this point a reanastomosis would lead to dehiscence or stricture. Therefore, this should be performed in an elective setting after 6–8 weeks.
- Cholangitis, which most often occurs within the first days after surgery, should be treated by antibiotics. If obvious obstruction is observed and no reoperation is considered, it should be treated by drainage through PTC or ERCP.
- A restenosis would clinically be evident by recurrent icterus and intermittent cholangitis. As the results of reoperations are poor, the placement of a stent should be considered.
- Enterocutaneous fistula (leakage from the blind end of the jejunum) should be treated in a conservative way.
- In case of pancreatitis, conservative treatment usually suffices.
- Delayed gastric emptying and/or ileus should always be taken seriously, since it may be a sign of other problems (as mentioned above) and a CT scan may be indicated. Beware of aspiration pneumonia!

Tricks of the Senior Surgeon

- Preoperative stenting (endoprosthesis through ERCP by the gastroenterologist or PTC by the radiologist) may help perioperative localization of the hepatic duct in case of proximal biliary obstruction.
- If PTC is in place, it is wise to make the skin incision away from the drain. This enables the surgeon to keep the drain for later cholangiography. In an end-to-side choledochojejunostomy, the hole in the jejunum should be very small because it always ends up larger than anticipated. Collection of bile during the procedure enables the surgeon to treat the patient with a targeted antibiotic therapy in case of infectious complications.

Choledochoduodenostomy

Ted Pappas, Miranda Voss

Introduction

This procedure was first performed by Riedel in 1888 for an impacted common bile duct stone. The main principle of the procedure is that a side-to-side anastomosis is designed to allow free flow of bile from the common bile duct into the duodenum.

Advantages Over Choledochojejunostomy

- It provides a more physiologic conduit
- Relatively quick and simple with fewer anastomotic sites
- Ease of access for future endoscopic interventions

Indications and Contraindications

Indications

Biliary dilatation resulting from:
- Benign distal biliary strictures not suitable for transduodenal sphincteroplasty
- Indeterminate biliary stricture in the head of the pancreas where a preoperative decision has been made not to resect if malignancy cannot be confirmed on exploration and open biopsy
- Unresectable malignant stricture where the duodenum comfortably reaches the dilated biliary tree
- Primary or recurrent common duct stones where endoscopic management has failed or is not available
- Impacted common duct stone

Contraindications

- Narrow common bile duct (<8mm)
- Active duodenal ulceration
- Malignancy when the duodenum does not comfortably reach the dilated bile duct

Preoperative Investigation and Preparation

Clinical:	Associated symptoms of gastric outlet obstruction
	History of duodenal ulceration
	Coagulopathy or biliary sepsis
	Evidence of dehydration
Laboratory:	Bilirubin
	Coagulation parameters
	Creatinine, electrolytes
Radiology:	Ultrasound to confirm site of obstruction and diameter of common bile duct (minimal investigation). Other investigations determined by underlying pathology
Preparation:	Adequate hydration
	Antibiotic prophylaxis

What We Should Not Do

Preoperative biliary stenting may decompress the common bile duct, which will make the anastomosis more difficult. It also increases the risk of wound infection. If the time to surgery is compatible with the patient's symptoms and cholangitis is not present, stenting should be avoided.

Procedure

Access
Right subcostal incision or midline (see Sect. 1, chapters "Positioning and Accesses" and "Retractors and Principles of Exposure").

Exposure and exploration: installation of retractor (Bookwalter). The colon is reflected inferiorly.
Kocherization of the duodenum as shown in the chapter "Resection of Gallbladder Cancer, Including Surgical Staging". Kocherization allows mobility of the duodenum that is essential for this procedure.

Cholecystectomy as shown in the chapter "Laparoscopic Cholecystectomy, Open Cholecystectomy and Cholecystostomy."

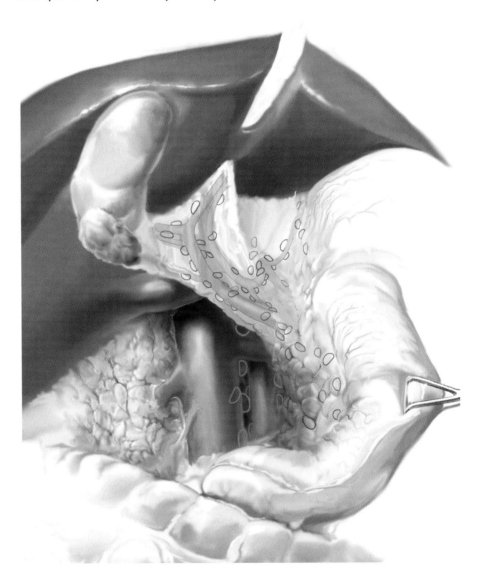

STEP 2   **Definition of common bile duct**

Incision of hepatoduodenal ligament to expose the common bile duct (A).
  Site of common bile duct confirmed with "seeker needle (B)."
  3-0 silk stay-sutures are placed in the common bile duct (C).

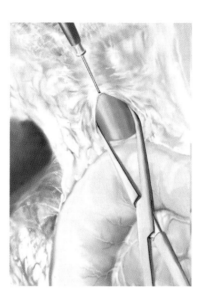

A

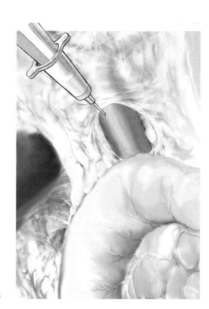

B

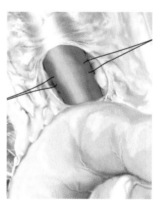

C

STEP 3   **Opening of bile duct and duodenum**

A 2-cm choledochotomy is performed. The distal extent of the choledochotomy should be in close proximity to the superior border of the mobilized duodenum, so that the duodenum comfortably reaches the choledochotomy.

A longitudinal duodenotomy is then performed. The duodenotomy should be approximately 70% of the length of the choledochotomy.

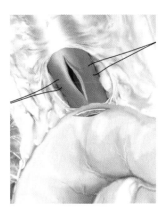

STEP 4   **Posterior wall anastomosis**

The anastomosis is performed using interrupted 3-0 absorbable sutures with knots in the lumen for the posterior wall. It is a mistake to place too many sutures; 12 are usually sufficient and the anastomosis may be visualized as a clockface.

The first suture should be placed in the 6 o'clock position (A). Traction on this suture aids in exposure for subsequent posterior wall sutures.

A further three sutures are placed out to the 3 o'clock position and three to the 9 o'clock position. All sutures are placed before tying (B).

The silk stay-sutures are removed. The anastomotic sutures are tied and all but the corner sutures are cut (C).

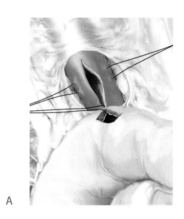

A

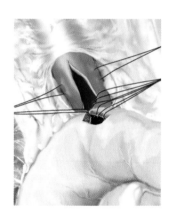

B

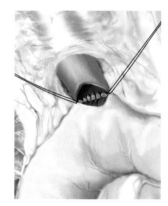

C

STEP 5   **Anterior wall anastomosis**

Traction on the corner sutures ensures that the corner is inverted. The corner may then be cut.

Sutures are placed from outside to in (A).

All are placed before tying (B).

The enterotomy should be shorter than the choledochotomy as the small intestine always stretches during creation of the anastomosis. This can cause a size mismatch (C).

Do not stent the anastomosis.

[Editor's variation: An even more facile method of completing this anastomosis is to place two absorbable sutures (3-0 vinyl) at the 6 o'clock position (D). The two sutures are then sewn in a running manner from 6 o'clock to 12 o'clock (E) and tied (F).]

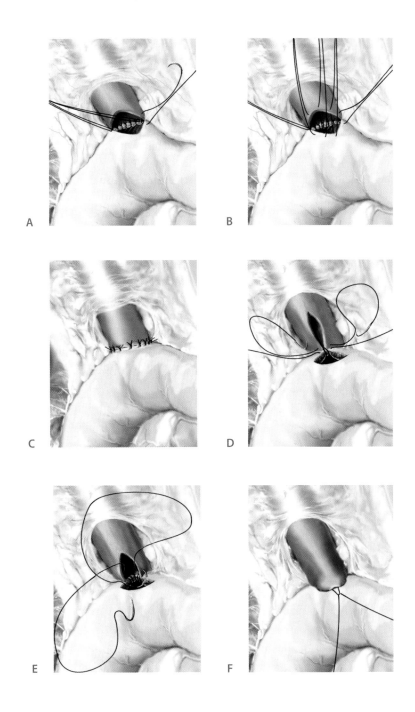

Postoperative Tests

- Bilirubin and alkaline phosphatase

Local Postoperative Complications

- Short term:
  - Wound infection; increased incidence where the bile duct has been stented.
  - Bile leakage: excessive drainage fluid with high bilirubin content; rare and usually indicates a technical problem. Priorities are to establish controlled fistula and to determine whether there is unobstructed biliary enteric continuity. CT scan and fistulogram via drain are initial investigations. Most will heal spontaneously if there is no downstream obstruction.
- Medium-long term:
  - Recurrent cholangitis; pain, jaundice and right upper quadrant pain with evidence of sepsis. These are most commonly the result of anastomotic stricture, but may also result from sump syndrome, development of hepato- or choledocholithiasis or disease in the upstream biliary tree. A CT scan will define the site of obstruction. Endoscopic retrograde cholangiopancreatography (ERCP) is necessary to define the anatomy of the biliary tree and for endoscopic treatment of several of the causes.
  - Anastomotic stricture. The usual presentation is with cholangitis, but it may present with progressive jaundice. More likely if choledochotomy <2 cm. It may respond to endoscopic balloon dilatation, but otherwise requires conversion to Roux-en-Y.
  - Sump syndrome: presents with pain, cholangitis, jaundice, less commonly pancreatitis months to years postoperatively. Diagnosis is made at ERCP where the blind end of the common duct is found to be full of food debris or calculi. Initial treatment is endoscopic.
  - Cholangiocarcinoma: usually occurs in patients with a long history of repeated episodes of cholangitis 10–20 years postoperatively. Early symptoms are non-specific with pain, weight loss and cholestasis. Cholangitis is unusual. Work-up of suspected cholangiocarcinoma is detailed elsewhere.

Tricks of the Senior Surgeon

- Anticipate a 50% stenosis and make the choledochotomy at least 2 cm long.
- Position the choledochotomy and the enterotomy to minimize tension.
- Generous kocherization should be performed to ensure there is no undue tension on the anastomosis.

Reconstruction of Bile Duct Injuries

Steven M. Strasberg

Introduction

Bile duct injuries have become more common since the introduction of laparoscopic surgery and are a major source of morbidity and litigation. Bile duct injuries may take many forms. Simpler injuries such as types A and D may be treated in the community setting when discovered intraoperatively or by endoscopic or percutaneous techniques when they present in the postoperative period. Some more complex injuries such as E1 and E2 types may also be treated by nonsurgical techniques when they present as strictures. This chapter deals with the more complex injuries that require hepaticojejunostomy for repair (types B and C injuries and most to type E injuries).

The figure illustrates the classification of injuries to the biliary tract. Type E injuries are subdivided according to the Bismuth classification. Types B and C injuries almost always involve aberrant right hepatic ducts. The notations >2 cm and <2 cm in types E1 and E2 injuries indicate the length of common hepatic duct remaining.
The injuries with an isolated right duct component and the subject of this paper are types B, C, E4 and E5.

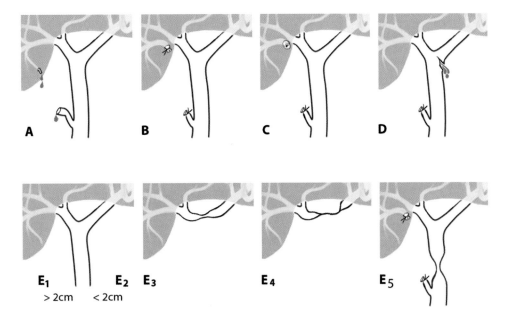

Timing of Repair

Factors favoring immediate repair are: (1) early referral, (2) lack of right upper quadrant bile collection, (3) simple injuries, (4) no vascular injury and (5) a stable patient. Factors favoring delayed repair are: (1) late (less than 1 week after injury) referral, (2) complex injuries (types E4, E5), (3) thermal etiology and (4) concomitant ischemic injury.

Preoperative Investigation and Preparation for the Procedure

- Communication with previous surgeon
- Previous surgical report
- Laboratory tests: bilirubin, alkaline phosphatase, ALT, AST, albumin, coagulation parameters, white blood cell count

Principles of Repair

- Anastomosis should be tension free, with good blood supply, mucosa to mucosa and of adequate caliber.
- Hepaticojejunostomy should be used in preference to either choledochocholedocotomy or choledochoduodenostomy.
- An anterior longitudinal opening in the bile duct with a long side-to-side anastomosis is preferred.
- Dissection behind the ducts should be minimized in order to minimize devascularization of the duct.

Use of Postoperative Stents

- There is no evidence that they are helpful if a large caliber mucosa-to-mucosa anastomosis has been achieved.
- We use them when very small ducts have been anastomosed.
- Transhepatic tubes can be left through the anastomosis in order to perform postoperative cholangiography.

More Radical Solutions

- When ductal reconstruction to a part of the liver is impossible, then resection should be performed.
- Occasionally prior failure of reconstruction leads to secondary biliary cirrhosis, end-stage liver failure, and a need for liver transplantation.

Procedure

Incision

The usual incision is a J-shaped right upper quadrant incision shown as a solid line. The vertical length of the incision should be at least 6 cm. The incision can be extended to the left (dotted line for increased exposure in large individuals). A midline incision may be suitable for thin persons. A large ring retractor is placed after clearing adhesions to the anterior abdominal wall.

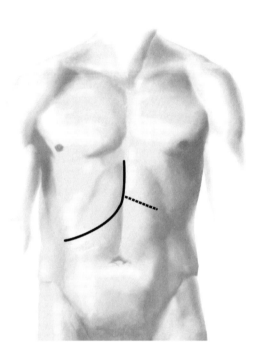

STEP 1

Schematic of the principles of the Hepp-Couinaud approach. This approach is adequate for types E1–E3 lesions. The dissection is started at the liver edge and carried down the face of segments 3–5 until portal structures are encountered. The dissection is continued directly on segment 4 in the plane shown (**A**). The end point of the dissection is entry into liver tissue in this plane. The liver plate (Wallerian sheath) is divided and the left bile duct identified just below this level. The left duct is accessed because it has a long extrahepatic length as opposed to the right. The left duct may lie horizontally as shown here or more vertically, in which case the dissection is more difficult. This dissection is facilitated by division of the bridge of liver tissue between segments 3 and 4 (**B**) and by reopening the gallbladder fossa when it has sealed at its lips. Resection of the inferior portion of segment 4 may also be helpful (see below).

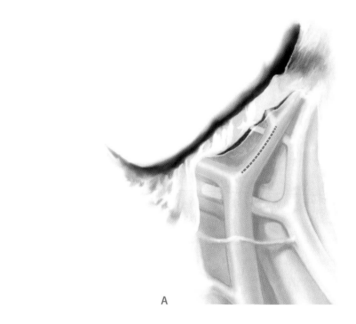

A

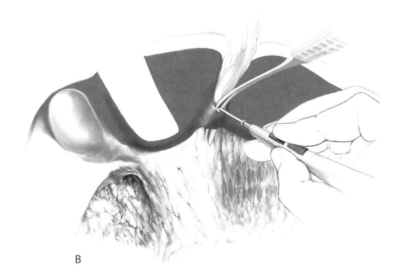

B

STEP 2

At this point a stent in the left duct can be palpated and the duct opened on its anterior surface. A 2-cm opening is adequate. Care should be taken not to extend the incision too far to the left, as the hepatic artery to segment 4 may be injured. Segment 4 is pulled up, the liver plate divided and the left hepatic duct identified. A Roux-en-Y loop has been prepared. The loop is laid up as shown. The double-headed arrows indicate the sites of openings that are made in the duct and the bowel.

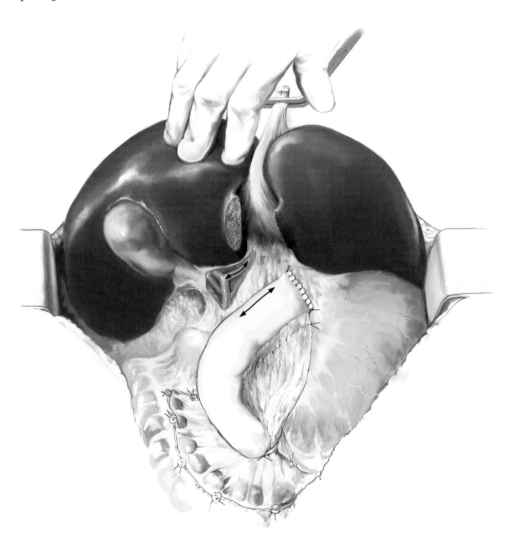

STEP 3

The anastomosis is performed with synthetic absorbable interrupted sutures (5-0 sutures are preferred by the author). The anterior row in the bile duct is placed first, then the posterior row in both structures is placed and tied, and finally the anterior row is placed in the bowel and tied (see chapter on biliary-enteric anastomosis: pages). A single suction drain is left. Stents are used only when the bile ducts are very small 2 mm or less; this is very uncommon.

Cases of Isolated Right Hepatic Duct

In types E4 and E5 and B and C injuries the Hepp-Couinaud approach alone will not suffice, as there is an isolated portion of the biliary tree on the right side. The key to dissection is based on the fact that the main right and left bile ducts lie in the same coronal plane, invested in fibrous Wallerian sheaths. Also of importance is that the gallbladder plate, a layer of fibrous tissue on which the gallbladder normally rests, attaches to the anterior surface of the sheath of the main right portal pedicle. To find the bile duct within the sheath of the pedicle the cystic plate must be detached from the anterior surface of the sheath of the right portal pedicle.

STEP 1

The liver capsule is divided toward the right until the cystic plate is met where it attaches to the sheath of the right portal pedicle. It is a stout ribbon of fibrous tissue about 2 mm in thickness and 5–8 mm in breadth.

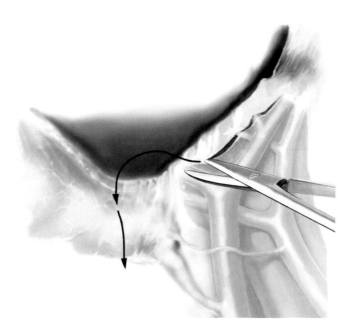

STEP 2

After dividing the cystic plate the liver lifts off the right portal pedicle. The division of the liver capsule is carried about 1 cm beyond the cystic plate. Now the liver (segment 5) may be dissected off the portal pedicle, by lifting and coring the base of segment 5. This exposes the anterior surface of the sheath of the right portal pedicle. The position of the right duct(s) in the pedicle is evident from the position of the stent (not shown). To prepare the right bile duct for anastomosis it is opened on the anterior surface (inset). Ideally, the duct(s) is opened 1 cm. The entire anastomosis is then performed to the anterior surface of the duct as described above for the left duct. When performing two (or more) anastomoses the anterior row in the bile ducts should be placed first and then the posterior row placed and tied, completing all anastomoses together by placement of the anterior row sutures in the bowel and tying of all anterior row sutures.

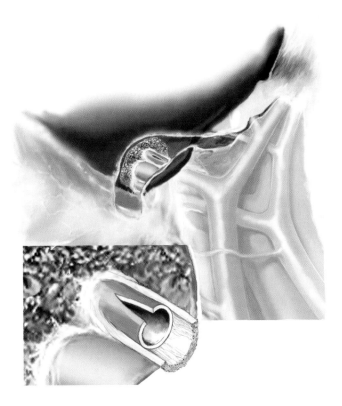

Access to Intrahepatic Ducts Provided by Partial Hepatectomy

In some cases, especially those in which there have been repeated bouts of cholangitis and the liver has become swollen and fibrotic, a condition most frequently seen after failed hepaticojejunostomy, segment 4 may overhang the upper bile ducts. In these cases resection or coring of segment 4 is also a useful adjunct. Resection provides excellent access to the upper part of the porta hepatis without relying on forceful retraction on the liver and provides room for the bowel to rest when the hepaticojejunostomy is performed. This maneuver is not restricted only to operations in which a portion of the right biliary tree has been isolated. It is also useful for types E3 and some E2 injuries. Bile ducts with stents may be seen at the bottom of the picture.

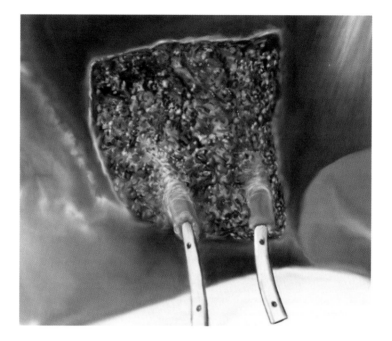

Close-up of bile ducts. Type E4 injury in which the right bile ducts have been exposed by dividing the gallbladder plate as described and segment 4 has been partially resected. Preoperatively placed stents are emanating from the ducts, and the ducts have been incised on their anterior surfaces for 1.5 cm. Sutures have been placed in the anterior row of the proposed anastomosis along with a few in the posterior row (A).

In figure B it was chosen to do a "cloacal" anastomosis rather than a double-barreled anastomosis because the ducts were close and the intervening scar small. Although the center of the anastomosis may scar, the long lateral horns are mucosa to mucosa and effectively a double-barreled anastomosis results.

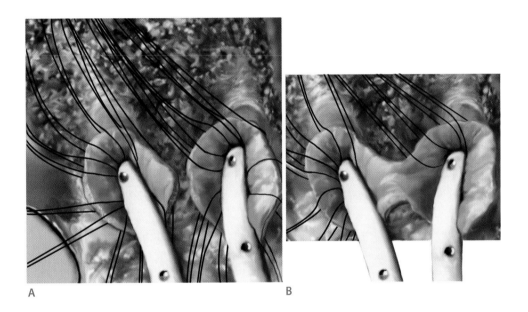

A   B

Operative Treatment of Choledochal Cysts

Benjamin N.J. Thomson, O. James Garden

Introduction

The earliest description of choledochal cysts is by Douglas in 1952 of a 17-year-old girl with jaundice, fever and a painful mass in the right hypochondrium. Choledochal cysts in Western countries have an incidence of around 1 in 200,000 live births. There is a higher incidence in Asia. Presentation is usually in childhood and 25 % are diagnosed in the first year. Frequent association with other hepatobiliary diseases, such as hepatic fibrosis, has been noted. There is an association with an aberrant pancreaticobiliary duct junction.

Surgical resection is required to prevent episodes of sepsis and pain and because of the association with cholangiocarcinoma. In the Western literature the incidence of cholangiocarcinoma is lower than in Japanese series. Cyst-enterostomy should no longer be performed. Classification is by Alonso-Lej et al.

- Type I Solitary cyst characterized by fusiform dilatation of the common bile duct (most common) (A)
- Type II Diverticulum of the common bile duct (B)
- Type III Choledochocoele (C)
- Type IV Intrahepatic cysts in association with a choledochal cyst (second most common) (E)
- Type V Caroli's disease. Intrahepatic cystic disease with no choledochal cyst (F)
  (Adapted from Todani et al. *Am J Surg* 1977; 134:263–269.)

Patients may also have a combination of intrahepatic and extrahepatic cysts (D).

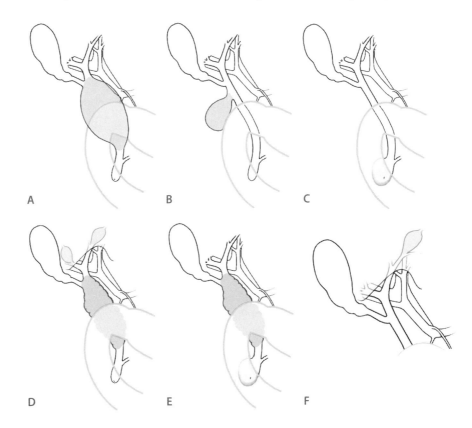

A   B   C

D   E   F

Indications and Contraindications

Indications
- Symptoms (jaundice, pain, cholangitis)
- Suspected or established malignancy
- Type I choledochal cyst
- Type II choledochal cyst
- Type IV choledochal cyst
- Previous cyst-enterostomy

Contraindications
- Severe liver disease (e.g., Child-Pugh C cirrhosis)
- Severe portal hypertension
- Coagulopathy

Investigation/Preparation

Clinical:	Chronic liver disease
Laboratory tests:	Bilirubin, alkaline phosphatase, ALT, albumin, prothrombin time, platelets
Radiologic tests:	Non-invasive; ultrasound, abdominal CT scan, invasive MRCP; ERCP if intrahepatic ducts are not visualized on MRCP
Operative preparation:	Antibiotics to cover biliary pathogens

Procedure

STEP 1	**Right subcostal incision, with extension to the left rectus if required**

Exposure with Doyen's blades (see figure on page 644).
  Omnitract retractor for retraction of the liver.
  Duodenum kocherized.

STEP 1a

The incision needs to be smaller if: (a) there is no apex to the wound, (b) the incision needs to be moved superiorly, (c) there is a wider blade on the retractor or (d) less liver is needed on view.

STEP 1b

Intraoperative ultrasound is performed to identify the anatomy and extent of the cyst, to assess cyst wall thickness and intrahepatic extension, and to identify frequently found intracyst calculi.
  Retrograde dissection is done of the gallbladder with division of the cystic artery.
  The cystic duct is followed to its insertion into the common bile duct/cyst.
  Mobilization of the cyst is performed from the portal vein and hepatic arteries.
  This dissection may be difficult due to dense inflammatory adhesions. The key is to avoid intramural (cyst) dissection by dissection in the adventitial plane around the vessels from which the cyst (and nodes) are dissected.
  The gallbladder is left in continuity to facilitate retraction of the cyst. This may be further aided by the placement of a vessel loop around the cyst.

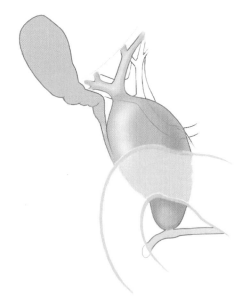

STEP 2   **Kocherization and mobilization of porta-hepatis**

A full kocherization is performed to allow access to the lower bile duct and
a retropancreatic approach.

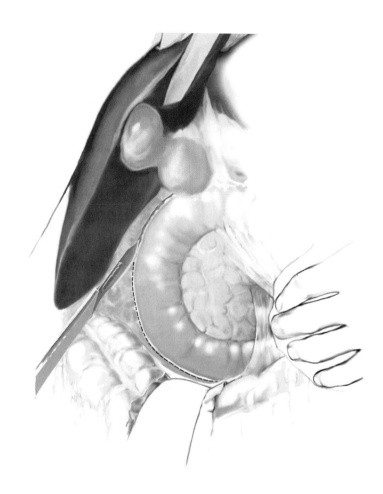

STEP 3

The cyst is now mobilized inferiorly to its lowest extent into the head of the pancreas avoiding damage to the pancreatic duct.

Intraoperative ultrasound may have provided useful information in this regard.
Ultrasonic dissection (CUSA) may aid in dissecting the cyst from the pancreas.
Multiple small vessels may be divided with diathermy.

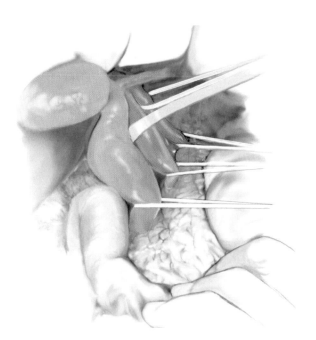

STEP 4

Opening the choledochal cyst

The cyst may require to be opened to enable visualization of the pancreatic duct, at its insertion into the common bile duct.

The cyst is controlled at its lower end above the junction of the bile duct and the pancreatic duct, which is preserved carefully (**A**). A view is shown looking into the pancreas with a partly mobilized cyst (**B**).

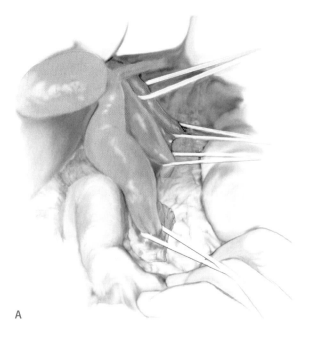

A

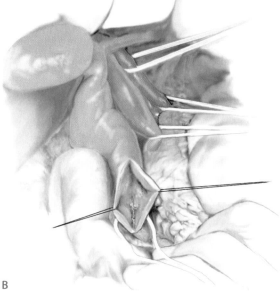

B

STEP 5   **Repair of the distal common bile duct**

If residual cyst lining remains it can be cauterized cautiously with diathermy current.

The lower common bile duct is repaired with interrupted 5-0 PDS sutures just at its junction with the pancreatic duct, damage to which is avoided carefully. The divided distal duct is seen with the pancreatic duct on view and closure started.

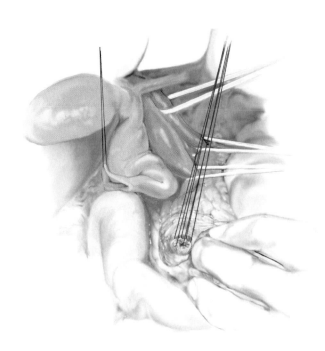

STEP 6

The cyst is mobilized superiorly to the confluence of the right and left hepatic ducts.

Assess carefully for aberrant ducts, which may need to be divided separately.

The dissection may need to be extended along the extrahepatic course of the left duct if it is ectatic.

Some advocate extended liver resection for cysts extending into the left or right duct.

It is possible to anastomose to the cyst at the confluence of the ducts, if this extends more proximally, rather than performing liver resection.

A hepaticojejunostomy is performed in an end-to-side manner with a single layer of interrupted 4-0 PDS sutures. A Roux-en-Y limb of 70 cm of proximal jejunum should be used.

A drain should be left adjacent to the hepaticojejunostomy. The cyst is removed and the hepaticojejunostomy started (A, B).

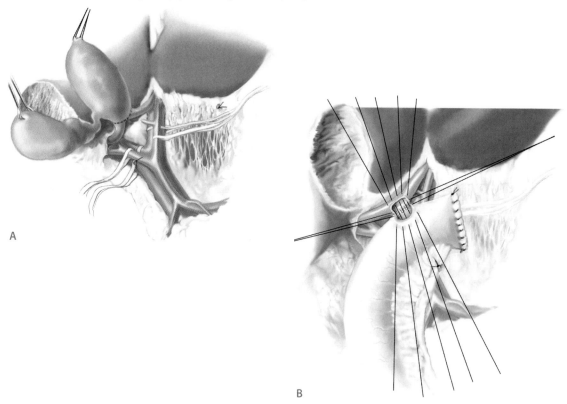

A

B

Complications

Biliary Leak

- A small amount of bile drainage can be expected in the first 48 hours, and will usually settle.
- Continuing leakage should be managed conservatively with drainage.
- Keep an eye open for amylase-rich fluid if there is difficult pancreatic dissection and/or persistent nonbile leak.

Late Complications

- Cholangitis (20–40%) usually in association with an anastomotic stricture.

Portal Hypertension

J. Michael Henderson

Introduction

J. Michael Henderson

Surgical operations for prevention of recurrent variceal bleeding have significantly diminished over the past decade. This section illustrates the different surgical options for managing variceal bleeding with total, partial, and selective shunts, and devascularization procedures. The peak of non-transplant surgical intervention for variceal bleeding was in the 1970s to 1980s when other management options were not available. What has happened since that time is that the pathophysiology has been better defined for portal hypertension, and there have been technological advances in endoscopy and radiology.

The pathophysiology of portal hypertension follows the sequences of an initial obstruction to portal venous flow, an increase in portal pressure, development of collaterals, splanchnic hyperemia, and a hyperdynamic systemic circulation. Pharmacologic intervention with non-cardioselective beta-blockade to moderate these pathophysiology changes has been successful in preventing initial bleeding, and in reducing the risk of re-bleeding. Reduction of splanchnic hyperemia with somastostatin or its analogues is effective in the acute setting.

Endoscopy has dramatically improved in the last two and a half decades with the universal adoption of videoendoscopy. For managing esophageal varices, treatment has evolved from an almost blind stick of a bleeding esophageal varix of three decades ago to sophisticated multiband-like ligators for both acute and elective management of gastroesophageal variceal bleeding. The lower complication rates with banding as opposed to sclerotherapy have established this as the primary treatment option for acute bleeding and initial prevention of recurrent bleeding.

The radiological evolution of hepatic imaging and ability to access the portal vein has led to transjugular intrahepatic portal systemic shunts (TIPS) over the past decade. TIPS can decompress varices successfully. High stenosis rates with bare stents have been reduced with the evolution of covered stents, but pseudointimal hyperplasia does remain a problem with a requirement for long-term monitoring of TIPS to maintain decompression.

Liver transplantation has also evolved dramatically over the last two decades, becoming the main surgical option for patients with variceal bleeding and advanced liver disease, and the only therapy that has significantly impacted mortality. For these patients, liver transplant is the best treatment option.

Is there still a role for the operations for portal hypertension described in this section? These procedures may be useful in some patient populations and are among the treatment options in different parts of the world. It should be recognized that all of the operations described in this section can work very well for some patients. While there is no doubt that the overall use of these procedures has markedly diminished, they should not be lost from the repertoire of surgeons managing complex hepatobiliary disease and should remain part of the repertoire of liver transplant surgeons where there is refractory variceal bleeding with well-preserved liver function. This chapter presents excellent descriptions of these operations from recognized experts with technical details and tips that make the operations possible for other surgeons with expertise in hepatobiliary surgery.

Distal Splenorenal Shunt

J. Michael Henderson

Introduction

The distal splenorenal shunt (DSRS) is widely known as the Warren shunt, and was introduced in 1966 by W. Dean Warren when he worked in Miami. Its development in conjunction with Drs. Zeppa and Foman brought together expertise in decompression of varices and devascularization procedures. The concept of selective decompression of the gastroesophageal segment to control variceal bleeding was combined with maintenance of portal hypertension in the portal vein to keep portal perfusion to the liver. The principle of the procedure is, therefore, that the shunt will control variceal bleeding, and maintenance of portal perfusion will preserve hepatic function.

Indications and Exclusion Criteria

Indications

- Variceal bleeding refractory to first line treatment with endoscopic and pharmacologic therapy
- Patients with well-preserved hepatic function (Child's Class A and B patients)

Contraindications

- Advanced liver disease
- Splenic vein thrombosis with no shuntable vessels
- Intractable ascites

Relative Contraindications

- Progressive liver disease in patients likely to come to transplant in the next 2–3 years
- Small splenic vein, but there is probably no absolute size contraindication in that the vein can be spatulated to a larger diameter anastomosis

Investigation/Preparation

- Focus on the varices, the vasculature, and the underlying liver disease.
- Clinical picture: recurrent variceal bleeding that is refractory or not amenable to appropriate endoscopic therapies.
- Laboratory studies to calculate Child's classification.
- Radiologic workup with vascular ultrasound, but arteriography is advisable in reaching a final decision to proceed with DSRS. Superior mesenteric and splenic arteriography followed through the venous phases defines portal venous anatomy and collaterals. The left renal vein should be directly studied because 20 % of the population have abnormal left renal veins.
- Timing and preparation:
    - DSRS should not be performed as an emergency procedure, but patients stabilized and brought to elective operation.
    - Ascites should be diuresed with appropriate salt restriction and diuretics prior to surgery.
    - Nutritional status should be optimized.
    - Coagulation status should be corrected.
    - Preoperative and perioperative fluid management is important, particularly with limitation of free sodium. Patients should be run "dry" to minimize the risk of postoperative ascites.
    - Appropriate perioperative antibiotic prophylaxis should be used.

Procedure

STEP 1

Positioning and access

The patient is positioned with slight left side elevation and the table broken 15° to 20° at the costal margin. This positioning improves access to the retropancreatic space for dissection of the splenic vein.

The incision is a bilateral subcostal incision, primarily on the left side and extended well laterally. Retraction requires a fixed retractor system elevating the left costal margin. Other blades of the retractor are used to aid exposure as indicated below.

Figures **A-1** and **A-2** illustrates the incision and the area of dissection for DSRS.

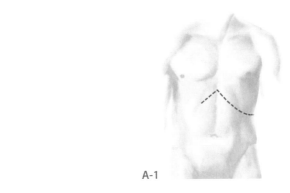

A-1

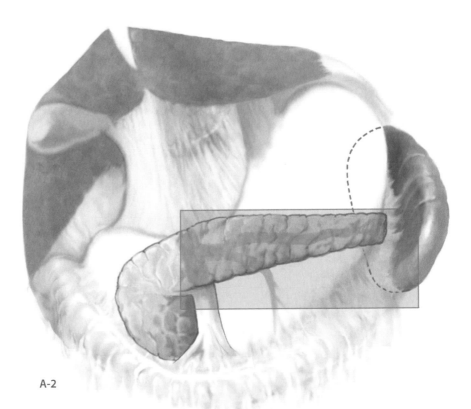

A-2

STEP 2   **Mobilization**

The figure illustrates the initial exposure, which requires mobilization of the greater curve of the stomach from the pylorus to the short gastric vessel. The gastroepiploic vessels should be interrupted and ligated. Access is further enhanced by taking down the splenocolic ligament and mobilizing the splenic flexure of the colon inferiorly. These two moves are also a component of the devascularization that separates the low pressure shunt from the high pressure portal venous system. Once this mobilization has taken place, inferior retractors can be placed on the colon, which improves exposure and access to the retropancreatic plane. The stomach should be retracted superiorly.

Dissection then focuses along the inferior margin of the pancreas, which is mobilized from the super mesenteric vein out to the splenic hilus.

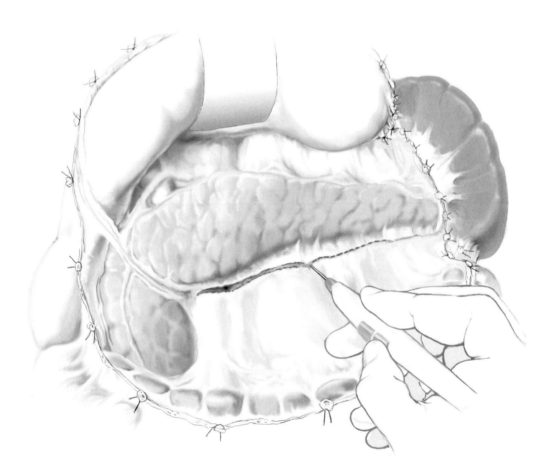

STEP 3   **Exposure and dissection of the splenic vein**

The splenic vein is initially identified by a combination of palpation and vision. In an obese patient the vein may not be readily seen on the posterior surface of the pancreas, but it can always be felt. Initial dissection of the splenic vein is started where it is most easily seen or palpated. The goal is to mobilize all the overlying adventitia along the inferior and posterior surface of the splenic vein from the superior mesenteric vein to the splenic hilus.

The inferior mesenteric vein enters the splenic vein in 50% of patients and the superior mesenteric vein in the other 50%. This is a useful landmark as it is always the first significant vein coming inferiorly as dissection proceeds from left to right. It should be ligated and interrupted.

The other key plane in this phase of the procedure is the posterior plane at the splenic superior mesenteric venous junction, as illustrated in the Figure. This is a safe plane to open with a finger or the tip of the sucker. The value of opening this plane is if any bleeding is encountered as the anterior dissection of the splenic vein is started, it can always be controlled by finger compression of the vessels.

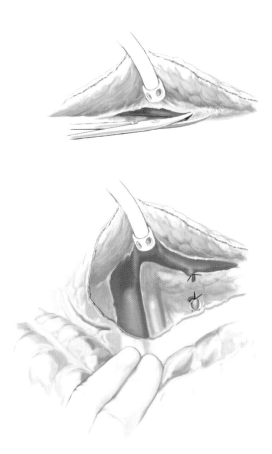

STEP 4   **Dissection of pancreatic tributaries to the splenic vein**

Pancreatic tributaries to the splenic vein always lie on the superior and anterior surface of the splenic vein. The trick in dissecting these small and fragile vessels is to open the plane on each side of these by spreading directly in the line of the small vessels. They can then be surrounded with a small right-angled clamp, and they should be ligated on the splenic vein side and clipped on the pancreatic side. This is the most delicate and difficult part of this procedure and requires considerable patience. It is facilitated by the step described in the Figure of fully mobilizing the posterior and inferior border of the splenic vein before commencing this dissection.

Sufficient splenic vein needs to be fully mobilized to allow for subsequent positioning of the vessel down to the left renal vein. The splenic vein should not be divided at this point.

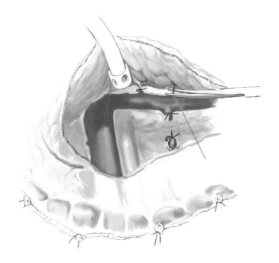

STEP 5

Exposure and dissection of the left renal vein

The left renal vein crosses in front of the aorta and behind the superior mesenteric artery. Palpation of these landmarks aids identification of the renal vein at this point. The retroperitoneum is bluntly opened until the vein is identified and then dissection is carried out along the anterior surface of the left renal vein. Tissue should be ligated at this point as it contains numerous lymphatics that if left open may cause chylous ascites. The renal vein is mobilized over sufficient length to allow it to come up comfortably into a Satinsky clamp for subsequent anastomosis. The left adrenal vein should be ligated as it always acts as an inflow to the renal vein. The left gonadal vein should be left intact as it often acts as an outflow tract and helps accommodate increased renal vein flow after the shunt is open.

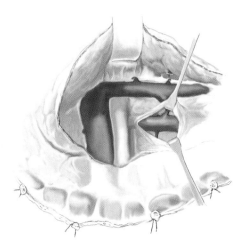

STEP 6   **Preparation of the splenic vein**

Once the left renal vein has been dissected and is ready for the anastomosis, the splenic vein is ligated flush at the superior mesenteric vein. Experience has shown that this is best achieved with a silk tie on the splenic vein stump and a large clip placed behind that. This is given the lowest instance of mesenteric venous thrombus at this site.

The splenic vein can then be moved downwards as shown in Fig. A-1, A-2, its relationship to the left renal vein confirmed, and the vein trimmed to an appropriate length for comfortable anastomosis. The goal is to have the splenic vein come down to the left renal vein without any kinking as the splenic vein emerges from the pancreas.

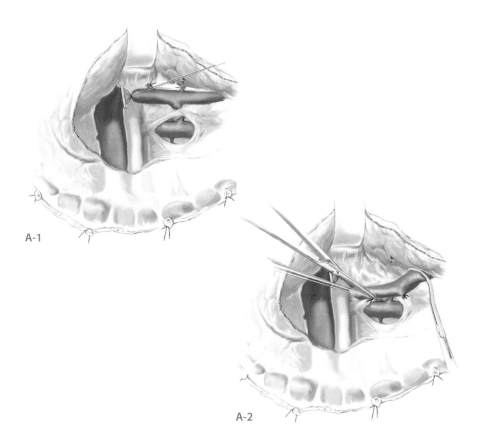

A-1

A-2

STEP 7   **Anastomosis:**

The anastomosis is made with a running suture to the posterior wall and interrupted sutures to the anterior wall. This is the preferred method to minimize the risk of a purse-string effect at this anastomosis. Suture material should be the surgeon's preference. We use a running 5-0 Ethibond stitch on the posterior wall and interrupted 5-0 silks to the anterior wall. This has proved very satisfactory with a low rate of thrombosis.

This can be a difficult anastomosis because it is sewn in a deep hole, particularly in the obese patient. Minimizing the movement at the depth of this hole aids in the completion of the anastomosis. The left renal vein clamp needs to be held forward by an assistant in the left upper quadrant and the splenic vein clamp may need to be held to keep the tension off the anastomosis. Careful positioning, with stability of these clamps, is key at this stage.

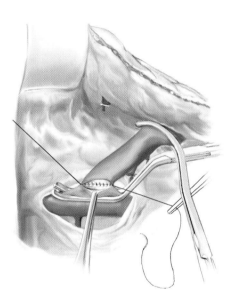

STEP 8   **Completion of the anastomosis**

Clamps are removed on completion of the anastomosis and the pancreas allowed to come down toward the left renal vein. A small amount of bleeding is usually controlled with some Surgicel and light packing for several minutes. Checking the position of this anastomosis is important to make sure there is no kinking or twisting of the splenic vein.

Completion of devascularization. The left gastric vein is identified if possible either as it joins the splenic vein or as it joins the portal vein. If it can be clipped at this site, it should be. It is also identified at the superior margin of the pancreas as shown in this figure and completely interrupted at this site.

Completion of the procedure at this point has now created a low pressure decompression of the spleen, gastric fundus, and distal esophagus, while maintaining portal hypertension and portal flow in the superior mesenteric and portal venous system.

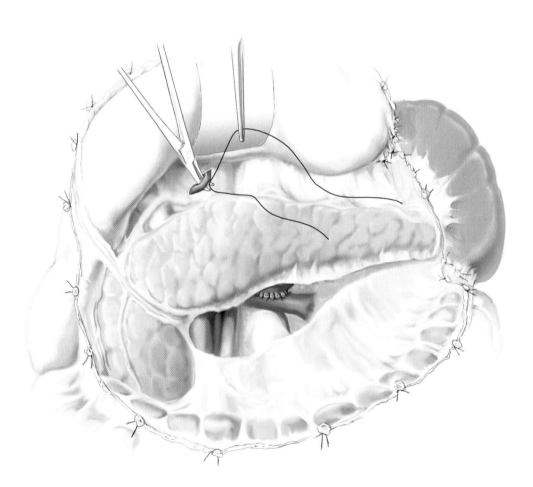

Postoperative Tests

- Follow liver labs on alternate days and electrolytes daily for 1 week.
- Diet: low sodium (2 g/day) and low fat diet (30 g/day) for 6 weeks. The latter is necessary because of the disruption of lymphatics around the left renal vein that can lead to a chylous ascites.
- Radiologic shunt study: direct catheterization of the shunt at 5–7 days to document patency and no significant pressure gradient.

Postoperative Complications

- Early:
  - Liver decompensation
  - Ascites
  - Shunt thrombosis
  - Managing these is primarily based on prevention. Careful patient selection will select good risk patients that should tolerate this operative procedure. Ascites is minimized by careful fluid management perioperatively and diet restrictions postoperatively. Shunt thrombosis is low risk (1–4%) and is minimized if the operative steps outlined above are followed.
- Late:
  - Progressive liver disease. These patients should be kept in long-term follow-up, primarily for monitoring of their cirrhosis.
  - Late shunt thrombosis is unusual, but any recurrence of bleeding requires documentation of shunt patency, usually by catheterization with pressure measurements.

Tricks of the Senior Surgeon

- Proper positioning of the patient helps later exposure.
- Exposure is critical – see Step 2.
- The posterior surface of the splenic vein is the safe dissection plane.
- Mobilize enough splenic vein for it to come down to the left renal vein easily.
- The left renal vein is best located by palpation as described in Step 5.

Low-Diameter Mesocaval Shunt

Miguel A. Mercado, Hector Orozco

Introduction

The mesocaval shunt decompresses portal hypertension with an interposition graft between the superior mesenteric vein (SMV) and the inferior vena cava (IVC). Popularized by Drapanas in the 1970s, it has had several proponents since, and most highlight that it is a shunt performed remote from the hepatic hilus. Similar in physiology to a side-to-side portacaval shunt, a mesocaval shunt diverts all portal flow if ≥12 mm diameter, while if 8–10 mm diameter some prograde portal flow is maintained.

Indications and Contraindications

Indications

- Variceal bleeding refractory to endoscopic treatment
- Child's A and B patients

Contraindications

- Advanced liver disease (Child's C)
- Mesenteric venous thrombosis

Investigations

History:	variceal bleeding
	Absence of advanced liver disease
Laboratory studies:	Child's A/B class
Vascular imaging:	Ultrasound with Doppler
	Angiography with venous phase imaging if SMV patency is questioned

Preparation

- Elective operation preferred
- Stabilize from acute bleed
    - Correct coagulation
    - Diurese ascites
    - Improve nutrition status

Procedure

| STEP 1 | Access and mobilization |

The abdomen is entered through a large median or transverse incision, to obtain adequate exposure of the whole cavity. A retractor (Thompson, Omni-Tract) is placed with blades that expose the root of the mesentery in the inframesocolic compartment. Traction of the transverse colon up and forward of the mesentery (caudal) exposes the third portion of the duodenum. The peritoneum is incised, in a semicircular fashion, from the root of the mesocolon to the ligament of Treitz. Only lax adhesions are usually found with occasional small veins that need electrocoagulation. The duodenum is freed completely.

The peritoneum is cut at the root of the mesentery, exposing the lymphatics (usually dilated and hypertrophied) that surround the mesenteric vessels. Chronic lymphatic hypertension produces fibrosis that makes dissection difficult. It is necessary to ligate all these structures in order to avoid postoperative lymph leakage. Also, small dilated veins can be found.

Complete dissection of the anterior and right lateral aspect of the superior mesenteric vein is done. All the vessels from the uncinate process of the pancreas (variable in length, diameter and distribution) are carefully dissected and ligated. The dissection is continued cephalad to the neck of the pancreas. The middle colic vein is ligated. Caudally, the dissection is continued down to the confluence of the ileocolic branch (which in many instances can be preserved). In some instances the ileocolic artery crosses over at this level; it can usually be retracted, but if necessary it can be ligated. It is necessary to dissect free the mesenteric vein 4–5 cm in length. Also, it is important to dissect the whole circumference of the vessel in order to comfortably place the vascular clamp.

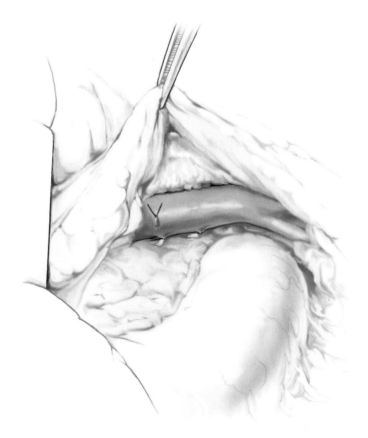

STEP 2   **Preparation of the inferior vena cava**

The infrarenal IVC is dissected free, after removing the lax areolar tissue that surrounds it. Some small veins are found that have to be suture ligated. It is not necessary to dissect the vessel in its whole circumference since it is easy to place the vascular clamp on the anterior wall of the IVC due to its width and low intravascular pressure.

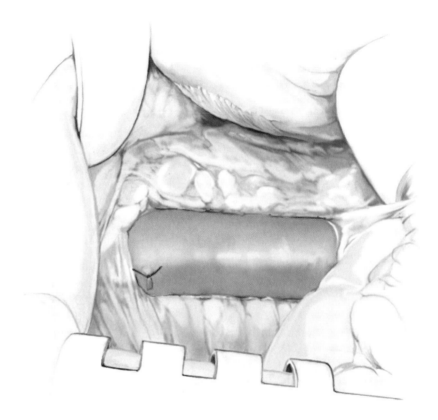

STEP 3

Venotomy of the vena cava

Retractors are placed to separate the duodenum (cephalad), the right colon (lateral) and the small intestine (caudal). Lymph nodes around the aorta can be observed; this is the limit of the medial dissection.

A Satinsky clamp is placed and a longitudinal venotomy is done approximately 12–14 mm in length using DeBakey scissors, in order to obtain an oval venotomy.

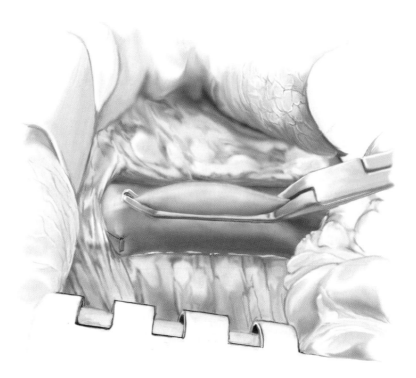

STEP 4

Suture on the caval side

A ring reinforced polytetrafluoroethylene (PTFE) 10-mm graft is cut in tangential fashion in order to obtain a 12 - to 14-mm opening for anastomosis. If the decision to place a wider graft has been made, a wider venotomy must be performed.

Using a 5-0 vascular Prolene suture placed at each angle, the graft is sewn with a running suture (Figure 4). The suture is placed from outside. An everted suture is advised at this point in order to minimize exposure of rough areas in the vascular lumen.

When the suture is completed, the graft is filled with heparinized saline.

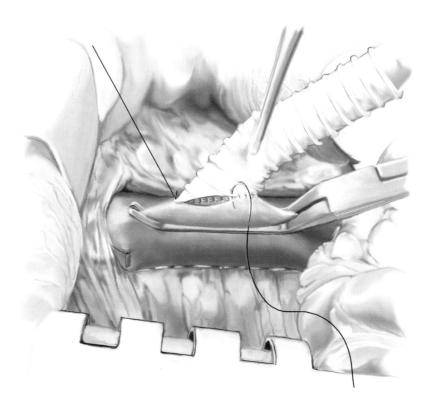

STEP 5   **Preparation and suture on the mesenteric side**

A Satinsky clamp is placed on the superior mesenteric vein and a semicircular cut of the vein is done with Potts scissors (Figure 5). This incision favors the position of the graft in the right and slightly posterior aspect of the vein. Using a 5-0 Prolene suture, each angle is placed and the PTFE graft is approximated close to the vein. The length of the graft has to be cut according to the position of the duodenum.

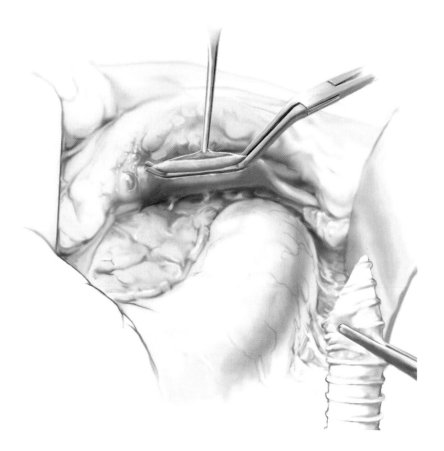

STEP 6

Completing the suture

The anastomosis is completed using a continuous suture. The posterior layer is done from within the lumen, so that the first stitch places the needle inside the lumen (Figure 6). When the posterior aspect is completed, the needle is brought outside and then the anterior layer of the anastomosis is done. An everted suture is advised.

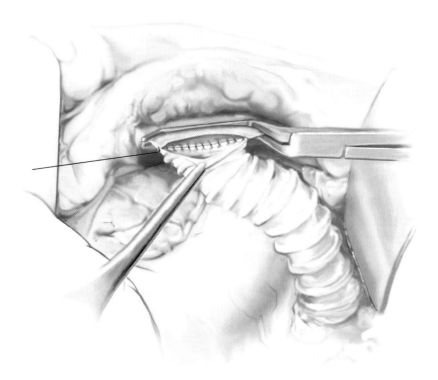

STEP 7

Release of the clamps

When the suture is complete, the vascular clamp in the inferior vena cava is released first followed by the vascular clamp in the mesenteric vein. Usually a small amount of bleeding at the suture line is observed. This resolves spontaneously with the application of dehydrated cellulose and mild pressure.

STEP 8

Final position

The final position of the graft. The duodenum is allowed to rest over the graft and the peritoneum is closed over the graft. No drainage is left and the abdominal wall is closed in standard fashion.

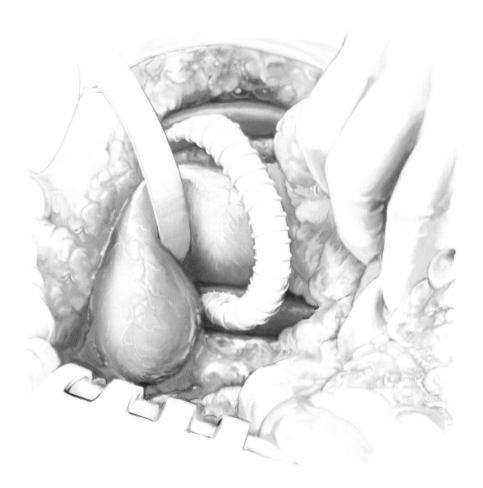

Postoperative Tests

- Daily laboratory studies
- Shunt study prior to discharge
  - Ultrasound
  - Possible angiography

Postoperative Complications

- Early:
  - Liver failure
  - Shunt thrombosis
- Late:
  - Liver decompensation
  - Encephalopathy
  - Shunt thrombosis

Tricks of the Senior Surgeon

- Injection of water around the vessels, through a small orifice when the vessel is identified, allows separation of dissection planes, making the dissection easier.
- Circumferential dissection of the mesenteric vein permits an easier mobilization of the vessel. Fixed segments of the wall can produce small tears of the vessel at the time of clamping and when traction to the vessel is done.
- When the posterior face of the mesenteric anastomosis is performed, it is important to maintain the graft close to the vein. Traction to the graft when the first stitches are placed can produce tears in the vein wall and loss of substance.
- When bleeding is observed at the anastomotic suture line, it is better to wait until it stops spontaneously. Placing new stitches can be troublesome because the wall is under tension and a larger hole can be made.

8MM Interposition Portacaval Shunt

Alexander S. Rosemurgy II, Dimitris P. Korkolis

Indications and Contraindications

Indications

- Control of acute hemorrhage from esophageal varices not amenable to or failing medical therapy, e.g., pharmacotherapy, balloon tamponade, endoscopic variceal sclerotherapy, in patients with liver cirrhosis and portal hypertension
- Control of bleeding gastric or intestinal varices
- Prevention of recurrent variceal bleeding after initial control
- Complicated Budd-Chiari syndrome

Contraindications

- Portal vein thrombosis, even with recanalization (cavernomatous transformation)
- Inferior vena cava thrombosis
- Extensive adhesions from previous operative procedures in the right upper quadrant (relative contraindication)
- Severe medical comorbidities (e.g., mitral regurgitation, severe aortic stenosis, etc.)

Preoperative Investigation and Preparation for the Procedure

History:	Alcohol consumption and alcohol withdrawal syndromes, hepatitis and hepatotoxic medications
Clinical evaluation:	Variceal bleeding, ascites, hypersplenism, hepatic encephalopathy, jaundice, nutritional status, signs of portal hypertension (e.g., caput medusa)
Laboratory tests:	ALT, AST, bilirubin, alkaline phosphatase, albumin, coagulation profile (PT, INR, platelets), tumor markers and serologies (e.g., hepatitis), when indicated. Electrolyte and acid-base profile
Color-flow Doppler ultrasound and visceral angiography:	Assessment of portasplanchnic patency, as well as patency of the inferior vena cava

Determination of Child-Pugh score

Procedure

Positioning, Access and Mobilization

Initially, the patient is positioned supine on the operating table. A nasogastric tube is placed only if gastric distension requires it. Neither vasopressin nor octreotide need to be given perioperatively, unless active bleeding is occurring. Otherwise, the operation can be undertaken with minimal blood loss and almost always without blood transfusion. The patient is then rolled into a 30-degree left lateral decubitus position by means of a bed sheet rolled tightly and placed just to the right of the spine.

The patient is operated on through a right transverse upper abdominal incision. The exact placement of this incision depends on the size of the liver, which is often palpable below the right costal margin. The incision is placed over the liver edge. It does not generally cross the midline and includes only a small portion of the musculature lateral to the rectus muscle.

If the falciform ligament is divided during the incision, it should be divided carefully, as it may contain large collateral vessels. Suture ligation of the falciform ligament at the time of the division is usually undertaken.

STEP 1	Kocherization and preparation of the vena cava

Optimum exposure of the right upper quadrant of the peritoneal cavity should be achieved, with as little dissection as possible. The foramen of Winslow is the key landmark. A limited Kocher maneuver is undertaken, always maintaining orientation with the foramen of Winslow. Visible venous collaterals, as well as large lymphatic channels, should be ligated before division. Cautery is liberally applied. The Kocher maneuver does not need to be extensive but just enough to adequately expose 5 cm of the subhepatic inferior vena cava and enable the placement of a side-biting vascular clamp.

The exposed segment of the inferior vena cava should include the portion that forms the dorsal border of the foramen of Winslow. The cephalad area of this segment of the cava may lie dorsal to the inferior tip of the caudate lobe of the liver. If necessary, this portion of the caudate lobe should be excised with electrocautery.

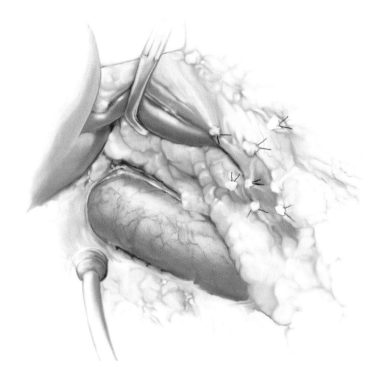

STEP 2   **Exposure of portal vein**

It is very important that the inferior vena cava is well exposed medially and laterally so
a vascular clamp can be placed. Exposure of at least one-half circumference of the 4- to
5-cm segment of the inferior vena cava is usually necessary to facilitate secure clamp
placement and anastomosis. After the inferior vena cava is adequately exposed, one or
two traction sutures are placed into the loose tissue adjacent to the right side of the cava.
These sutures are further placed into the lateral abdominal wall to retract laterally and
optimize exposure.

The gallbladder is retracted toward the patient's left shoulder. This lifts and rotates
the gallbladder and the common bile duct ventrally and medially. The hepatoduodenal
ligament is then dissected posteriorly and laterally, along its whole length with attention
to minimize chances of duct injury, as well as injury to an accessory or replaced right
hepatic artery, if present. The common bile duct should be retracted ventrally and
medially with a vein retractor to facilitate exposure of the portal vein. As the portal
vein comes into view, a Russian forceps is used to grasp it and a plastic Yankauer sucker
is utilized for circumferential dissection of the vein. The portal vein is then controlled
by a vessel loop. This vessel loop may be helpful if bleeding develops because it can
provide secure control of the portal vein.

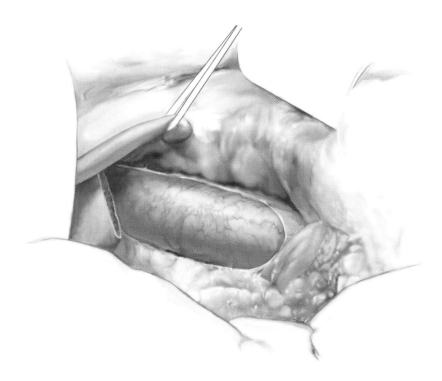

STEP 3   **Caval anastomosis**

A segment of 8 mm externally reinforced polytetrafluoroethylene (PTFE) graft is used for the portacaval shunt. The graft is 3 cm long from toe to toe and 1.5 cm from heel to heel. The bevels of the graft are oriented at 90 degrees to each other because the portal vein is not parallel to but rather oriented approximately 60 degrees to the inferior vena cava.

The graft is placed in heparinized saline and negative pressure is applied in order to remove any air bubbles. A side-biting Satinsky clamp is then securely placed on the anterior surface of the vena cava. Hypotension is virtually never a problem because of this clamping. A window must then be cut in the vena cava so that outflow from the graft is adequate; merely opening the cava is not sufficient. When the vena cava is opened, the ex vivo portion of the vein should be approximately 4 mm long and 1–2 mm wide. This will provide an adequate opening in the vena cava.

The graft is placed on the vena cava so that its bevel allows it to lean cephalad. The anastomosis is undertaken with 5-0 Prolene in a running fashion. This anastomosis is initiated with a horizontal mattress suture so that sewing is always from "inside-out" on the vein and "outside-in" on the graft (Figure 3). The back wall is completed first. Before the knot is tied, a suture is reversed so that the knot is secured across the anastomosis.

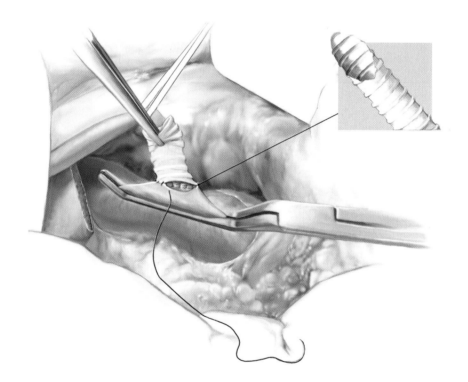

| STEP 4 | **Testing the caval anastomosis** |

Once the anastomosis has been completed and the knot tied, a right-angled clamp is placed across the graft, and the side-biting clamp is removed. This tests the anastomosis; it should not leak and it should only bleed at needle holes and then only minimally (Figure 4). The Satinsky clamp is repositioned on the vena cava and the right-angled clamp removed from the graft. The graft is then vigorously irrigated with heparinized saline through an 18-gauge angiocatheter.

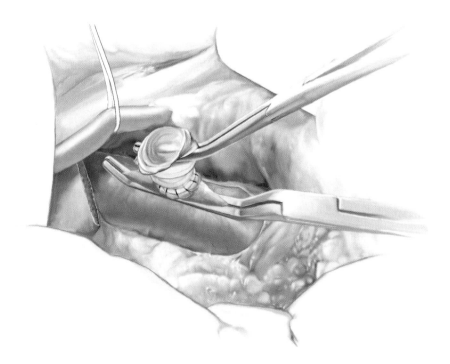

STEP 5   **Exposure of the portal vein**

The portal vein anastomosis is now constructed. The common bile duct and accessory right hepatic artery, if present, are retracted ventrally and medially, exposing the dissected portal vein. The bevel of the portal vein end of the graft is at 90° to the IVC level as shown here.

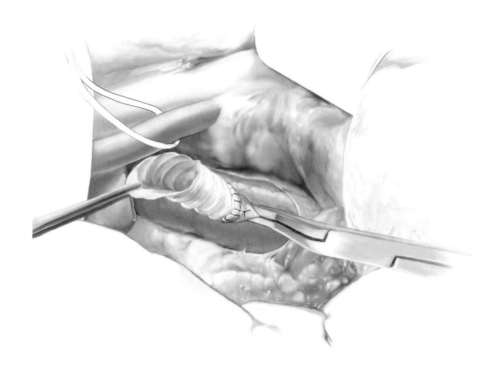

| STEP 6 | **Preparation of the portal anastomosis** |

A right-angled side-biting clamp is then placed across the portal vein. This clamp does not have to occlude all the portal flow, but it must be placed securely enough to prevent bleeding once the vein is opened. Once the Satinsky clamp is placed, the posterolateral surface of the portal vein is incised with a No. 11 knife blade. Potts scissors are then used to lengthen the opening in order to accommodate the placement of the graft. In contrast to the inferior vena cava, a window does not usually need to be cut in the portal vein. A 5-0 Prolene suture is placed in the ventral edge of the opening in the portal vein to act as a retraction suture, so as to "open up" the hole in the vein.

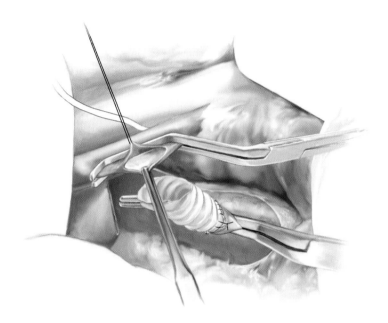

STEP 7

Portal anastomosis

With this exposure, the posterior wall of the portal vein is then sewn to the graft with a 5-0 Prolene suture. The anastomosis is initiated by placing a horizontal mattress suture in the midportion of the posterior wall of the portal vein. Thereafter, all sewing of this anastomosis is "inside-out" on the portal vein and "outside-in" on the graft. As sewing is carried around both the cephalad and caudad corners of the anastomosis, the sutures along the back wall are drawn taut with a nerve hook. As the sewing continues toward the middle of the anterior portion of the anastomosis, the clamp on the portal vein is momentarily opened so that clot and debris within the vein will be blown out. Heparinized saline is again applied liberally through the anterior defect of the anastomosis into the graft.

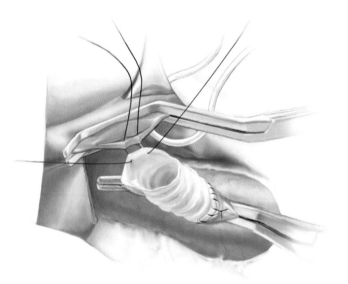

| STEP 8 | **Completing the anastomosis** |

The anastomosis is then completed, with one of the sutures reversed so that the knot is tied across the anastomosis. The clamp on the vena cava is released first, and then the clamp on the portal vein is removed. There should be a thrill in the vena cava, just cephalad to the anastomosis.

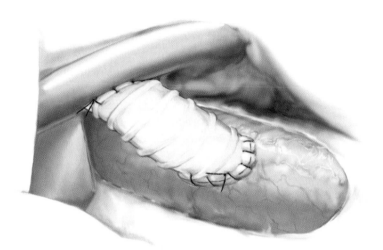

Postoperative Tests

- Postoperative surveillance in an appropriate hospital setting.
- Remove nasogastric tube, if present, as soon as possible.
- Attention should be given to avoid dehydration. Low urinary output during the first 24–48 h predisposes to graft thrombosis.
  If hypovolemia is diagnosed, rehydration with normal saline and use of intravenous mannitol are recommended.
- Liver function tests (including SGOT), coagulation parameters, and hemoglobin should be checked for at least 48 h, postoperatively.
- Daily assessment of clinical signs of liver failure, such as jaundice and encephalopathy.
- Ascites can be controlled with fluid and salt restriction, as well as with judicious use of diuretics.
- The shunt should be evaluated with transfemoral cannulation, in order to document patency and to measure the portal vein-inferior vena cava pressure gradients at 3–6 days postoperatively.

Complications

- Intra-abdominal bleeding
- Recurrence of gastrointestinal hemorrhage due to shunt thrombosis
- Hepatic failure
- Changes in cardiopulmonary dynamics (increased cardiac index)
- Ascites
- Portal-systemic encephalopathy
- Bile duct injury
- Injury to an accessory right hepatic artery
- Wound infection
- Shunt failure

Summary

Pressures within the portal vein and inferior vena cava are measured early in the operation, before the vessels are clamped. These pressures can be recorded with a 25-gauge needle and a pressure-transducing setup. A portal-caval pressure gradient is determined. On completion of the shunt, pressures are measured again. In a satisfactorily completed shunting, we look for a decrease in portal pressure of ≥10 mmHg and a gradient between the portal vein and the inferior vena cava of less than 10 mmHg.

The vena cava-graft anastomosis is marked with large Hemoclips placed on tissue adherent to the cava and secured both cephalad and caudad to the anastomosis. These clips allow the radiologist to identify and cannulate the inferior vena cava-graft anastomosis during the routine postoperative assessment of the shunt.

After copious irrigation of the operative field, the wound is closed along anatomic layers using #2 Prolene suture. The skin is reapproximated with a running nylon suture, in order to minimize any postoperative ascitic leak.

Tricks of the Senior Surgeon

- Identify the foramen of Winslow. The Kocher maneuver should be limited.
- Cut a window in the inferior vena cava.
- Begin each anastomosis with a horizontal mattress suture.
- Check the graft-inferior vena cava anastomosis before proceeding with the portal vein-graft anastomosis.
- If there is significant bleeding when a portion of the caudate lobe is removed, apply pressure and most of the bleeding will drop within minutes.
- Bleeding from either anastomosis is generally best managed by using a figure-of-eight technique.

Portacaval Shunts: Side-To-Side and End-To-Side

Marshall J. Orloff, Mark S. Orloff, Susan L. Orloff

Indications and Contraindications

Indications

- Bleeding esophageal or gastric varices (BEV or BGV) due to portal hypertension caused by cirrhosis, or, much less commonly, caused by other liver diseases (e.g., schistosomiasis)
- Bleeding from portal hypertensive gastropathy unresponsive to pharmacologic therapy
- Budd-Chiari syndrome with patent inferior vena cava
- Intractable ascites unresponsive to nonsurgical therapy
- Failed transjugular intrahepatic portasystemic shunt (TIPS)

Contraindications

- Thrombosis of the portal vein without liver disease (extrahepatic portal hypertension)
- In patients with liver disease, thrombosis of the portal vein that is long-standing and not amenable to venous thrombectomy
- Occlusion of the hepatic artery (e.g., due to hepatic arterial infusion chemotherapy)

Timing Considerations

- *Prophylactive* portacaval shunt in patients with esophageal or gastric varices that have never bled – practiced by some surgeons but not recommended by the authors
- *Elective* therapeutic portacaval shunt in patients who have recovered from an episode of BEV or BGV. This is the most widely used form of portacaval shunt
- *Emergency* portacaval shunt within 48 h of the onset of BEV or BGV, strongly advocated by the authors

Diagnosis of BEV or BGV

- History and physical examination to confirm diagnosis
- Blood studies for complete evaluation
- Esophagogastroduodenoscopy
- Doppler ultrasonography to determine portal vein patency and absence of gross liver tumors
- Other studies occasionally necessary:
  a) Visceral arteriography with indirect portography and inferior vena cavography with pressure measurements – usually not necessary in cirrhosis but essential in extrahepatic portal hypertension and Budd-Chiari syndrome
  b) Hepatic vein catheterization with venography and wedged hepatic vein pressure measurements
  c) Percutaneous liver biopsy – usually not necessary in cirrhosis but helpful in Budd-Chiari syndrome

Preoperative Preparation During Acute Bleeding

- Temporary hemostasis with intravenous infusion of octreotide (50 mcg/h) or vasopressin (0.2–0.4 units/min)
- Temporary hemostasis during endoscopy by injection sclerotherapy or banding of esophageal varices
- Restoration of blood volume by transfusion of packed red blood cells and fresh frozen plasma through large-bore intravenous catheters
- Prevention of portasystemic encephalopathy by instillation via nasogastric tube of neomycin (4 g), lactulose (30 ml), and cathartics (60 ml magnesium sulfate)
- Correction of hypokalemia and metabolic alkalosis by intravenous administration of large quantities of potassium chloride
- Intravenous administration of hypertonic glucose solution containing therapeutic doses of vitamins K, B, and C
- Preoperative administration of antibiotics
- Frequent monitoring of vital functions by an arterial catheter for blood pressure, a central venous catheter, and a urinary bladder catheter. Serial measurements of hematocrit, arterial pH and blood gases, and rate of blood loss by continuous suction through a nasogastric tube

Procedure

STEP 1

Position of patient

The patient is placed on the operating table with the right side elevated at an angle of 30° to the table by two sandbags placed underneath the right posterior trunk. The costal margin is at the level of the flexion break of the table, the right arm is suspended from an ether screen with towels, and the left arm is extended on an arm board cephalad to the ether screen. The table is "broken" at the level of the costal margin and at the knees so as to widen the space between the right costal margin and right iliac crest, and to make it possible to perform the operation easily through a right subcostal incision (A1, A-2). The incision extends from the xiphoid to well into the flank and is made two finger breadths below the costal margin. The skin is incised superficially with the scalpel and the other layers with the electrocautery, which greatly reduces the blood loss and shortens the operating time. When the electrocautery is used, it is usually unnecessary to clamp any blood vessels with hemostats. The right rectus abdominis, external oblique, and transverse abdominis muscles are completely divided and the medial 3–4 cm of the latissimus dorsi muscle is incised. The peritoneum often contains many collateral veins and is incised with the electrocautery to obtain immediate hemostasis.

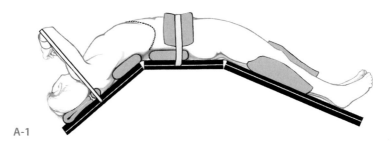

A-1

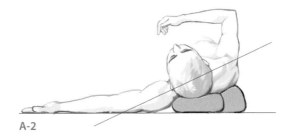

A-2

STEP 2   **Exposure of operative field**

The operative field is exposed by retraction of the viscera with three Deaver retractors positioned at right angles to each other. The inferior one retracts the hepatic flexure of the colon toward the feet, the medial one displaces the descending duodenum medially and the superior retractor retracts the liver and gallbladder toward the head. Alternatively, a self-retaining retractor may be used to accomplish the same exposure. The posterior peritoneum is often intensely "stained" with portasystemic collateral veins.

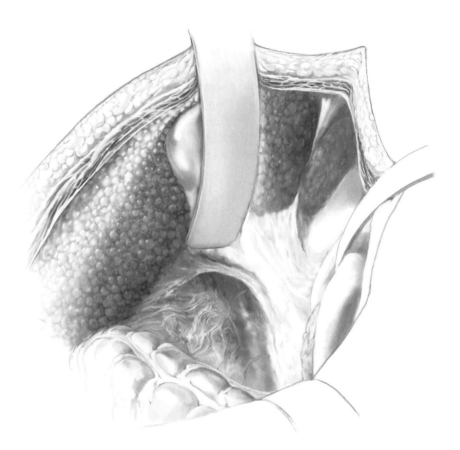

STEP 3

Isolation of inferior vena cava

The inferior vena cava (IVC) lies behind the descending duodenum. The posterior peritoneum overlying the IVC is incised with the electrocautery by an extended Kocher maneuver just lateral to the descending duodenum, and the retractors are repositioned to retract the head of the pancreas medially and the right kidney caudally. The peritoneum is often greatly thickened and contains many collateral veins. Bleeding usually can be controlled with the electrocautery but sometimes requires suture ligatures. The anterior surface of the IVC is cleared of fibroareolar tissue, and the IVC is isolated around its entire circumference by blunt and sharp dissection from the entrance of the right and left renal veins, below, to the point where it disappears behind the liver, above. The IVC is encircled with an umbilical tape. To accomplish the isolation, several tributaries must be ligated in continuity with fine silk ligatures and then divided. These tributaries often include the right adrenal vein, one or two pairs of lumbar veins that enter on the posterior surface, and the caudal pair of small hepatic veins from the caudate lobe of the liver that enter on the anterior surface of the IVC directly from the liver.

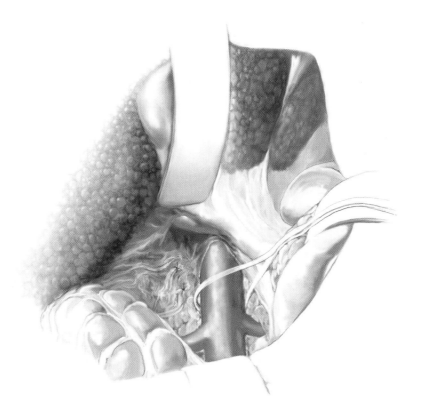

STEP 4

Testing adequacy of IVC mobilization

When the IVC has been mobilized completely, it can be lifted up toward the portal vein. Failure to isolate the IVC circumferentially is one major reason for the erroneous claim that the side-to-side portacaval shunt often cannot be performed because the portal vein and IVC are too widely separated.

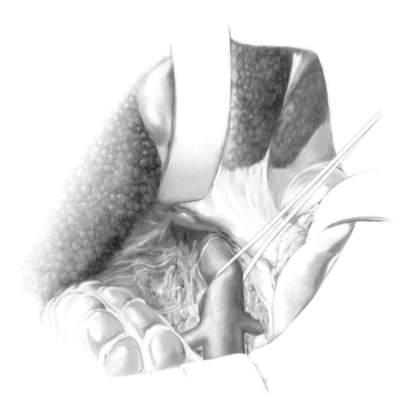

STEP 5

Isolation of portal vein

The superior retractor is repositioned medially so that it retracts the liver at the point of entrance of the portal triad. The portal vein is located in the posterolateral aspect of the portal triad and is approached from behind. The fibrofatty tissue on the posterolateral aspect of the portal triad, which contains nerves, lymphatics, and lymph nodes, is divided by blunt and sharp dissection. This technique is a safe maneuver because there are no portal venous tributaries on this aspect of the portal triad. As soon as the surface of the portal vein is exposed, a vein retractor or Gilbernet retractor is inserted to retract the common bile duct medially. The portal vein is mobilized circumferentially at its midportion and is encircled with an umbilical tape. It then is isolated up to its bifurcation in the liver hilum. Several tributaries on the medial aspect are ligated in continuity with fine silk and divided.

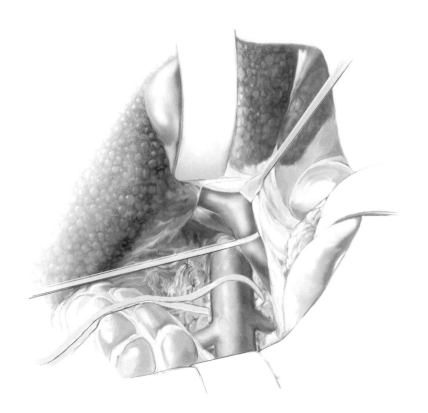

STEP 6   Mobilization of portal vein behind pancreas

Using the umbilical tape to pull the portal vein out of its bed, the portal vein is cleared to
the point where it disappears behind the pancreas. The tough fibrofatty tissue that binds
the portal vein to the pancreas must be divided. Several tributaries that enter the medial
aspect of the portal vein and one tributary that enters the posterolateral aspect are
divided. It is usually not necessary to divide the splenic vein. Wide mobilization of the
portal vein is essential for performance of a side-to-side portacaval anastomosis. Failure
to mobilize the portal vein behind the pancreas is a second major reason for difficulty in
accomplishing the side-to-side shunt. In some patients, it is necessary to divide a bit of
the head of the pancreas between right-angled clamps to obtain adequate mobilization
of the portal vein. Bleeding from the edges of the divided pancreas is controlled with
suture ligatures. Division of a small amount of the pancreas is a very helpful maneuver
and we have never observed postoperative complications, such as pancreatitis, from its
performance. Before incising the pancreas, the surgeon should insert his or her index
finger into the tunnel between the portal vein and the pancreas to determine by palpation if there is a replaced common hepatic or right hepatic artery arising from the superior mesenteric artery and crossing the portal vein. Since the portal venous blood flow
to the liver is diverted through the portacaval shunt, ligation of the hepatic arterial
blood supply may be lethal.

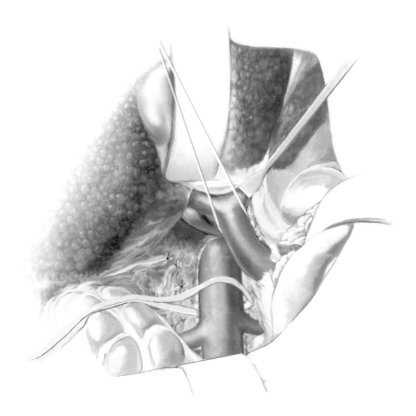

STEP 7

Testing adequacy of mobilization of portal vein and IVC

To determine the adequacy of mobilization of portal vein and IVC, the two vessels are brought together by traction on the umbilical tapes that surround them . It is essential to determine that the two vessels can be brought together without excessive tension. If this cannot be done, it is almost always because the vessels have not been adequately mobilized, and further dissection of the vessels should be undertaken. Resection of part of an enlarged caudate lobe of the cirrhotic liver, recommended by some surgeons to facilitate bringing the vessels together, is associated with some difficulties and, in our opinion, is neither necessary nor advisable.

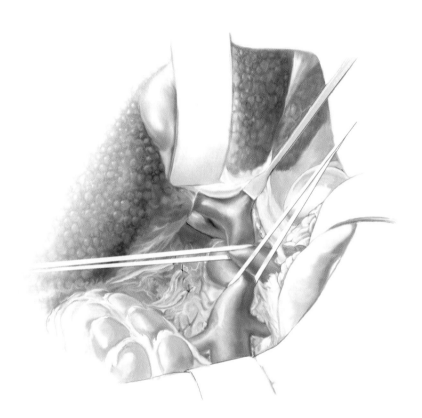

STEP 8   **Measurement of venous pressures**

Pressures in the IVC and portal vein are measured with a saline (spinal) manometer by direct needle puncture before performance of the portacaval anastomosis. For all pressure measurements, the bottom of the manometer is positioned at the level of the IVC, which is marked on the skin surface of the body with a towel clip (A-1 to A-5). All portal pressures are *corrected* by subtracting the IVC pressure from the portal pressure. A portal vein-IVC pressure gradient, also known as the corrected free portal pressure, of 150 mm saline or higher, represents clinically significant portal hypertension. Most patients with bleeding esophageal varices have a portal vein-IVC gradient of 200 mm saline or higher. The pressure measurements include:

- IVCP – inferior vena caval pressure
- FPP – free portal pressure
- HOPP – hepatic occluded portal pressure, obtained on the hepatic side of a clamp occluding the portal vein
- SOPP – splanchnic occluded portal pressure, obtained on the intestinal side of a clamp occluding the portal vein

In normal humans, HOPP is much lower than FPP, and SOPP is much higher. In patients with portal hypertension, the finding of an HOPP that is higher than the FPP suggests the possibility that blood flow in the portal vein is reversed because of severe hepatic outflow obstruction.

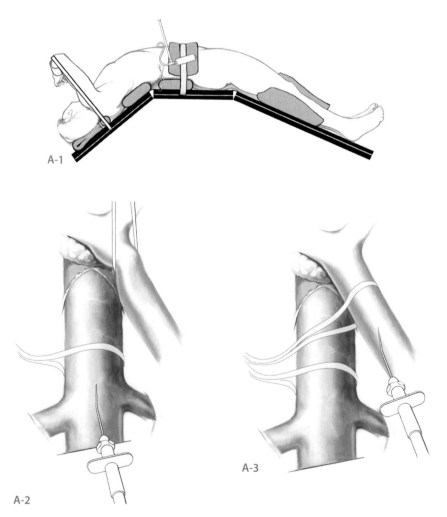

A-1

A-2

A-3

Measurement of venous pressures

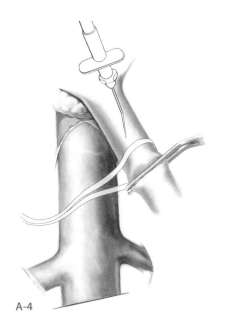

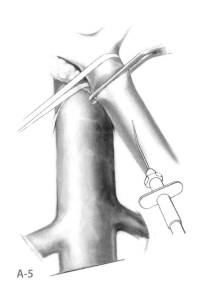

STEP 9   **Side-to-side portacaval anastomosis**

A Satinsky clamp is placed obliquely across a 5-cm segment of the anteromedial wall of the IVC in a direction parallel to the course of the overlying portal vein and the IVC is elevated toward the portal vein (A-1). A 5-cm segment of the portal vein is isolated between two angled vascular clamps and the portal vein is depressed toward the IVC, bringing the two vessels into apposition.

A 2.0- to 2.5-cm-long strip of the IVC and a 2.0- to 2.5-cm-long strip of the portal vein are excised with scissors (A-2). It is important to excise a longitudinal segment of the wall of each vessel rather than simply to make an incision in each vessel. A retraction suture of 5-0 silk is placed in the lateral wall of the IVC opening and is weighted by attachment to a hemostat to keep the IVC orifice open. The clamps on the portal vein are momentarily released to flush out any clots and then the openings in both vessels are irrigated with saline.

The anastomosis is started with a posterior continuous over-and-over suture of 5-0 vascular suture material (A-3). The posterior continuous suture is tied at each end of the anastomosis.

The anterior row of sutures consists of an everting continuous horizontal mattress stitch of 5-0 vascular suture material started at each end of the anastomosis (A-4). The suture started at the inferior end of the anastomosis is discontinued after three or four throws and is deliberately left loose so that the interior surface of the vessels can be visualized as the anastomosis is completed. In this way inadvertent inclusion of the posterior wall in the anterior row of sutures is avoided. The suture started at the superior end of the anastomosis is inserted with continuous tension until the inferior suture, at which point the inferior suture is drawn tight and the two sutures are tied to each other. Before drawing the inferior suture tight, the clamps on the portal vein are momentarily released to flush out any clots, and the anastomosis is thoroughly irrigated with saline (A-5).

Upon completion of the anastomosis, a single interrupted tension suture is placed just beyond each end of the anastomosis to take tension off the anastomotic suture line. The clamp on the IVC is removed first, the clamp on the hepatic side of the portal vein is removed next, and finally the clamp on the intestinal side of the portal vein is removed. Bleeding from the anastomosis infrequently occurs; it can be controlled by one or two well placed interrupted sutures of 5-0 vascular suture material.

Pressures in the portal vein and IVC must be measured after the anastomosis is completed. Usually the postshunt pressures in the portal vein and IVC are identical. A pressure gradient of >50 mm saline between the two vessels indicates an obstruction in the anastomosis, even when no obstruction can be palpated. In such circumstances, the anastomosis should be opened to remove any clots and, if necessary, the entire anastomosis should be taken down and redone. It is essential that there be no more than a 50-mm saline gradient between the portal vein and IVC to achieve permanently adequate portal decompression and to avoid ultimate thrombosis of the shunt.

STEP 9 (continued)   Side-to-side portacaval anastomosis

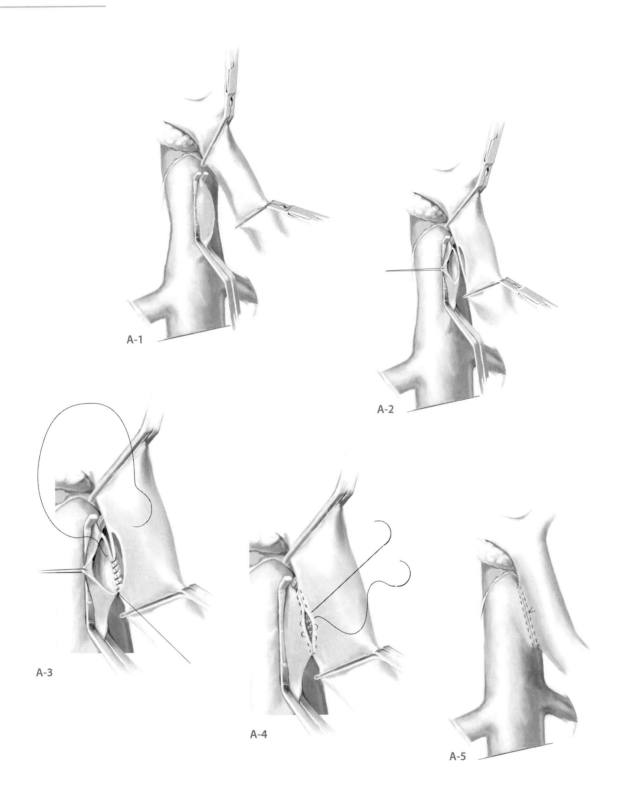

A-1

A-2

A-3

A-4

A-5

STEP 10   **Multiple steps in sewing an end-to-side portacaval anastomosis**

The end-to-side portacaval anastomosis is a satisfactory alternative to the side-to-side shunt in most cases, and some surgeons believe that it is somewhat less difficult to perform. It is not essential to isolate the IVC around its entire circumference, and it is often not necessary to clear as long a segment of the portal vein as in the lateral anastomosis. The disadvantage is that the liver sinusoids are not decompressed.

The Satinsky clamp on the IVC is placed obliquely on the anteromedial wall in the direction that will receive the end of the portal vein at an angle of about 45°. A 2-cm-long strip of the IVC is excised and a retraction suture is placed in the lateral wall (A-1). The portal vein is doubly ligated with a free ligature and a suture ligature of 2-0 silk just before its bifurcation in the hilum of the liver. An angled vascular clamp is placed across the portal vein near the pancreas, and the portal vein is divided obliquely just proximal to the ligation site.

In order to maximize the size of the anastomosis, the portal vein is transected tangentially so that the anterior wall is longer than the posterior wall at the transected end (A-2). After transection the clamp on the portal vein is momentarily released to flush out any clots before starting the anastomosis. This maneuver is repeated just before the final sutures in the anterior row of the anastomosis are placed.

The end-to-side anastomosis is performed with a continuous, over-and-over 5-0 vascular suture in the posterior row and a second 5-0 vascular suture in the anterior row (A-3). It is important that the portal vein describes a smooth curve in its descent toward the IVC and that it is attached to the IVC at an oblique angle. Twisting and kinking of the portal vein are the most common causes of a functionally unsatisfactory anastomosis. After the anastomosis is completed, pressure measurements are performed according to the guidelines described for the side-to-side shunt.

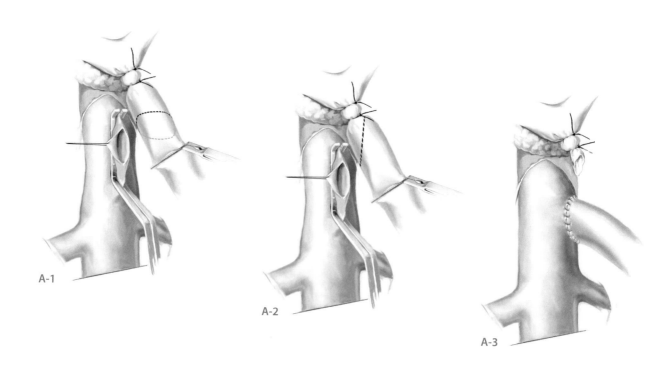

A-1

A-2

A-3

Liver Biopsy
A wedge liver biopsy is always obtained.

Postoperative Care

All patients should be admitted to an intensive care unit with equipment and personnel geared to managing the complicated problems associated with hepatic disease.

Monitoring
Careful monitoring of vital signs, central venous pressure, urine output, arterial pH, arterial and alveolar gases, fluid balance, body weight, and abdominal girth is essential.

Postoperative Complications

- Early:
    - Hepatic failure
    - Renal failure
    - Infection
    - Gastric acid hypersecretion
    - Delirium tremens
    - Ascites
    - Gastrointestinal bleeding
- Late:
    - Portasystemic encephalopathy (PSE)
    - Liver failure
    - Shunt thrombosis
    - Hepatocellular carcinoma

Tricks of the Senior Surgeon

- The position of the patient on the operating table is crucial and can make the difference between an easy and difficult operation.
- A long subcostal incision is associated with many fewer postoperative complications than a thoracoabdominal incision and is much to be preferred.
- Use of the electrocautery throughout the operation substantially reduces the operating time and the blood loss.
- Bleeding from the many portasystemic collateral vessels is best managed by pressure with gauze sponge packs, particularly as most of the bleeding stops as soon as the portacaval anastomosis is completed and the portal hypertension is relieved. Attempts to control each of the bleeding collaterals with ligatures and sutures prolong the operation and increase the blood loss. The objective is to decompress the portal system as rapidly as possible.
- Circumferential mobilization of the inferior vena cava between the entrance of the renal veins and the liver is essential for the side-to-side anastomosis and is neither hazardous nor difficult to perform. Apposition of the two vessels is greatly facilitated by elevation of the vena cava toward the portal vein.
- Mobilization of a long segment of portal vein, which includes division of the tough fibrofatty tissue that binds the portal vein to the pancreas and sometimes includes division of a bit of the head of the pancreas, is essential for the side-to-side anastomosis and sometimes for the end-to-side anastomosis.
- Beware of the replaced hepatic artery crossing the portal vein behind the head of the pancreas. Palpate it with the index finger in the funnel between the head of the pancreas and portal vein. Ligation of the hepatic artery may be lethal.
- Resection of an enlarged caudate lobe of the cirrhotic liver to facilitate apposition of the two vessels is hazardous and unnecessary.
- Pressures in the IVC and portal vein should always be measured after completion of the portacaval shunt. A pressure gradient of greater than 50 mm saline is unacceptable and requires revision of the anastomosis.

Gastroesophageal Devascularization: Sugiura Type Procedures

Norihiro Kokudo, Seiji Kawasaki (Thoracoabdominal Approach with Splenectomy),
Hector Orozco, Miguel A. Mercado (Complete Porto-azygos Disconnection
with Spleen Preservation),
Markus Selzner, Pierre-Alain Clavien (Abdominal Approach Only with Splenectomy)

Introduction

To improve the effect of Walker's simple esophageal transection, Sugiura and colleagues refined the technique of esophageal transection, adding the extensive paraesophageal devascularization via abdominal and thoracic incisions. The resulting procedure has been known as the Sugiura procedure. Three different approaches will be described including a spleen preserving procedure as well as a procedure with an abdominal approach only (i.e., without thoracotomy).

Indications and Contraindications

Indications	■ Bleeding or risky esophagogastric varices
	■ Esophagogastric varices resistant to endoscopic treatment
	■ Child-Turcotte (Pugh) Class A or B patients
Contraindications	■ Child-Turcotte (Pugh) Class C patients

Preoperative Investigation and Preparation for the Procedure

History:	Alcohol, hepatitis, recent overeating or overdrinking
Clinical evaluation:	Hematemesis, melena, encephalopathy, ascites, jaundice, nutritional status, splenomegaly, bleeding tendency
Laboratory tests:	Blood cell count, bilirubin, albumin, ALT, AST, prothrombin time, ammonia, total bile acid, indocyanine green test
Endoscopy:	Assessment of esophagogastric varices and portal hypertensive gastropathy, searching for the bleeding point
CT scan, ultrasound, or MRI:	Assessment of collateral vessels, portal flow, ascites, searching for hepatoma
In emergency cases:	Volume resuscitation, placement of Sengstaken-Blakemore tube, intratracheal intubation (when indicated)

Postoperative Tests

- Postoperative surveillance in an intensive or intermediate care unit
- Blood cell count, bilirubin, albumin, ALT, AST, and prothrombin time for at least 48h
- Check daily for clinical signs of gastrointestinal bleeding, liver failure, or pneumonia

Postoperative Complications

- Short term:
  - Liver failure
  - Gastrointestinal bleeding
  - Anastomotic leakage
  - Pleural effusion
  - Ascites
  - Portal vein thrombosis
  - Subphrenic abscess
  - Pancreatic leakage
- Long term:
  - Esophageal stricture
  - Remnant varices

Procedure 1:
Thoracoabdominal Approach with Splenectomy

Norihiro Kokudo, Seiji Kawasaki

Outline of the Procedure

Thoracoabdominal esophageal transection: The Sugiura procedure is a transthoraco abdominal esophageal transection, which consists of paraesophageal devascularization, esophageal transection and reanastomosis, splenectomy, and pyloroplasty. These thoracic and abdominal operations are performed in one or two stages depending on the surgical risk of the patients. The most important and unique feature of this procedure is an extensive devascularization from the level of the left pulmonary vein to the upper half of the stomach 6–7 cm along the lesser curvature below the cardia.

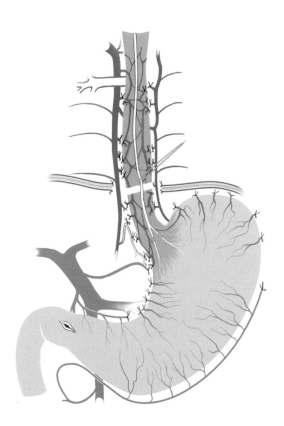

STEP 1   Incision and exposure of the thoracic esophagus

A standard left lateral thoracotomy incision is made, entering via the 7th intercostal space. The inferior mediastinum is opened at the anterior portion of the descending aorta.

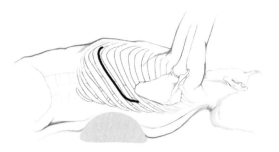

STEP 2   Paraesophageal devascularization

Using a curved Kelly forceps, the thoracic esophagus is isolated and taped at a level where collateral veins are scant. In emergency cases, lifting of the tape facilitates hemostasis inside the esophagus. Lifting the esophagus, paraesophageal devascularization is performed. Many dilated collateral veins resembling a vein plexus can be recognized around the esophagus. They are parallel to the vagus nerves and have many shunts to the esophagus. All of these shunting veins must be completely ligated and divided, with care taken not to damage the truncus vagalis and collateral veins. There are usually about 30–50 shunting veins to be ligated. The length of devascularization of the thoracic esophagus is about 12–18 cm. The upper edge of the devascularization is the inferior pulmonary vein, and the lower edge is where preperitoneal adipose tissue is exposed .

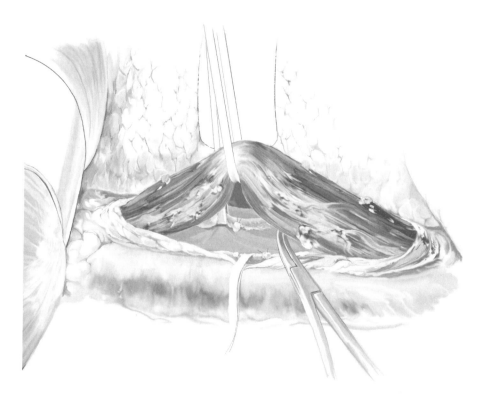

STEP 3

Esophageal transection 1

Upon completion of devascularization, the esophagus is doubly clamped with pairs of specially ordered esophageal clamps of the noncrushing, nonslipping type similar to Botallo's forceps ("Sugiura's clamp"). The distance between the two clamps is approximately 4 cm. The two clamps are jointed with a thumbscrew in the mid-portion.

Esophageal transection is performed at the level of the diaphragm. The anterior muscular layer is divided with a knife and a tape passed around the submucosal layer.

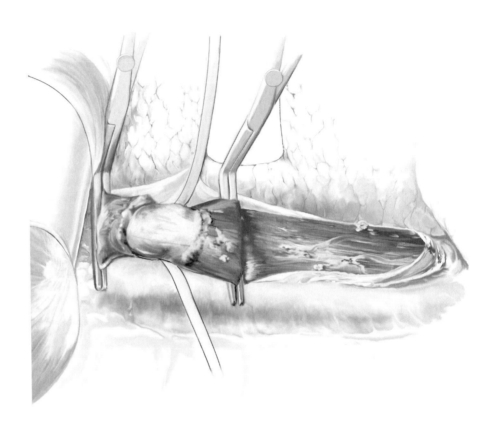

STEP 4   **Esophageal transection 2**

The mucosal layer of the esophagus is completely divided, with the posterior muscular layer left intact (A-1). The posterior muscle layer is preserved to prevent twisting, stricture, and leakage. The divided esophageal varices should not be ligated, because ligation of the divided varices may cause postoperative stenosis.

Posterior mucosal layer is sutured using 4-0 or 5-0 Vicryl (A-2).

Anterior mucosal layer is sutured (A-3). About 50–70 interrupted sutures are placed in total, and the divided varices are occluded with sutures.

After the muscle layer of 4-0 Ti-Cron is completed, a nasogastric tube is left in the stomach (A-4).

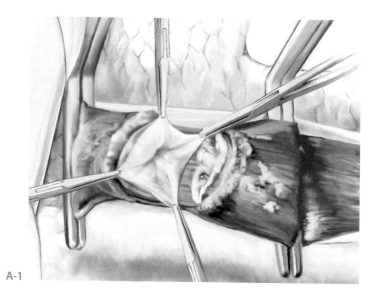

A-1

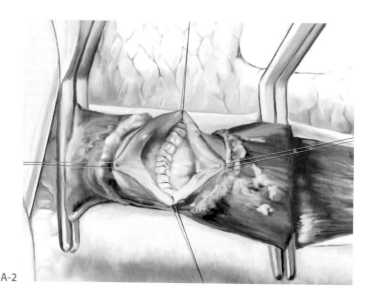

A-2

Esophageal transection 2

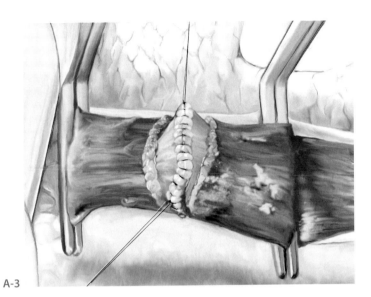

A-3

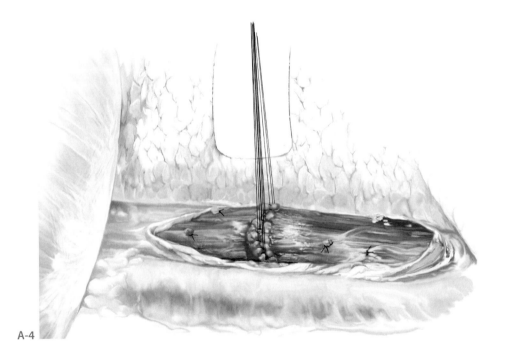

A-4

STEP 5   **Diaphragmatic incision**

After completion of esophageal transection, the diaphragm is incised, with care taken
not to damage the phrenic nerve and pericardiacophrenic vessels.

The spleen is then exposed and the left triangular ligament of the liver is divided and
ligated.

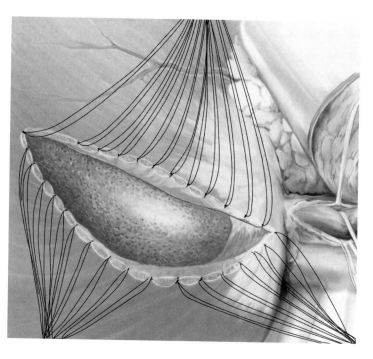

STEP 6   **Splenectomy 1**

The splenophrenic, splenorenal, and splenocolic ligaments are divided and the spleen is
completely mobilized. The gastrosplenic ligament is divided and short gastric vessels are
transected. The dissection is directed toward the hilus of the spleen.

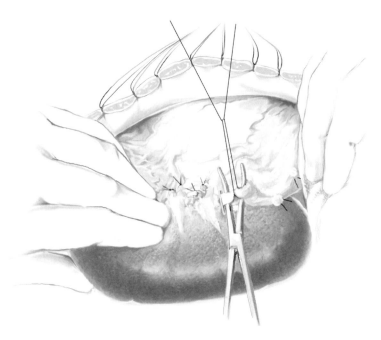

STEP 7   **Splenectomy 2**

After the ligamentous attachments and short gastric vessels have been divided, all that remains are the main splenic artery and vein. They are doubly ligated and divided. Care should be taken not to damage pancreatic tissue, because even a small tear may cause pancreatic leakage.

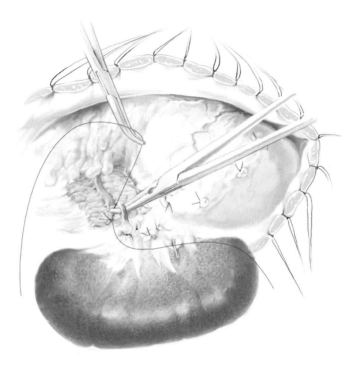

STEP 8   **Paraesophagogastric devascularization**

The abdominal esophagus and the cardia are devascularized from the greater curvature and the posterior of the stomach to the esophagus. The posterior gastric vagus nerve is divided by this procedure because the nerve runs very close to the stomach. Devascularization of the lesser curvature of the stomach and the abdominal esophagus follows, and the cardioesophageal branches of the left gastric vessels are ligated and divided. The length of devascularization is about 7 cm at the lesser curvature of the cardia. The esophagus and the cardia are completely mobilized and freed from the adjacent structures. A common pyloroplasty is performed because the gastric vagus nerves are divided.

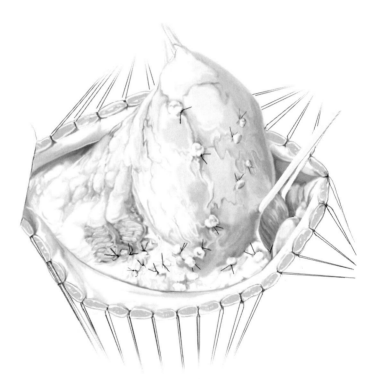

STEP 9

Closure

A drain is inserted in the left subphrenic space and the diaphragm is closed with 2-0 Vicryl (A-1).

The mediastinum is closed with 4-0 Ti-Cron (A-2), and the chest is closed after inserting a chest drain. A tight closure of the mediastinum may prevent thoracic empyema when a minor anastomotic leakage occurs.

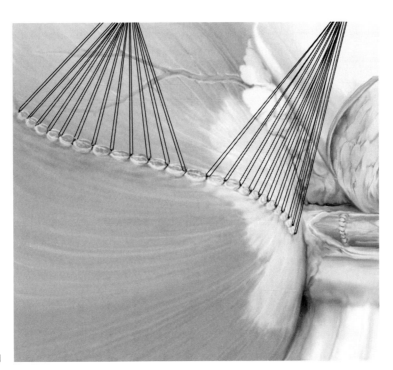

A-1

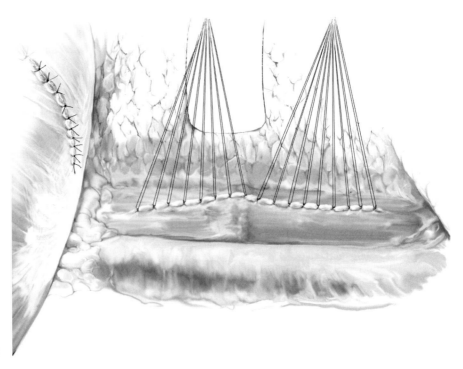

A-2

Tricks of the Senior Surgeon

- During the devascularization procedure, every shunting vein between the dilated paraesophageal collateral veins and esophageal wall should be ligated. Care should be taken not to damage the truncus vagalis and collateral veins, which are theoretically very important in preventing variceal recurrence. Although this is not always practically achievable, collateral channels in the mediastinum are believed to be preserved during the operation.
- A lasting extirpation of esophageal varices after nonshunting operation may depend on the portosystemic collateral changes that take place after the operation. Preserved paraesophageal and mediastinal collateral channels after the Sugiura operation are expected to function as a spontaneous shunt.

Acknowledgements
The authors thank Dr. Shunji Futagawa (Professor Emeritus of the 2nd Department of Surgery, Juntendo University) for supplying original drawings for this chapter.

Procedure 2:
Complete Porto-azygos Disconnection
with Spleen Preservation

Hector Orozco, Miguel A. Mercado

Introduction

Complete porto-azygos disconnection requires both abdominal and thoracic procedures. The following series of illustrations offers the alternative of a spleen preserving abdominal devascularization.

Indications, testing, and preoperative management are the same as for the full thoracoabdominal procedure described in the previous chapter.

Overview of the Abdominal Procedure

The abdominal part of the procedure includes the following components:
- Dividing the gastrohepatic ligament – gastrocolic ligament – left gastric artery and vein.
- Ligature the right gastric artery and vein over the lesser curvature.
- Ligature the right gastroepiploic vein.
- Devascularization of the great curvature with preservation of the spleen.
- Devascularization of the abdominal esophagus and transection of the main vagus nerves.
- Pyloroplasty.

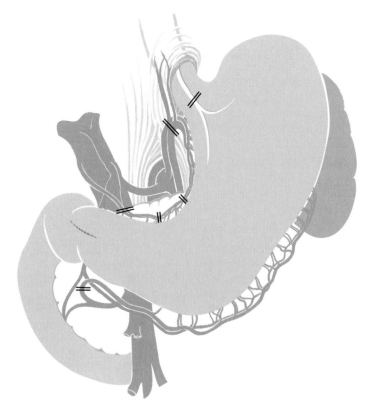

STEP 1   **Devascularization of the greater curvature**

From the left side, showing the complete devascularization of the greater curvature of
the stomach, with all vessels divided from the pylorus up to the esophagus. The short
gastric vessels are divided, leaving the spleen in situ.

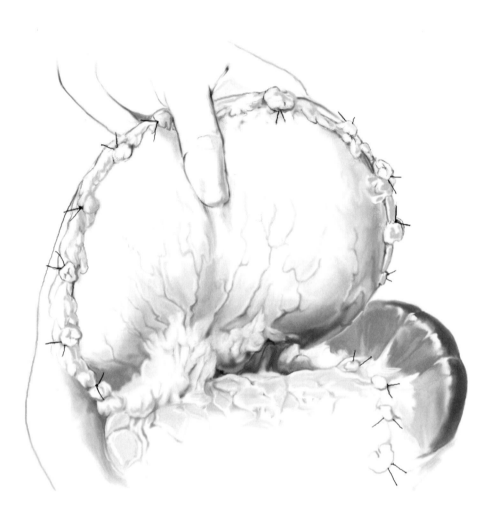

STEP 2

Completion of the devascularization of the lesser curvature

Complete devascularization of the stomach from the right side of the patient. This shows the upper two-thirds of the lesser curvature devascularized up to the esophagus.

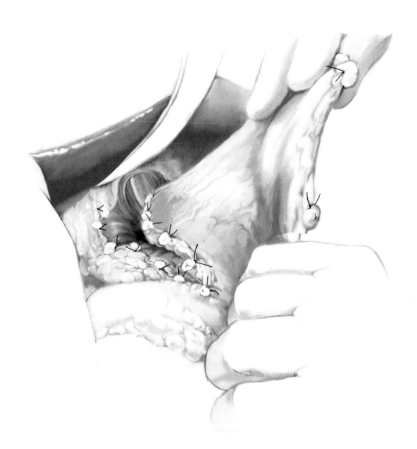

STEP 3   **Devascularization of the esophagus**

Complete devascularization of the esophagus and stomach viewed from behind, from
the left side of the patient. The esophagus is circumferentially devascularized for 7 cm
above the gastroesophageal junction. The preservation of the spleen can be seen.

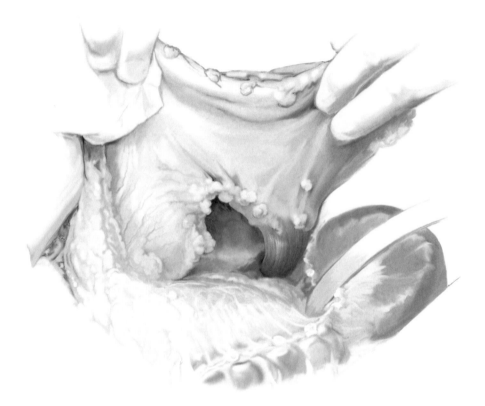

STEP 4	Ligation of the right gastroepiploic vein

The right gastroepiploic vein is ligated below the pylorus while the right gastroepiploic artery is preserved.

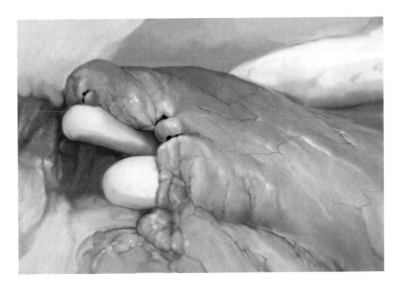

STEP 5	Pyloroplasty

Pyloroplasty is performed with a single layer of interrupted sutures as in the first procedure.

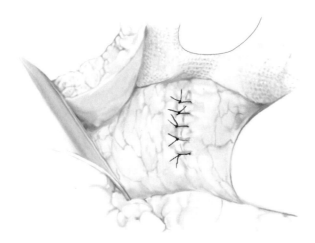

Procedure 3:
Abdominal Approach Only with Splenectomy

Markus Selzner, Pierre-Alain Clavien

STEP 1	Access and mobilization

A Thompson retractor is installed after left transverse incision and midline extension. A transverse upper abdominal incision is performed at the left side with a midline extension up to the xyphoid. Both rectum muscles are transsected and the abdominal cavity is entered to the left of the midline. The abdominal cavity has to be opened with care since enlarged veins might be present in the setting of portal hypertension.

STEP 2	Isolation of the spleen

The splenectomy in the setting of portal hypertension is often the most challenging part of the procedure. The vessels along the large gastric curvature are divided to expose the short gastric vessels, which are isolated and separated. Then the posterior adhesions of the spleen are divided. Afterwards the left colon flexure is retracted downwards and the adhesions between colon and spleen are divided (A).

The hilus of the spleen is isolated and the splenic artery and vein are identified whenever possible. The hilar structures are clamped with large Kelly clamps, divided and suture-ligated. Removal of the enlarged spleen results in more space in the left upper abdomen and often facilitates the further preparation of the stomach and the esophagus (B).

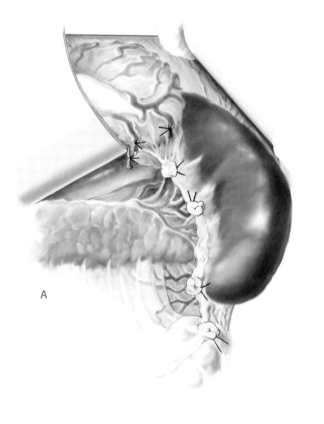
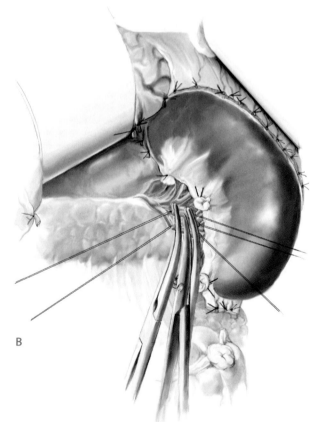

STEP 3   **Devascularization of the lesser and larger gastric curvature**

The preparation of the stomach is similar to the spleen preserving technique and has been described in the previous chapters. Briefly, the upper two-thirds of the stomach are isolated. The gastric vessels are ligated close to the stomach wall. Unlike in the spleen preserving procedure, care must be taken to preserve the right gastric artery and vein as well as the left gastric vein. It is important to perform the gastric isolation close to the stomach wall in order to preserve vessels draining to the azygos veins.

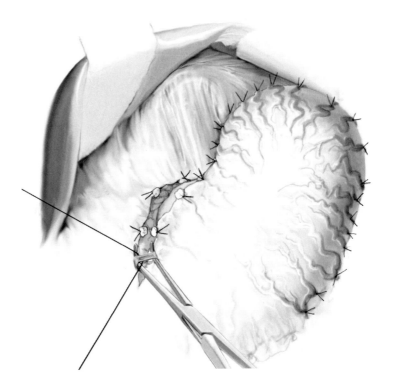

STEP 4   **Isolation of the distal esophagus**

The lower 12 cm of the esophagus is isolated. The venus plexus directly on the esophagus are transsected. The vagus nerve is also divided during this maneuver. All transverse vessels to the esophagus must be separated and ligated. It is important to preserve longitudinal vessels parallel to the esophagus, which drain in the azygos system.

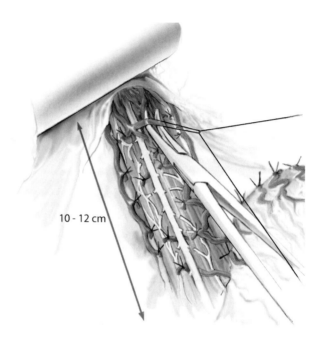

STEP 5   **Transsection of the esophagus:**

A transverse incision is performed in the well vascularized distal part of the stomach.
An end-to-end anastomosis (EEA) stapler is introduced and advanced to the lower
esophagus. A ligature is placed around the EEA stapler and the esophagus is transsected
5 cm above the gastro-esophageal junction. After firing the EEA stapler an intact mucosa
ring must be present in the head of the EEA.

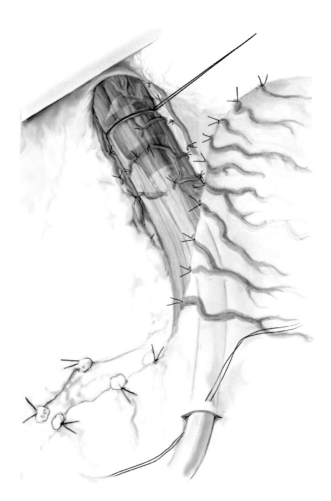

STEP 6   **Pyloroplasty**

As in the first two procedures, an extramucosal pyloroplasty according to Mikulic is performed. The muscles of the pylorus are divided longitudinally without opening the mucosa. The incision is closed with transverse single sutures (PDS 2-0).

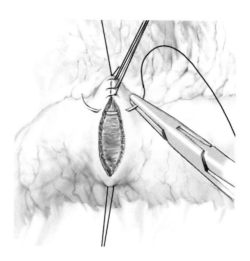

Tricks of the Senior Surgeon

- Preserve the blood flow to the azygos system (left gastric vein).
- Perform gastric devascularization after splenectomy.
- Introduce the EEA stapler in the distal nonischemic stomach.

Pancreas

Michael G. Sarr

Introduction

Michael G. Sarr

The last two decades have witnessed the escalating evolution of surgical thought/approach toward pancreatic diseases. New operations, new approaches, new techniques, and maybe even new philosophies of the operative management of pancreatic disease have been embraced based on a better understanding of etiopathogenesis of pancreatic diseases (e.g., necrotizing pancreatitis), introduction of new technology (laparoscopy, minimal access approaches, interventional radiology/endoscopy), and the vast advances in both diagnosis (computed tomography, endoscopic ultrasonography, magnetic resonance imaging, positron emission tomography) and critical care medicine. Indeed, even a new disease has been described (intraductal papillary mucinous neoplasm); though it had always been there, we just never recognized it! With these advances, experience with certain operations has increased markedly (e.g., pancreaticoduodenectomy) as operative morbidity and mortality have decreased, convincing our internal medicine/gastroenterologic colleagues that aggressive resectional approaches to the pancreas (in experienced centers) are associated with operative mortalities of <5% and are no longer complicated by the mortality rates of 20–25% of the 1960s and 1970s.

New operations have appeared:
- Chronic pancreatitis
  - Duodenum-preserving head resection (Beger/Frey procedures)
  - Thoracoscopic splanchnicectomy
- Necrotizing pancreatitis
  - Aggressive necrosectomy with several different techniques of peripancreatic drainage
  - Minimal access necrosectomy (not just drainage)
- Recurrent pancreatitis
  - Sphincterotomy/septectomy
- Pancreas transplantation
  - Islet cell, segmental, whole organ
- New technology
  - Laparoscopic approaches to enucleation of pancreatic islet cell neoplasms, distal pancreatectomy, internal (enteric) drainage of pseudocyst, gastrojejunostomy, even necrosectomy for necrotizing pancreatitis
- New philosophies
  - Laparoscopic staging of pancreatic malignancies to avoid non-therapeutic celiotomies

But, other basic techniques, approaches, and operations have not changed dramatically and require the same careful, systematic exposure, and operative skills.

This section deals with both the old and the new. Each topic is written by an expert and includes his or her tricks that facilitate, speed, or improve the exposure and conduct of the operations involved.

The next two decades will continue this relentless evolution in surgery of the pancreas. It will be interesting to watch how the current state-of-the-art changes – won't it?

Drainage of Pancreatic Pseudocysts

Gerard V. Aranha, Lawrence W. Way, Scott G. Houghton

Introduction

The goals of surgical treatment of most pancreatic pseudocysts are to provide a pathway of internal (enteric) drainage of the "leaking" exocrine secretions to allow the pseudocyst cavity to collapse, thereby either "sealing off" the ductal leak or creating a permanent internal fistula for drainage. Internal drainage includes cystogastrostomy, cystojejunostomy, and less commonly cystoduodenostomy. Internal drainage can also be accomplished by endoscopic cystogastrostomy or cystoduodenostomy in selected patients.

Indications and Contraindications

Indications

- Cystogastrostomy: symptomatic or very large pseudocysts of the pancreas adherent to the posterior wall of the stomach, i.e., the posterior wall of the stomach forms the anterior wall of the pseudocyst
- Cystojejunostomy: a pseudocyst not adhering to the posterior gastric wall in any location in the pancreas – head, body, or tail or Pseudocysts that bulge through the transverse mesocolon
- Cystoduodenostomy: a pseudocyst of the head of the pancreas anatomically placed so that only a cystoduodenostomy is possible

Contraindications

- Cystogastrostomy: Pseudocyst in the head or tail of the pancreas not adherent to stomach, or a pseudocyst that bulges through the transverse mesocolon only partially adherent to the stomach
- When the surgeon is not entirely certain that the cystic mass is a pseudocyst of the pancreas
- Grossly infected pseudocysts
- Cystojejunostomy: Pseudocysts more amenable to cystogastrostomy or cystoduodenostomy
- Cystoduodenostomy: Pseudocyst not immediately adjacent to duodenum, or concern about disrupting pancreatic ductal entry into duodenum (major or minor ampulla)

Preoperative Investigations and Preparation for the Procedure

History:	Vague abdominal or back pain after an attack of acute pancreatitis, nausea, vomiting, and weight loss
Clinical:	Fullness or mass in the epigastrium
Laboratory tests:	Persistent increase in serum amylase after attack of acute pancreatitis
Diagnostic imaging:	CT can identify one or more pseudocysts in the pancreas and may help to differentiate a cystic neoplasm from a pseudocyst
ERCP	Rarely used but can differentiate a pseudocyst that communicates with the main pancreatic duct from a cystic neoplasm, which should not occur unless it is an IPMN (intraductal papillary mucinous neoplasm)
Preoperative preparation:	NPO two to four hours before operation. A perioperative prophylactic I.V. antibiotic is repeated depending on the duration of operation

Procedures

Open Cystogastrostomy

STEP 1

Exposure of pseudocyst

A bilateral subcostal incision is preferred; alternatively, a midline incision may be used.

After routine abdominal exploration, a mechanical ring retractor is placed to retract the liver and abdominal wall.

The pseudocyst adherent to the posterior gastric wall is visualized or palpated transgastrically.

Seromuscular stay sutures are placed in the anterior gastric wall over the cyst.

A long gastrotomy is made, and the anterior gastric wall is retracted using stay sutures.

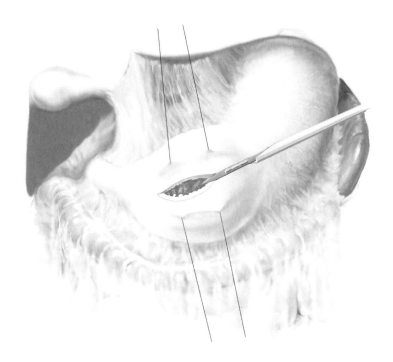

STEP 2

Transgastric opening of pseudocyst

The cyst is palpated through the posterior gastric wall.

The cyst is aspirated using a 22-gauge needle; usually, clear, opalescent, or brownish fluid is obtained; if thick mucoid fluid is obtained, the diagnosis of cystic neoplasm must be entertained (A-1).

After aspiration, the syringe is removed from the needle, which is left in place and secured with a hemostat.

A #11 blade knife is used to enter the cyst alongside of the needle (A-2).

Once the cyst is entered, the needle is removed and a right-angled clamp is inserted into the opening, elevating the posterior wall to enlarge the opening to at least 3–4 cm or longer if possible.

Biopsy of the cyst wall using a long-handled, #15 blade knife should be imperative (A-3).

The cyst is probed with a finger, loculations gently broken down, and contents aspirated. Thick debris is removed carefully with packing forceps.

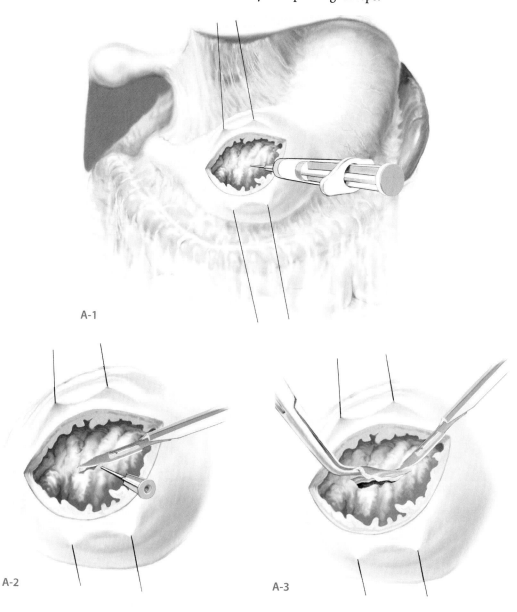

A-1

A-2

A-3

STEP 3

Oversewing of cystogastrostomy

The posterior common cyst/gastric wall is oversewn ("reefed") with running 3-0 silk suture. One suture is run from 3 o'clock to 9 o'clock and tied, the other suture is run from 9 o'clock to 3 o'clock; this avoids a "pursestring" effect on the opening and allows the cyst to communicate freely with the stomach.

The gastrotomy is closed in two layers; the inner, running 3-0 polyglyconate suture is placed in a Connell fashion to invert the mucosa and obtain hemostasis; the outer layer consists of interrupted 3-0 silk seromuscular sutures.

The abdomen is closed without drainage using running 1-0 polydioxanon for the anterior and posterior rectus fasciae for a subcostal incision and 1-0 polyglycolic acid for a midline incision.

The skin incision is closed with staples.

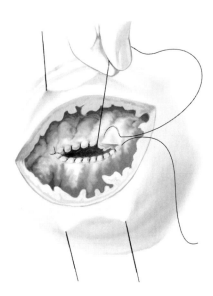

Open Cystoduodenostomy

STEP 1

Specific indications include a pseudocyst in the head of the pancreas anatomically placed so that only a cystoduodenostomy is possible.

The same approach/setup as for cystogastrostomy above.

The pseudocyst is visualized and palpated.

The cyst is aspirated with a 22-gauge needle.

A clear, opalescent, or brownish fluid should be obtained; mucoid fluid suggests a cystic neoplasm.

The syringe is removed from the needle, and a #11 blade knife is used to enter the cyst along the needle.

A right-angled clamp is inserted to elevate the cyst wall, for enlarging the opening to at least 2–3 cm of longer; a biopsy is taken of the cyst wall.

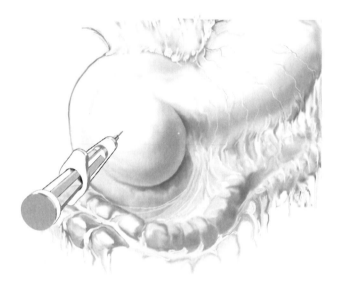

STEP 2

The duodenum is well Kocherized.

In this depiction, a lateral-to-lateral or side-to-side cystoduodenostomy is shown.
Creation of an anterior vertical duodenotomy of at least 2–3 cm is carried out (A-1).

Posterior sutures between the cyst and the duodenum are placed in a single interrupted layer using 3-0 silk (A-2).

Sutures are placed from the duodenum to the cyst to create an anterior wall using a single layer of interrupted 3-0 silk (A-3).

If a transduodenal cystoduodenostomy can be used, it is similar to cystogastrostomy. However, pseudocyst drainage into the posterior duodenum is done into the first or third portion of the duodenum to avoid injuring the common duct; staying in the midline of the posterior duodenal wall avoids injury to the gastroduodenal and pancreaticoduodenal vessels. Intraoperative ultrasonography can be used to identify the common bile duct and vessels if necessary.

Abdominal incision closed as for cystogastrostomy.

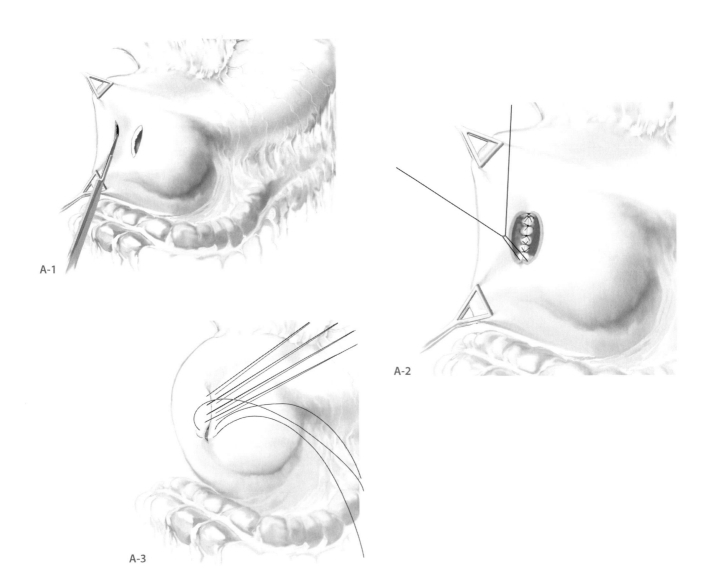

A-1

A-2

A-3

Open Cystojejunostomy

Exposure of pseudocyst

Specific indications include a pseudocyst not adhering to the posterior gastric wall in any location in the pancreas – head, body, or tail and those pseudocysts that bulge through the transverse mesocolon.

　　We prefer a bilateral subcostal incision with a mechanical ring retractor.

　　The pseudocyst is intimate with the transverse mesocolon.

　　Aspirate the cyst with a 22-gauge needle.

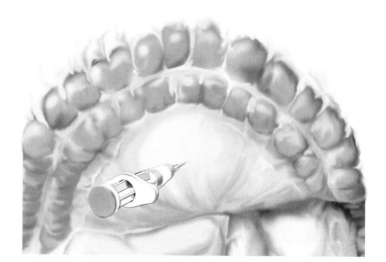

STEP 2

The jejunum is transected with a mechanical stapler 20 cm from the ligament of Treitz.

The distal end is oversewn and brought up to the cyst as a Roux limb.

3-0 interrupted silk sutures are placed between the cyst wall and midway between the antimesenteric and mesenteric borders of the posterior jejunal wall for 4–5 cm or longer and tied down after all sutures are placed (A-1).

A cystotomy is made in similar fashion as for cystogastrostomy and cystoduodenostomy; a biopsy is taken of the cyst wall (A-2).

An interrupted single layer of 3-0 silk sutures is placed between the cyst and the jejunum to create an anterior wall (A-3).

The cystojejunostomy is completed as for side-to-side cystoduodenostomy (A-4).

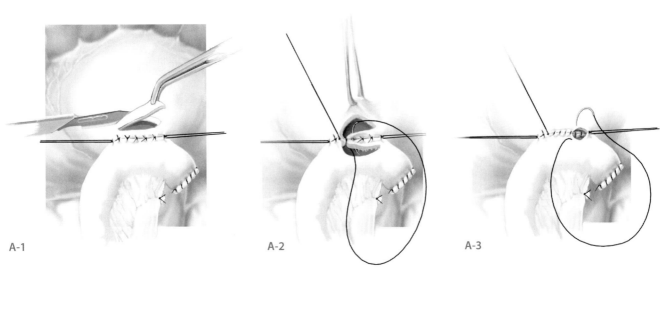

A-1 A-2 A-3

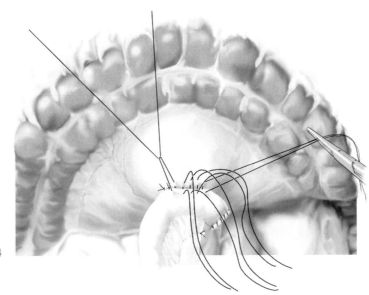

A-4

STEP 3

The proximal jejunum is anastomosed to the Roux limb 60 cm distally.

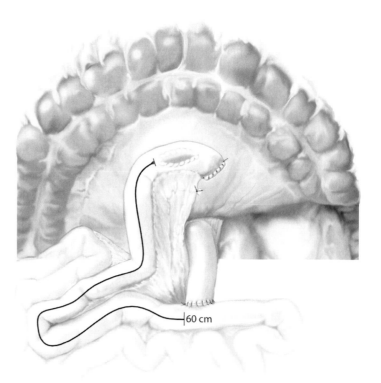

STEP 4

When the pseudocyst does not bulge through the mesocolon and is not adherent to the stomach or duodenum, the gastrocolic ligament is taken down to enter the lesser sac.

The Roux limb is brought retrocolic either to the right or left of the mesocolic vessels.

The anastomosis of the pseudocyst is done as in Step 2.

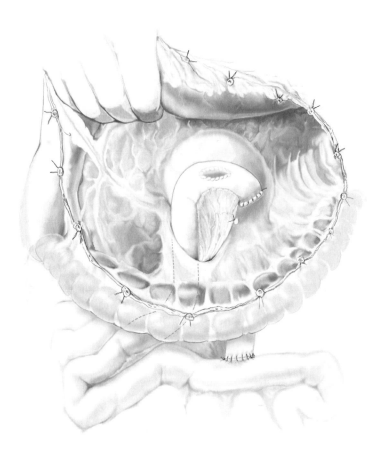

Laparoscopic Cystogastrostomy

STEP 1

Alternatives to open cystogastrostomy include either a totally endoscopic approach to cystogastrostomy or a less-well standardized, percutaneous, radiologic, transgastric cystogastric tube placement attempting to accomplish the same overall goals. The laparoscopic approach provides another "access route" that allows a better visualization as well as the ability to use laparoscopic surgical techniques not limited to the narrow access port of the gastroscope. Two trocars are placed into the lumen of the gas-distended stomach to provide the access for the cystogastrostomy. The gastric lumen becomes the counterpart of the gas-filled peritoneal cavity used for conventional laparoscopic operations (A-1).

The operation begins by placing a periumbilical trocar for introduction of a laparoscope (5 mm or 10 mm). Two additional trocars are inserted in the mid clavicular line several centimeters rostrally on either side of the camera trocar.

A nasogastric tube is passed into the stomach and attached to a laparoscopic insufflator. CO_2 gas is instilled to inflate the gastric lumen until the anterior gastric wall comes within a few millimeters of the anterior abdominal wall as visualized via the laparoscope. A radially expanding 10-mm trocar is inserted into the stomach as follows. First, pass the trocar through the abdominal wall where the anterior surface of the stomach abuts the abdominal wall, usually in the left epigastrium. Then poise it at the desired entry site on the anterior gastric wall and pop it into the stomach using a quick snap of the wrist. Pass a 5-mm, 30 degree laparoscope down the trocar and look into the gastric lumen; because the gastric walls reflect light so well, the view is bright and full of detail. Insert a second trocar into the stomach 6–10 cm from the first one. Check that positioning is satisfactory for intragastric surgery by passing the 5-mm scope down each of the trocars. The radially expanding trocars create snug, gas-tight puncture wounds in the stomach; conventional cutting trocars make wounds that leak (A-2).

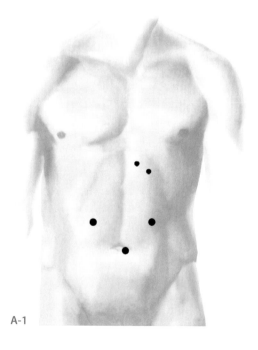

A-1

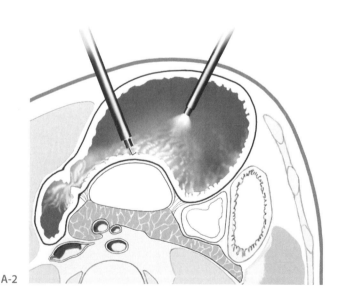

A-2

Next, shut off gas insufflation into the peritoneal cavity and open the valves on these trocars to room air to allow any small amount of gas that might leak from inside the stomach around the gastric trocars to escape instead of accumulating in the peritoneal cavity and competing for space with the distended stomach. The insufflation pressure in the gastric lumen should be set at $20\,cm/H_2O$ with insufflation connected to one of the trocars.

It is usually possible to see a convexity on the posterior gastric wall created by the pseudocyst. To localize the pseudocyst, pass a long aspirating needle through the back wall of the stomach into the cyst and aspirate some cyst fluid. If fluid is not found, either the needle is not in the cyst or the cyst contents are too thick to aspirate. The latter is uncommon, however, so the first alternative is most likely. Check the CT, recalculate the cyst location, and try again. In our experience, finding the cyst has rarely been difficult and has never required use of laparoscopic ultrasonography; however, use of this technique may prove helpful.

Having located the cyst, use the hook monopolar electrocautery (at a high power setting) to cut a hole through the posterior gastric wall into the pseudocyst; do not make the full cystogastrostomy incision, just a 1-cm hole (A-3).

Next, aspirate the cyst contents and pass the scope into, or almost into, the cyst cavity. After determining where your entry hole lies in relation to the cyst's circumference and area of contact with the stomach, extend the cystogastrostomy incision so it involves the center of the common wall between cyst and stomach and spans one-third to one-half of the cyst diameter. Check for bleeding and control with further electrocautery or suture ligation.

Remove semi-solid necrotic debris from within the cyst lumen and temporarily deposit this material in the dependent fundus of the stomach; the debris should be pushed through the pylorus into the duodenum before removing the gastric trocars. Do not try to "debride" the wall of the pseudocyst.

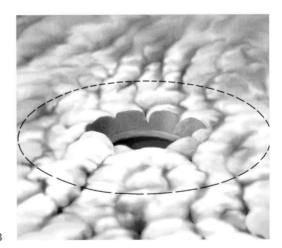

A-3

STEP 2

The intragastric scope and any other instruments are withdrawn from the gastric trocars, the pneumoperitoneum reinstated, and a laparoscope is inserted in the periumbilical trocar. The gastric trocars are withdrawn from the stomach under direct vision, but not pulled out of the abdomen because the port sites will leak gas. Decompress the stomach through the nasogastric tube.

Using intracorporeal suturing and knot tying (or alternatively an endoscopic stapler), place two interrupted Lembert stitches of 2-0 silk to close the puncture sites in the anterior gastric wall. All five trocars and the nasogastric tube can be removed (A-1, A-2).

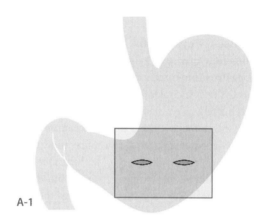

A-1

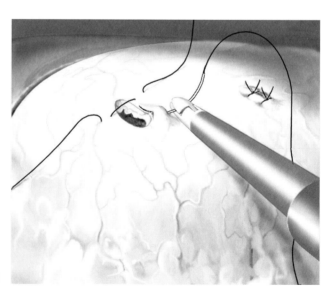

A-2

Postoperative Care

- Observation in the Intensive or Intermediate Care Unit is required only in selected patients.
- Nasogastric suction for 48 h.

Local Postoperative Complications

- Early:
    - Upper GI bleeding – usually from the anastomotic site
    - Anastomotic leak and/or intra-abdominal abscess
    - Beware alcohol withdrawal
- Late:
    - Recurrent pseudocyst
    - Error in diagnosis, i.e., mistaking a cystic neoplasm of pancreas for a pseudocyst; this leads to a persistent recurrent cyst with symptoms

Tricks of the Senior Surgeon

Open internal drainage of pseudocysts:

- Always make sure that the cyst contents are that of a pseudocyst; i.e., clear, opalescent or brownish and not mucoid as in a cystic neoplasm.
- Leave the aspirating needle in place to enter the cyst with a knife alongside the needle.
- Use a right-angled clamp to elevate the cyst wall to make an adequate sized opening.
- Virtually always biopsy the cyst wall.
- If the cyst contents appear purulent, send the fluid for gram stain. If only white cells are seen, then internal drainage can be done; however, if numerous bacteria are seen and the fluid is purulent, external drainage is preferable.
- Use intraoperative ultrasonography liberally, because it can identify and locate more than one cyst. It can also locate the common bile duct and pancreatic duct. Finally, it can reveal the relationship of the pseudocyst to adjacent visceral and vascular structures.

Laparoscopic cystogastrostomy:

- This laparoendoscopic approach recapitulates the open transgastric cystogastrostomy. While others have described a side-to-side cystogastrostomy via a laparoscopic approach using a linear endoscopic stapler, the risk of an intraperitoneal "anastomotic leak" is avoided by the approach we have described.
- The initial short cystogastrostomy can be lengthened using an endoscopic linear stapler or even the harmonic scalpel, but we have not found this necessary and these techniques just increase the cost of the procedure.
- Carefully inspect the site of the cystogastrostomy; if there is any bleeding, the incision can either be reefed/oversewn intragastrically via the two trocars using a 2-0 silk suture or further controlled with electrocautery.
- Beware of the patient with a large "pseudocyst" of the pancreatic body after an episode of necrotizing pancreatitis. Be certain to exclude the presence of splenic vein compression/occlusion and gastric varices; these varices can be quite large and lead to severe hemorrhage during the cystogastrostomy.

Denervation: Pain Management

Michael G. Sarr, Keith D. Lillemoe (Intraoperative Chemical Splanchnicectomy),
Bhugwan Singh, J.E.J. Krige, Philip C. Bornman (Thoracoscopic Splanchnicectomy)

Introduction

The pain of both benign and malignant pancreatic disease can be incapacitating.
Attempts to relieve pancreatic pain by extensive operative denervation have proved not
to be effective. Newer, less-invasive techniques of selective denervations appear effective
as shorter medium-term palliation.

Indications and Contraindications

Indications

- Epigastric and back pain related to:
  unresectable pancreatic, periampullary, and other upper GI cancers,
  chronic pancreatitis not amenable to other operative therapy

Contraindications

- Non-response to other attempts at percutaneous or endoscopic chemical
  splanchnicectomy

Procedures

Intraoperative Chemical Splanchnicectomy
Michael G. Sarr, Keith D. Lillemoe

Intraoperative chemical splanchnicectomy can be useful, especially in patients who are found at the time of exploration for resection to have unresectable pancreatic cancer. Rather than having these patients undergo percutaneous or endoscopic chemical splanchnicectomy postoperatively, an intraoperative approach is easy, effective, and warranted.

Procedure

- The celiac plexus contains visceral afferent (pain) nerves from the stomach, pancreas, hepatobiliary tree, kidneys, and mid gut.
- There are one to five ganglia on each side of the celiac and superior mesenteric arteries which lie anterior to the diaphragmatic crura and medial to the adrenal glands.
- Supplies needed include a 10- or 20-ml syringe, a 20-gauge spinal needle, and 40 ml of a 50% alcohol or 5% phenol solution.
- The lesser curvature of the stomach is retracted caudally.
- The first two fingers of the surgeon's left hand "straddle" the aorta.
- The index finger palpates the pulse of the splenic artery, while the second finger palpates the thrill of the common hepatic artery.
- The surgeon's right hand controls the syringe with the neurolytic agent.
- The spinal needle is advanced into the right para-aortic region just rostral to the hepatic artery, and is clamped by the assistant to prevent displacement.
- The surgeon aspirates the syringe; if no blood is obtained (i.e., needle in vessel), 10 ml of the neurolytic agent is injected, the needle removed, and the area compressed with a gauze pack.
- The syringe is re-filled, and the same maneuver is carried out just below the common hepatic on the right para-aortic area and rostral and caudal to the splenic artery in the left para-aortic region.

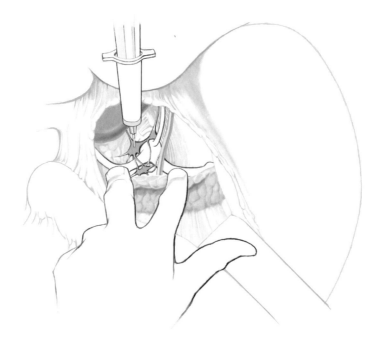

Thoracoscopic Splanchnicectomy

Bhugwan Singh, J.E.J. Krige, Philip C. Bornman

STEP 1

With the introduction of minimal access thoracostomy, interest and experience with a thoracoscopic approach to splanchnic nerve transection has grown. This procedure avoids the need for a major thoracotomy.

A standard general anesthetic is administered using a single lumen endotracheal tube.

The patient is positioned in a prone position; pillows support the epigastric and sternal areas to facilitate breathing.

The arms are abducted and elbows flexed.

A pneumothorax is induced using a Veress needle placed in the intercostal space adjacent to the inferior scapular angle (usually 5th intercostal space); the pneumothorax is maintained with carbon dioxide insufflation to an intrapleural pressure of 8 cm water; total lung collapse is not necessary because an 8 cm pressure pneumothorax is adequate to visualize the splanchnic nerves.

A 5-mm cannula is introduced in the 7th intercostal space in the posterior axillary line; a laparoscope/"thoracoscope" is passed through this cannula, connected to a video monitor, and is passed into the pleural space.

A second 5-mm cannula, inserted at the site of Veress needle placement, provides access for the dissecting instrument.

On the right side, the procedure commences at the 4th intercostal space at the level of the azygous vein, which is usually the origin of the most proximal splanchnic root.

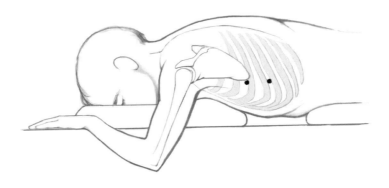

STEP 2

Accurate identification of the splanchnic nerves is the critical initial step in this procedure (A-1, A-2).

Splanchnic nerves [greater (GSN), lesser (LSN) and least (lsn)] have their origin medially from the sympathetic chain, usually from the lower eight ganglia.

Whereas the GSN is consistently present, presence of the LSN and the lsn is more variable, ranging from 86% to 100% and from 16% to 98% respectively.

The GSN is usually formed by contributions from the 5th to 9th ganglia, but contributions range widely from the 3rd to 11th thoracic ganglia.

Variable intersplanchnic connections occur between the splanchnic roots and nerves and provide an alternate neural pathway for transmission of pancreatic pain.

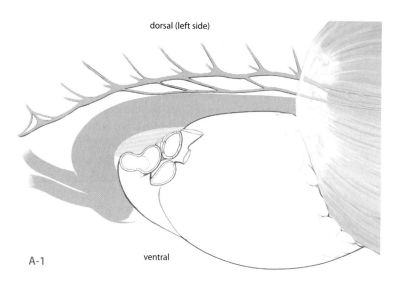

A-1

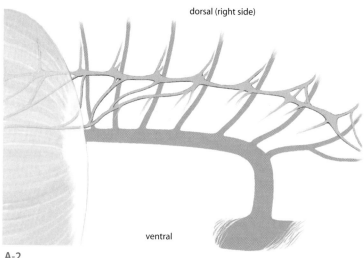

A-2

STEP 3

Using an electrosurgical hook, the parietal pleura is entered approximately 10 mm medial to the sympathetic chain; the pleura is stripped off the posterior chest wall up to the diaphragmatic recess so that a 10-mm-wide longitudinal pleurotomy is achieved.

Commencing from the most proximal contribution to the GSN and working distally, all branches passing medially from the sympathetic chain are mobilized sequentially using the hook dissector and transected using cautery; in this fashion all roots to the GSN, LSN and lsn (if present) are transected. When there is any doubt, gentle traction on the sympathetic chain confirms complete dissection of splanchnic nerves.

On the left side, the procedure commences at the 4th intercostal space at the level of the aortic arch, usually the origin of the most proximal splanchnic root; the principles of this technique are the same as on the right side.

Extension of peri-pancreatic inflammation to the retropleural space may cause thickening of the pleura, impairing visualization and impeding easy dissection of the sympathetic chain and splanchnic nerves.

Troublesome bleeding can be controlled by judicious use of cautery.

After completion of the neurotomy, carbon dioxide insufflation is stopped and gentle suction applied through the dissecting port with positive end expiratory pressure applied by the anesthetist.

Intercostal chest drains are not placed, provided lung reexpansion is present up to the intercostal musculature.

A chest radiograph is taken when respiratory distress, progressive desaturation, or unremitting surgical emphysema develops.

The patient may be discharged after overnight hospital stay.

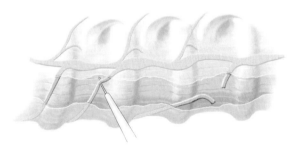

Postoperative Tests

Thoracoscopic Splanchnicectomy
- Surveillance in an intermediate care unit with oxygen saturation monitoring
- Routine chest radiograph to exclude residual pneumothorax

Local Postoperative Complications

Intraoperative Splanchnicectomy
- Short term:
  - Intra-arterial injection of neurolytic agent – this can be prevented by aspirating the syringe containing the neurolytic agent *before* injecting
  - Retroperitoneal bleeding – unusual, minimized by applying topical pressure after instillation of neurolytic agent
  - Transient orthostatic hypotension – unusual, lasts only 1–2 days
  - Very rare, anecdotal case reports of paraplegia secondary to intrathecal injection of neurolytic agent – this is preventable with careful technique
- Long term:
  - Recurrent pain

Thoracoscopic Splanchnicectomy
- Short term:
  - Pulmonary: pneumothorax, hemothorax, and hemo-pneumothorax – treat by closed intercostal chest drainage. Less common is chylothorax, requiring ligation of the thoracic duct.
  - Transient ileus – managed conservatively.
  - Inadvertent injury or transection of sympathetic chain may predispose to retrograde ejaculation.
- Long term:
  - *Recurrence of pain*

Tricks of the Senior Surgeon

Intraoperative splanchnicectomy:
- Use a 20-gauge spinal needle (longer than a regular needle).
- Use of a smaller volume syringe allows the surgeon to hold the needle/syringe in one hand.
- Do not disrupt the peritoneum overlying the retroperitoneum in the region of the celiac plexus.
- Two minutes of topical pressure will prevent hematomas.

Thoracoscopic splanchnicectomy:
- Meticulous positioning of the ports aids visibility of the entire sympathetic chain.
- Total collapse of the lung is unnecessary; an 8-cm water pressure pneumothorax is also usually adequate to identify the splanchnic nerves.
- The proximal contribution to the GSN is identified by tracing the sympathetic chain distally as it courses over the necks of the proximal ribs.
- Gentle traction on the sympathetic chain brings the splanchnic branches into profile.
- Troublesome bleeding from an intercostal vein can be controlled with pressure, cautery, or clip.
- Accurate placement of ports in the intercostal spaces avoids postoperative intercostal neuralgia.

Enteric Ductal Drainage for Chronic Pancreatitis

William H. Nealon

Introduction

The concept of draining an apparently obstructed main pancreatic duct was first addressed by opening either the proximal end of the pancreatic duct at the ampulla by doing a sphincterotomy or at the distal end of the pancreatic duct by removing the tail (Duval procedure). Puestow is credited with the concept of a longitudinal incision along the main pancreatic duct through the body and the head of the pancreas. This procedure was first described as a modification of a Duval procedure and therefore included resection of the pancreatic tail. Partington and Rochelle determined that a tail resection was unnecessary and carried out only a side-to-side lateral pancreaticojejunostomy. The principle of the procedure is to decompress an apparently obstructed main pancreatic duct (and maybe to also decompress the pancreatic parenchyma – the pancreatic compartment syndrome suggested by Reber). This assumption is based on the fact that the pancreatic duct is markedly dilated, suggesting a restriction to flow.

Indications and Contraindications

Indications	
	■ Chronic persistent pain
	■ To prevent episodes of acute exacerbations in chronic pancreatitis
	■ To facilitate resolution of symptomatic pancreatic pseudocyst
	■ To prevent further loss of pancreatic exocrine and endocrine function

Contraindications	
	■ "Small duct" (<5 mm) chronic pancreatitis
	■ Extrahepatic venous obstruction, because of the risk of hemorrhage
	■ Suspicion of malignancy
	■ Advanced cirrhosis

Preoperative Investigations and Preparation for Procedure

History: History of chronic, unremitting epigastric abdominal pain
                              or acute exacerbations of typical pancreatic pain, history
                              of ethanol abuse or other possible causes of chronic pancre-
                              atitis

Clinical evaluation: Establish presence or absence of narcotic usage and require-
                              ment (if narcotic addicted, entertain the concept of postopera-
                              tive detoxification), frequency of hospitalizations, nutritional
                              status, pancreatic functional status (endocrine and exocrine),
                              ASA risk status

Laboratory tests: Serum amylase and/or lipase, albumin, alkaline phosphatase,
                              GGT, bilirubin coagulation parameters, CA 19–9, glucose

Imaging: CT or MRI/ MRCP, ERCP if indicated

Preparation for surgery: Maximize endocrine status (insulin), maximize exocrine
                              status (enzyme replacement), bowel preparation if necessary,
                              perioperative prophylactic antibiotics

Procedure: Lateral Pancreaticojejunostomy
(Modified Puestow Procedure)

STEP 1

Exposure and exploration are facilitated by insertion of a retractor (Thompson)

First, the lesser sac is entered by separating the attachments between the gastrocolic omentum and the transverse colon.

Any "congenital" or acquired adhesions between the posterior surface of the stomach and the anterior surface of the pancreas are transected widely, exposing the anterior surface of the pancreas, including the head of the pancreas – take care to identify and exclude the right gastroepiploic artery and vein, which are situated between the head of the pancreas and the pylorus.

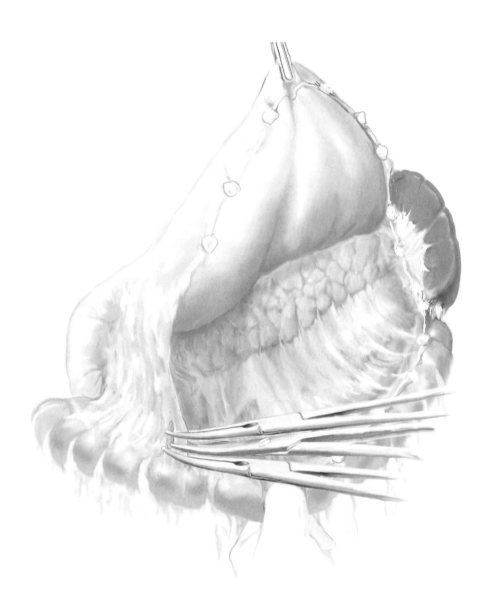

STEP 2   **Mobilize the inferior border of the body of the pancreas**

Identify and avoid the inferior mesenteric vein to the left of the spine.

Extend the dissection from the body toward the head of the pancreas. This facilitates bimanual examination and palpation of the anterior surface of the gland.

Place a broad curved retractor beneath the posterior wall of the stomach and retract superiorly.

Palpate and determine the location of the main pancreatic duct.

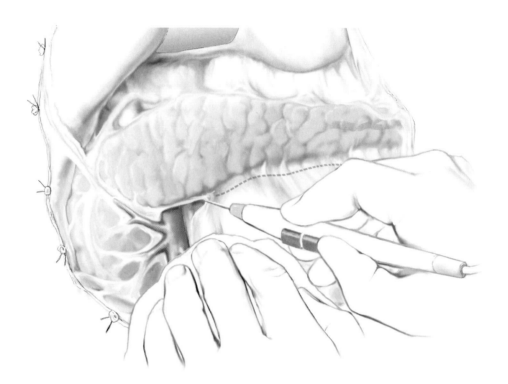

STEP 3

The pancreas should be easily appreciated because of its hard, fibrotic texture.
The dilated main pancreatic duct feels a bit like a large vein on the arm with a ballotable texture and a definite "trough."

The superior and inferior borders of this softer area feel like a canyon or a cliff and this represents the fibrotic pancreas on both sides.

Once the palpation is conclusive, a 22-gauge needle is passed through the anterior surface of the pancreas and into the pancreatic duct; on removing the needle, you should see clear fluid return, confirming that the main pancreatic duct has been accessed. The purpose of this maneuver is to avoid incising into the splenic vein or another structure mistaken for the main pancreatic duct.

Once pancreatic juice is determined, then electrocautery is utilized to incise the anterior surface of the body of the pancreas into the pancreatic duct parallel and adjacent to the needle, which is left in the pancreatic duct as a guide.

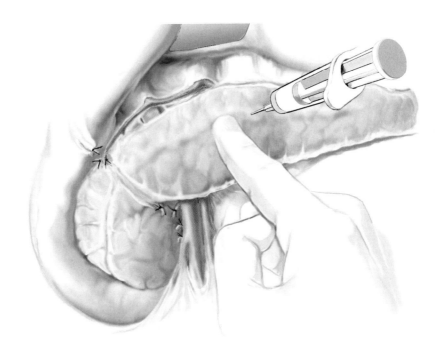

STEP 4

A right angle clamp will facilitate using the electric cautery to open widely the duct out to the tail of the pancreas laterally and toward the head of the pancreas. As you reach the genu of the main pancreatic duct it is important to extend the incision through the genu and toward the ampulla. This maneuver requires not only turning the incision inferiorly but also considerably increasing the depth of incision through the parenchyma of the pancreas in the head of the gland because the duct goes more posteriorly. This area also has a rich blood supply, and some amount of hemorrhage may be encountered during this incision. Success rates are thought to depend on in great part on an adequate drainage into the head of the pancreas in this manner. There appears to be less significance to the extent of drainage into the tail of the pancreas except in patients who have more localized disease in the tail of the pancreas.

Once adequate space is established, a Seurat clamp may be utilized. All stones encountered should be removed from the duct; any secondary ductular stones should also be removed.

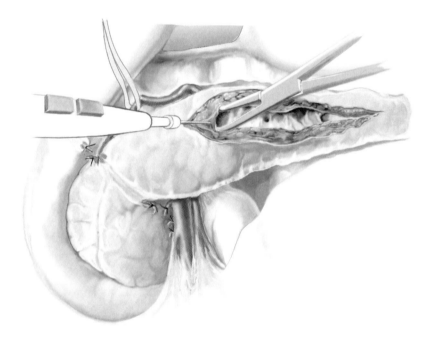

STEP 5

Roux-en-Y jejunal preparation

An area is chosen approximately 15 cm distal to the ligament of Treitz in a position which will facilitate easy performance of the jejunojejunostomy. The mesenteric attachments are divided between clamps to mobilize the Roux limb. A GIA stapling device is utilized to divide the jejunum at this site.

The avascular area is then chosen in the left transverse mesocolon. A window is created through which the distal divided end of jejunum may be brought. It is important to avoid undue tension at the mesentery; at times, it is necessary to divide the truncal branches of the jejunal mesenteric vessels below the arcade to permit a flexible limb. The divided end of jejunum is aligned toward the head of the pancreas, and a side-to-side approach is established.

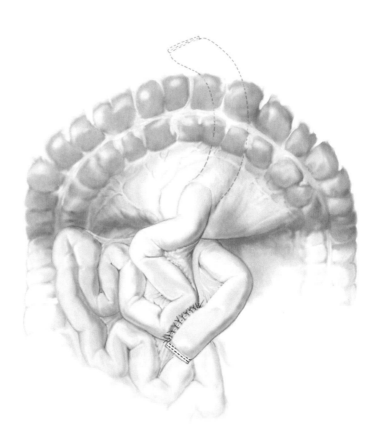

STEP 6   **Pancreaticojejunostomy**

The anastomosis is performed using a single layer of nonabsorbable suture. We use two, separate, 3-0 silk sutures. The posterior suture line is placed first before opening the jejunum (A-1.1). It is important to make smaller advances in the jejunum than is made in the open pancreatic duct. The first suture is placed just at the corner of the ductal incision in the tail of the pancreas and each suture is placed progressionally toward the head of the pancreas (A-1.2). The advance on the jejunum may be no more than 3 mm, whereas the advance on the pancreatic duct may be 6 mm. The depth of insertion of the needle into the pancreatic body into the duct depends upon the pancreas. In a relatively thin parenchyma, the sutures are placed into the duct itself. On occasion a very thick pancreatic parenchyma is better managed by placing sutures into the capsule of the pancreas, but they may be tied above the epithelium of the main pancreatic duct. Sutures are not tied until each suture has been placed over to the corner toward the head of the pancreas.

At this point, the limb of jejunum is lowered and placed in its position for anastomosis, and all sutures are tied.

An incision is then made in the jejunal limb to match the size of the pancreatic duct incision. The reason for placing the sutures more closely on the jejunum is the fact that once the jejunum is opened it typically dilates, and you may be left with a very poor match in sizes for your anterior suture line.

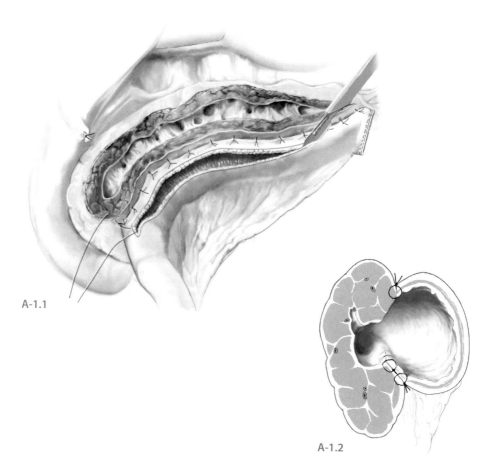

A-1.1

A-1.2

Pancreaticojejunostomy

The anterior suture line is performed by first burying the corner stitch from the posterior suture line by drawing that suture toward the pancreatic ductal incision and placing a Lembert suture in the jejunal limb at the very corner. A transition is made from the sutures being placed "outside-in" on the posterior suture line to "inside-out" on the anterior row. The sutures should be placed at both corners, and the suture from the corner on the posterior suture line may be cut. In contradistinction to the posterior suture line, each of the sutures are tied after being placed in the anterior suture line. This is particularly helpful to assure alignment and a proper size match for the anastomosis (A-2).

After the two corner sutures have been placed, a Lembert suture is placed in the jejunal limb halfway between the left and right borders of the pancreatic duct incision to establish alignment of the jejunal limb. Finally, halfway between this center suture and the two corners, another similar suture is placed in the jejunum and fixed to the incision on the superior border of the pancreatic ductal incision. After this, it is easy to complete the gaps between these sutures which have already been placed in order to complete the anastomosis with interrupted 3-0 silk suture.

The point where the jejunum passes through the transverse mesocolon should be fixed to the mesocolon using an interrupted 3-0 silk stitch; this obliterates the internal hernia defect.

Finally, 40 cm distal to the pancreaticojejunostomy, a jejunojejunostomy is performed in an end-to-side fashion. We prefer a hand-sewn anastomosis with an outer layer of interrupted 3-0 silk sutures and an inner suture line of continuous absorbable suture such as polyglycolic acid.

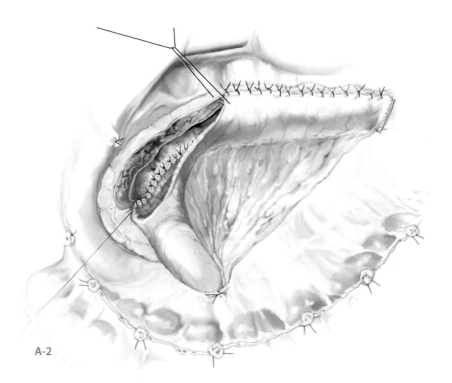

A-2

Postoperative Tests

- First 24h, monitor for hemorrhage
- Monitor serum glucose concentrations for possible glucose intolerance even in patients who had not required insulin preoperatively
- Reinforce the need for a progressive reduction in narcotic analgesic (this continues after discharge from hospital)
- Although the final outcome is determined only when the patient is free of narcotic use, pain scales may be of some value

Local Postoperative Complications

- Short term:
  - Intra-abdominal hemorrhage
  - Pancreatic ductal leak (persistent drain output)
  - Glucose intolerance resulting from the stress of operation
  - Alcohol withdrawal syndrome
  - Wound infection
- Long term:
  - Failure to resolve pain
  - Ongoing narcotic addition
  - Recurrent episodes of pancreatitis
  - Progressive loss of pancreatic function

Tricks of the Senior Surgeon

- It may be difficult to palpate the duct, and various maneuvers may help.
- Kocherize the duodenum and palpate carefully the head of the pancreas.
- Perform intraoperative ultrasonography.
- Choose an area in the mid body of the pancreas and perform a vertical incision in hope of bisecting the duct.
- Once some incision has been made in the parenchyma, the surgeon may safely massage the tail and proximal body of the pancreas in hope of expressing pancreatic juice.
- Avoid trying to access the pancreatic duct directly over the superior mesenteric vein/portal vein/splenic vein junction – too deep an incision may lead to serious bleeding.
- Concentrate on getting a good size match between the ductal incision and the jejunal incision; mismatches in size can lead to pancreatic leak.

Resection for Neoplasms of the Pancreas

Tina W.F. Yen, Douglas B. Evans (Proximal Resection),
Sergio Pedrazzoli, Claudio Pasquali, Cosimo Sperti (Central Resection),
Eric Nakakura, Mark Duncan, Frederick Eckhauser (Distal Pancreatectomy)

Introduction

With the increased experience of centers of expertise in pancreatic diseases, pancreatectomy for neoplasms has become routine, with acceptable morbidity and mortality. Improvements in imaging modalities and heightened awareness of less well-appreciated pancreatic neoplasms (non-functional neuroendocrine neoplasms, the spectrum of primary cystic neoplasms of the pancreas, and especially intraductal papillary mucinous neoplasms) has increased the visibility of formal pancreatectomy. The following sections address specific types of anatomic pancreatic resections.

Proximal Resection

Tina W.F. Yen, Douglas B. Evans

Introduction

Kausch was the first to describe a pancreatoduodenectomy, but Whipple, who described pancreaticoduodenectomy for pancreatic head adenocarcinoma in 1935 as a two-stage operation, has largely been given credit by the eponym. Waugh and Clagett modified the operation in 1946 to its current one-stage procedure. The operation involves the en bloc removal of the pancreatic head, duodenum, gallbladder, and bile duct, with the gastric antrum. Traverso and Longmire popularized the pylorus-preserving technique. The goal of the operation is complete removal of the neoplasm (R0 resection). There are no data to support debulking (R2 resection) in patients with adenocarcinoma of the pancreas. Therefore, the preoperative assessment of local tumor resectability is of critical importance.

Indications and Contraindications

General Principles

- We advocate objective, anatomic criteria for defining resectability based on high quality CT images.
- Local tumor resectability [relationship of the neoplasm to the celiac axis, superior mesenteric artery (SMA) and superior mesenteric-portal vein (SMPV) confluence] cannot be determined accurately at laparotomy before gastric and pancreatic transection; thus, preoperative assessment of critical tumor-vessel relationships is mandatory.

Indications

- Resectable neoplasms have the following CT characteristics:
  - Normal fat plane between the low-density tumor and the superior mesenteric artery and superior mesenteric vein (SMV)
  - Absence of extrapancreatic disease
  - Patent SMPV confluence (assumes ability of the surgeon to resect and reconstruct isolated segments of the SMV or SMPV)
  - No direct tumor extension to the celiac axis or SMA
- "Borderline" resectable neoplasms include:
  - Short segment occlusion of the SMPV confluence with an adequate vessel for grafting above and below the site of occlusion (assumes the technical ability to resect and reconstruct the SMV or SMPV)
  - Neoplasms which demonstrate short-segment (usually <1 cm) abutment of the common or proper hepatic artery or the SMA on high-quality CT

Absolute Contraindications

- Extrapancreatic metastatic disease

- Neoplasms encasing the celiac axis or SMA (anything more than short-segment abutment)

Preoperative Investigations and Preparation for the Procedure

Predisposing factors:	Tobacco, obesity, impaired glucose tolerance, smoking, family history (~10%), associated syndromes [familial pancreatitis, Peutz-Jeghers syndrome, familial atypical multiple-mole melanoma (FAMMM) syndrome, hereditary nonpolyposis colon cancer (HNPCC)]
Physical examination:	Jaundice, left supraclavicular adenopathy, ascites, nutritional status (weight loss), cardiovascular health, performance status (most important for assessment of operativel risk)
Laboratory tests:	CA 19–9, CEA, liver function tests, coagulation profile, complete blood count
Chest X-ray:	To rule out metastatic disease
Multislice or multidetector abdominal CT:	To assess resectability; relationship of the tumor to the right lateral wall of the SMA is the most critical aspect of the staging evaluation
Endoscopic ultrasound scan (EUS):	Indicated if a low-attenuation pancreatic head mass is not visualized on CT
EUS-guided fine needle aspiration (FNA):	Needed to establish a tissue diagnosis which is necessary in patients being considered for protocol-based, preoperative systemic therapy and/or chemoradiation; if no neoadjuvant therapy is indicated, a preoperative biopsy only delays exploration
ERCP:	To allow endobiliary decompression when operative intervention is delayed (poor performance status, need for further investigation of medical co-morbidities, or for neoadjuvant therapy).

Mechanical bowel preparation

Prophylactic IV antibiotics prior to operation

Procedure: Pancreatoduodenectomy

| STEP 1 | Isolation of the infrapancreatic SMV |

We use a bilateral subcostal or midline incision, usually performing laparoscopy prior to laparotomy under the same anesthetic. Exposure is optimal with a Thompson retractor or another self-retaining retractor. When opening the abdomen, preserve the falciform ligament for later coverage of the stump of the gastroduodenal artery (GDA) prior to abdominal closure.

Evaluation for extrapancreatic metastatic disease:

- Biopsy-proven liver or peritoneal metastases are a contraindication to pancreatoduodenectomy
- Intraoperative ultrasonography of the liver is used selectively in patients whose CT is indeterminate
- Lymph node biopsy for frozen-section analysis remains controversial. In a good-risk patient with localized, resectable pancreatic cancer, lymph node metastases are not an absolute contraindication to pancreatoduodenectomy when performed as part of a multimodality approach to pancreatic cancer with an oncologic-type node dissection, not just "berry picking." In a high-risk patient (medical comorbidities or oncologic concerns), a grossly positive regional lymph node is a contraindication to pancreatoduodenectomy.

First, enter the lesser sac by elevating the greater omentum off the transverse colon.

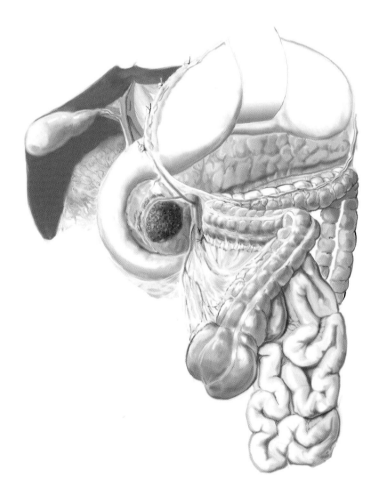

STEP 1 (continued)

Isolation of the infrapancreatic SMV

- Mobilize the right colon and hepatic flexure to expose the entire duodenal sweep. This step mobilizes the root of the small bowel mesentery by incising the visceral peritoneum to the ligament of Treitz.
- Incise the retroperitoneal peritoneum along the inferior border of the pancreas from the patient's left of the middle colic vessels toward the patient's right to expose the junction of the middle colic vein and the SMV.
- Divide the middle colic vein prior to its junction with the SMV to allow greater exposure of the infrapancreatic SMV; this minimizes the risk of traction injury to the SMV.
- We do *not* attempt to develop a plane of dissection between the anterior surface of the SMV and the posterior surface of the pancreatic neck as the pancreatic head neoplasms involve the posterolateral aspect of the SMV or SMPV confluence *not* the anterior surface of these vessels. We rarely divide the gastroepiploic vein at this time (unless it is coming off of a common trunk with the middle colic vein); this vessel is much easier to divide after the pancreatic transection.

STEP 2

Extended Kocher maneuver

Begin the Kocher maneuver at the transverse portion of the duodenum by dissecting the inferior vena cava (IVC).

Elevate all fibrofatty and lymphatic tissue medial to the right ureter and anterior to the IVC with the specimen (we usually preserve the gonadal vein as it courses anterior to the right ureter because it is a good landmark to avoid inadvertent injury to the right ureter).

Fully mobilize the pancreatic head and duodenum to the cephalad aspect of the left renal vein as it crosses the aorta. The SMA origin can often be exposed at this level by medially rotating the pancreatic head and duodenum and incising the perineural tissue lateral to the first 2 cm of the SMA origin.

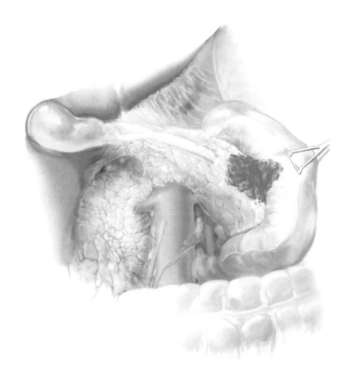

| STEP 3 | Dissection of the porta hepatis |

Expose the common hepatic artery (CHA) by removing the lymph node that lies directly anterior to the CHA proximal to the right gastric artery and the GDA; the portal vein (PV) lies posterior to the inferior border of the CHA just proximal to the GDA origin.

Ligate and divide the right gastric artery and the GDA. If the tumor extends to within a few millimeters of the GDA origin, do not attempt bluntly to dissect the origin of the GDA; instead, obtain proximal control of the CHA and distal control of the proper hepatic artery and then divide the GDA flush at its origin. The hepatic artery is fragile; aggressive blunt dissection may create an intimal flap. We close the arteriotomy at the GDA origin with 6-0 polypropylene suture often with a small vascular pledget.

Perform cholecystectomy and transect the common hepatic duct (CHD) at its junction with the cystic duct, thereby exposing the underlying PV. Careful palpation prior to division of the bile duct should alert one to the possibility of a replaced right hepatic artery coming off the SMA traveling posterior to the lateral aspect of the bile duct. Note: if the foramen of Winslow was closed due to adhesions, it should have been reestablished at the time of the Kocher maneuver. Access to the foramen of Winslow is necessary to palpate the porta hepatis and appreciate a replaced right hepatic artery.

When possible, place a gentle bulldog clamp on the transected CHD to prevent bile spillage until the bile duct reconstruction.

Divide the loose connective tissue anterior to the PV caudally to the junction of the PV and the neck of the pancreas. The PV should not be extensively mobilized at this point, as iatrogenic injury to the PV prior to gastric and pancreatic transection results in excessive blood loss due to inadequate vascular exposure.

Be aware of anomalous hepatic arterial circulation. Rarely, the hepatic artery (distal to the origin of the GDA) courses posterior to the PV. An accessory or replaced right hepatic artery may also course posterolateral to the PV but would arise from the proximal SMA, not the celiac axis. The right hepatic artery should be preserved. The entire common hepatic artery may also arise from the SMA.

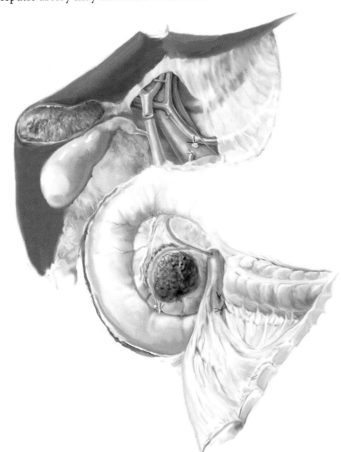

STEP 4

Transection of the gastric antrum (or the duodenum if pylorus preservation is planned)

Ligate and divide the terminal branches of the left gastric artery along the lesser curvature of the stomach prior to gastric transection.

Transect the antrum of the stomach with a linear cutting stapler at the third or fourth transverse vein on the lesser curvature and at the confluence of the gastroepiploic veins on the greater curvature (A-1).

Divide the omentum at the site of transection of the greater curvature transection.

Pylorus preservation may be considered in patients with small periampullary neoplasms. It should not be performed in patients with bulky neoplasms of the pancreatic head, neoplasms involving the first or second portions of the duodenum, or lesions associated with grossly positive pyloric or peripyloric lymph nodes (A-2).

Divide the gastroepiploic arcade and the duodenum at least 3 cm beyond the pylorus whenever possible. However, at the time of reconstruction, we trim another 1.0–1.5 cm off of the duodenum to create the duodenojejunostomy 1.0–1.5 cm from the pylorus to ensure an adequate blood supply to the duodenum.

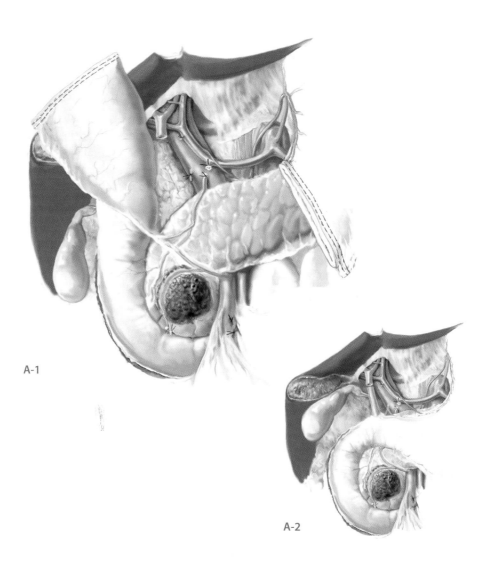

A-1

A-2

| STEP 5 | Transection of the jejunum |

Take down the loose attachments of the ligament of Treitz with care to avoid the inferior mesenteric vein

Transect the jejunum with a linear cutting stapler about 10 cm distal to the ligament of Treitz, and ligate and divide the mesentery (A-1). We prefer to tie the vessels on the mesenteric side (staying side) and use the harmonic scalpel on the serosal (jejunal/duodenal) side.

Continue this dissection to involve the fourth and third portions of the duodenum.

Reflect the devascularized duodenum and jejunum beneath the mesenteric vessels (A-2).

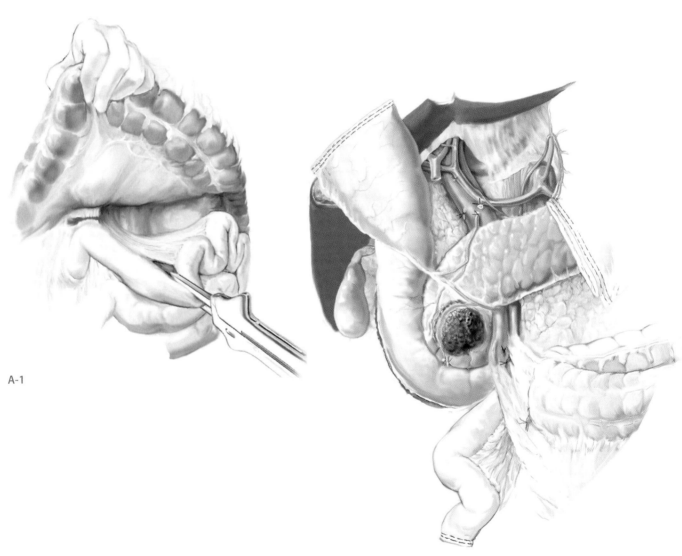

A-1

A-2

STEP 6   **Transection of the pancreas and completion of the retroperitoneal dissection**

The most important and difficult part of the operation involves complete mobilization
of the SMPV confluence and separation of the specimen from the right lateral border
of the SMA.

Place traction sutures on the superior and inferior borders of the neck of the
pancreas. This is important along the inferior border of the pancreas, where a small
artery will be found in most patients.

Transect the pancreas with electrocautery down to the anterior surface of the SMPV
confluence.

If there is evidence of tumor adherence to the PV or SMV, the pancreas can be
divided at a more distal location (along the left or medial border of the SMPV confluence) in preparation for segmental venous resection.

Reflect the specimen to the patient's right and separate it from the PV and SMV by
ligation and division of the small venous tributaries to the uncinate process and pancreatic head. Note: The relationship of the tumor to the lateral and posterior walls of the
SMPV confluence can be directly inspected only after gastric and pancreatic transection.
This relationship cannot be accurately assessed intraoperatively by simply developing a
plane of dissection between the anterior surface of the SMPV confluence and the posterior aspect of the neck of the pancreas (which is why this age-old maneuver is no longer
performed earlier in the operation).

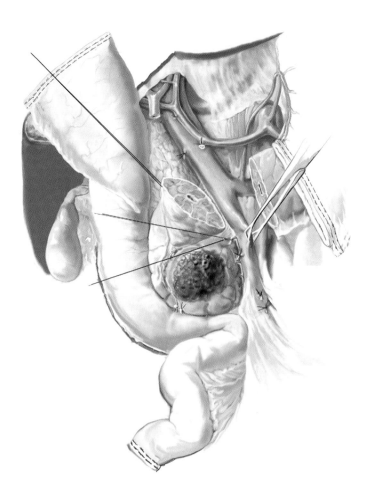

STEP 7   **Removal of uncinate process**

Complete removal of the uncinate process from the SMV and its first jejunal branch (which courses posterior to the SMA) is required for mobilization of the SMPV confluence and identification of the SMA. The first jejunal branch of the SMV, which originates from the right posterolateral aspect of the SMV (at the level of the uncinate process), travels posterior to the SMA, and enters the medial (proximal) aspect of the jejunal mesentery, giving off one or two branches directly to the uncinate process that need to be divided. If tumor involvement of the SMV here prevents dissection of the uncinate process from the SMV, the first jejunal branch can be divided (in which case we expose the SMA medial to the SMV). Injury to the SMV at the level of the first jejunal branch, or a tangential laceration in the first jejunal branch (as it courses posterior to the SMA), is hard to control and represents the most frequent cause of iatrogenic SMA injury as one attempts to suture a venous injury prior to exposure of the SMA.

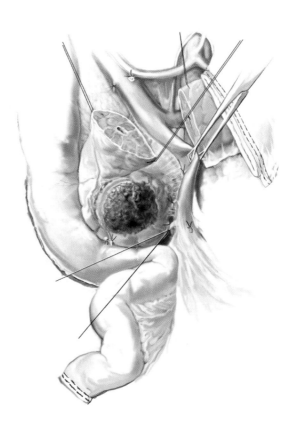

| STEP 8 | **Freeing of right side of SMV** |

Medial retraction of the SMPV confluence allows identification of the SMA lateral to the SMPV confluence and facilitates dissection of the pancreatic head and soft tissues off of the right lateral wall of the proximal SMA. Failure to fully mobilize the SMPV confluence and expose the SMA usually results in a positive resection margin due to incomplete removal of the uncinate process and the mesenteric soft tissue adjacent to the SMA.

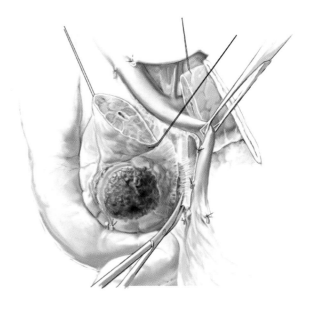

| STEP 9 | **Ligation of inferior pancreatoduodenal artery** |

In addition, incomplete mobilization of the SMPV confluence can result in iatrogenic injury to the SMA due to poor exposure. Failure to individually dissect and ligate the inferior pancreaticoduodenal artery is the major cause of postoperative retroperitoneal hemorrhage as these vessels may retract (if ligated with a large amount of mesenteric soft tissue) and bleed in the postoperative period.

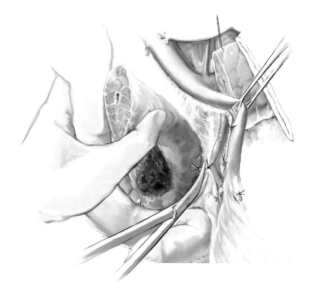

STEP 10   **Retroperitoneal margin**

Properly orient the specimen to enable accurate assessment of the retroperitoneal margin and other standard pathologic variables. The soft tissue adjacent to the proximal 3–4 cm of the SMA represents the retroperitoneal margin and is inked by the pathologist for permanent-section evaluation. A grossly positive retroperitoneal margin should not occur if high-quality preoperative imaging is performed. A microscopically positive retroperitoneal margin will occur in 10–20 % of resections (R1 resection).

Perform frozen section analysis of pancreatic and CHD transection margins.

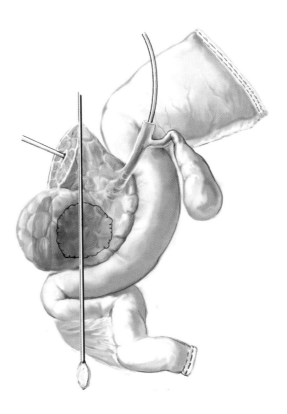

STEP 11   **Vascular reconstruction**

Steps 1 through 5 of the pancreatoduodenectomy are completed as described above.
Tumor adherence to the lateral wall of the SMPV confluence prevents dissection of the
SMV and PV off the pancreatic head and uncinate process, thereby inhibiting medial
retraction of the SMPV confluence (and lateral retraction of the specimen). The standard technique for segmental venous resection involves transection of the splenic vein.
Division of the splenic vein allows complete exposure of the SMA medial to the SMV
and provides increased SMV and PV length (as they are no longer tethered by the
splenic vein) for a primary venous anastomosis. The retroperitoneal dissection is
completed by sharply dividing the soft tissues anterior to the aorta and to the right of
the exposed SMA; the specimen is then attached only by the SMPV confluence. Vascular
clamps are placed 2–3 cm proximal (on the PV) and distal (on the SMV) to the involved
venous segment, and the vein is transected, allowing tumor removal (A-1). A generous
2- to 3-cm segment of SMPV confluence can be resected without need for interposition
grafting if the splenic vein is divided. Venous resection is always performed with inflow
occlusion of the SMA to prevent small bowel edema (which makes pancreatic and biliary
reconstruction more difficult). Systemic heparinization is usually employed prior to
occluding the SMA. The free ends of the vein are reapproximated using interrupted
sutures of 6-0 polypropylene (A-2).

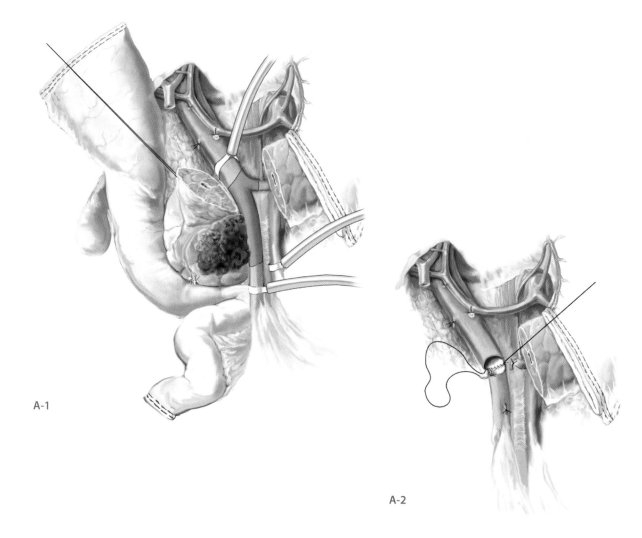

A-1

A-2

STEP 12   **SMV reconstruction**

When tumor involvement is limited to the SMV, we preserve the splenic vein-PV junction. Splenic vein preservation is possible only when tumor invasion of the SMV or PV does not involve the splenic vein confluence. Preservation of the splenic vein-SMV-PV confluence significantly limits the mobility of the PV and prevents primary anastomosis of the SMV (after segmental SMV resection) unless segmental resection is limited to less than 2 cm (A-1). Therefore, in most patients who undergo SMV resection with splenic vein preservation, an interposition graft using the internal jugular vein is necessary. Preservation of the splenic vein adds significant complexity to venous resection because it prevents direct access to the most proximal 3–4 cm of the SMA (medial to the SMV). Venous resection and reconstruction can be performed either before the specimen has been separated from the right lateral wall of the SMA or after complete mesenteric dissection by separating the specimen first from the SMA (A-2). Both techniques require significant experience with pancreatoduodenectomy.

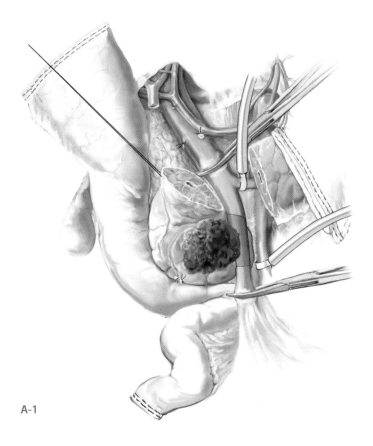

A-1

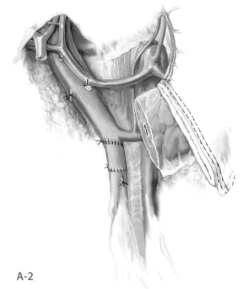

A-2

STEP 13   **Pancreatic reconstruction**

The pancreatic remnant is mobilized from the retroperitoneum and splenic vein for a distance of 2–3 cm to allow suture placement for the pancreaticojejunal anastomosis.

We bring the transected jejunum retrocolic through a generous defect in the transverse mesocolon to the left of the middle colic vessels.

We prefer a two-layer, end-to-side pancreaticojejunostomy with a small stent when the pancreatic duct is not dilated. The outer row consists of interrupted 4-0 seromuscular monofilament sutures. The inner row consists of 4-0 or 5-0 interrupted monofilament sutures approximating full-thickness pancreatic duct to full-thickness jejunum. Posterior knots are tied on the inside, while the lateral and anterior knots are tied on the outside. If a stent is used, prior to securing the anterior sutures, the stent is placed across the anastomosis so that it extends into the pancreatic duct and small bowel for a distance of approximately 2 cm, respectively.

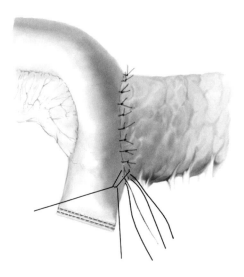

STEP 14	Biliary reconstruction

Distal to the pancreaticojejunostomy, we create a one-layer, end-to-side hepaticojejunostomy with 4-0 absorbable monofilament sutures (this anastomosis is not stented even when the CHD is of normal size).

Align the jejunum with the bile duct to avoid tension on the pancreatic and biliary anastomoses.

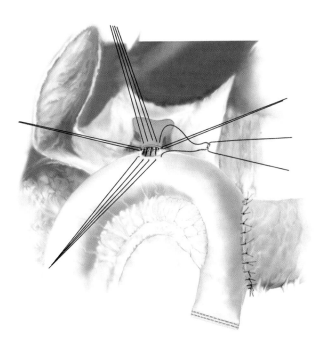

STEP 15   **Gastric or duodenal reconstruction**

The gastrojejunostomy is placed antecolic and is hand-sewn in two layers (**A**).
When the pylorus is preserved, the duodenojejunostomy is created in an end-to-side
fashion with a single layer, hand-sewn technique using monofilament absorbable sutures
(**B**). The distance between the biliary and gastric/duodenal anastomoses is 50 cm to
prevent reflux of gastric content.

A 10-Fr. feeding jejunostomy tube for postoperative enteral feeding is placed distal
to the gastrojejunostomy using the Witzel technique.

The falciform ligament is placed between the CHA and the afferent jejunal limb
to cover the stump of the GDA. This strategy may help to prevent pseudoaneurysm
formation at the GDA stump in the event of a pancreatic anastomotic leak and resulting
abscess formation.

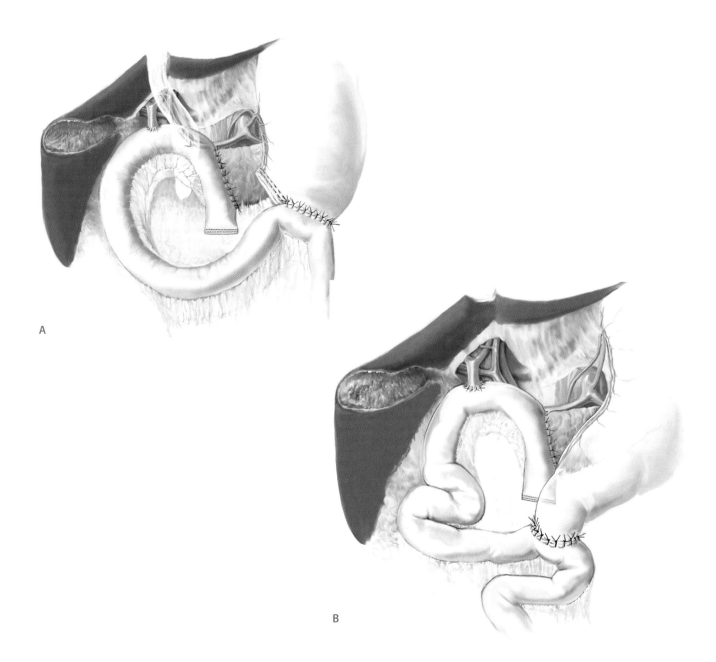

A

B

Postoperative Tests

- Hgb, WBC, platelet count
- Electrolytes/creatinine
- Serum amylase activity
- Amylase activity in drain fluid
- Total serum bilirubin
- CT for fever, leukocytosis, or sepsis – most likely cause is a leak at the pancreato-jejunostomy

Local Complications

- Short term:
  - Intra-abdominal abscess/pancreatic anastomotic leak
    - Fever, leukocytosis, ileus, abdominal distention, usually after postoperative days 4–5
    - Abdomen/pelvic CT
    - CT-guided aspiration and percutaneous catheter drainage if an infected fluid collection develops
  - GDA-enteric fistula
    - Gastrointestinal or drain tract bleeding rare before postoperative day 10
    - Usually due to pancreatic anastomotic leak with surrounding infection and inflammation resulting in GDA stump blowout
    - Treatment of choice is angiography with hepatic artery stenting or embolization, not operative exploration unless as a last resort
  - Delayed gastric emptying
    - Jejunostomy tube placement allows use of enteral feeding which prevents the need for intravenous alimentation if poor gastric emptying occurs
- Long term:
  - Recurrent pancreatic cancer – local in bed of pancreas; distal in liver, lungs or peritoneum
  - Development of pancreatic exocrine insufficiency (~40%) or endocrine insufficiency (~20%)
  - Pancreatic anastomotic stricture with recurrent pancreatitis or pancreatic pain
  - Small intestinal obstruction

Tricks of the Senior Surgeon

- Assess resectability preoperatively; the relationship between the tumor and the SMV/SMA is difficult and usually impossible to assess accurately before gastric and pancreatic transection.

- Do not attempt blunt dissection of the GDA origin as an intimal dissection may result in occlusion of the hepatic artery. When the tumor extends close to the origin of the GDA, obtain proximal and distal control of the hepatic artery and sharply divide the GDA at its origin; the resulting arteriotomy can be closed with 6-0 polypropylene with or without a vascular pledget.

- Always fully mobilize the SMPV confluence and expose the SMA. The SMA will not be injured if it is in direct vision.

- Bring the jejunum retrocolic and not retroperitoneal (in the bed of the resected duodenum) for pancreatic and biliary reconstruction. The incision in the transverse mesocolon should be to the patient's left of the middle colic artery.

Central Resection

Sergio Pedrazzoli, Claudio Pasquali, Cosimo Sperti

Introduction

In 1959, Letton and Wilson reported the first non-resective treatment of traumatic rupture of the neck of the pancreas. The right stump of the pancreatic head was over-sewn, and a Roux-en-Y loop of jejunum was anastomosed to the left body/tail of the pancreas. In 1984, Dagradi and Serio reported the first central pancreatectomy for an insulinoma, and in 1988, Fagniez, Kracht, and Rotman reported two central pancreatectomies performed for an insulinoma and a serous cystadenoma. At least 150 central pancreatectomies have been reported so far without mortality. Central pancreatectomy involves anatomic removal of benign or borderline lesions of the neck and/or proximal body of the pancreas together with 1 cm of normal tissue on both sides. The goal is to preserve at least 5 cm of the normal pancreatic tissue of the body/tail of the pancreas that would otherwise be removed with a complete left pancreatectomy.

Indications and Contraindications

Indications	■ Small, centrally located lesions (<5 cm in diameter) not amenable to enucleation
	■ Traumatic transection of the neck of the pancreas
	■ Benign, borderline, or low grade malignant lesions (selected neuroendocrine neoplasms, serous or mucinous cysticneoplasms, solid pseudopapillary neoplasms, branch type intraductal papillary mucinous neoplasms, solitary true cysts, parasitic cysts, etc.)
	■ Maintenance of a distal pancreatic stump of at least 5 cm in length
Contraindications	■ Malignant pancreatic lesions
	■ Involvement of the pancreas by contiguous malignant neoplasms
	■ Insulin-dependent diabetes
Relative Contraindications	■ Advanced age (>70 years)
	■ High-risk patient
	■ Non-insulin-dependent diabetes (NIDD)

Preoperative Investigations and Preparation for the Procedure

History:	Endocrine syndrome (hypoglycemia, acute pancreatitis, upper abdominal pain)
Clinical evaluation:	Exclude diarrhea secondary to exocrine insufficiency, diabetes, and signs of portal hypertension
Laboratory tests:	Amylase, lipase, and/or peptide hormones (insulin, gastrin, glucagon, vasoactive intestinal polypeptide, pancreatic polypeptide, somatostatin, chromogranin A), tumor markers (CA 19–9, CEA, MCA, etc.). If an endocrine neoplasm is suspected, store a preoperative sample of serum and/or plasma for specific assays based on histologic and immuno-histochemical characterization of the resected lesion
Imaging:	Differential diagnosis and assessment of resectability based on ultrasonography, computed tomography, magnetic resonance imaging, or endoscopic ultrasonography
	– 111In-pentetreotide scintigraphy (OctreoScan): endocrine neoplasms
	– Positron emission tomography (PET): differentiates between benign and malignant lesions
Preoperative preparation:	– Somatostatin analogues: no specific study on central pancreatectomy
	– Perioperative antibiotics: as for any clean-contaminated operation

Procedure: Central Pancreatectomy

STEP 1   **Exposure of central part of pancreas**

Optimal access is via a midline incision

The pancreas is exposed by detaching the greater omentum from the transverse colon and freeing the superior aspect of the middle colic vessels until the anterior aspect of the pancreas is exposed completely; stomach is retracted rostrally.

The superior mesenteric vein is identified, and its anterior surface cleared below the neck of the pancreas; care must be taken not to injure venous tributaries; occasionally a middle colic branch of the superior mesenteric vein requires division, especially if it joins in a V-shaped way with the right gastroepiploic vein. Gastroepiploic vessels are preserved, unless the lesion reaches the right border of the superior mesenteric-portal vein (A-1).

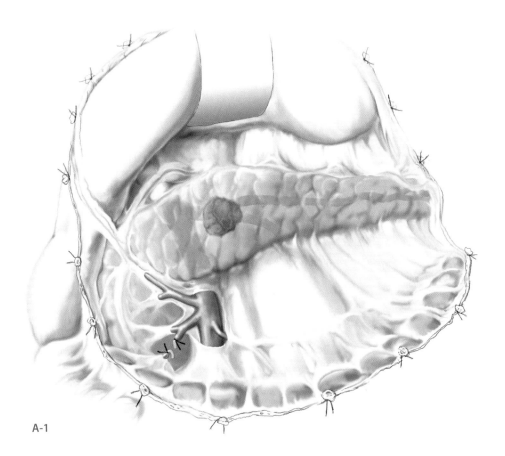

A-1

Exposure of central part of pancreas

Evaluate the extent of the lesion by intraoperative ultrasonography (IOUS); this technique is particularly useful for small, deeply located lesions. Mark with electrocautery the exact extent of the planned central pancreatectomy including 1 cm of normal pancreatic tissue on both sides (A-2).

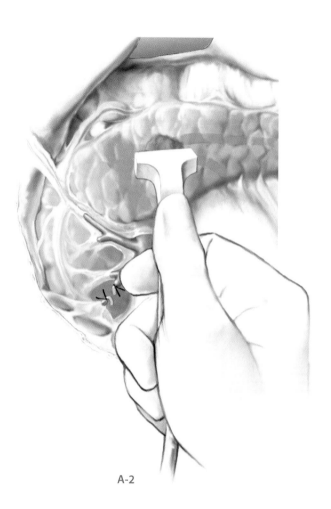

A-2

STEP 2   **Mobilizing pancreas to be resected**

The posterior peritoneum is incised with electrocautery along the inferior border of the part of the pancreas to be removed until the splenic vein is visualized. Attention should be paid to ligate and divide an often present, small artery and vein that lies between the left side of the superior mesenteric vein and the inferior border of the pancreas (A-1).

Lymph node(s) anterior to the common hepatic artery are removed, and the common hepatic artery is detached from the superior border of the pancreas extending from the celiac axis to the gastroduodenal artery.

The hepatic artery is retracted rostrally (A-2).

When the tumor extends to the left of the origin of splenic artery, the splenic artery should first be mobilized and retracted rostrally, taking care to divide the dorsal artery.

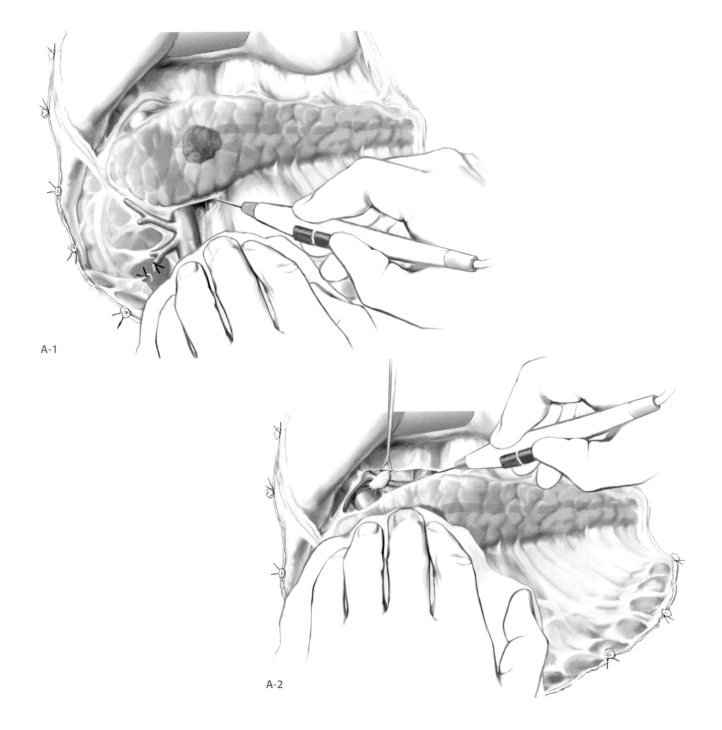

A-1

A-2

STEP 3   **Mobilization of superior mesenteric and splenic vein**

The plane between the superior mesenteric/portal vein and the neck of pancreas is gently teased apart; usually no veins transgress this space. In the rare event of a pancreatic vein joining the anterior surface of the portal vein, the pancreas can be transected progressively from below, until the vein is exposed allowing division of the vein between ties.

The pancreas is encircled with a tape and retracted anterorostrally, allowing visualization and ligation of the veins from the posterior pancreas (to be resected) entering the splenic vein (A-1).

The splenic vein is then separated carefully from the pancreas to be resected.

Transection of the proximal pancreas (right side) begins 1 cm proximal to the lesion; anterior retraction of the left pancreas may allow better visualization and ligation of the veins from the posterior pancreas to the splenic vein (A-2).

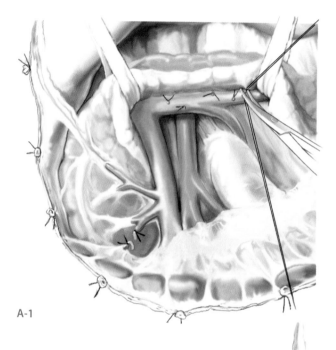

A-1

A-2

STEP 4	Removal of central pancreas

Transection of pancreas: Stay sutures are placed on the superior and inferior pancreatic margins just to the right and left of the proximal and distal lines of division to occlude the superior and inferior pancreatic vessels running transversely in the parenchyma.

The pancreas is divided by scalpel using a V-shaped incision on the right side of the tumor to facilitate closure in a fish-mouth fashion; the pancreas is transected 1 cm to the left of the tumor with suture ligation of the larger arterial bleeders in the cut edge (A-1).

The pancreatic duct in the right side of the remnant gland is suture-ligated with 5-0 non-absorbable monofilament, and the pancreatic tissue closed in a fish-mouth fashion with interrupted 3-0 synthetic absorbable sutures (A-2).

A very thin neck of pancreas can also be closed with a stapler and bleeding from small arteries controlled with absorbable synthetic stitches; the pancreatic duct is still identified and suture-ligated individually with 5-0 non-absorbable monofilament (A-3).

The right-sided limit of a central pancreatectomy is the left side of the gastroduodenal artery; transecting the pancreas to the right of the gastroduodenal artery can injure the common bile duct.

The specimen is sent to the pathologist for frozen section examination and for checking the right and left resection margins. A stitch on one margin will orient the specimen for the pathologist.

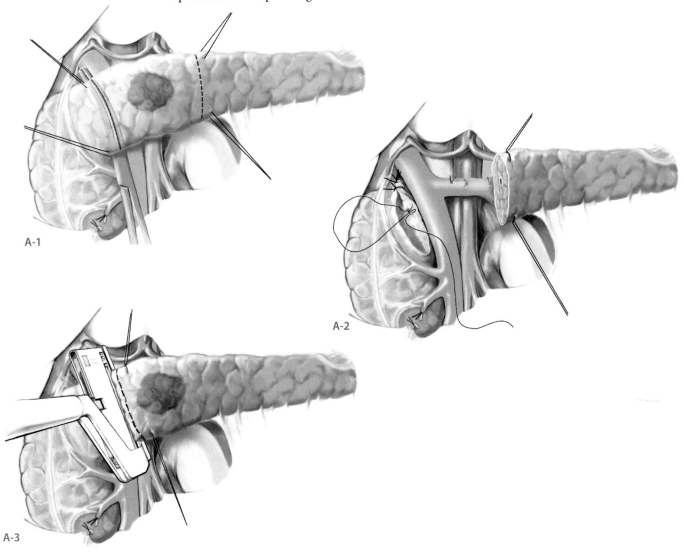

A-1

A-2

A-3

STEP 5 **Invagination/dunking pancreatojejunostomy**

The left pancreatic stump is mobilized distally for 2.5–3 cm; the first layer of interrupted 3-0 absorbable monofilament is placed between the jejunum and posterior aspect of the pancreatic stump 2 cm from the transected edge; the second layer of continuous 3-0 absorbable monofilament approximates the cut end of the jejunum and the transected edge of the pancreatic stump (A-1).

An anterior layer of interrupted 3-0 absorbable monofilament is applied between the seromuscular layer of the jejunum and the pancreatic capsule 2 cm from the pancreatic border. By means of this layer, the first 2 cm of the pancreatic stump progressively invaginates into the jejunum (A-2).

When a difficult invagination is expected due to a large, fat pancreatic stump, one trick to complete the procedure safely involves excising the muscular layer of the last 2 cm of jejunum (A-3).

Invagination as described above leaves an inner cylinder only of mucosa and a full thickness external cylinder (A-4).

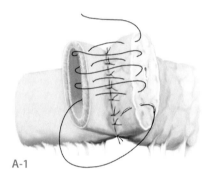

A-1

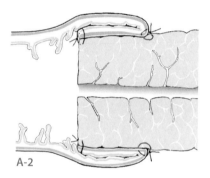

A-2

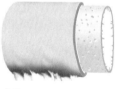

A-3

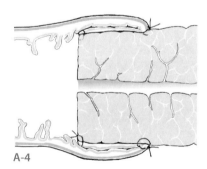

A-4

| STEP 6 | Alternative: duct-to-mucosal pancreaticojejunostomy |

The left pancreatic stump is not mobilized beyond the stay sutures; the end of jejunum is stapled and oversewn.

A small opening calibrated to the diameter of the pancreatic duct is made in the jejunum on the antimesenteric border 3–4 cm from the stapled end; the mucosa is everted and fixed to the seromuscular layer with 6-0 absorbable monofilament (A-1).

A mucosa-to-mucosa anastomosis is performed with 5-0 or 6-0 double-armed monofilament absorbable sutures knotted outside the lumen; magnification aids this procedure greatly.

Anterior (A-2) and posterior (A-3) layers of interrupted 3-0 absorbable monofilament approximate the jejunum and the anterior and posterior aspects of the pancreatic stump.

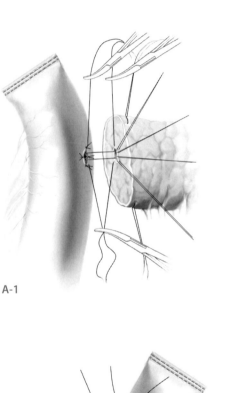

A-1

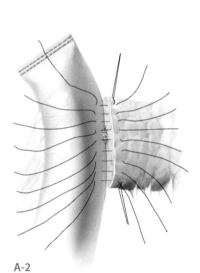

A-2

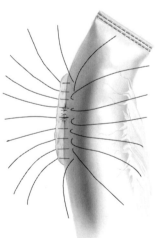

A-3

Postoperative Care and Tests

- Postoperative surveillance in an intensive care unit
- Serum amylase and/or lipase activity
- Check for amylase and lipase activity in drain fluids

Local Postoperative Complications

- Short term:
  - Anastomotic disruption
  - Pancreatic fistula
  - Peripancreatic abscess
  - Intra-abdominal bleeding
  - Acute pancreatitis
  - Subdiaphragmatic abscess
  - Splenic-portal vein thrombosis
  - Pleural effusion
- Long term:
  - Pancreatic pseudocyst
  - Pancreatic ascites
  - Pancreatitis
  - Diabetes

Tricks of the Senior Surgeon

- If the approach to the superior mesenteric portal trunk is difficult, Kocherization of the head of the pancreas is advisable; control of bleeding will be easier.
- If the superior mesenteric/portal trunk or one of its branches is injured, do not panic and use instruments blindly! Compress the venous trunk between the fingers inserted posteriorly (after the Kocher maneuver) behind the head of the pancreas and the thumb on the anterior aspect of the pancreas; suture the tear with 5-0 polypropylene.
- If the pancreas is too large for an invagination/dunking pancreatojejunostomy, choose either a duct-to-mucosal anastomosis or a pancreaticogastrostomy. Closure of the left pancreatic stump is followed by gland fibrosis that compromises endocrine secretion, nullifying the long term benefits of the central resection.

Distal Pancreatectomy

Eric Nakakura, Mark Duncan, Frederick Eckhauser

Introduction

Unlike cancer of the head of the pancreas, ductal adenocarcinoma of the pancreas is less often resectable because of the delay in symptoms and diagnosis. However, when feasible, the survival after R0 resection of a distal ductal cancer is similar to that of proximal resections. With the improvements in imaging as well as screening of more high-risk populations, the number of distal pancreatectomies for malignancy appears to be increasing. Moreover, cystic neoplasms of the pancreas and non-functional neuroendocrine neoplasms also occur in the body/tail of the pancreas and are more commonly "resectable."

Indications and Contraindications

Indications
- Ductal adenocarcinoma of the body and tail of pancreas

Contraindications
- Major visceral vessel encasement (celiac axis, proximal splenic or hepatic artery), widespread local metastatic disease, or distant metastases [liver, peritoneum, distal nodes (celiac, superior, mesenteric or para-aortic)]
- Local extension to spleen, stomach, colon, or left kidney is not always a contra-indication

Preoperative Investigation and Preparation for the Procedure

History:	Weight loss, abdominal or back pain, pancreatitis, new onset diabetes mellitus, family history of pancreatic cancer
Clinical evaluation:	Jaundice, nutritional status, ascites, palpable left supraclavicular node, signs of sinistral portal hypertension (splenomegaly, gastric varices)
Laboratory tests:	Tumor markers (i.e., CA19–9, CEA), liver function tests
ERCP, EUS, CT:	Assessment of resectability (no distant metastases, no major visceral vessel encasement), staging extent of tumor
Other considerations:	Preoperative vaccination against pneumococcus, meningococcus, and *Haemophilus influenzae*; staging laparoscopy (before vs at time of proposed resection)

Procedure: Distal Pancreatectomy

Access: An upper midline or left subcostal incision is best, depending on the angle of the costal margin.

STEP 1

The exposure and exploration are aided markedly by installation of a fixed blade retractor.

A careful, systematic exploration of the abdomen is performed to detect distant metastases (peritoneum, liver, distant nodal basins).

The lesser sac is entered through the gastrocolic ligament to expose the entire ventral surface of the pancreas from the gastroduodenal artery medially to the splenic hilum laterally.

The splenic flexure of the colon is mobilized inferiorly; cephalad retraction of the stomach and caudad retraction of transverse colon exposes the pancreatic bed.

Vessels along the greater curvature of the stomach, including the vasa brevia, are ligated with fine silk ties and divided.

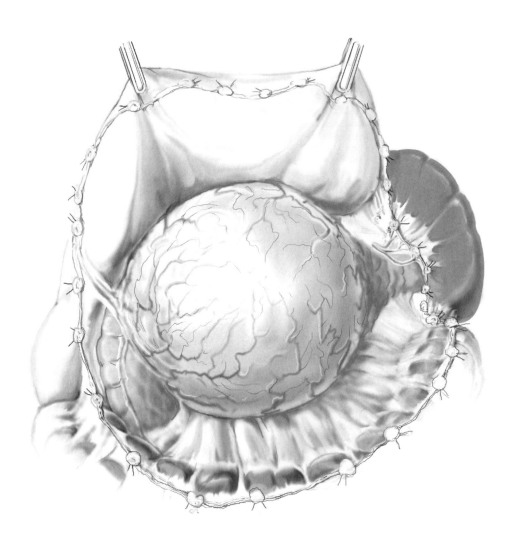

STEP 2

Deliver the pancreas and spleen from the retroperitoneum
(see also chapter "Distal Pancreatectomy")

The peritoneum along the inferior border of the pancreas is incised sharply or with electrocautery, maintaining a margin between the edge of the tumor mass.

The spleen is then mobilized laterally and posteriorly by dividing its peritoneal attachments.

The splenocolic ligament is next divided carefully to prevent injuring the splenic flexure of the colon. A thorough bimanual palpation of the pancreas is performed to assess mobility of the mass and the tumor stage.

If the tumor is adherent to the stomach, diaphragm, mesocolon/colon, retroperitoneum, adrenal gland or kidney, an en bloc resection is advised.

The spleen and pancreas are mobilized anteromedially from the retroperitoneum using either blunt or sharp dissection depending on tumor extension.

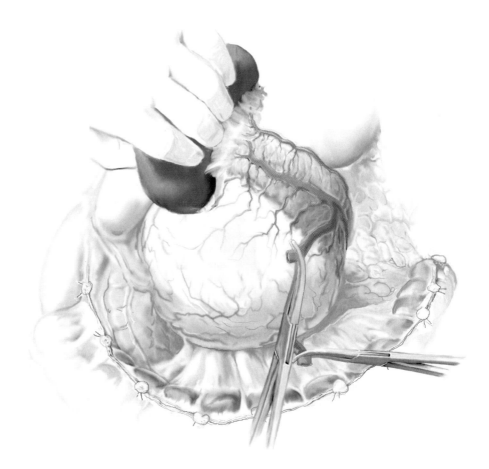

STEP 3   **Isolate and secure the splenic vasculature**

The splenic artery is identified and suture ligated as it passes along the posterosuperior border of the body and tail of the pancreas.

The splenic vein is generally identified inferior and posterior to the splenic artery, where it is ligated and divided; if the inferior mesenteric vein joins the splenic vein near the confluence of the splenic and superior mesenteric veins, it may be preserved – otherwise, it can be ligated with impunity.

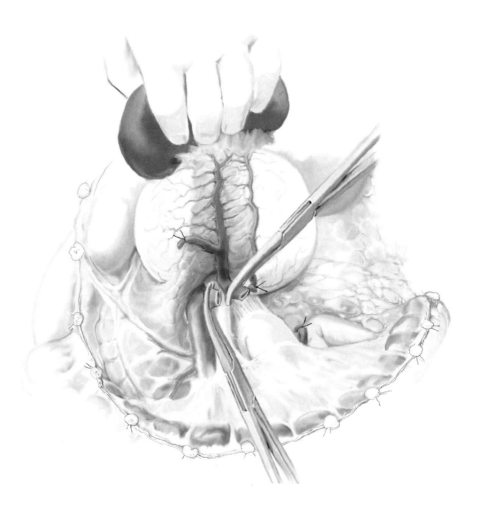

STEP 4

Divide the pancreas (A-1, A-2)

Stay sutures are placed through the superior and inferior margins of the pancreas on both sides of the transection margin to provide hemostasis and traction.

The pancreas is divided sharply to minimize the effects of cautery artifact on the frozen section of the proximal margin, which is imperative to check for tumor involvement.

Alternatively, the pancreas can be divided using a linear stapler at the margin of the pancreatic remnant provided the pancreas is not too thick (≥1 cm).

The resected specimen of the distal pancreas and spleen is sent for frozen section evaluation of the proximal pancreatic margin.

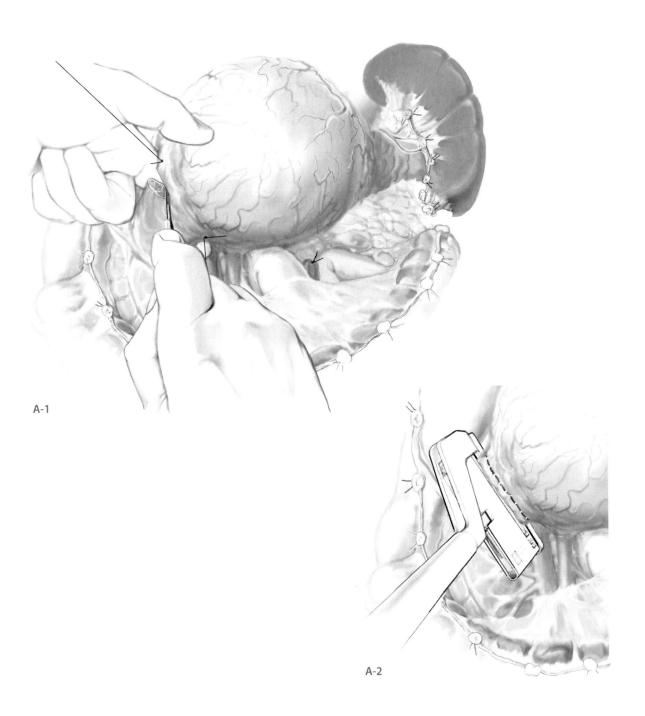

A-1

A-2

STEP 5   **Close the pancreatic duct**

The transected pancreatic duct is closed specifically with a fine, polypropylene suture placed either as a figure-of-eight or as a U stitch proximal to the divided open end of the duct; when the pancreas is divided with a stapler technique, suture closure of pancreatic duct is not necessary (A-1).

The divided end of the pancreatic remnant is closed with interrupted, partially overlapping 3-0 polypropylene mattress sutures.

When a stapling instrument used, it is not necessary to oversew the divided end of pancreas; some surgeons, however, prefer a continuous suture of fine polypropylene to reinforce the staple suture. If the pancreas is thick, however, a staple closure is not suggested (A-2).

A closed suction drain is placed in the bed of the resected gland in proximity to but not in direct apposition with the divided end of the pancreas.

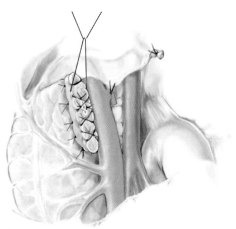

A-1

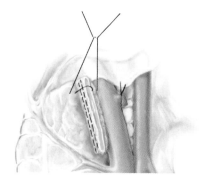

A-2

Postoperative Care and Tests

Postoperative surveillance in an intermediate care or general care unit; intensive care unit monitoring should not be necessary

Monitor hemoglobin, coagulation parameters, and acid/base and electrolyte balance at regular intervals

Postoperative Complications

- Short term:
    - Intra-abdominal bleeding
    - Pancreatic fistula
    - Peripancreatic fluid collection
    - Subphrenic abscess
    - Pleural effusion
    - Diabetes mellitus
    - Portal vein thrombosis
    - Ascites (differentiate pancreatic from non-pancreatic origin)
- Long term:
    - Pancreatic exocrine insufficiency
    - Diabetes mellitus
    - Local or distant recurrence
    - Pancreatic pseudocyst

Tricks of the Senior Surgeon

- The position of the patient is important; a moderate reverse Trendelenberg position with the patient rolled slightly toward the right facilitates the exposure by dropping the pancreas and spleen away from the left hemidiaphragm and by dropping the left transverse and splenic flexure of the colon away from the operative field.
- When easily accessible, the proximal splenic artery should be secured prior to completely mobilizing the pancreas and spleen from the retroperitoneum; this enables a rapid, secure, immediate hemostasis if the splenic capsule is torn during mobilization.
- The splenic artery and vein are suture ligated and divided individually rather than securing both together with a mass ligature; this approach decreases the risk of postoperative splenic arteriovenous fistula.
- Whenever possible, monofilament suture material rather than silk should be used to close the divided end of the pancreas. Monofilament, such as polypropylene, has a lower slip coefficient and can be pulled more easily (and potentially with less trauma) through tissue; monofilament lacks interstices and may be more resistant to infection than polyfilamentous sutures.

Enteric Drainage of Pancreatic Fistulas with Onlay Roux-en-Y Limb

Peter Shamamian, Stuart Marcus

Introduction

The majority of pancreatic fistulae will resolve with conservative measures, including improving pancreatic duct drainage through the ampulla, nutritional support, and somatostatin analogues. When pancreatic fistulae result from pancreatic ductal disruption and pancreatic secretions produced in a portion of the pancreas do not flow into the GI tract, operative intervention is indicated.

Indications and Contraindications

Indications in Non-Resolving Fistulae

- Pancreatic ductal disruption secondary to pancreatic trauma
- Fistulae following debridement of pancreatic necrosis
- Fistulae from complications of pancreatic surgery (i.e., enucleation of endocrine neoplasms)
- Fistulae from pancreatic injury during surgery on juxtapancreatic organs (i.e., stomach, colon, left kidney, left adrenal, spleen)
- Fistulae secondary to external drainage of pancreatic pseudocysts
- Fistulae associated with pancreatic ascites
- Pancreato-pleural fistulae

Contraindications

- Ongoing acute pancreatic inflammation
- Pancreatic abscess
- Undrained peri-pancreatic fluid collection

Preoperative Investigation and Preparation for the Procedure

History:	Pancreatitis, pancreatic trauma, pancreatic pseudocyst, prior pancreatic surgery, prior non-operative therapy with internal or external drains; exclude alcohol abuse, cirrhosis, portal hypertension
Clinical evaluation:	Quantify fistula output, optimize nutritional status, provide adequate external drainage, protect the skin from pancreatic secretions
Laboratory tests:	Serum electrolytes, amylase, lipase, and liver chemistries, bacterial culture, cytology and amylase of any drained peritoneal or pleural fluid

Preoperative Imaging

- CT: exclude presence of undrained collections or abscess
- ERCP: delineate pancreatic ductal anatomy, site of duct disruption, obstructing strictures or calculi
- Fistulogram: anatomy of pancreatic segment from which fistulous tract originates; adequate external preoperative drainage is essential.
- Angiogram: if suspicion of a pseudoaneurysm

Procedure

STEP 1

Access: incision, midline or bilateral subcostal depending on patient habitus (see Sect. 1, chapter "Positioning and Accesses").

The first step involves exposure to the lesser sac and installation of the mechanical retractor (see Sect. 1, chapter "Positioning and Accesses").

The preoperative fistulogram helps to locate the disrupted pancreatic duct.

Carefully trace the external drainage catheter into the lesser sac; dissection continues through the peripancreatic inflammatory tissue to the anterior surface of the pancreas (A-1).

It is often possible to directly visualize the fistulous tract as it exits the pancreas parenchyma.

Intraoperative secretin (SecreFlo, ChiRhoClin, Inc. Silver Springs, MD, USA) 0.2 µg/kg (after a 0.2-µg test dose) given intravenously stimulates pancreatic secretion and assists identification of the ductal disruption when it is not visualized clearly (A-2).

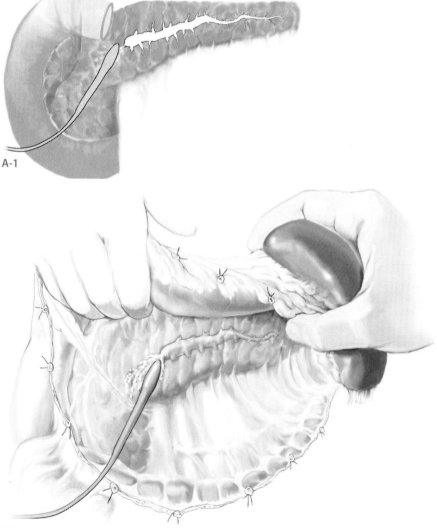

A-1

A-2

STEP 2

If possible, a catheter or probe is passed through the fistulous tract into the pancreatic duct.

If the pancreatic duct is identified, opening the anterior wall (spatulating the duct) increases the effective diameter of the anastomosis and facilitates the conduct of the anastomosis.

Pancreatography can be obtained if not done already.

The pancreatic duct should be imaged proximally and distally.

The jejunum is transected about 15 cm distal to the ligament of Treitz.

The blind end of the jejunum is closed by a stapling device or sutures.

Enteric continuity is reestablished by end-to-side jejunojejunostomy at least 60 cm from the closed end of the Roux limb.

The anastomosis is constructed by suturing the side of the jejunum to the pancreatic duct or the rim of scarred tissue at the fistulous tract at its point of origin on the pancreas. For details of construction of the Roux-en-Y limb see Sect. 2, chapter "Subtotal Gastrectomy, Antrectomy, Billroth II and Roux-en-Y Reconstruction and Local Excision in Complicated Gastric Ulcers."

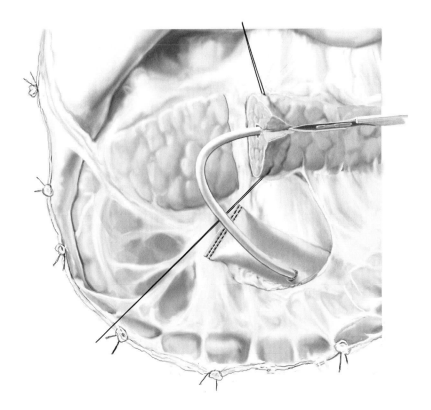

STEP 3

A posterior row of Lembert-type sutures is placed using 4-0 silk.

Next a row of absorbable sutures (4-0 or 5-0 polyglycolic acid) are placed full thickness through the pancreatic duct and the jejunum.

A catheter can be left as a stent through the anastomosis and brought out of the anterior abdominal wall, allowing the anastomosis to be studied postoperatively through the catheter if indicated.

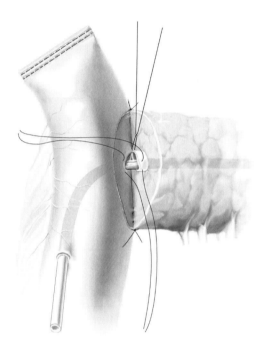

STEP 4

If the pancreatic duct cannot be identified definitively, the jejunum can be sewn over the fistulous tract as an onlay anastomosis to the pancreatic parenchyma; it would be optimal to keep a stent across this onlay anastomosis.

A soft closed suction drain is placed adjacent to the anastomosis.

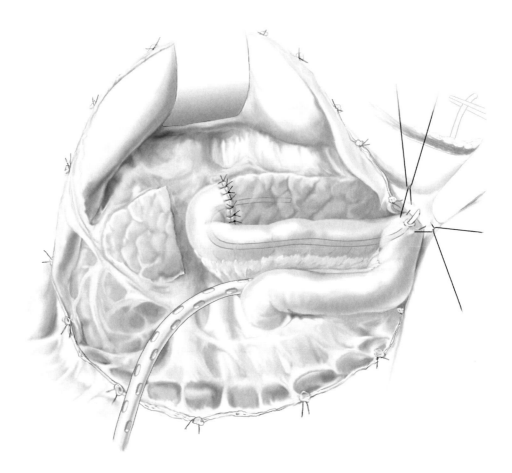

Postoperative Tests

- Hemodynamic and respiratory monitoring in intensive or intermediate care unit.
- Measure daily drain output; note changes after beginning oral intake. Drains are removed after resumption of oral intake and output is <50 ml/day.
- Measure drain amylase if persistent significant drainage >50 ml/day. If fluid is amylase rich, convert drains from closed suction drains to passive drains after 7 days, then advanced 1–2 cm/day.

Local Postoperative Complications

- Anastomotic leak, possible recurrent fistula
- Abscess
- Pancreatitis
- Pancreatic pseudocyst
- Intra-abdominal hemorrhage

Tricks of the Senior Surgeon

- Patience, adequate drainage, and complete pre- or intraoperative imaging is paramount for definition of the fistula and associated ductal anatomy; should marked disease remain in the duct, an alternative procedure, e.g., resection or lateral pancreaticojejunostomy, might be a better choice.
- One goal of fistula drainage is to preserve pancreatic endocrine and exocrine function. If the fistula arises from the tail of the pancreas, resection of the distal pancreas may be the best option if minimal loss of functional pancreatic tissue is anticipated.
- Spontaneous closure of the pancreatic fistula can be aided with a somatostatin analogue; success may be predictable based on radiographic evaluation. Fistulae that arise from a divided duct will not resolve.
- Closure of fistulae that radiographically connect to the GI tract may be facilitated by transpapillary pancreatic stents and by ensuring that strictures and obstructing calculi are addressed.
- Internal drainage of the fistulous tract into the stomach is not suggested; rather a defunctionalized Roux limb of jejunum is preferred when resection is not the best option.
- Sew to the pancreatic parenchyma at the point of origin of fistula and not to the fistulous tract; the parenchyma is usually thickened and scarred.
- If internal drainage is not possible (high operative risk or anatomic considerations), chronic external drainage is the best option.
- Amylase-rich fluid in the drain signifies breakdown of the anastomosis; management is considerably easier if a stent is placed across anastomosis at operation. The anastomosis can be evaluated radiographically; as the output decreases, the stent is converted from closed suction to passive drainage and then advanced 1 cm/day.
- Early intra-abdominal hemorrhage is best treated by reoperation and direct vessel ligation. Late hemorrhage may be a sentinel bleed from a pseudoaneurysm; immediate angiography and vessel embolization are indicated.

Sphincteroplasty for Pancreas Divisum

Andrew L. Warshaw

Indications and Contraindications

Indications

- Strong: recurrent episodes of documented acute pancreatitis (typical pain, increased serum amylase) in patients with congenital pancreas divisum or other variants of a dominant dorsal duct (absent duct of Wirsung, filamentous communication to duct of Wirsung)
- Weak: patients with pancreas divisum and episodic "obstructive pancreatic pain" (pain with characteristics and location attributable to a pancreatic origin but without objective substantiation by hyperamylasemia or pancreatic edema).

Contraindications

- Chronic pancreatitis (fibrosis, major duct dilation, pseudocyst, segmental duct obstruction, calcification)
- Pancreatitis from alcoholism, hypercalcemia, hyperlipidemia, gallstones, or trauma
- Recent severe acute pancreatitis, significant residual inflammation/swelling

Preoperative Investigation and Preparation for the Procedure

History:	Recurrent episodes of epigastric pain, especially with radiation through to the mid back; pain starts sporadically, with bouts months apart, but may become frequent and even constant; attacks are usually mild, more common in young women; mean onset is at 34 years but can occur in childhood, onset is uncommon after age 50 years.
Clinical evaluation:	May have tenderness over the pancreas.
Laboratory tests:	Serum amylase and/or lipase.
Imaging:	ERCP or MRCP to elucidate pancreatic ductal anatomy; ERCP must include opacification of the dominant dorsal duct via accessory papilla. Caution: acquired obstruction of the duct of Wirsung by tumor in the pancreatic head can mimic pancreas divisum.
Functional tests:	Transabdominal ultrasonography, endoscopic ultrasonography, or MRCP with secretion stimulation – demonstrates abnormally delayed return of principal pancreatic duct to normal size after hyperstimulation of pancreatic secretion. Impaired emptying through stenotic accessory papilla results in persistent (15- to 30-min) duct dilation.

Procedure

STEP 1

Exposure of minor papilla

An upper midline or right subcostal incision depends on patient habitus.

Extensive mobilization of the duodenum and the head of the pancreas (extended Kocher maneuver) facilitates exposure.

Cholecystectomy is performed if the gallbladder is still present; passage of a biliary Fogarty® catheter via the cystic duct or common duct through the major ampulla into the duodenum aids localization of the accessory papilla.

A transverse duodenotomy is made just proximal to the papilla of Vater, which can usually be felt transduodenally or with the aid of the biliary Fogarty® catheter.

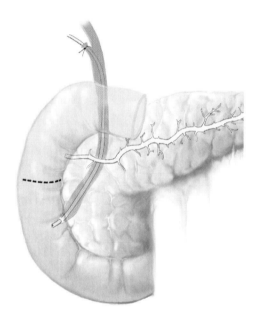

STEP 2   **Location of minor papilla intraduodenally**

Locate the accessory (minor) papilla 2–3 cm proximal and anteromedial to the papilla of Vater; minimize trauma to the duodenal mucosa.

Secretin (1 U/kg intravenously) helps locate the papilla by inducing visible flow of pancreatic juice and sometimes by ballooning out the papilla.

Grasp the duodenal mucosa just distal to the minor papilla to fix its position; insert a fine probe or Angiocath into the orifice. (It may be necessary to pierce the membranous tip of the papilla when the orifice is miniscule.)

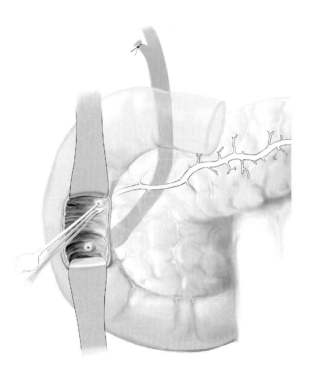

STEP 3   **Sphincterotomy of minor duct**

Fine traction sutures are placed at the distal margins of the accessory papilla; the papilla
is incised over a probe in the duct. Pancreatic juice should gush forth, and a dilated
vestibule proximal to the papillary membrane should be immediately apparent. The
smooth light pink mucosa lining the pancreatic duct is easily distinguished from the
duodenal mucosa.

The incision is extended about 1 cm, only as far as necessary to lay the duct vestibule
widely open.

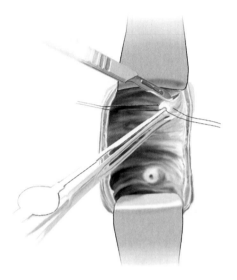

STEP 4   **Sphincteroplasty of minor duct**

The duodenal mucosa and the pancreatic duct epithelium are approximated with fine
absorbable synthetic sutures for hemostasis and to facilitate healing without re-stenosis.

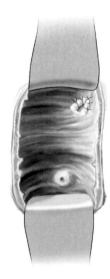

STEP 5	**Duct drainage and duodenal closure**

A small catheter (e.g., 5-French pediatric feeding tube) is passed through the duodenal wall and into the pancreatic duct to insure against postoperative duct obstruction. The catheter is inserted within the duodenal wall through a 14-gauge needle or commercial catheter fitted on a trocar, tunneled within the duodenal wall, and closed with a double-purse-string absorbable suture (A-1). The catheter is brought out through the abdominal wall for postoperative drainage and remains in place for 2–3 weeks before removal (A-2, A-3).

The duodenotomy is closed transversely in two layers; no right upper quadrant drain is needed.

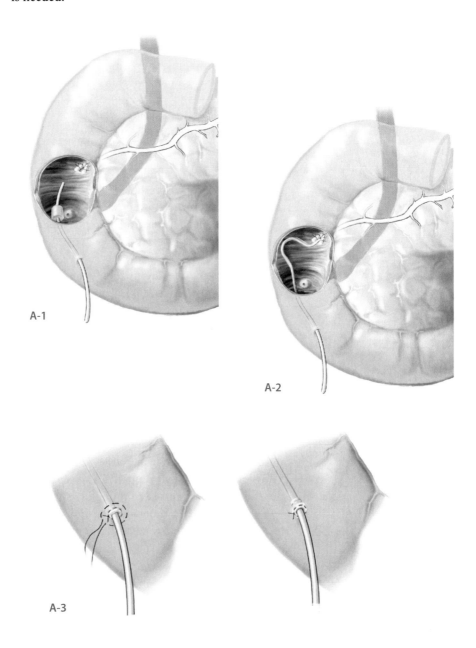

Postoperative Tests

- Routine postoperative surveillance.
- Serum amylase is not necessary unless there is a specific clinical indication.

Local Postoperative Complications

- Short term:
  - Acute pancreatitis
  - Duodenal obstruction
  - Duodenal leak
- Long term:
  - Recurrent papillary stenosis
  - Recurrent symptoms, pancreatitis
  - Failure to cure preoperative pain syndrome

Tricks of the Senior Surgeon

- The major papilla (ampulla) of Vater is often palpable through the duodenal wall even without a transcholedochal (e.g., via cystic duct) catheter through the Ampulla of Vater.
- The accessory papilla is proximal in the duodenum, perhaps only 3 cm from the pylorus; a prominent vessel on the lateral duodenal wall is often noted at this point.
- The transverse duodenotomy provides adequate exposure and is less likely to cause postoperative duodenal stenosis than a longitudinal suture line.
- The accessory papilla may be difficult to find by visual inspection, it is often small, protrudes minimally from the duodenal surface and is located more easily by gentle palpation of the medial wall of the duodenum. It feels like a small "bump" or nipple.
- Application of methylene blue to the duodenal mucosa may help to locate the pancreatic duct orifice; pancreatic secretions, especially after secretin, wash off the blue dye at the orifice.
- After cannulating the orifice, do not remove the probing instrument until the incision into the papilla has been completed. Local trauma may make rediscovery of a small, traumatized orifice very difficult.
- The dorsal duct of Santorini follows a perpendicular course through the duodenal wall (in contrast to the oblique path of the duct of Wirsung); the sphincteroplasty is therefore necessarily short. Going past the thin membrane of the first centimeter makes the apex of the sphincteroplasty difficult to suture.

Sphincterotomy/Sphincteroplasty for Papillary Dysfunction: Stenosing Papillitis

Frank G. Moody

Introduction

Simple division (5 mm) of the anterior surface of the sphincter of Oddi (sphincterotomy) was utilized extensively in the mid 20th century for presumed biliary-pancreatic pain from biliary dyskinesia. Lack of success led to a more generous longer (2–3 cm) division of the sphincter with formal sphincteroplasty with only marginal improvement in outcome. Our group and others have utilized a generous sphincteroplasty with division of the transampullary septum to include division of the pancreatic component of the sphincter; with this extended approach, we have achieved good to excellent results in appropriately selected patients. The rationale for the procedure is to allow free egress of bile and pancreatic juice into the duodenum after stimulation from ingestion of a meal. Stenting of even the septotomy can now be accomplished after endoscopic sphincteroplasty in experienced hands.

Indications and Contraindications

Indications

- Persistence or recurrence of severe episodes of right upper quadrant or epigastric pain after cholecystectomy

Contraindications

- Absolute contraindications: alcoholism, chronic pancreatitis, and depression
- Relative contraindications: unwillingness to pursue a trial of supervised detoxification (chemical withdrawal) from narcotics

Preoperative Investigations and Preparation for Procedure

Clinical:	Episodic, mid-epigastric pain, often young women, 25–40 years old, usually after cholecystectomy
Physical examination:	Lack of jaundice or epigastric tenderness, essentially normal abdominal examination
Laboratory evaluation:	Hemoglobin, amylase/lipase; one-third of patients with papillary stenosis will have *transient* increase in biliary or pancreatic enzymes but only *during* the episode of pain; cardiorespiratory evaluation as indicated
Imaging:	Ultrasonography to exclude cholecystolithiasis and choledocholithiasis; ERCP probably should be attempted in all patients; deformity of papilla or dilation of bile or pancreatic ducts is present in 25%; cannulation of pancreatic duct is possible only in 50%
Other:	Transpapillary manometry, when performed, shows high resting pressures in the pancreatic and biliary ducts
Psychologic/psychiatric consultation:	*All* candidates for operative approach, a viable attempt preopeatively at narcotic detoxification should be entertained (almost never successful)

Preoperative Preparation

■ A serious discussion with and commitment by the patient for postoperative narcotic detoxification is strongly suggested
■ Perioperative antibiotics (clean-contaminated procedure)
■ Perioperative prophylactic heparin and sequential compression devices (SCDs) to minimize venous thrombosis

Procedure: Transduodenal Spincteroplasty with Transampullary Septectomy

STEP 1

The abdomen is entered through the incision for prior cholecystectomy or through a midline incision.

Exposure is optimized by a Thompson retractor or some similar mechanical retractor.

After exploration, the duodenum and head of the pancreas are mobilized by a generous Kocher maneuver; the hepatic flexure of the colon is mobilized inferiorly, with care not to enter Gerotta's fascia. The head of the pancreas is mobilized from the underlying vena cava and the aorta in the avascular plane behind the duodenum.

This wide mobilization allows access to the cystic duct remnant, common bile duct, and anterior surface of the junction of the middle and lower third of the 2nd part of the duodenum where the papilla of Vater resides; the papilla is usually readily palpable through depressing the lateral duodenal wall against the medical wall.

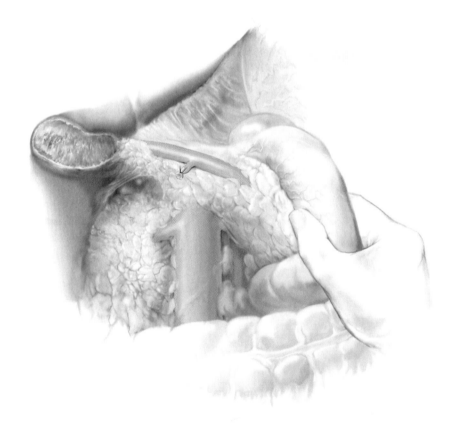

STEP 2

The biliary tree is intubated to accurately locate the papilla.

Access to the biliary tree is gained through a small opening in the cystic duct remnant or, if necessary, the common bile duct; the latter access can be avoided if you can confidently locate the ampulla by transduodenal palpation.

A 3-Fr. tapered, urethral filiform probe (or a small biliary Fogarty catheter) is passed through the common bile duct and into the duodenum to locate the papilla.

Suspicion of a common bile duct stone may require formal bile duct exploration. Rigid probes (e.g. Bakes dilators) should not be used, because the bile duct is vulnerable to perforation when papillary stenosis is present. Note the operator's left hand supporting the intrapancreatic portion of the common bile duct as the filiform passes through the papilla.

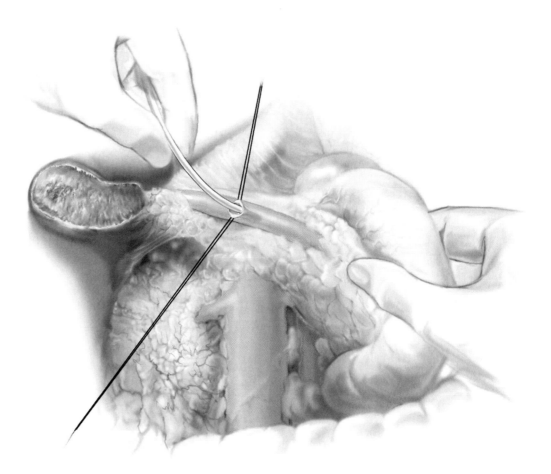

STEP 3

A 2-cm anterior duodenotomy is made directly over where the filiform leaves the papilla.

Stay sutures are placed at the 2 and 8 o'clock position to elevate the papilla up to the level of the duodenotomy.

An incision is made along an 11 o'clock plane on the anterior surface of the papilla; use of small iris scissors facilitates transection of the sphincter – cautery should be avoided, because it obscures recognition of the mucosal edges.

Approximating the bile duct epithelium to the duodenal mucosa is carried out in sequential fashion with 5-0 polyglycolic acid sutures; the length of the sphincteroplasty (2–3 cm) should be determined by a point where the bile duct separates from the duodenal wall. Care must be taken to precisely approximate the bile duct epithelium and duodenal mucosa in this area.

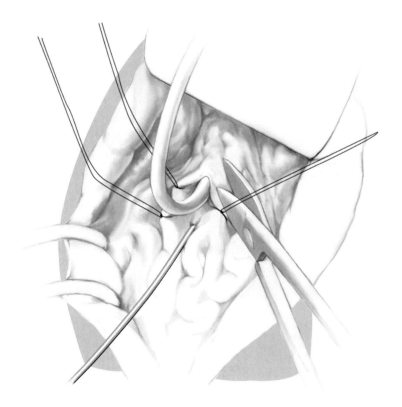

STEP 4

Papillary stenosis often is associated with marked deformity of the transampullary septum (the tissue that separates the intrapancreatic bile duct from the pancreatic duct within the papilla of Vater).

The ostia of the duct of Wirsung can be difficult to visualize; it may be necessary to gently probe the inferior lip of papilla with the smallest of lacrimal probes.

Once cannulated, the ostia should be dilated with one or two larger probes.

The septum can then be divided safely by a sharp scalpel incision (11 blade) for at least 1 cm or to the point where the pancreatic duct measures at least 3 mm; deformity or scarring in this region may make this difficult.

A pancreatogram should be obtained at this point if not already done.

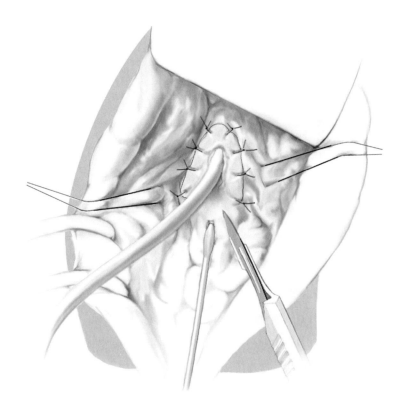

STEP 5

The mucosa of the pancreatic duct is approximated to the bile duct epithelium with interrupted 7-0 polyglycolic acid suture utilizing a small ophthalmic needle; this figure reveals what the papilla *should* look like at completion of the operation. Note that the anterior surface of the papilla has been effaced, and that the bile duct and duct of Wirsung enter the duodenum through separate openings.

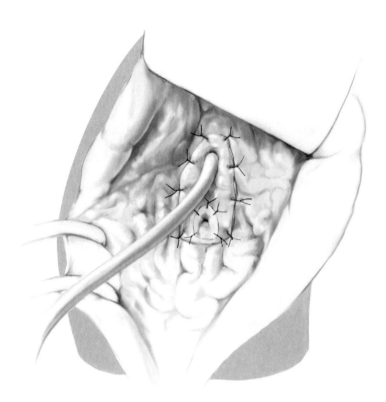

STEP 6

The duodenum is closed in two layers with an inner row of a fine absorbable suture, placed in a running Connell, mucosal-inverting fashion, and the outer layer of interrupted seromuscular non-absorbable sutures are placed in interrupted Lembert fashion.

A Jackson-Pratt or similar type of silicon closed-suction drain is positioned in the retroperitoneal bed of the duodenum, and a tag of omentum is sutured over the duodenotomy.

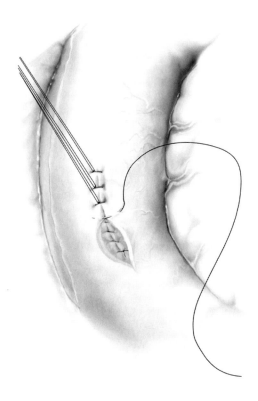

Postoperative Tests

- Hemogram, WBC, serum amylase
- Monitor drain output
- Cholangiogram if T-tube is present on postoperative day 6
- A nasogastric tube is not necessary
- Resumption of oral intake as soon as tolerated

Local Postoperative Complications

- Early:
  - Pancreatitis – usually postoperative day 1 – fever, abdominal pain, increased serum amylase
  - Atelectasis – usually postoperative day 2 – fever, abnormal chest X-ray
  - Cholangitis – usually postoperative day 3 – fever, jaundice
  - Bilious drainage – usually postoperative day 3–7 – duodenal leak
  - Wound infection – postoperative day 4–7 – fever, increased WBC, tender red wound
  - Pulmonary embolus – postoperative day 7–10 – shortness of breath
  - Gastrointestinal bleeding may occur from the sphincteroplasty site
- Late:
  - Recurrent pain
  - Recurrent stenosis of bile or pancreatic duct (± pancreatitis)
  - Persistent narcotic dependence

Tricks of the Senior Surgeon

- Select your patients carefully.
- Wear a headlight and use optimal magnification (loops).
- Handle the papilla gently and with great respect.
- Insist on postoperative narcotic detoxification.
- Be kind and empathetic toward the patient with this form of addictive postcholecystectomy pain.

Pancreatic Enucleation

Geoffrey B. Thompson (Open Enucleation),
Michel Gagner (Laparoscopic Enucleation)

Introduction

Enucleation of functioning neuroendocrine neoplasms (insulinomas, selected gastrinomas) and non-functioning, well-circumscribed neuroendocrine neoplasms <2 cm has been shown to be appropriate therapy for these benign neoplasms. Overtly malignant neuroendocrine neoplasms require a formal anatomic pancreatic resection.

Indications and Contraindications

Indications

- Insulinomas
- Selected gastrinomas, somatostatinomas
- Non-functional neuroendocrine neoplasms, usually <2 cm, well-circumscribed, no signs of malignancy

Contraindications

- Glucagonoma (these are usually malignant and require an anatomic resection)
- Recent acute pancreatitis
- Uncontrolled coagulopathy/severe thrombocytopenia
- Co-morbidities dramatically limiting life expectancy
- Active peptic ulceration (gastrinoma patients)
- Signs of malignancy – multiple enlarged lymph nodes, liver metastases

Preoperative Investigations and Preparation for Procedure

- History:
  - Insulinoma: "spells" associated with hypoglycemia, Whipple's triad
  - Gastrinoma: peptic symptoms, gastroesophageal reflux disease (GERD), diarrhea, unusual location of duodenal ulcers (distal to 1st portion of duodenum)
- Clinical history:
  - Insulinoma: documented neuroglycopenic episodes (confusion, amnesia, double vision, blurred vision, coma), symptoms relieved by glucose administration (Whipple's triad)
  - Gastrinoma: increased serum gastrin, and gastric acid secretion
- Laboratory tests:
  - Insulinoma:
    - Supervised 72-h fast; endpoint – neuroglycopenia and plasma glucose <45 mg/dl
    - Increased C-peptide level (>200 pmol/l)
    - Increased insulin level ≥3 (immunochemiluminometric assay, ICMA)
    - Increased proinsulin level
    - Negative sulfonylurea screen in urine
    - Negative insulin antibodies
  - Gastrinoma (off antisecretory medication)
    - Increased serum gastrin (>500 pg/ml)
    - Gastric pH<3
    - Positive secretin provocative test (when available) or calcium stimulation test
- Localization:
  - Spiral CT with triple-phase contrast
  - Magnetic resonance imaging
  - Transabdominal ultrasonography
  - Endoscopic ultrasonography ± fine-needle aspiration
  - Selective arterial calcium stimulation test (insulinomas, gastrinomas)
  - Selective use of octreotide scintigraphy

Procedures

Open Enucleation
Geoffrey B. Thompson

STEP 1

Setup, transverse epigastric incision, exploration, entry into lesser sac

Plasma glucose concentrations should be checked every 20–30 min with the patient off all glucose-containing fluids (insulinoma patients only).

The patient is best positioned supine with arms tucked at sides.

A transverse epigastric incision is best. A third-arm mechanical retractor facilitates the exposure and allows a thorough abdominal/pelvic exploration to be carried out.

First, the gastrocolic omentum is mobilized off the transverse colon from left to right, entering the lesser sac; the stomach and the omentum are held cephalad by the second assistant, and the transverse colon is retracted caudad, exposing the pancreas.

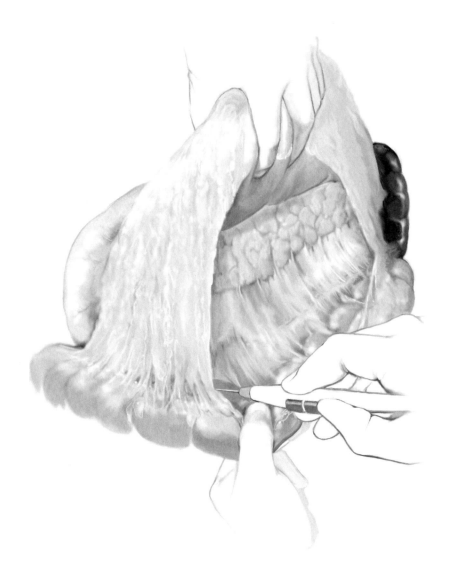

STEP 2   **Kocherization, mobilization body and tail, inspection, and palpation**

Before further mobilization, the pancreas is inspected and palpated carefully. If the tumor is readily apparent on the surface or edge of gland and its location is consistent with preoperative localization studies, further mobilization may be limited to the involved portion of the pancreas, unless there is a familial syndrome or other concerns predisposing the patient to multiple neoplasms.

For tumors in the head and uncinate region, the duodenum is widely Kocherized out to and including the ligament of Treitz; division of the right gastroepiploic vessels on the anterior surface of the pancreatic head and the anterior inferior pancreatoduodenal vein to the uncinate facilitates exposure of the head and uncinate and reduces the risk of inadvertent vascular injury and bleeding during further dissection; transpancreatic palpation of the head and uncinate allows localization of tumors in this region.

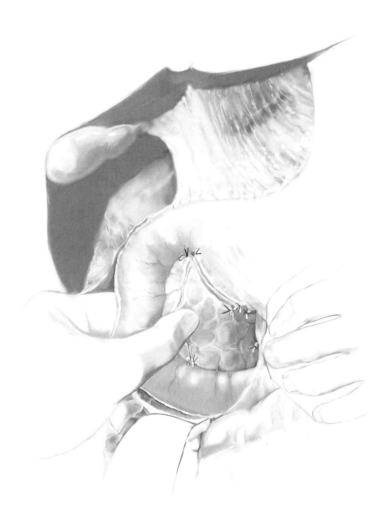

STEP 3

When the tumor is in the neck of the pancreas, a plane is developed between the underside of the neck of the gland and the underlying portal vein – the superior mesenteric vein junction. After exposing the superior mesenteric vein at the inferior edge of the neck of the pancreas, gentle blunt dissection with an index finger or a small cherry-tipped sucker completes the dissection under direct vision; care is taken to stay directly on top of the vein throughout the dissection to avoid injury to lateral venous tributaries to the uncinate. In patients with insulinoma, this is usually an easy dissection.

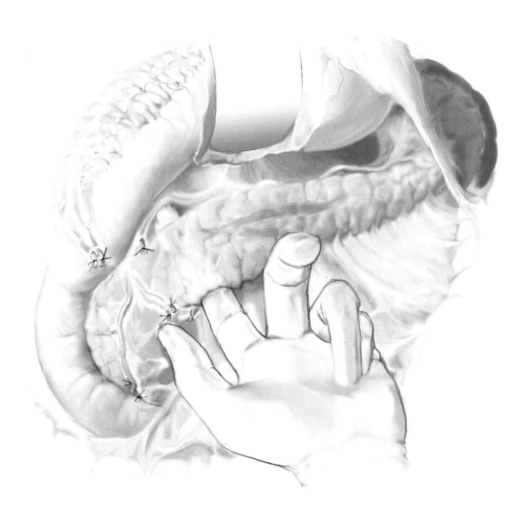

STEP 4

When the tumor is in the body of the pancreas, dissection continues along the avascular inferior border of the body of the gland. After incising this plane, the body of the pancreas is mobilized from the inferior to superior border (A-1).

When the tumor is in the tail of the pancreas, mobilization of the spleen by incising its lateral peritoneal attachments to the kidney and diaphragm usually allows best exposure. Short gastric vessels are not divided until the decision is made regarding splenic-preservation (A-2).

When the tumor is occult, all these maneuvers should be performed prior to intra-operative ultrasonography (IOUS); bimanual and bidigital palpation allow the gland to be examined from head to tail; suspicious lymph nodes are excised for frozen section analysis (A-3).

Real-time IOUS is next performed using a 6-mHz transducer in the longitudinal and transverse axes. Islet cell neoplasms appear as hypoechoic masses within the pancreatic parenchyma, are more firm in texture than the surrounding parenchyma, and are tan to reddish-brown.

Islet cell neoplasms typically have a rim of vascular enhancement not seen with lymph nodes on color-flow Doppler examination.

Further palpation of lesions on ultrasonography often reveals subtle thickening within the pancreas not appreciated during the initial exploration.

If doubt of the findings exists, ultrasonography-guided fine-needle aspiration provides immediate cytologic evaluation; this is especially important for occult islet cell neoplasms deep within the head of gland abutting the pancreatic and/or bile ducts; this situation requires pancreatoduodenectomy, and absolute cytologic confirmation of an islet cell neoplasms is essential.

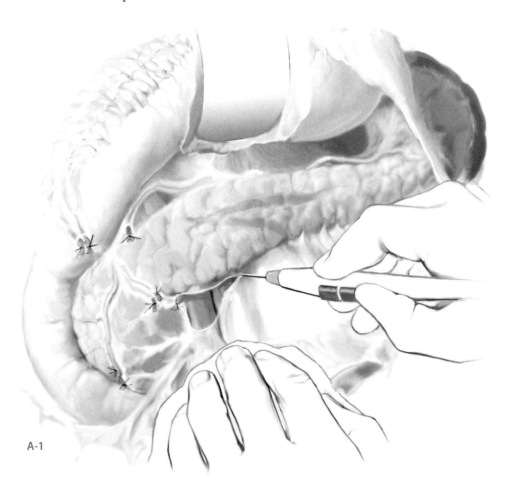

A-1

STEP 4 *(continued)*

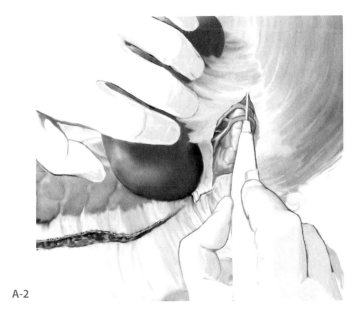

A-2

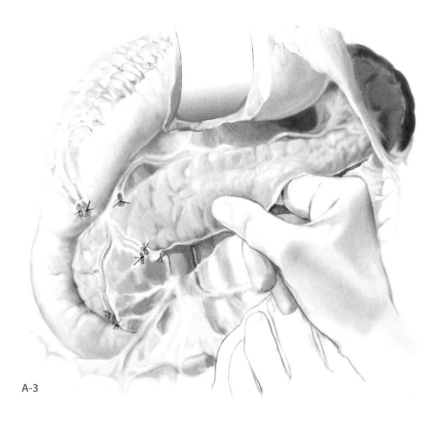

A-3

STEP 5   **Enucleation**

Once the site of the tumor is ascertained and no other abnormalities are noted, a decision must be made regarding enucleation versus resection; over two-thirds of insulinomas can be enucleated safely with attention to detail.

For palpable tumors on the edge of the gland, anterior surface, or posterior surface, the very thin operculum of pancreatic tissue overlying the tumor is carefully incised using a combination of bipolar cautery and a fine-tipped hemostat, the underlying insulinoma exposed, and a traction suture is placed deep into the tumor in figure-of-eight fashion to avoid fracture. Constant gentle elevation of the traction suture allows direct visualization of the small feeding vascular tributaries, which can be managed with bipolar cautery but infrequently require fine metallic clips. The pancreatic parenchyma is dissected away from the tumor using a fine endarterectomy spatula. Near the base of the enucleation, the endarterectomy spatula really helps to push the parenchyma away from the adenoma, especially when enucleating tumors are abutting the pancreatic duct.

Once enucleation is complete, ultrasonography confirms the integrity of the main pancreatic duct. In the past, secretin was administered to dilate the pancreatic duct to demonstrate major leaks from the enucleation site.

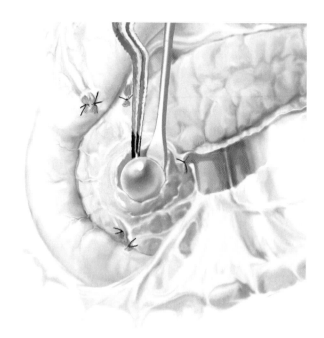

Enucleation

When the spleen is sizable or the patient is thin, the splenic artery and vein can be freed from the pancreas by individually dividing venous and arterial tributaries with fine metal clips and/or a harmonic scalpel; concern regarding patency of the splenic vein should lead to splenectomy or arterial and venous ligation, leaving the spleen based on short gastric vessels; the former is essential for a larger spleen. This avoids future development of left-sided portal hypertension and gastric varices.

All malignant islet cell neoplasms require oncologic principles with distal pancreatectomy and splenectomy or pancreatoduodenectomy including regional lymphadenectomy.

After enucleation/resection, the abdomen is irrigated and hemostasis assured.

The stomach and greater omentum are draped over the colon and the abdomen closed.

Major ductal disruption in the body and tail of the gland is best managed with immediate distal pancreatectomy.

A major ductal injury in the head of the pancreas is managed by (1) suture closure of the duct with fine absorbable suture and drainage, (2) closure of the hole over a tiny silastic stent passed across the papilla with placement of the Roux limb over the enucleation site, or (3) pancreatoduodenectomy (<2% of patients). External drainage is strongly suggested in all patients.

Once the insulinoma is removed, plasma glucose concentrations are drawn every 15 min; increases in serum glucose concentration by 20 mg/dl in the first 30 min after excision usually indicate a cure, but false positive and false negative studies are possible; in some centers, rapid insulin assays are available.

The enucleation site is left open and drains are placed nearby.

Tumors larger than 2 cm centralized within the body or tail of the pancreas are probably best managed by distal pancreatic resection with or without splenectomy unless they are located excentrically .

For tumors in the tail of the gland, it is usually easy to separate the splenic artery and vein from the gland, and the pancreatic tail is removed using a stapling device; the staple line is reinforced with a row of absorbable horizontal mattress sutures that incorporate the pancreatic duct. Drains are placed.

For larger tumors in the body of the pancreas, splenic preservation can be accomplished in two ways. In obese patients, the splenic artery and vein are divided 1–1.5 cm outside the splenic hilum, leaving the spleen based on the short gastric vessels provided the spleen is not enlarged. Once the spleen and blood supply are separated from the pancreas, the splenic artery is re-divided and ligated at its origin. The splenic vein is also re-divided and ligated at its junction with the superior mesenteric/portal vein junction, and the body and tail are removed with a stapler.

Laparoscopic Enucleation
Michel Gagner

STEP 1

Operative room positioning/trocar placement

The patient is placed under general anesthesia with orotracheal intubation.

A nasogastric tube and Foley urinary catheter are put in place.

Prophylactic parenteral antibiotics are given.

The patient is positioned in the lithotomy position with a wedge under the left flank (45° of elevation).

The surgeon stands between the patient's legs, the first assistant to patient's right, and the scrub nurse to the patient's left.

Two monitors are positioned at each of the patient's shoulders.

A five-trocar technique is used (10-mm trocar at umbilicus for 10 mm, 30° laparoscope); the size and position of the other four trocars vary with patient habitus, but a 12-mm trocar in the left mid-axillary line is used to introduce the linear stapler.

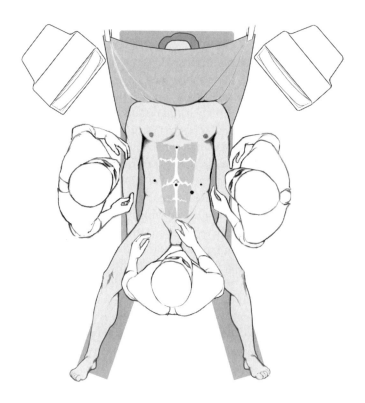

STEP 2	**Pancreatic exposure and mobilization**

Exploratory laparoscopy is performed first to exclude local or distant extension of the neoplasm.

The small bowel is removed from the operative field and the table rotated/inclined with the left side up and in reverse Trendelenberg to obtain the best exposure.

The lesser sac is exposed by opening the gastrocolic ligament widely inferior to the gastroepiploic arcade using an ultrasonic scalpel (Ultracision, United States Surgical Co., CT) or electrothermal bipolar vessel sealing device (LigaSure Lap, Tyco Healthcare, CO). The splenic flexure of the colon is mobilized inferiorly to expose the pancreatic tail; if further exposure is needed, the short gastric vessels are transected.

The retroperitoneum is incised along the inferior and superior border of the body/tail of pancreas; the mesenteric vessels are identified at the uncinate process, as well as the splenic artery at the superior border of the pancreas.

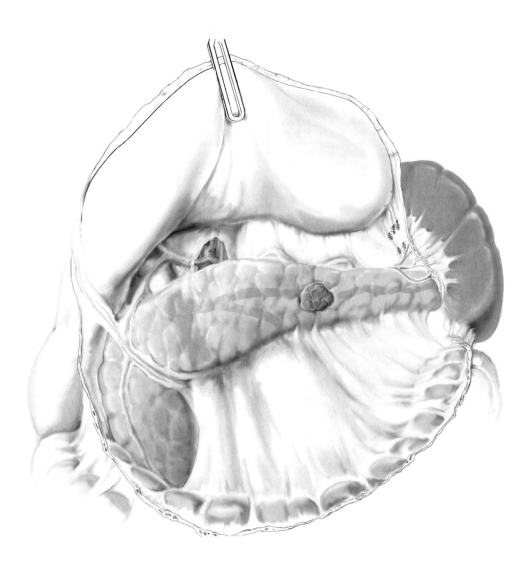

STEP 3   **Ultrasonography**

Endoscopic ultrasonography is performed routinely; the aim is to localize the tumor, define resection margin, exclude secondary lesion (both hepatic or pancreatic), and define the relationship with the main vessels and pancreatic duct.

The probe we use fits through a 10-mm trocar; its tip can be angulated for maximal surface contact. For small lesions, a water balloon is placed between the probe and the pancreatic body to improve resolution.

The ideal treatment is enucleation; however, with a larger tumor or one deep or localized too close to the main vessels or pancreatic duct, a pancreatic tail resection, with or without splenectomy, is preferred.

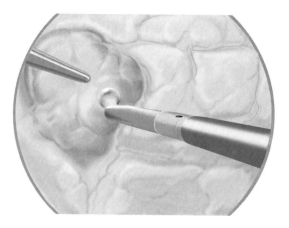

STEP 4   **Enucleation of pancreatic tumor**

A pancreatotomy is performed in a circle a few millimeters from the edge of the tumor.

An ultrasonic scalpel is used to dissect the tumor from the normal parenchyma.

As the plane of dissection goes deeper, small vessels are cauterized or ligated with ultrasonic energy.

An irrigation-suction cannula keeps the field free of blood; if hemorrhage occurs, pressure is applied for several minutes.

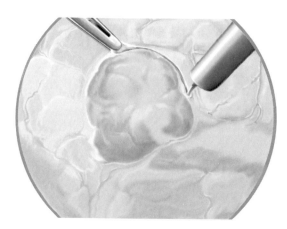

STEP 5

Enucleation of pancreatic tumor

Larger vessels feeding the tumor are controlled using 5- or 10-mm vascular clips.

The resected tumor is placed in a retrieval bag and extracted through the 12-mm trocar.

Frozen sections confirm the histology and assess resection margins.

Intraoperative insulin assays are obtained before/after resecting the insulinoma.

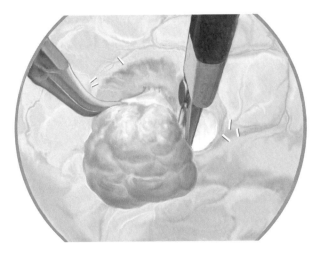

STEP 6

Hemostasis and drainage

The bed of the tumor is covered with fibrin glue to prevent pancreatic exocrine leakage.

A closed suction drain is left in the lesser sac near the resection site.

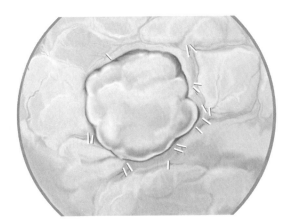

Postoperative Tests

Hold all glucose for 24h (insulinoma)
   Plasma glucose every 6–8h for 48h then twice daily until oral intake resumes
(insulinoma)
      Every other day CBC, electrolytes, amylase
      Drain fluid amylase if fluid becomes cloudy

Local Postoperative Complications

- Short term:
  - Pancreatic leak
  - Acute pancreatitis
  - Bleeding
  - Intra-abdominal abscess
  - Wound infection
  - Persistent hypoglycemia, hypergastrinemia
- Long term:
  - Chronic pancreaticocutaneous fistula
  - Pancreatic ascites (internal fistula)
  - Pancreatic pseudocyst
  - Diabetes mellitus
  - Recurrent peptic ulcer disease (gastrinoma)
  - Recurrent hypoglycemia secondary to missed insulinoma, unrecognized factitious hypoglycemia, nesidioblastosis, multiple endocrine neoplasia syndrome

Tricks of the Senior Surgeon

Open Enucleation
- Minimize mobilization of the pancreas if the tumor is readily apparent (use IOUS to look for multiple tumors).
- IOUS guides tumor removal (enucleation versus resection); use IOUS to check the continuity of the main pancreatic duct after enucleation.
- Avoid sutures and unipolar electrocautery; utilize a traction suture, bipolar cautery, fine clips, and an endarterectomy spatula during enucleation to avoid major ductal injury.
- Leave the enucleation sites open.
- Fibrin glue and octreotide do not prevent pancreatic fistulas.
- Always leave drain(s).

Laparoscopic Enucleation
- A 5-mm hook cautery can be very useful to dissect the deep plane between the pancreas and insulinoma.
- Reuse the laparoscopic ultrasound probe to monitor enucleation.
- If the enucleation plane is difficult, perform a laparoscopic or open distal pancreatectomy.
- Clip the last deeper posterior centimeter of the pancreatic parenchyma to control posterior vessels feeding the tumor and possible pancreatic ductules.

Transduodenal Resection
of Periampullary Villous Neoplasms

Michael L. Kendrick, Michael B. Farnell

Introduction

Halsted reported the first ampullary resection of a periampullary carcinoma in 1899.

This approach offers a decreased operative risk and potential complications compared to more radical procedures; however, the disadvantages include a high incidence of recurrence and the need for ongoing endoscopic surveillance.

Indications and Contraindications

Indications

- Benign periampullary villous neoplasm
- Prohibitive operative risk for pancreatoduodenectomy
- Patient preference or refusal of pancreatoduodenectomy

Contraindications

- Presence or suspicion of malignancy
- Pancreatic or common bile duct tumor extension greater than 1.5 cm
- Large tumor (>2.5 cm) precluding adequate margins for reconstruction and closure

Preoperative Investigations and Preparation for Procedure

Endoscopy with Biopsy
- Mandatory in all patients
- With high suspicion or biopsy-proven malignancy, especially with tissue invasion, strong consideration should be given for radical resection
- Findings suggesting malignancy include: bile and/or pancreatic ductal dilation, hard or ulcerated tumor, or high-grade dysplasia
- Cautionary notes:
    - Endoscopic biopsy misses diagnosis of malignancy in 40%
    - Most accurate diagnostic method for invasion is complete excision with pathologic analysis

Endoscopic Retrograde Cholangiopancreatography
- The gold standard
- Determines ductal extension

Computed Tomography
- Excludes evidence of local complications (ductal dilation, pancreatitis, etc.) or metastatic disease

Endoscopic Ultrasonography
- Can (in experienced hands) delineate transmural invasion, ductal extension, or nodal involvement
- Very operator-dependent

Procedure: Transduodenal Resection of Periampullary Neoplasm

STEP 1

Access and exposure

Incision: a right subcostal incision is usually preferable in the majority of patients.

Exploration: first, one must exclude metastatic disease to the liver, nodes, or peritoneum (these are extremely rare).

Exposure: a fixed mechanical, upper abdominal retractor markedly facilitates operation.

- After mobilization of the hepatic flexure inferiorly, a wide Kocher maneuver is performed mobilizing the duodenum medially (A-1).
- Next, assessment of the posterior duodenum is performed (A-2).
- The lesion and ampulla are localized by palpation medially from the lateral duodenal wall (A-3).

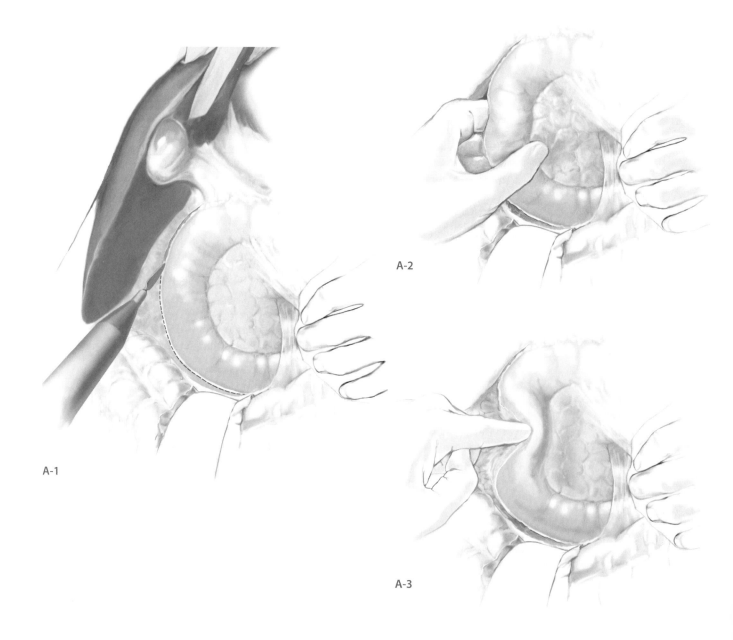

A-2

A-1

A-3

STEP 2   **Duodenotomy and setup (A-1.1)**

An anterolateral oblique duodenotomy is made (A-1.2).

Cholecystectomy is performed in routine fashion. A flexible catheter (e.g., biliary Fogarty® catheter) is placed antegrade from the cystic duct distally through the papilla into the duodenum, which assists localization of the ampulla.

A 5- to 10-mm margin is scored circumferentially in the mucosa around the adenoma with electrocautery. Sutures placed at the margins assist with retraction. A mixture of saline and epinephrine (1:100,000) is injected submucosally to elevate the mucosa and the tumor to facilitate resection.

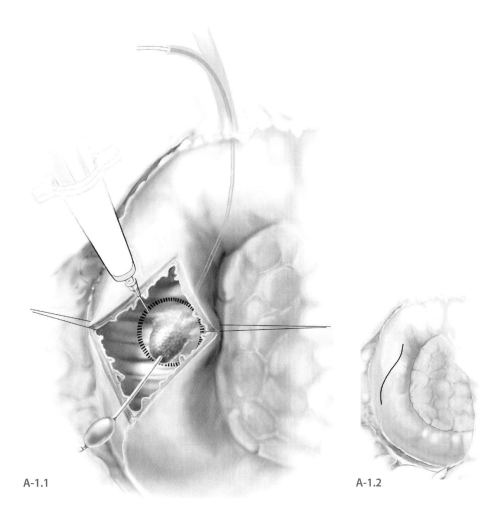

A-1.1   A-1.2

STEP 3   **Resection**

The extent and depth of the excision are based on the preoperative and intraoperative assessment; submucosal excision may be adequate for superficial lesions not involving the ducts. Full thickness "ampullectomy" is necessary for lesions with transmural invasion or ductal extension (A-1).

"Needle-point" electrocautery is used to excise the lesion with the rim of normal tissue (A-2). More extensive resection including the margin of pancreas, and the pancreatic and common bile ducts is necessary to ensure adequate margins; the specimen is examined carefully, oriented, and margins marked for frozen section. Optical magnification assists this step as well as the reconstruction (A-3).

If carcinoma in-situ or invasive carcinoma is identified, conversion to a formal pancreatoduodenectomy in acceptable risk patients is best.

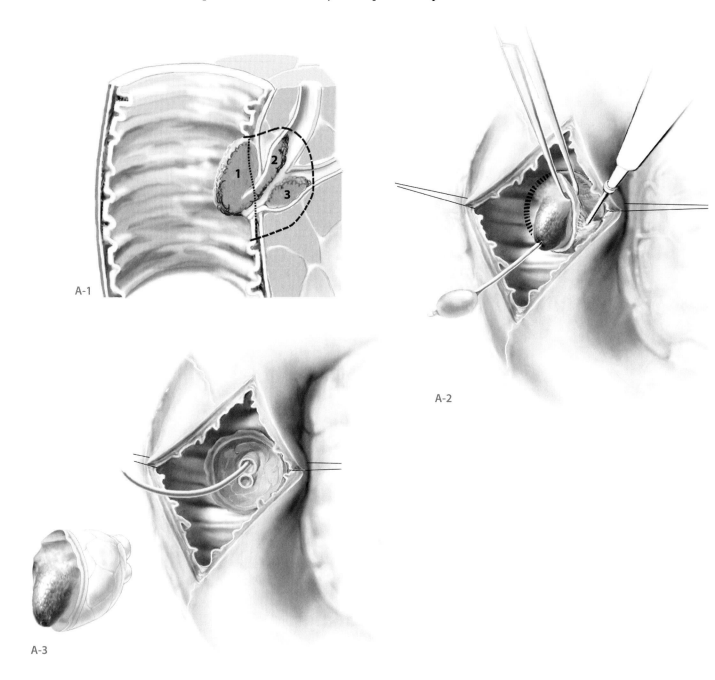

A-1

A-2

A-3

STEP 4   **Reconstruction**

Once the lesion is confirmed to be benign, local reconstruction is initiated; the method of reconstruction depends on the extent of resection and ductal anatomy.

Submucosal excisions are reconstructed using interrupted absorbable suture to approximate the mucosa of the ampulla to that of the duodenum. Care is taken not to obliterate the orifice of the pancreatic duct located at the caudal aspect of the transected ampulla. Intravenous secretin (0.25 µg/kg) is used to identify the pancreatic duct if the orifice is uncertain (A-1).

Ampullectomy is reconstructed by approximating the adjacent portion of the pancreatic and bile duct (inset) with interrupted 5-0 or 6-0 absorbable suture followed by reconstruction of the entire complex, as for submucosal excisions to duodenal mucosa (A-2).

Ampullectomy or more extensive resection of the pancreatic and bile ducts may require separate reconstruction (A-3).

- Assessment of ductal patency is imperative and is done with a small probe.
- The lateral duodenotomy is closed in a two-layer fashion.
- A paraduodenal drain is placed in Morrison's pouch and brought out through the right lateral abdominal wall.

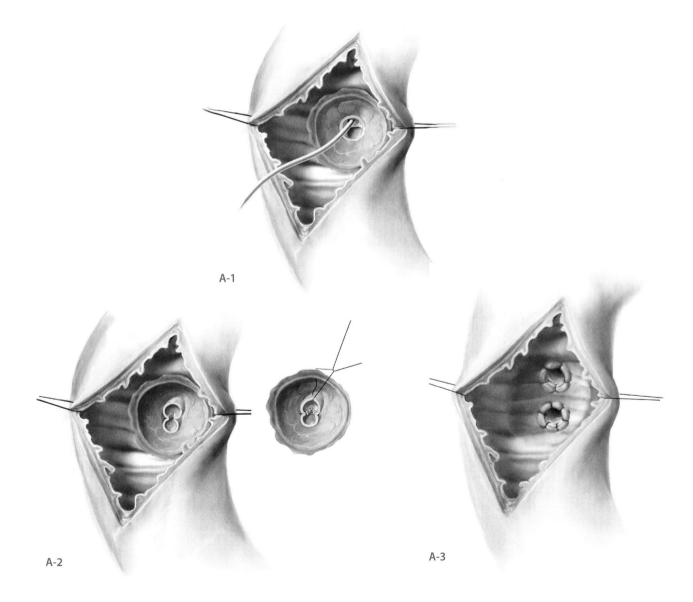

A-1

A-2   A-3

Postoperative Care

- The nasogastric tube is removed the night of or morning after operation.
- Routine postoperative tests and imaging are unnecessary.
- The drain is removed when the patient can tolerate oral intake and is without evidence of any complications.

Local Postoperative Complications

- Short term:
  - Transient increases in of serum liver function studies and pancreatic enzymes (infrequently clinically significant)
  - Duodenal, pancreatic, or biliary leak
  - Intraduodenal hemorrhage
  - Pancreatitis
- Long term:
  - Common bile duct or pancreatic duct stricture
  - Duodenal stricture
  - Recurrent villous adenoma (est. ~40% at 10 years of follow-up)
  - Development of ampullary carcinoma (malignant recurrence) is possible and thus requires regular surveillance

Postoperative Surveillance

- Endoscopic gastroduodenoscopy with a side-viewing instrument should be performed 6 months postoperatively, biannually for 2 years, and then annually.
- Strictures are interrogated for recurrent neoplasm and ideally treated with pancreatoduodenectomy.

Tricks of the Senior Surgeon

- A subcostal incision provides excellent lateral exposure, greatly facilitating access for the dissection.
- An anterolateral oblique duodenotomy gives ideal exposure, allows further extension if needed, and a two-layer closure does not compromise duodenal lumen.
- An extended Kocher maneuver is imperative.
- A folded laparotomy pad placed behind the duodenum displaces the operative field anteriorly.
- A catheter placed antegrade via the cystic duct provides assurance in locating and protecting the retroduodenal common bile duct, especially when a full thickness excision is performed.
- Placement of sutures at the margin of the specimen assists exposure and dissection.
- Optical magnification is very helpful for resection and reconstruction.

Pancreas Transplantation

Nicolas Demartines, Hans Sollinger

Introduction

The aim of pancreas transplantation is to restore normal glycemia in diabetics and to attempt to stop the vascular pathophysiology of diabetes, i.e., microangiopathy and, whenever possible, to reverse established renal, ophthalmologic, and neurologic complications of microangiopathy. Pancreas transplantation can be performed either simultaneously with or sometimes after a previous kidney transplant, or less commonly as a primary procedure alone.

The operative technique of the pancreas transplantation has evolved from a segmental organ transplantation to a complete (pancreatoduodenal) transplantation. Similarly, the original method of drainage of the exocrine pancreas into the bladder has also evolved into enteric drainage. In many centers, enteric drainage has been shown to be safe and efficient and has largely replaced bladder drainage.

The question about the benefit of portal venous drainage versus caval (systemic) drainage remains unresolved, and both techniques will be described.

Indications and Contraindications

Indications

Indications for Pancreas Transplantation
- Type 1 diabetes mellitus

Indications for Simultaneous Pancreas and Kidney Transplantation
- Diabetic nephropathy
- End-stage renal disease

Indication for Pancreas Transplantation After Kidney Transplantation
- Functioning kidney graft

Indication for Pancreas Transplantation Alone (Severe Complications of Diabetes)
- Instability of glycemia – unstable, "brittle", insulin-dependent diabetes
- Progressive retinopathy
- Progressive neuropathy

Contraindications
- Coexistent cancer (excluding squamous or basal cell carcinoma of skin)
- Severe infection
- Psychiatric disease (psychosis)
- Peripheral arteriopathy with infection
- Symptomatic coronary artery disease

Preoperative Investigations and Preparation for the Procedure

- Routine evaluation for transplantation with appropriate serum cross-match
- Evaluation of renal function unless on preoperative hemodialysis
- Clinical cardiovascular evaluation, further cardiac workup if clinically indicated
- Clinical exclusion of concurrent infection

Procedure

Back-table preparation

We prefer to completely prepare the pancreas for transplantation during cold ischemia. All connective tissues around the pancreas are divided with 2-0 or 4-0 silk ligatures placed close to the pancreas. The spleen is resected and the splenic vessels carefully ligated with 0 silk. The superior mesenteric artery and vein distal to the pancreatic vessels are divided in one of two ways: either with a vascular stapler close to the pancreas or by ligating the vessels with 0 silk and oversewing them with polypropylene running sutures. A 12-cm segment of the second portion of the duodenum containing the entrance of the pancreatic duct is isolated using a gastrointestinal stapler. The staple lines are oversewn for hemostasis with a running suture of resorbable suture. The portal vein is usually left short at the procurement; this permits a very short portal anastomosis, which decreases the risk of venous thrombosis. The mesenteric and splenic arteries are connected with use of a Y-graft from the donor iliac bifurcation with running sutures of 6-0 polypropylene. The graft is now ready for implantation.

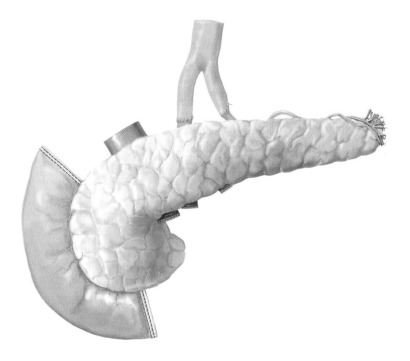

STEP 2   (A-1, A-2)

Access to the retroperitoneum for portocaval anastomosis is obtained with a midline incision. An Omnitract or Octopus retractor aids exposure. The cecum and right colon are mobilized medially to expose the vena cava. Care should be taken to avoid injury to the right ureter that may cross the iliac vessels on the right side at several different levels, either at the caval bifurcation or more laterally. The ureter is retracted laterally. During preparation of the vena cava for anastomosis (~5cm needed), the surgeon must remember the sacral vein located posteriorly, usually just cephalad to the iliac bifurcation. The right common iliac artery is prepared similarly. Lymphatic vessels should be ligated to avoid formation of a lymphocele.

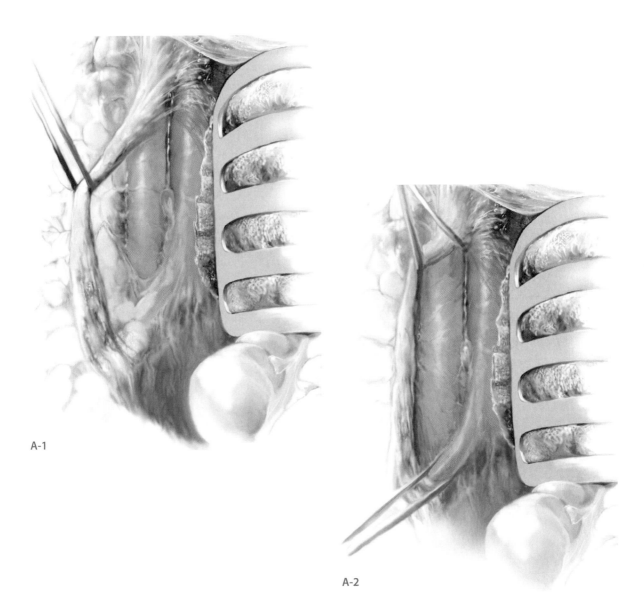

A-1

A-2

STEP 3   **Venous anastomosis (A-1, A-2)**

A Satinsky vascular clamp is placed on the vena cava for the venous anastomosis.
The type of clamp used on the common iliac artery depends on the site for anastomosis
and the presence/absence of arteriosclerosis, either a Satinsky clamp or two right angle
vascular clamps.

For the posterior aspect of the venous anastomosis, the cava is opened longitudinally
for 20–30 mm, corresponding to the size of the portal vein of the graft. A stay suture on
the left side of the opened vena cava maximizes exposure. After irrigating the lumen
with a heparin/saline solution, a 6-0 polypropylene running suture starts on the right
side of the cava and is carried around the posterior circumference. The technique for
the vascular anastomosis is also used for a portomesenteric venous anastomosis.

The anterior part of the anastomosis is performed next with the same running
suture, taking care not to include the posterior wall with the anterior suture layer.
Before completing the anastomosis by tying the two ends of the suture, a bulldog clamp
is placed on the portal vein and the anastomosis is tested by filling and distending the
cava and portal vein with a heparin/saline solution through a cannula. The bulldog
clamp should remain in place while the vascular clamp on the cava is removed.

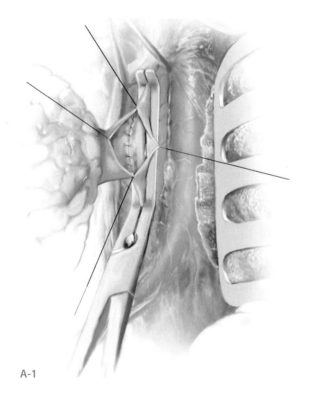

A-1

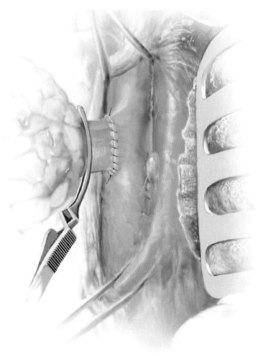

A-2

STEP 4   **Arterial anastomosis**

The right common iliac artery is opened, and a patch corresponding to the diameter
of the graft artery is resected. The vascular anastomosis is performed with two running
sutures of 6-0 polypropylene. A bulldog vascular clamp is placed on the arterial graft,
and the anastomosis is filled with heparin/saline solution.

After testing the arterial anastomosis for leak, the pancreas graft is ready to be
perfused. First, the venous clamp is removed and then the arterial one. The anesthesiologist should be warned about the possibility of cardiac dysrhythmias or hypotension
when the graft is first perfused. Also, it is not unusual for small vessels not ligated during
the back-table preparation to bleed during reperfusion; careful hemostasis is mandatory.

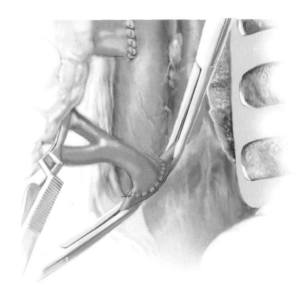

STEP 5   **Portomesenteric anastomosis**

Whenever possible, the venous anastomosis should be performed without an additional venous graft to decrease the risk of venous thrombosis. For this procedure, the colon is not mobilized. The small intestine is retracted to the left, and the superior mesenteric vein is located caudal to the transverse mesocolon. An incision is made about 20 mm lateral of the vein to allow a better control of this vein while positioning the pancreas graft. The venous anastomosis is performed with the same technique described above. For the arterial anastomosis, the common iliac artery is palpated medial to the ileocolic artery through the mesocolon, and the mesentery opened for 4–5 cm to expose the common iliac artery. The anastomosis is performed through the mesentery using the same technique as above.

This approach speeds the procedure and avoids complete mobilization of the right colon. The retroperitoneum is not opened, decreasing the risk of postoperative hemorrhage. Whether benefit is achieved through a portomesenteric versus systemic venous drainage is still debated.

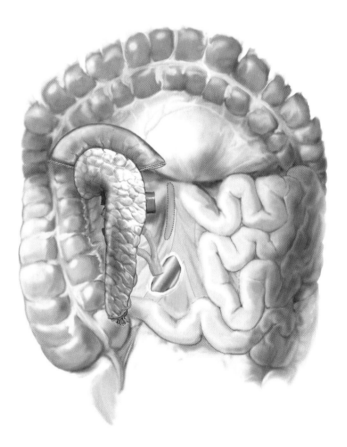

STEP 6

Duodenojejunostomy (A-1, A-2)

Exocrine drainage of the pancreas graft remains a major unsolved problem. The jejunum 40–50 cm distal to the ligament of Treitz is selected for a side-to-side duodeno-jejunostomy. With portomesenteric venous drainage, the entire graft is intraperitoneal. The anastomosis should be about 30–50 mm in length. The anastomosis is performed in two layers with the inner layer as a running 4-0 absorbable suture, including all layers of the gut wall. The outer layer is performed with interrupted 0 silk seromuscular sutures.

Second layer of the duodenal anastomosis: Once the running suture is achieved, the second layer of interrupted stitches of silk is performed. As an alternative, the second layer may be a running suture.

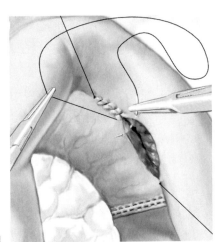

A-1

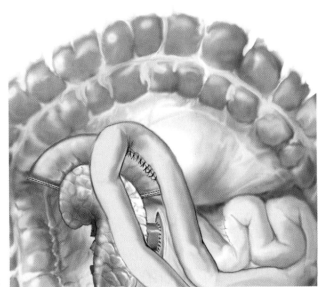

A-2

STEP 7   **Drainage and duodenal fixation**

An 18-Fr. closed suction drain is placed alongside the pancreas graft. The cecum is usually pexed or reperitonealized with either running or interrupted polypropylene sutures to avoid later cecal volvulus. Such lateral refixation is not necessary for portomesenteric venous drainage.

If a simultaneous kidney transplant is to be done, the same intra-abdominal access can be used to expose the iliac vessels transperitoneally or a separate contralateral retroperitoneal approach is an alternative.

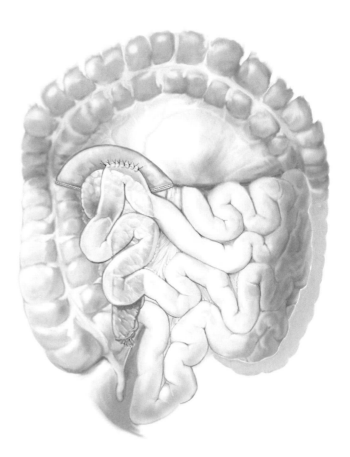

Postoperative Tests

The intraoperative glycemia monitoring shows usually normalization without additional insulin within 1–2h after the graft reperfusion.

■ Close postoperative management in an intensive or immediate care unit
■ Daily hemoglobin and kidney function
■ Blood sugar determination every 4h

Local Postoperative Complications

■ Short term:
    – Postoperative bleeding
    – Duodenal anastomotic leak
    – Ascites (R/O pancreatic ascites/anastomotic leak)
    – Portal vein graft thrombosis
    – Hypoglycemia
    – Acute rejection
    – Mild pancreatitis
■ Long term:
    – Chronic pancreas rejection
    – Adhesive small bowel obstruction

Tricks of the Senior Surgeon

■ Whenever possible, avoid the use of a venous graft on the donor portal vein.
■ Meticulous hemostasis at the end of the procedure is imperative to prevent delayed hemorrhage up to 2h after reperfusion.
■ The exocrine drainage must be tension-free, and the drainage catheter kept away from the anastomosis to avoid catheter erosion.

Chronic Pancreatitis

L. William Traverso (Proximal Pancreatectomy),
Charles F. Frey, Kathrin Mayer, Hans G. Beger, Bettina Rau, Wolfgang Schlosser
(Non-Anatomic Resections: The Frey and Beger Procedures)

Introduction

As our knowledge of the pathogenesis of pancreatitis-associated pain has matured and as experience with formal operative pancreatectomies has grown, the emphasis on operative treatment of patients with symptomatic chronic pancreatitis has switched from distal-based resections (60%→80%→95% pancreatectomies) to proximal based resections (pancreatoduodenectomy) and more recently to non-anatomic, duodenum-preserving subtotal resections. The following sections will address proximal and distal resections, respectively.

Proximal Pancreatectomy

L. William Traverso

The goals of a pylorus preserving Whipple procedure for chronic pancreatitis are twofold. The first goal is to remove the head of the pancreas, what Longmire referred to as the "pacemaker of pancreatitis", which serves as the source of chronic pain. In properly selected patients, relief of pain will occur in almost every patient, 75% of whom will remain pain-free. In the remaining patients, pain relief will have been achieved that yields substantial improvement that allows the patient to reenter daily life patterns.

The other goal is to minimize gastrointestinal dysfunction. To achieve the latter, the author has followed patients for over a decade to determine that these goals have been achieved using techniques described in this chapter. The anatomic approach is to preserve a *functioning* pylorus, the entire stomach, and the first 3–5 cm of the duodenum. Therefore, the neurovascular supply to the pylorus is protected and preserved by wide dissection; maintaining intact vagal innervation to the distal stomach appears to be mandatory for a functioning pylorus.

Indications and Contraindications

Indications **(Must Have All of Below)**	■ Disabling abdominal pain ■ Chronic pancreatitis – residual pancreatic damage, anatomic or functional, that persists even if the primary cause or other factors are eliminated ■ Cambridge Classification of Image Severity of "marked" chronic pancreatitis, i.e., main pancreatic duct stricture in head of gland (with or without stones, biliary stricture, or duodenal stenosis) or intrapancreatic head pseudocyst (with or without pseudoaneurysm) ■ Etiology has been remedied – gallstones or alcohol ■ Endotherapy failed with or without extracorporeal lithotripsy
Contraindications **(for Pylorus Preservation)**	■ Previous vagotomy and non-functional pylorus ■ Pancreatic cancer discovered intraoperatively in the area of the anterior superior head of gland ■ History of severe peptic ulcer disease ■ Occluded portal or superior mesenteric vein (SMV) (look for large collaterals in hepatoduodenal ligament on CT)

Preoperative Investigations and Preparation for the Procedure

■ The goal of imaging studies is to picture the anatomy, i.e., a "composite pancreas" from images of pancreas-protocol CT, endoscopic retrograde cholangiography (ERCP), and, if necessary, intraoperative pancreatography; if jaundiced, biliary decompression is usually indicated until bilirubin is almost normal.

■ Allow acute inflammation or infection to subside with minimally invasive drainage as necessary.

■ If CT shows an intrapancreatic pseudocyst in the head of the gland, arteriography is often indicated to investigate the presence of a pseudoaneurysm. If present, then preoperative embolization is needed.

■ Preoperative mechanical bowel preparation is used as are intravenous perioperative antibiotics.

Procedure: Pancreatoduodenectomy

STEP 1

Incision and mobilization, duodenum, pylorus, antrum (A-1, A-2)

An upper midline incision from the xiphoid to just below the umbilicus gives optimal exposure.

A mechanical retractor elevates and retracts the costal margins (Fowler retractor, Pilling Surgical, Horsham, PA) and an articulating Martin Arm retractor (Elmed, Inc., Addison, IL) retracts the liver off the hepatoduodenal ligament.

Division of the round ligament with excision of the abdominal portion optimizes exposure.

The duodenum is mobilized with a wide Kocher maneuver arounds to the superior mesenteric artery.

Next, the lesser sac is opened by dissecting the omentum rostrally off the transverse colon, leaving it attached to the stomach.

Wide dissection frees the cephalad superior surface of the duodenal bulb and pylorus from the hepatoduodenal ligament and the dorsal inferior surface from the head of the pancreas, right gastroepiploic artery, and the nest of veins entering the right gastroepiploic vein on the surface of the SMV. The neurovascular supply to the pylorus rostral and caudal to the duodenal bulb is carefully protected and preserved.

The following blood vessels are divided at their origins away from the pylorus: right gastric artery (if present, usually not one major vessel), superior duodenal vessels of Wilkie, and the gastroepiploic artery and vein at the inferior border of the pancreas.

Dissection of the duodenal bulb is continued for 3–5 cm to the junction of the first portion of the duodenum to the area where the duodenum and pancreas merge, to form an "angle"; distal to the angle, tiny shared blood vessels are encountered between the pancreas and duodenum.

The duodenum is divided with a stapling device at this angle; the stomach and stapled first part of the duodenum are now mobile and retracted toward the left upper quadrant.

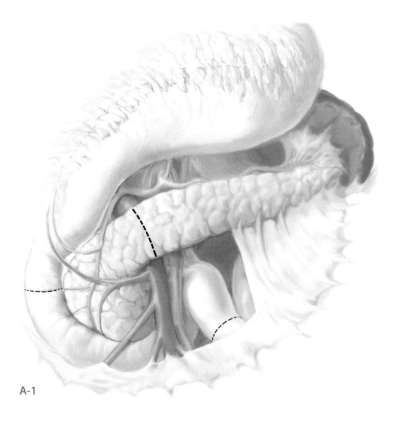

A-1

Incision and mobilization, duodenum, pylorus, antrum (A-1, A-2)

After placing stay-sutures along the superior and inferior edges of the neck of the pancreas, a plane is developed carefully behind the neck of the pancreas, but anterior to the superiormesenteric portal venous confluence. The neck of the pancreas is then divided carefully. In score patients with severe chronic inflammation, this maneuver may be very difficult.

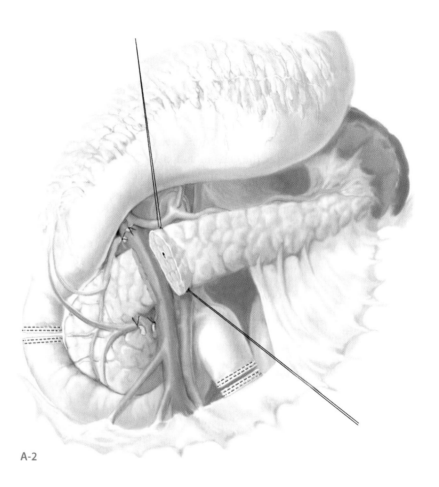

A-2

STEP 2   **Excision of pancreatic head, remaining duodenum, and distal common bile duct**

This resection is no different than resection for cancer except that nodal tissue along the right side of the superior mesenteric artery is not necessarily removed with the specimen. The uncinate process can be clamped on its surface to separate it from the SMV and the first jejunal vein that enters this area. To decrease blood loss, the surgeon on the left side of the patient compresses the pancreatic head and uncinate process between the fingers of the left hand to control vessels in lymphatic attachments to the superior mesenteric artery behind the portal vein.

Electrocautery is avoided when dividing the main pancreatic duct over the portal vein; cautery or harmonic scalpel (Ethicon Endosurgery, Cincinnati, OH) is useful in dividing the parenchyma.

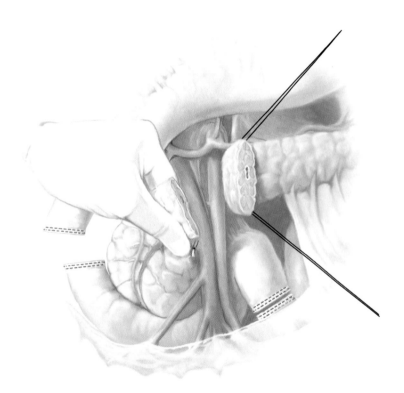

STEP 3   **Preparation of neoduodenum (A-1, A-2)**

Using a harmonic scalpel, the mesenteric vascular attachments to the proximal jejunum are divided; the jejunum is divided with a stapler 6–8 cm distal to the ligament of Treitz.

The avascular portion of the transverse mesocolon is opened just to the left of the middle colic vein.

The defect in the ligament of Treitz is closed to avoid internal hernia.

An intraoperative fluoroscopic pancreatogram of the pancreatic remnant is obtained if this area of the duct was not visualized by preoperative ERCP. A partial longitudinal incision with lateral pancreaticojejunostomy may be indicated to the body and tail of the gland if chain-of-lake strictures are seen on pancreatography.

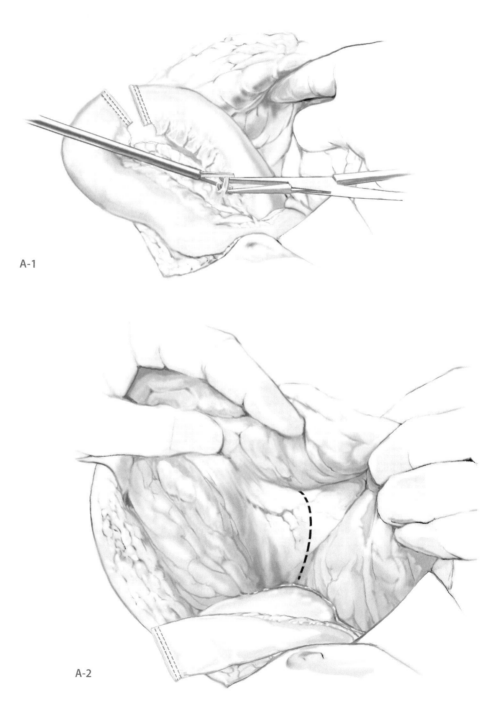

A-1

A-2

STEP 4

Reconstruction – pancreatic anastomosis

Pancreatic and biliary anastomoses are retrocolic; the duodenojejunostomy is antecolic; anastomoses are positioned to isolate potential leakage of bile and pancreatic anastomoses from the duodenojejunostomy to minimize delayed gastric emptying (8% in my last 215 resections).

The stump of the proximal jejunum is delivered into the supracolic space through a retrocolic defect in the mesocolon; the stomach with the preserved pylorus and duodenal bulb is brought antecolic over the left transverse colon, allowing for an anatomically remote duodenojejunostomy.

Patients with a normal 2- to 3-mm duct in the pancreatic remnant are more prone to anastomotic leak at the pancreaticojejunostomy.

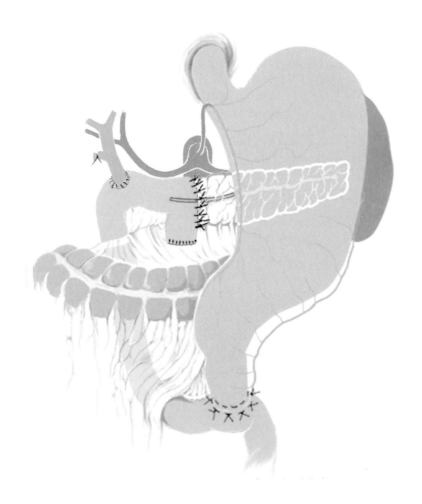

STEP 5   **Pancreaticojejunostomy**

The technique of the pancreaticojejunostomy involves a seromuscular envelope containing a stented, end-to-side, mucosa-to-mucosa anastomosis using optical magnification.

First the back wall of the outer 3/0 silk sutures is placed and tied anteriorly. A small enterotomy is made in the jejunal mucosa opposite the pancreatic duct (A-1, A-2). The mucosa-to-mucosa anastomosis is created with interrupted 6-0 polyglycolic suture with the knots tied on the outside of this inner layer. Exact placement of the mucosal suture is key and is performed using a ×12.5 surgical microscope (A-3). A 4-cm-long, 3-Fr. polytetrafluoroethylene, radiodense stent with multiple holes throughout the stent (Geenan stent – Wilson-Cook Medical, Inc. Winston-Salem, NC) is inserted into the duct just before placing the last (anterior) mucosa-to-mucosa stitch. Using 6-0 polyglycolic acid suture, the stent is attached loosely in its mid portion to the jejunal mucosa near the last anterior stitch. This stent, which insures apposition of mucosa and decompresses the pancreatic duct upstream from the mucosal sutures, passes spontaneously in about 2 weeks and can be checked for position with an abdominal X-ray; an anterior outer layer of 3-0 silk completes the anastomosis (A-4).

If chain-of-lakes-type ductal dilation is present in the remnant pancreas, then a longitudinal side-to-side technique is used (A-5).

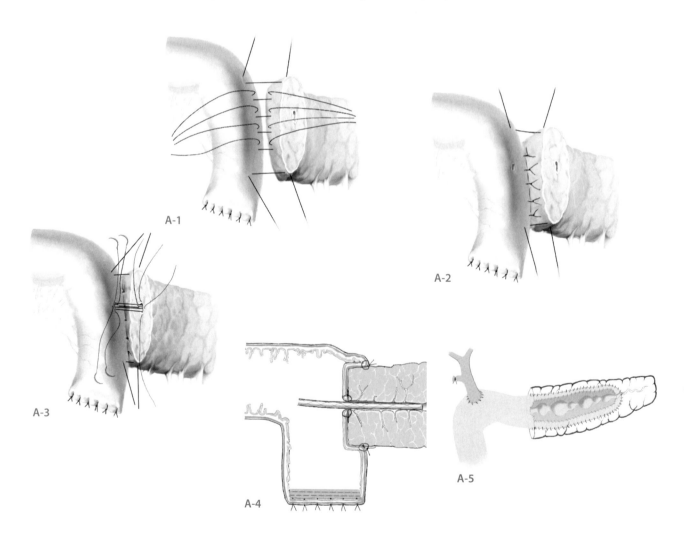

A-1

A-2

A-3

A-4

A-5

STEP 6   **Biliary anastomosis**

A single layer, end choledocho-to-side jejunal anastomosis is performed with inter-rupted 5-0 polydioxone with knots tied on the outside (to prevent stone formation on knots of delayed absorbable suture); no tube choledochostomy is needed.

The jejunal limb is tacked to the exit site through the transverse mesocolon with 3/0 silk sutures.

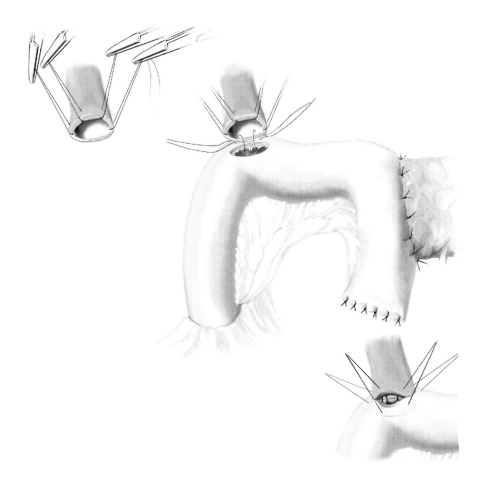

STEP 7

Antecolic duodenojejunostomy

The intact stomach, first part of the duodenum, and omentum are brought over the left side of the transverse colon. The jejunal limb (after it exits the transverse mesocolon downstream from the biliary and pancreatic anastomoses) is brought up to the end of the stapled duodenum, and an end duodenal-to-side jejunal anastomosis is performed in two layers 10 cm distal to the exit site of the jejunum from the transverse mesocolon. An inner layer of running 3-0 polyglycolic acid and an outer layer of interrupted 3-0 silk are put in place.

A 15-Fr. drainage catheter is placed under the biliary and pancreatic anastomoses from the right upper quadrant.

The midline fascia is closed with an interrupted figure-of-eight 0 polyglyconate suture.

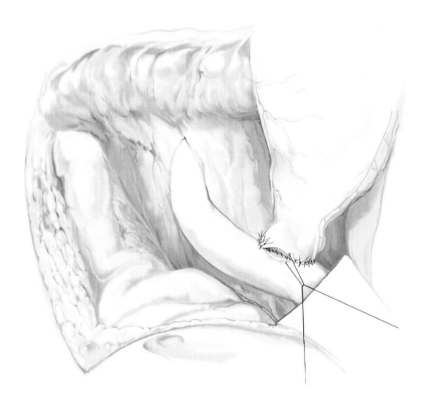

Postoperative Care

- The NG tube is removed 1–3 days postoperatively.
- Drains are removed when drainage volume is <30–50 ml/day with low amylase activity.
- Oral intake is allowed when tolerated.
- Early:
  - Intra-abdominal hemorrhage– examine specifically ligatures of named arteries for pseudoaneurysms and pancreatic remnant
  - GI hemorrhage – either from pancreaticojejunostomy or duodenojejunostomy
  - Delayed gastric emptying
  - Anastomotic leak – most likely at pancreaticojejunostomy but possible at choledochojejunostomy and duodenojejunostomy
  - Intra-abdominal abscess, usually related to transient or persistent anastomotic leak
  - Wound infection
  - Intestinal obstruction – exclude internal hernia
- Late:
  - Recurrent epigastric pain
  - Extrahepatic jaundice secondary to stricture at choledochojejunostomy
  - Pancreatic insufficiency either from progression of disease (chronic pancreatitis) or stricture at pancreaticojejunostomy
  - Adhesive intestinal obstruction
  - Stomal or duodenal ulcer at or near duodenojejunostomy
  - Pancreatic adenocarcinoma, estimated as high as up to 1% risk per year

Tricks of the Senior Surgeon

- The key to pain relief for chronic pancreatitis is pancreatic resection performed when the strict anatomic selection criteria described in this section are met.
- Excess blood loss results in increased morbidity. To accomplish this, all named vessels are triply ligated with non-absorbable suture. The ultrasonic scissors are utilized for dividing small veins and particularly those around the right gastroepiploic and supraduodenal vessels. This technique is also handy when separating the mesenteric vascular attachments to the proximal jejunum removed with the specimen in the area of the ligament of Treitz.
- The left hand of the surgeon standing on the left side of the patient can minimize blood loss during division of the attachments of the vascular lymphatics from the dorsal head of the pancreas to the area around the superior mesenteric artery. Pedicles of tissue are divided as the dissection proceeds along the superior mesenteric artery. Only one clamp is used for each pedicle on the patient side of the divided pedicle; the specimen side is not clamped and is compressed by the left hand.
- Preserve all of the greater omentum as this "watchdog" of the abdomen decreases postoperative infection.
- Use intraoperative fluoroscopic pancreatography to ensure that the pancreatic remnant is adequately drained. I use a cholangiocatheter with a balloon tip.
- When a small pancreatic duct is used for the pancreaticojejunostomy, the anastomosis is best done with magnification to avoid crossing the sutures. The duct-to-mucosa anastomoses can be done in a more exact fashion by seeing the needle pass in and out of a small pancreatic duct. I find the surgical microscope at 12.5 power useful to minimize pancreaticojejunostomy leak.
- The choledochojejunostomy should have all of the absorbable knots tied on the outside, and no absorbable suture should be exposed to bile flow.
- I use a single closed suction drain made of silicone rubber.
- An antecolic duodenojejunostomy has a marked decrease in delayed gastric emptying compared to the retrocolic method.

Non-Anatomic Resections:
The Frey and Beger Procedures

Charles F. Frey, Kathrin Mayer, Hans G. Beger, Bettina Rau, Wolfgang Schlosser

Introduction

Local (non-anatomic) resections of the head of the pancreas with longitudinal pancreaticojejunostomy (LR-LPY or Frey procedure) and the duodenum-preserving (anatomic) subtotal head resection (Beger procedure) share similar goals, i.e., relief of pain and management of local pancreatic complications (biliary, duodenal, or venous obstruction, provision of pancreatic ductal drainage, subtotal resection of inflammatory mass in head of pancreas). The rationale for this approach is that the pain of chronic pancreatitis is believed to arise from either a ductal or pancreatic parenchymal hypertensive "compartment" syndrome and/or from inflammatory neural "irritation". The head of the pancreas is thought to be the driver or "pacemaker" of the pain. Pancreatic subtotal resections can accomplish removal of the "pain pacemaker" region of the gland with a lesser operative morbidity as well as preserve gastroduodenal continuity.

Indications and Contraindications

Indications

- Incapacitating abdominal pain, usually of a continuous nature, and in selected patients also when intermittent and frequent or associated with recurrent attacks of acute pancreatitis
- Resolution of pancreatic and extrapancreatic structural complications associated with chronic pancreatitis
  - Extrapancreatic – common bile duct obstruction, duodenal obstruction, selected patients with compression of portal and/or superior mesenteric veins
  - Pancreatic
    - Parenchymal: scarring, multiple fibrous strictures of duct ("chain of lakes") with calcification, ductal hypertension, retention cysts, ductal stones
    - Ductal disruptions: contained – pseudocyst; uncontained – ascites; fistula – pleural or pericardial
- Inadequate pain relief after ductal drainage procedure or distal pancreatectomy
- Pancreas divisum causing chronic pancreatitis

Contraindications

■ Absolute contraindications:
  - Findings which raise concern of potential malignancy are absence of history of alcoholism, hyperlipidemia, hyperparathyroidism, recent history of onset of pain, and increased serum CA 19–9 level
  - If cancer cannot be excluded, a resective operation is suggested, i.e., pancreato duodenectomy or distal pancreatectomy
  - Complete thrombosis of superior mesenteric/portal venous junction with peripancreatic varices
■ Relative contraindications:
  - Disease limited to the body and tail of gland (infrequent)
  - Unrelenting narcotic addition or when the patient refuses the concept of postoperative detoxification
  - Inability to manage possible postoperative diabetes mellitus due to anticipated poor compliance
  - Obstruction of superior mesenteric/portal vein junction with mild to moderate portal hypertension

Other Considerations
not

■ The "small" pancreatic duct (<3–4 mm) in the head, body, or tail of the pancreas is

a contraindication.
■ Ducts in the pancreatic head (body or tail) are either resected or unroofed and thereby decompressed; a jejunal Roux limb can be sewn to the pancreatic capsule.

Preoperative Investigations and Preparation for the Procedure

- Exclude non-pancreatic pain.
- Maximize medical treatment including nutrition, enzyme replacement, and cessation of alcohol intake.
- Assess the extent of chemical dependency (narcotics, alcohol).
- Strive for a preoperative commitment to undergo postoperative alcohol and/or drug rehabilitation.

Preoperative Investigation

- History:
  - Exclude alcohol or drug addiction, gallstones, pancreatitis-inducing medications, hyperparathyroidism, hypercalcemia, and hyperlipidemia
  - Evaluate for steatorrhea and diabetes mellitus (glucose intolerance), especially the need for insulin
  - Severity of pain (Likert visual analog pain scale completed by patient)
  - Psychosocial stability
  - Quality of life survey (optional)
    - European Organization for Research and Treatment of Cancer QLQ-C30 (EORTC)
    - Medical Outcomes Trust Short-Form 36 (MOS SF-36)
  - Impact of pain on employment, family support, daily activities
- Clinical evaluation:
  - Jaundice, ascites, nutritional status, weight, physiologic health, co-morbidities
  - Baseline pancreatic exocrine and endocrine function if indicated
- Laboratory tests:
  - CA 19–9 (most useful if common bile duct patent), LFTs, HbAIC, glucose tolerance test
  - Fecal fat and secretin studies are only required rarely
  - Imaging
  - Triphasic helical CT to evaluate for:
    - Pancreatic masses
    - Portal and left-sided hypertension or thrombosis of the splenic vein
    - Involvement of adjacent organs
    - Extrapancreatic causes of pancreatitis (cholelithiasis)
  - ERCP to evaluate pancreatic and biliary ductal systems and esophagogastroduodenoscopy to exclude peptic ulcer disease
  - Endoscopic or intraoperative ultrasonography to evaluate for vascular involvement and biopsy if indicated

Preparation for the Procedure

- Broad spectrum, perioperative prophylactic antibiotics
- Full bowel preparation

Procedure: Local Resection of the Head of the Pancreas with Longitudinal Pancreaticojejunostomy (The Frey Procedure)

STEP 1

Exposure and exploration; assessment and mobilization of pancreas; entering the lesser sac

A bilateral subcostal incision is suitable for most patients; a midline incision from xiphoid to umbilicus is better for patients with vertically oriented costal arches.

Dividing the gastrocolic ligament between hepatic and splenic flexures exposes the lesser sac.

The right gastroepiploic artery and vein are ligated and divided to expose the anterior surface of the head and neck of the pancreas.

Cephalad retraction of the stomach and caudad retraction of the transverse colon expose the body and tail of the pancreas.

The inferior border of the body and tail of the pancreas are mobilized to completely expose the anterior surface of the pancreas.

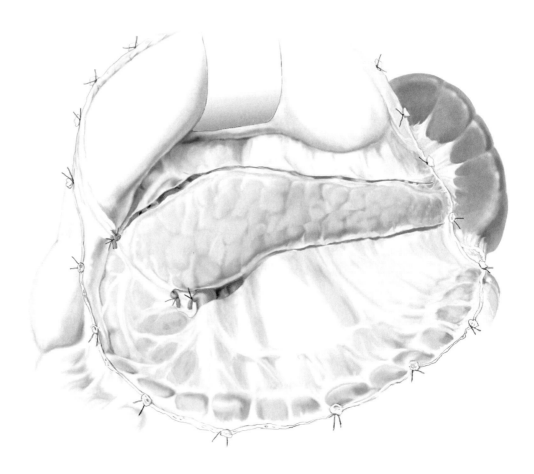

STEP 2   **Exposure of the head of pancreas**

The duodenum and head of pancreas are mobilized by an extended Kocher maneuver; this maneuver allows manual palpation of both sides of the pancreatic head to determine the thickness and consistency and to rule out a pancreatic mass.

The gastroduodenal artery may be encircled with a vessel loop should ligation be necessary for hemostasis (rare) during resection of the head of the gland.

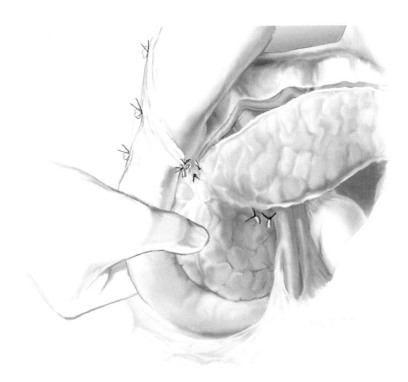

STEP 3   **Exposure of the SMV alongside the head of the pancreas**

Importantly, it is not necessary to free the portal vein beneath the neck of the pancreas.

The SMV should be exposed adjacent to the head and uncinate process of the pancreas to provide optimal exposure.

Exposing the head and uncinate process is important not only for the coring out process, but also to provide an adequate rim of pancreatic tissue to which the Roux-en-Y jejunal limb is to be sewn.

Free up the small veins and arteries from the head side of the SMV (arteriovenous tributaries).

Divide the venous tributaries to the SMV from the third portion of the duodenum inferiorly; note that the inferior pancreatoduodenal artery on occasion may run anterior rather than posterior to the SMV.

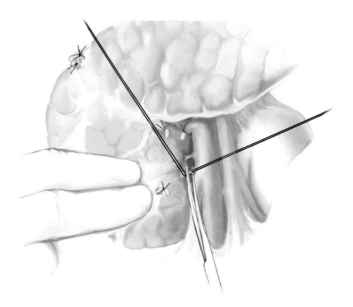

STEP 4 **Locating the main pancreatic duct (A-1, A-2)**

To find the pancreatic duct, the main duct in the body of pancreas is usually located eccentrically, closer to the superior border and deeper toward the posterior surface of the gland.

If large, the duct may bulge from the anterior aspect of the gland or, if smaller, palpated or balloted as a "groove" along the long axis of the gland.

To identify a small duct, we connect a 10-ml syringe to a 23-gauge butterfly needle aiming obliquely and posteriorly in the suspected direction of the duct; avoid the neck of the pancreas when searching/aspirating to minimize injury to the underlying SMV; aspiration of clear fluid is an indication the duct has been located.

Measure duct pressure by connecting the needle to the manometer; in our experience, average pancreatic ductal pressure in chronic pancreatitis patients is 33 cmH$_2$O (range: 20–47 cmH$_2$O), in contrast to a normal ductal pressure of ~10 cmH$_2$O.

Leave the needle in the duct.

The duct of Wirsung in the neck of the pancreas is usually eccentric and slightly superior and posterior (closer to the SMV/portal vein).

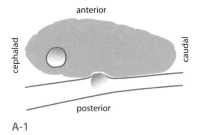

A-1

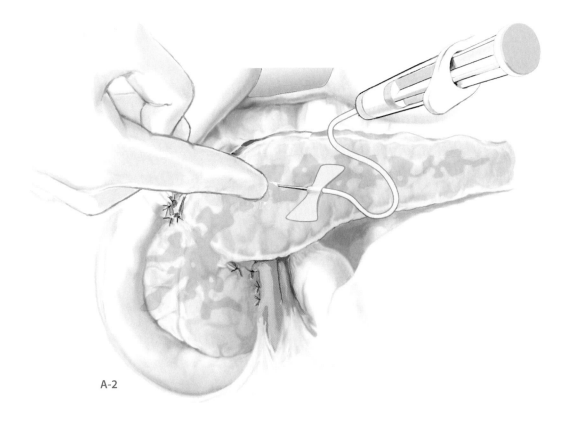

A-2

STEP 5   **Opening the pancreatic ductal system**

The anterior capsule of the pancreas is incised directly over the guide needle using electrocautery; a right-angle clamp is used to probe and define the direction of the duct.

The anterior aspect of the duct is opened to within 1.5 cm of the tail of the gland; the duct is opened in the opposite direction toward the duodenal wall, along the duct of Wirsung, and extended to within 0.5–1 cm of the ampulla of Vater (A-1).

The duct, after it crosses the portal vein, plunges posteriorly and then inferior-laterally, coursing in the head close to the posterior capsule of the gland.

The duct to the uncinate process from the duct of Wirsung (mid-head) also runs close to the posterior capsule of the gland and is opened using a right angle clamp to define the direction of the duct (A-2).

Pancreatic calculi in side branches are searched for, and all encountered in any ductal systems are removed.

To assess ampullary patency and the adequacy of head resection, the surgeon places a probe (a 2–3 mm Bakes dilator or the tip of the curved clamp) in the opened duct of Wirsung and pushes it against a finger indenting the duodenum.

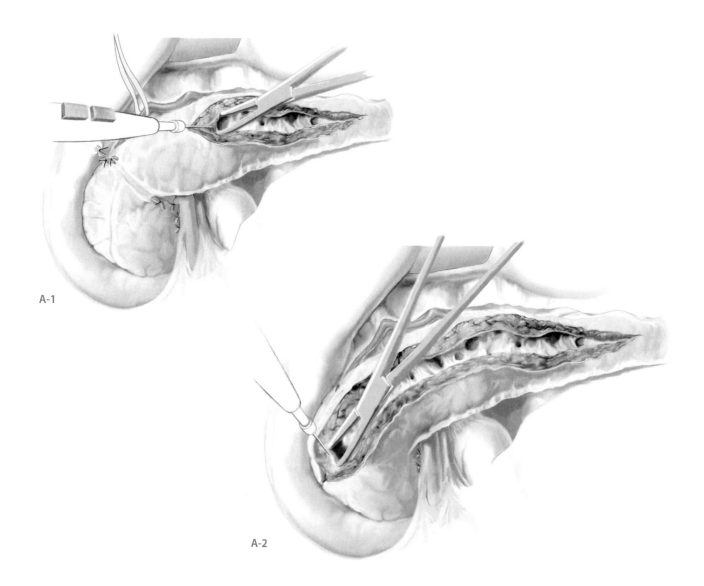

A-1

A-2

STEP 5 *(continued)*

Opening the pancreatic ductal system

The clamp should pass through the ampulla into the duodenum (A-3).

The pancreatic head containing the ampullary portion of the pancreatic duct invaginates into the duodenum; looking down from above on the anterior surface of the gland, the pancreaticoduodenal junction is *not* a guide to locating the ampulla.

The ampulla is 2–3 cm more lateral and posterior due to invagination of the pancreatic head into the duodenum. This consideration is important, because failure to the open main pancreatic duct down to the duodenum will leave a significant portion of the main pancreatic duct of Wirsung in the head of pancreas undrained along with its tributary ducts; the thicker the head of pancreas, the longer the undrained portion of pancreatic duct. This situation occurs when the anterior surface of the pancreatoduodenal junction is used as a guide to the position of the ampulla; unexcised small retention cysts associated with tributary ducts located deep within the fibrotic head of pancreas may be a source of persistent pain (A-4).

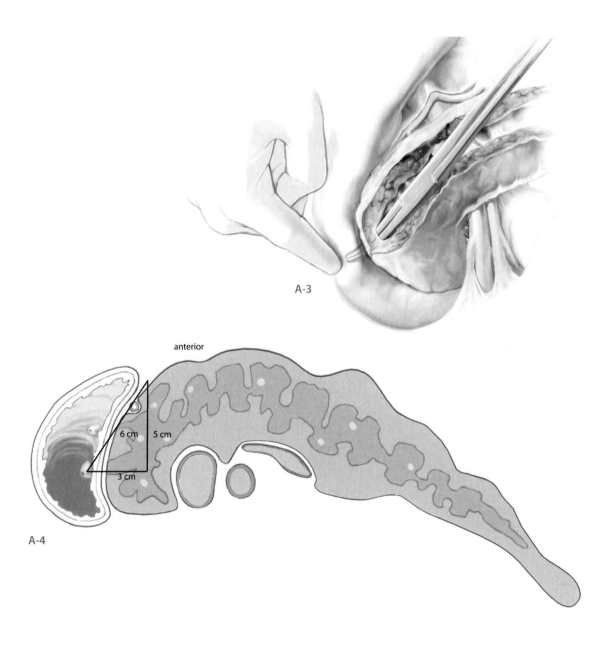

A-3

anterior

6 cm   5 cm

3 cm

A-4

Local resection of the head of the pancreas

Working onward from the opened pancreatic duct, full-thickness slices of pancreatic tissue are excised to remove the anterior capsule of the gland and all intervening parenchyma down to the duct of Wirsung; thickness of the remaining shell of the head of the pancreas is carefully assessed after each slice to determine the amount of tissue that needs to be removed.

The posterior wall of the pancreatic duct of Wirsung in the head of pancreas marks the posterior extension of resection because it is within a few millimeters of the posterior capsule of the gland.

The duct of Santorini and its tributaries are located anteriorly in the pancreatic head; these ducts and tissue anteriorly are excised. In contrast, the duct to the uncinate process and its tributaries and the duct of Wirsung lie posterior; these systems should be unroofed but not excised as the posterior capsule of pancreas might be breached and the retroperitoneum exposed.

Careful palpation of the cored-out head of the pancreas helps identify retention cysts or impacted calculi in tributary ducts that should be removed.

Only a rim of pancreatic tissue should be left anteriorly along the inner aspect of the duodenal curve and a margin of 5–10mm of pancreatic tissue to the right of the SMV to avoid vascular injury; care should be taken to preserve the pancreatoduodenal arcade.

Based on the weight of excised tissue, approximately 4–12g of fibrotic tissue should be removed. This is an underestimate of the total tissue removed; additional tissue is vaporized when taking multiple slices.

Should there be concern about possible malignancy, tissue should be submitted for frozen section, histopathologic examination; if positive, pancreatoduodenectomy should be performed.

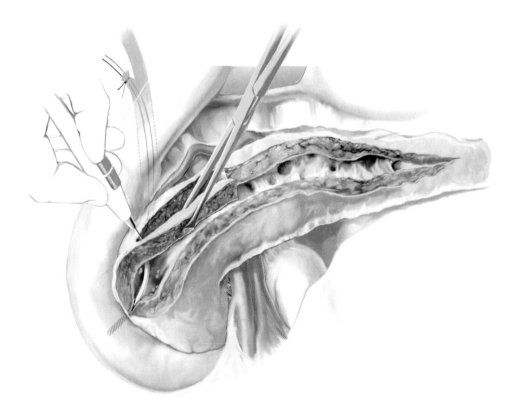

STEP 7   **Managing and avoiding injury to the common bile duct (CBD) – avoiding injury**

About 50 % of patients with chronic pancreatitis have radiographic evidence of anatomic tortuosity, kinking, and narrowing of CBD; with significant stricturing, 10 % of patients undergoing head resection have preoperative findings of CBD obstruction – biochemical or clinical jaundice.

During the coring out process, it is important to identify and free the intrapancreatic portion of the CBD from the inflamed, fibrotic periductal tissue.

The position of the CBD in the posterior pancreas is variable and either may be posterior to the pancreas, indenting the pancreas (on palpation a "groove" may be discerned), or traversing the pancreatic parenchyma; the latter site is most commonly associated with stricturing.

In patients with anatomic obstruction, a 3-mm Bakes dilator or biliary Fogarty® catheter is passed into the CBD to guide and protect the CBD during pancreatic resection.

If the CBD is injured or strictured or the obstruction is unable to be relieved, a choledochojejunostomy is an option.

An alternative method for coring out the head of the pancreas is excavation of the head with total resection of the main and secondary ducts. The ductal system is followed to the level of the ampulla or to where the pancreatic duct meets the intrapancreatic CBD; the pancreatic duct is divided; the proximal duct margin is sewn closed with a 4-0 nylon suture. Use of the Cavitron R Ultrasonic Aspirator (CUSA), System 200 (Valleylab, Norwalk, CT), facilitates conical removal of parenchyma in conjunction with electrocautery; the high-energy hand-piece at a setting of 70–80 % power permits clear visualization of tissue, ducts, and vessels in the head of pancreas. The proximal pancreatic duct is removed in total by transecting the dorsal duct at the pancreatic neck.

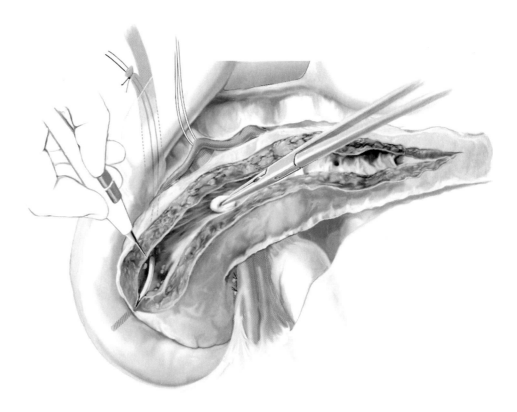

STEP 8   **Thumb-index measurement for depth**

The duct of Wirsung guides the proper depth of excavation/resection, ducts of Wirsung and the uncinate process are adjacent to the posterior capsule and are opened (decompressed); the duct of Santorini is excised.

   A limited cuff of pancreatic tissue may be left between the cored-out head of the pancreas and duodenum. Sufficient pancreatic tissue usually remains to preserve the important pancreatoduodenal arcade, which maintains the viability of the mid-duodenum.

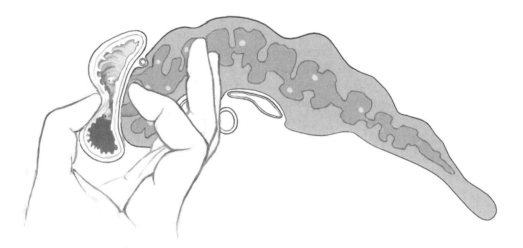

STEP 9

Reconstruction with Roux-en-Y drainage of the head of the pancreas with pancreaticojejunostomy – the outer layer of the anastomosis

The Roux limb is brought through the transverse mesocolon to lie over the entire pancreas.

A two-layer pancreaticojejunostomy is performed with an outer layer of interrupted, Lembert 3-0 silk sutures, approximating the jejunal serosa to the capsule of the pancreas; the wall of the duodenum may be included with the pancreas in this layer. Inflammation and edema may render distinction between the duodenum and the pancreas less well-defined.

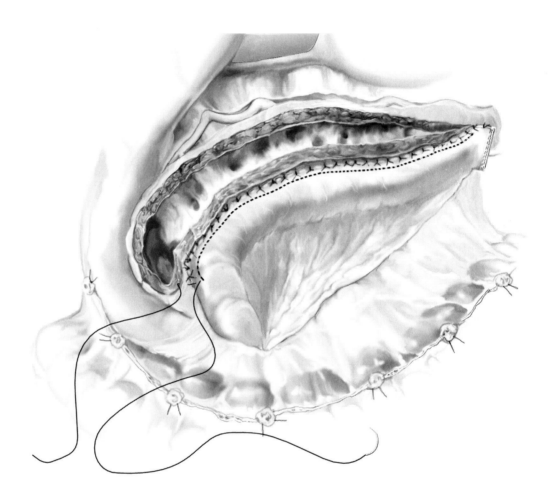

STEP 10   **Pancreaticojejunostomy – inner layer of anastomosis**

A running, 3-0 absorbable suture attaches the full thickness of the jejunum to the cut surface of the pancreas along the capsule, continuing along the cored-out head of pancreas; a formal pancreatic duct-to-jejunal anastomosis is not necessary.

Sewing the jejunum to the capsule of pancreas rather than to the pancreatic duct allows decompression of the ducts as small as 2–3 mm in diameter (relief of the pancreatic compartment syndrome).

If only the pancreatic head is diseased or if the patient has had a distal pancreatectomy, then only a coring out of the head is necessary with the head drained into the Roux limb.

The jejunal Roux limb is anchored to the transverse mesocolon to prevent internal herniation.

Continuity of the GI tract is reestablished by end-to-side jejunojejunostomy 60–70 cm distal to the pancreaticojejunostomy; all mesenteric defects are closed.

No drain is needed unless a choledochotomy has been performed.

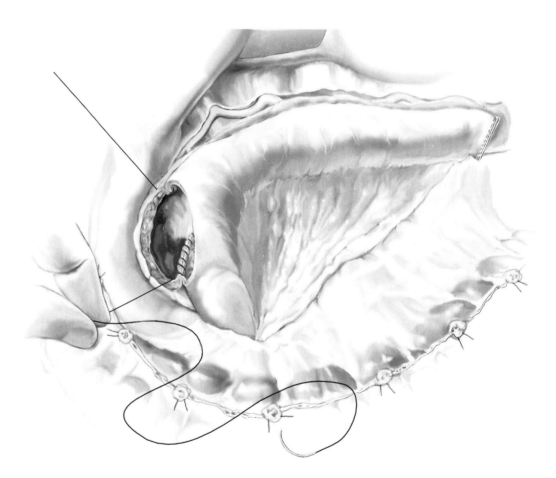

Procedure: Non-Anatomic Duodenum-Preserving Head Resection (The Beger Procedure)

Duodenum-preserving pancreatic head resection was first described by Beger in 1979. The aim of the operation is a subtotal resection of the pancreatic head with removal of the inflammatory mass while preserving the duodenum, extrahepatic common bile duct, gallbladder, and stomach, as well as preserving a portion of the pancreatic parenchyma of the head of the gland.

STEP 1

The head of the pancreas is exposed by dividing the gastrocolic ligament, with care taken to avoid injury to the gastroepiploic vessels. The duodenocolic ligament is transected and the transverse colon handled carefully. Subsequently, a Kocher maneuver is performed. Exposure of the portal vein and the superior mesenteric veins at the inferior margin of the pancreas follows.

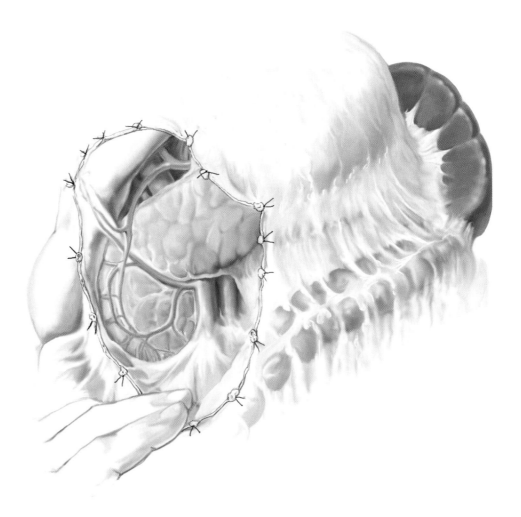

STEP 2

Ligation of feeding vessels

The gastroduodenal artery is ligated at the upper margin of the body of the pancreas. The common hepatic artery is prepared and banded with a loop. The common bile duct is exposed circumferentially at the upper margin of the pancreas in the hepatoduodenal ligament. Next, the plane between the anterior surface of the portal vein and the posterior aspect of the pancreatic head is developed either from above the neck of the gland starting at the portal vein or more commonly starting from below the neck of the gland at the superior mesenteric vein. This maneuver can be quite difficult, especially in cases of inflammatory and edematous reaction in the head of the pancreas.

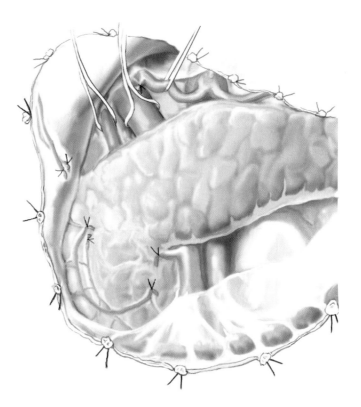

STEP 3

Transection of the neck of the pancreas

The subtotal resection of the pancreatic head is begun by transecting the neck of the
gland, starting near the duodenal edge of the portal vein in a sagittal plane as shown.
At the cut surface of the left pancreas, meticulous hemostasis using non-absorbable
5-0 or 6-0 monofilament sutures is mandatory.

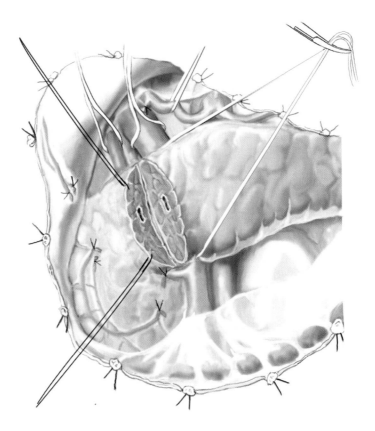

STEP 4   **Subtotal excision of the head of gland**

The head of the pancreas is rotated ventroinferiorly. This can be achieved by bluntly freeing the head of the pancreas from the portal vein. Small branches entering the portal vein directly must be ligated and divided. The head of the pancreas is released from the retroportal region with little technical difficulty as long as individual dissection of the vessels entering into the portal vein proceeds meticulously. Also, the pancreatic parenchyma is transected along the left lateral wall of the intrapancreatic portion of the distal common bile duct toward the papilla.

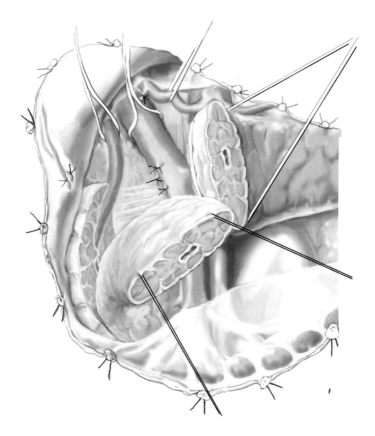

STEP 5

Subtotal resection of the pancreatic head is completed by including the tissue of the uncinate process. It is not necessary to preserve the gastroduodenal artery for adequate blood supply to the duodenum because the supraduodenal vessels, as well as duodenal vessels arising from the superior mesenteric artery, maintain sufficient perfusion of the duodenal wall. In most patients it is not difficult to dissect the pancreatic tissue along the wall of the intrapancreatic portion of the common bile duct towards the papilla and further down including the uncinate process. Removal of fibrotic tissue along the common bile duct results in decompression of the duct in most patients. In patients with inflammation in the wall of the common bile duct, the duct is opened by an incision in the lateral wall for an internal biliary bypass. After subtotal resection of the pancreatic head, a 5- to 8-mm shell-like remnant of the pancreatic head between the common bile duct and the duodenal wall remains.

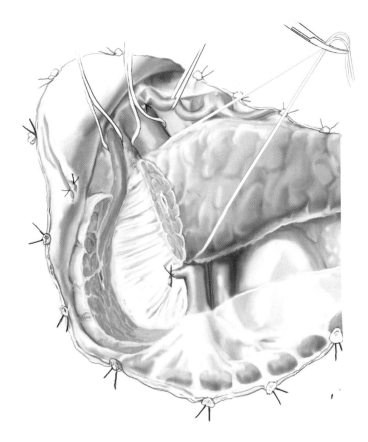

STEP 6 ## Pancreaticojejunostomy

Reconstruction after subtotal resection of the head of the pancreas is initiated by transecting the upper jejunum 40 cm distal to the ligament of Treitz. The Roux-en-Y jejunal limb is brought through a retrocolic mesenteric defect. An end-to-side anastomosis between the left pancreas and jejunum is performed (Warren-Cattell). In this instance, a duct-to-mucosa anastomosis between the pancreatic duct and the jejunal mucosa is performed first. The anastomosis is completed with a single-layer seromuscular suture between the jejunum and the capsule of the left pancreas.

A side-to-side anastomosis is made between the jejunal limb and the remnant of the pancreatic head for 5–8 cm. The jejunal incision for this anastomosis is 4–8 cm long. A single-layer anastomosis between the jejunum and the pancreas along the incision line serves as the inner layer; the outer layer is performed between the pancreatic capsule and the seromuscularis of the jejunum. For restoration of intestinal continuity, an enteroenterostomy is carried out 40 cm distal to the pancreaticojejunal anastomosis.

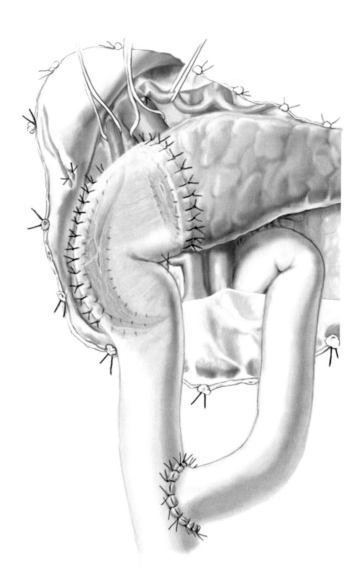

STEP 7   **Choledochojejunostomy**

For patients with a wide distal pancreatic body/tail remnant, an end-to-side pancreato-jejunostomy may be better. Similarly, the intrapancreatic protion of the common bile duct can be opened in the proximal pancreatic head remnant and included in the prox-imal side-to-side pancreatojejunostomy.

An additional anastomosis between the suprastenotic portion of the common bile duct and the jejunal limb is can be carried out in patients in whom the subtotal resec-tion of the head of the pancreas has not resulted in complete decompression of the intrapancreatic common bile duct and also when intraoperative examination reveals fibrotic involvement of the common bile duct proximal to the papilla. The side-to-side anastomosis between the common bile duct and the jejunum is sutured using a single-layer technique. In these patients, cholecystectomy is strongly suggested.

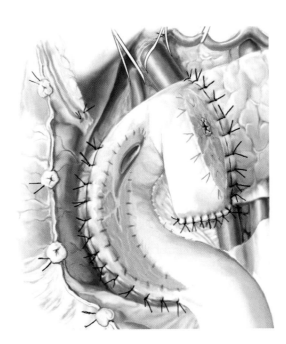

STEP 8   **Modification of pancreaticojejunostomy**

In patients with a dilated pancreatic duct or stenosis, the main pancreatic duct is incised longitudinally on its anterior surface extending toward the tail. In these patients, a side-to-side anastomosis is made between the jejunum and the longitudinally incised pancreas, similar to the Partington-Rochelle procedure (see page 758-761).

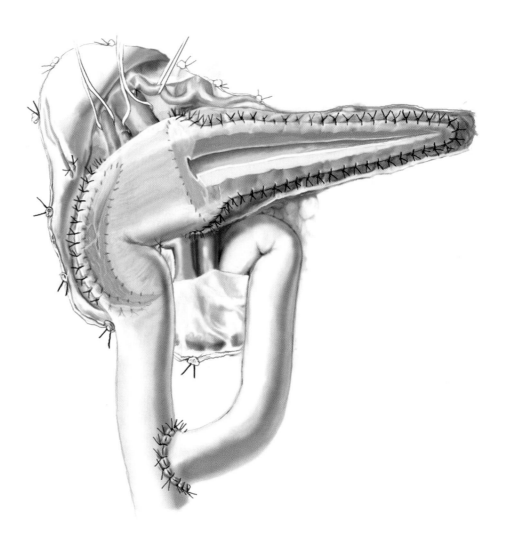

Postoperative Management

- Postoperative monitoring in an intensive care unit is only rarely required and is based on non-pancreatic co-morbidities
- Close monitoring of vital signs, fluid balance, and serum glucose concentrations
- Temporary nasogastric decompression
- No somatostatin analogue is recommended

Local Postoperative Complications

- Short term:
  - Pancreatic leak: ascites, fistula, local collection
  - Bile leak (uncommon)
  - Obstructive jaundice (e.g., due to operative injury to the common bile duct or perioperative inflammation and edema) (uncommon)
  - Jejunal leak
  - Intra-abdominal bleeding
  - Pancreatic leak:
    - Total parenteral nutrition and bowel rest; most leaks close spontaneously
    - CT-guided percutaneous drainage for fluid collections
    - If the patient is septic, reoperation may be indicated
- Long term:
  - Pseudocyst
  - Biliary stricture
  - Recurrence of pain
  - Pancreatic exocrine and/or exocrine insufficiency

Tricks of the Senior Surgeon

The Frey Procedure
- Don't try to "talk" the patient into an operation:
  - Explain the magnitude of the operation in detail and all long- and short-term complications, including failure to relieve pain.
  - Explain the natural history of chronic pancreatitis including the likelihood of endocrine or exocrine pancreatic insufficiency in the future.
- Technical:
  - Open the duct of Wirsung in the head of the pancreas down to the ampulla, creating a road map of the duct *before* resecting parenchyma; when the duct is impacted with calculi, a small bone curette, stone forceps, or right angle clamp may be helpful in removing calculi.
  - In patients with CBD obstruction, one must free up inflamed fibrotic tissue obstructing the duct; a groove can often be felt posteriorly in the location where the CBD traverses the pancreas. To avoid injury to the CBD, a Bakes dilator is placed into the CBD through a cystic or common bile ductotomy. The dilator within the duct is palpated between the index finger behind and the thumb in front of CBD through the surrounding inflamed, fibrotic tissue as the duct is freed up.
  - Due to inflammation and edema, sometimes it may be impossible to distinguish the exact margin between the duodenal wall and the pancreas when suturing the Roux-en-Y jejunal limb to the cored out pancreas. We have encountered no adverse effects aside from including some duodenal wall with pancreatic sutures.
- Patient follow-up: continue to follow patients yourself postoperatively; patients look to you (the surgeon) for physical and emotional support rather than to the gastroenterologist or primary care physician.

The Beger Procedure
- Tunneling of the pancreatic head along the portal vein groove starts with the preparation of the superior mesenteric vein on the caudal border of the pancreatic neck. Blunt dissection begins in front and along the mesenteric aspect of the portal vein toward the cranial border of the pancreatic neck. To facilitate this step a suture at this level in the lower border of the pancreas allows lifting the pancreatic neck segment anteriorly. If severe bleeding should occur, compression of the pancreas towards the spinal column interrupts the blood flow from the splenic vein. Transection of the head anterior to the portal vein exposes the portal vein for repair of the vessel wall.
- Placing a hand behind the head of the pancreas when the subtotal excision of the pancreatic head is to be performed helps to minimize blood loss.
- If the intrapancreatic wall of the common bile duct is not palpable or visible, a Kehr-Sonde or a biliary Fogarty® catheter can be passed via a choledochotomy or preferably through the cystic duct to help palpate the intrapancreatic common bile duct.
- Frozen section of the inflammatory mass is necessary, because about 5% of patients with an inflammatory mass have pancreatic cancer.
- Accidental incision of the intrapancreatic wall of the common bile duct need not be sutured; this part can be included into the anastomosis between the shell of the pancreatic head remnant and the jejunal loop (side-to-side anastomosis).
- If there is marked stenosis of the intrapancreatic common bile duct, an additional biliary anastomosis is necessary. A single layer anastomosis between the jejunal loop and the common bile duct using absorbable suture material should suffice.

Exploration of the Gastrinoma Triangle

Jeffrey A. Norton

Introduction

Gastrin-secreting neoplasms were first described by Zollinger and Ellison in 1955. These unusual neoplasms can be either benign or malignant. The diagnosis of the Zollinger-Ellison syndrome depends on an increased fasting serum gastrin concentration (>100 pg/ml), increased basal acid output (>10 mEq/l), and an abnormal secretin test (increase of >200 pg/ml in serum gastrin concentration after 2 U/kg of intravenous secretin). While originally believed to be primarily neoplasms of the pancreas, today we know that most "curable" gastrinomas arise in the wall of the proximal duodenum. Gastrinomas can occur as sporadic (non-familial) neoplasms or as one of the manifestations of multiple endocrine neoplasia-1 syndrome (MEN-1); MEN-1 includes neoplasms of the pituitary and parathyroids, neuroendocrine neoplasms of the duodenum and pancreas, and carcinoid neoplasms of the foregut and midgut.

Indications and Contraindications

Indications	■ Zollinger-Ellison syndrome without evidence of unresectable metastatic disease

Contraindications	■ "Falsely" increased serum gastrin concentration secondary to:
	  – Pernicious anemia
	  – Medications that inhibit acid production, e.g., H_2 receptor inhibitors, proton pump inhibitors
	■ G-cell hyperplasia

Preoperative Investigations and Preparation for the Procedure

History:	– Peptic ulcer disease (PUD), watery diarrhea, gastroesophageal reflux disease (GERD) and possibly a family history of the associated endocrinopathies, primary hyperparathyroidism, prolactinoma, insulinoma, Cushing's syndrome, carcinoid tumors or carcinoid syndrome.
Clinical evaluation:	– Upper gastrointestinal endoscopy with/without endoscopic ultrasonography.
Laboratory tests:	– Fasting serum concentration of gastrin, basal acid output off all acid secretory inhibitors for at least 3–7 days, secretin test.
	– When indicated, serum concentrations of intact PTH, total or ionized calcium, prolactin, fasting glucose, pancreatic polypeptide, chromogranin A, and serotonin, 24-h urine excretion of free cortisol, and if indicated 5-hydroxyindole acetic acid (HIAA).
Medical management:	– Appropriately high doses of proton pump inhibitor to stop acid hypersecretion and control PUD, GERD, and diarrhea. Often up to 80–120 mg pantoprazole two or three times a day or 20–40 mg of omeprazole. Pantoprazole can be given at the same dose either intravenously or orally and is indicated in the perioperative period.
Radiologic localization studies:	– CT or MR to image pancreas, duodenum, and liver, and to exclude liver metastases.
	– Somatostatin receptor scintigraphy, the so-called Octreo-Scan, is the best imaging study which images 90% of gastrinomas; although it will detect distant metastases, it frequently misses the small duodenal gastrinomas.
	– Endoscopic ultrasonography can detect small tumors within the pancreas, but may miss duodenal gastrinomas.

Procedure: Exploration of the Gastrinoma Triangle

STEP 1   **Exposure of the pancreas**

The gastrinoma triangle is defined as the region that includes the head of the pancreas and the duodenum in which over 85% of gastrinomas arise.

Most gastrinomas arise in the proximal duodenum, especially the occult neoplasms, but gastrinomas also occur in the pancreatic head, especially in association with the multiple endocrine neoplasia (MEN) syndrome.

Several "primary" lymph node gastrinomas have been reported to occur within the gastrinoma triangle with long-term cure after lymphadenectomy alone.

Sporadic gastrinomas are usually solitary and often (~50%) metastatic to lymph nodes.

In the familial MEN-1 setting, gastrinomas are usually multiple within the duodenum and pancreas and can metastasize as well. In all instances, the duodenal gastrinomas are most frequently missed, and thus opening the duodenum for transmural palpation is critical for their operative detection.

Access is best obtained via a bilateral subcostal division of the falciform ligament, and installation of a mechanical retractor (we prefer the Thompson retractor).

Next, the surgeon opens the lesser sac widely by dividing the gastrocolic ligament from the hepatic flexure to the splenic flexure, thereby exposing the entire neck, body, and tail of the pancreas. The tissue along the inferior border of the pancreas is opened to allow the surgeon to palpate tumors within the pancreas between the thumb and forefingers.

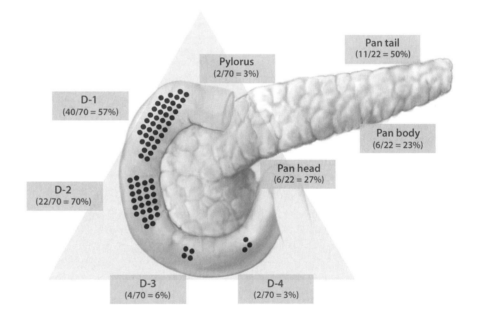

Extended Kocher maneuver

The next maneuver involves an extended Kocher maneuver by mobilizing the entire right colon and the proximal as well as the distal duodenum; this allows palpation of the head of the pancreas and, equally important, the wall of the duodenum.

Intraoperative ultrasonography is performed in a systematic fashion with a near-field, high-resolution transducer. Small neoplasms within the pancreas are identified by their sonolucent nature compared to the more echo-dense pancreas. Although intra-operative ultrasonography of the duodenum is also performed, duodenal gastrinomas, if small, are often missed by this procedure.

Finally, the liver is also evaluated for metastases.

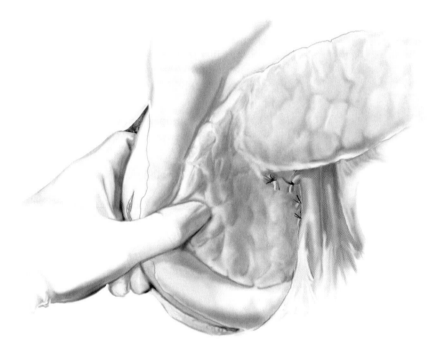

STEP 3

Lymphadenectomy of gastrinoma triangle

All lymph nodes within the gastrinoma triangle are excised in a systematic fashion for pathologic analysis starting with a lymphadenectomy of the hepatoduodenal ligament. Lymph nodes from the porta hepatis to the duodenum are excised, labeled, and sent for pathologic analysis, as are nodes from both the anterior and posterior border of the head of the pancreas.

Neuroendocrine neoplasms identified within the head of the pancreas are enucleated with palpation or via ultrasonographic control. When a tumor is enucleated from the head of the pancreas, 5 ml of fibrin glue is applied to the site of enucleation, and a closed suction drain is placed nearby.

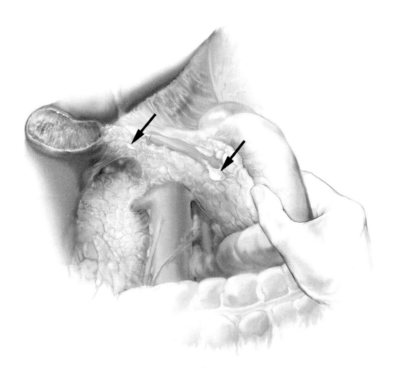

STEP 4   **Opening the duodenum to identify and remove duodenal gastrinomas (A, B)**

If the location of the tumor is not known, a duodenotomy is essential, because duodenal gastrinomas often may only become detectable by this method. The surgeon can palpate the tumor within the wall of the duodenum between the index finger within the duodenal lumen and the thumb on the serosal side.

If the duodenal tumor has been identified, the duodenal incision used to remove the duodenal gastrinoma can be used to explore the remainder of the duodenum.

Because the neoplasm arises from the submucosa and can invade the mucosa, the gastrinoma should be excised via a full thickness specimen with a rim of normal duodenal wall around the tumor. In patients with MEN-1, multiple duodenal neoplasms may be present, and the surgeon must carefully palpate and inspect the remainder of the inner surface of the duodenum after it is open to exclude the presence of other neoplasms. Do not confuse the ampulla of Vater or the entrace of the minor pancreatic duct with a gastrinoma. After excising a duodenal gastrinoma, the duodenum is closed with a single-layer, full-thickness, monofilament absorbable suture in a transverse direction so as not to narrow the lumen. If a long duodenotomy is necessary, a longitudinal closure is performed. A periduodenal or peripancreatic closed suction drain is left.

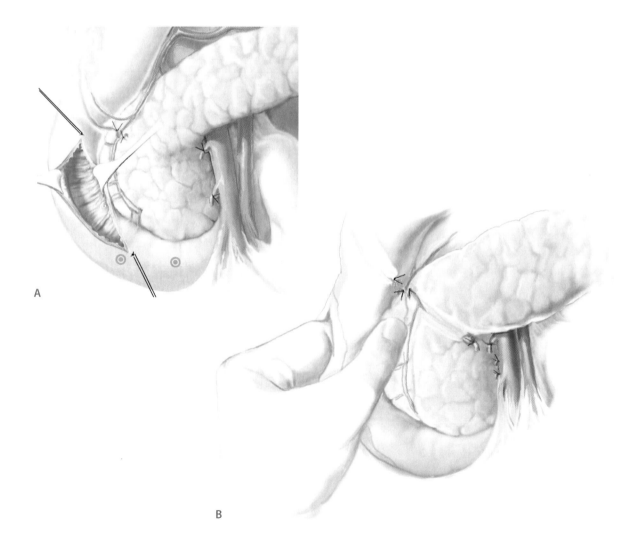

A

B

Postoperative Tests

- The patient is kept on the same dose of proton pump inhibitor postoperatively for 1–3 months as the preoperative dose; parietal cell hypertrophy as occurs with Zollinger-Ellison syndrome may take approximately 3–6 months to involute.
- A postoperative fasting serum gastrin measurement should be compared to the preoperative level. For selected patients, fasting serum gastrin, basal acid output, and secretin stimulated gastrin are not done 3–6 months postoperatively.
- On occasion, we often obtain a CT with oral contrast on postoperative day 5 to rule out a duodenal leak and a peripancreatic fluid collection.
- The drain is removed when the patient is eating a regular diet, drainage fluid is low in amylase activity, and the volume is less than 20 ml/day for 2 consecutive days. We may discharge the patient with a drain in place to be removed later.

Local Postoperative Complications

- Short term:
  - Duodenal leak
  - Pancreatic leak and/or abscess
  - Pancreatic fistula
  - Intra-abdominal bleeding
  - Pancreatitis
  - Duodenal ulcer bleeding
- Long term:
  - Duodenal stricture
  - Recurrent hypergastrinemia
- Other manifestations of MEN-1 (hypothalamic, parathyroid, carcinoid)

Tricks of the Senior Surgeon

- Do not cut corners; do the same operation every time regardless of the preoperative localization studies.
- Develop a dedicated team approach; an ultrasonographer willing to take the time and effort to find the gastrinoma is crucial.
- Beware of the ampulla and the pancreatic duct on the medial wall of the duodenum as these can feel like nodules and have been mistaken for a duodenal gastrinoma. I remove the gallbladder and pass a catheter through the cystic duct into the duodenum if there is any question about the location of ampulla. On occasion, I have given secretin intraoperatively to stimulate pancreatic secretion if there is a question that I may be identifying the pancreatic duct orifice.
- Exclude MEN-1 preoperatively by screening for other endocrinopathies and questioning family history.
- Remember that patients with both Zollinger-Ellison syndrome and MEN-1 generally have multiple pancreatic and duodenal neuroendocrine neoplasms, and thus cure-rate is very low. If a patient also has primary hyperparathyroidism, do the parathyroid operation first as this may ameliorate the manifestations of Zollinger-Ellison syndrome.
- Be sure to continue the patient on an aggressive pharmacologic acid suppressive medication during the perioperative and postoperative period.

Necrosectomy

Waldemar Uhl, Oliver Strobel, Markus W. Buchler
(Open Necrosectomy with Closed Postoperative Lavage),
Carlos Fernández-del Castillo (Necrosectomy and Closed Packing),
Gregory G. Tsiotos, Michael G. Sarr (Planned Repeated Necrosectomy),
C. Ross Carter, Clement W. Imrie (Percutaneous Necrosectomy)

Introduction

Severe acute pancreatitis remains a life-threatening disease. The first phase (about 10–14 days) is characterized by formation of pancreatic and peripancreatic necrosis and development of a systemic inflammatory response syndrome. This systemic response to the pancreatic inflammation/necrosis causes early organ failure that necessitates intensive care therapy. In the second phase (after 2 weeks), the leading cause of morbidity and mortality is superinfection of necrosis with development of septic multiple organ failure. In the last 2 decades, treatment has evolved considerably, and with improved intensive care management, there is a worldwide trend toward a more conservative strategy with operative intervention initiated primarily because of the local and systemic manifestations of infected necrosis and less so for sterile necrosis. However, today, septic complications caused by pancreatic infection account for 80% of the mortality, and infected necrosis therefore usually remains an absolute indication for same form of invasive intervention.

The goals of operative necrosectomy are to remove the necrotic and infected tissue and to minimize injury to viable tissues. In addition, each technique described below also aims to minimize the accumulation of exudative fluid and extravasated pancreatic exocrine secretions from the operative bed, because if undrained, infection invariably occurs.

This section will discuss four operative techniques of necrosectomy and drainage. All have similarities in their ultimate goal of complete debridement of necrotic tissue, but all tend to achieve this goal differently. Indeed, individual patients may be best treated selectively.

Indications and Contraindications

Indications

- Pancreatic and/or peripancreatic necrosis (based on contrast-enhanced dynamic CT scan) complicated by documented infection (guided FNA culture or extraluminal retroperitoneal gas).
- Sterile necrosis with progressive clinical deterioration despite maximal medical treatment; an aggressive operative approach in the absence of documented infection is, however, controversial.
- *Timing*: Necrosectomy should be undertaken as late as possible after onset of disease, when the necrotic process has ceased, viable and nonviable tissues are well demarcated, and the infected necrotic tissues are better organized and "walled off."
- Operative necrosectomy for patients greater than 3–4 weeks after onset of disease who are not improving and cannot eat but who have documented "sterile necrosis" remains controversial – some groups maintain that recovery is speeded with necrosectomy; others maintain a nonoperative approach ultimately proves safer.
- Massive hemorrhage or bowel perforation (colon, duodenum).

Contraindications

- Pancreatic and/or peripancreatic necrosis without evidence of infection or clinical deterioration.
- Early operation (within 1 week from onset of acute pancreatitis) before the systemic inflammatory response syndrome (SIRS) has subsided and maximal intensive medical treatment is still necessary. Hemodynamic and metabolic instability early after necrotizing pancreatitis is secondary to SIRS and not to bacterial sepsis.

Preoperative Investigation and Preparation for Procedure

- The diagnosis of acute pancreatitis is one of exclusion (exclude other surgical conditions) based on history, physical examination, and biochemistry.
- Initial assessment and continuous intensive care unit monitoring of severity (APACHE-II score).
- Laboratory assessment – CBC and electrolytes, liver function tests, and coagulation profile; some groups utilize serum C-reactive protein as a diagnostic/prognostic guide.
- Cardiovascular, respiratory, and metabolic resuscitation; aggressive management of SIRS for the first 10–14 days of acute pancreatitis.
- Contrast-enhanced dynamic CT about 1 week from onset of acute pancreatitis to assess the presence and extent of pancreatic and/or peripancreatic tissue necrosis, as well as extraluminal retroperitoneal gas.
- Early "prophylactic" administration of appropriate antibiotics (Imipenem) to prevent pancreatic superinfection from the gut is adopted by most, but not all, surgeons; use of oral antifungal agents is favored.
- Initiation of parenteral nutrition with early conversion to intrajejunal feeding (using a nasojejunal tube with its tip distal to the fourth portion of the duodenum); if possible, intragastric feeding may be effective.
- In severe gallstone pancreatitis, if choledocholithiasis is present, early endoscopic sphincterotomy and stone removal decreases morbidity and mortality.
- When operation is planned, the preoperative CT serves as the "road map" for necrosectomy to delineate all fluid collections in areas remote from the pancreas, especially for the retroperitoneal paracolic gutters and perinephric spaces.

Procedures

Open Necrosectomy with Closed Postoperative Lavage
Waldemar Uhl, Oliver Strobel, Markus W. Büchler

STEP 1

Exposure

Our technique of necrosectomy involves a primary, organ-preserving local debridement of necrotic tissue, accompanied by continuous removal of infected necrotic debris, ongoing necrosis, peripancreatic exudate, and extravasated pancreatic exocrine fluid by continuous peripancreatic lavage/debridement. We believe that our technique represents a lesser invasive strategy with results comparable to other techniques.

Midline vertical incision allows assessment of the entire abdominal cavity, generalized irrigation, and diverting ileostomy when the necrotic process involves the mesocolon and mesenteric area.

The lesser sac is entered bluntly and opened by dividing the duodenocolic and gastrocolic ligaments close to the greater curvature of the stomach inferior to the gastroepiploic vessels; this approach avoids injury to the colonic vessels and transverse mesocolon (A-1).

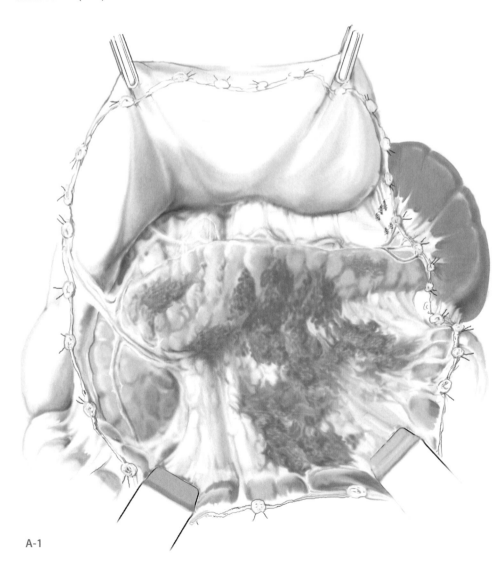

A-1

Exposure

Caution is necessary because of inflammatory adhesions between the pancreas, transverse mesocolon, and posterior wall of the stomach.

The pancreatic area is fully exposed; necrotic areas are darker and more woody-feeling than viable tissue.

Necrosis is usually not limited to the pancreas but also involves the peripancreatic and retroperitoneal fatty tissue as well; pancreatic parenchymal necrosis is usually patchy and superficial with deeper parts of the pancreas still perfused and viable (A-2).

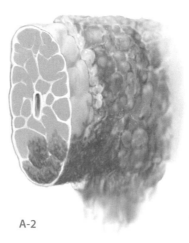

A-2

STEP 2	Blunt dissection of necrotic tissue

All fluid collections (defined by CT images) must be opened and evacuated by suction.

Removal of necrotic pancreatic and peripancreatic fatty tissue accomplished by blunt digital dissection or careful use of instruments and irrigation is the goal; sharp dissection is specifically avoided specifically to prevent uncontrollable hemorrhage.

Necrotic tissue is systematically sought in the retroperitoneum behind the transverse, ascending, and descending colon, and down to Gerota's fascia; all areas of necrosis are removed by blunt dissection.

Necrotic tissue and fluid from the operation room are sent for culture.

After necrosectomy, the pancreatic area and the retroperitoneal cavity are irrigated generously with 4–10l of normal saline.

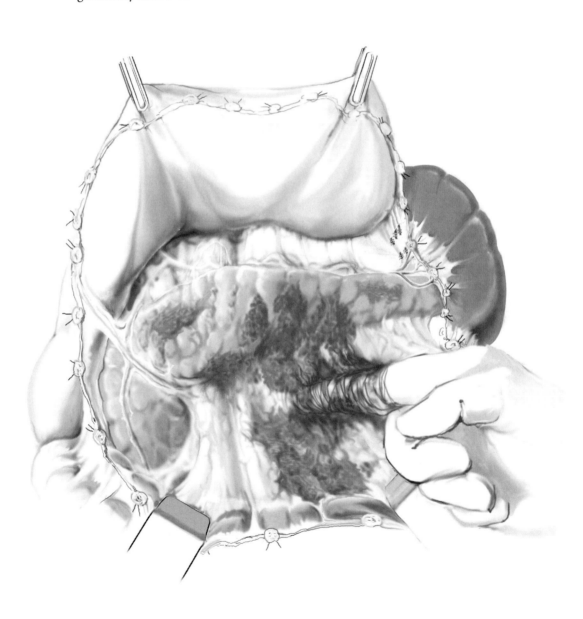

STEP 3   **Hemostasis after necrosectomy**

A careful blunt technique removes devitalized tissue and preserves the viable pancreatic parenchyma.

Bleeding from the pancreas is controlled by transfixion sutures using nonabsorbable, monofilament suture material.

The spleen is usually not involved specifically in the necrotic process, and thus the need for splenectomy should be very rare.

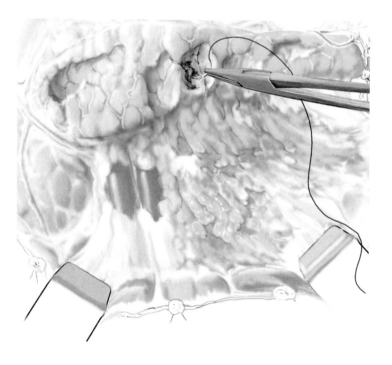

STEP 4   **Placement of catheters for postoperative closed lavage**

Four drainage catheters, two from each side, are directed to the contralateral side of the
peripancreatic space and placed with the tip of the catheter at the head and tail of the
pancreas behind the ascending and descending colon. Two of these four catheters
(sump-like tubes, 20-24 Fr.) have two lumens – a smaller one for inflow of lavage fluid
and a wider one for outflow; other drains (silicon tubes, 28–32 Fr.) have one lumen of
larger diameter to allow evacuation of both fluid and necrotic debris.

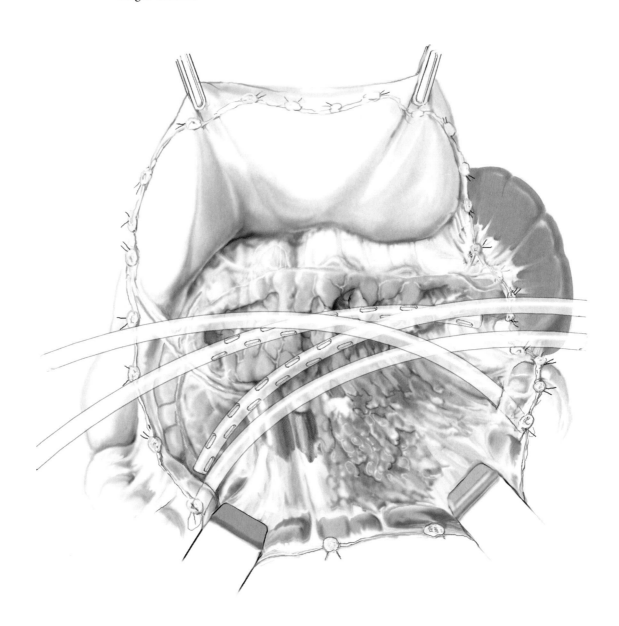

STEP 5   **Closure**

Gastrocolic and duodenocolic ligaments are re-sutured together to create a closed peripancreatic compartment to allow for contained postoperative lavage of the lesser sac and involved retroperitoneum.

With marked meso- and retrocolic necrosis threatening the viability of the transverse colon, a diverting ileostomy is created in the right lower quadrant.

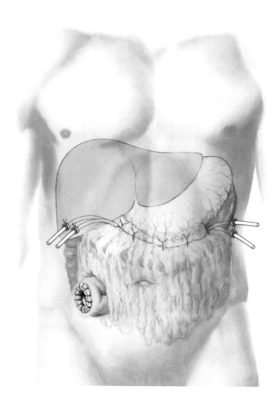

Necrosectomy and Closed Packing

Carlos Fernández-del Castillo

STEP 1   **Exposure and entry into the lesser sac, pancreatic and peripancreatic necrosectomy**

In any surgical approach to necrotizing pancreatitis, the goal is to remove the necrotic tissue and to minimize accumulation of exudative fluid and extravasated pancreatic exocrine secretions. Reoperation in this setting can be difficult and can lead to increased morbidity. The principle of necrosectomy and "closed packing" is to perform a single operation, with thorough debridement and removal of necrotic and infected tissue, while minimizing the need for reoperation or subsequent pancreatic drainage.

For most patients, a midline incision allows better exposure and optimal placement of drains.

The transverse colon is elevated anteriorly and access to the lesser sac is gained via the left mesocolon. When necrosis is extensive, often there is bulging of the necrotic process at this site and entry should be made bluntly with a clamp or finger. Fluid is evacuated and sent for culture.

The opening is enlarged, and with two fingers the cavity is explored. Depending on the extent and location of necrosis, an incision can also be made in the right mesocolon and, if necessary, the middle colic vessels are clamped and ligated.

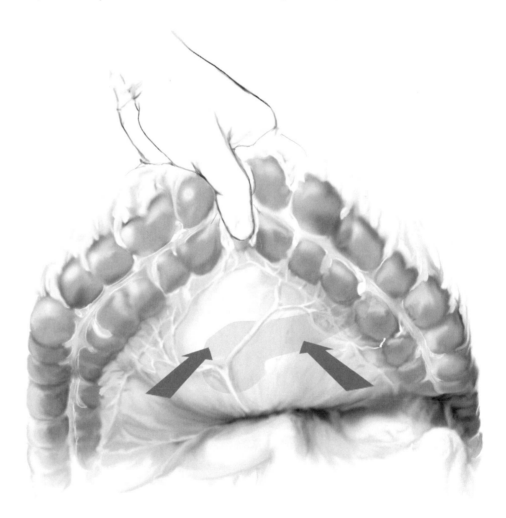

STEP 2   **Pancreatic and peripancreatic necrosectomy/debridement**

Debridement and removal of the necrotic tissue (necrosectomy) is done bluntly with the fingers or with a sponge. It is important to break into all the recesses of the cavity as guided by the CT to thoroughly remove the debris and necrotic material, a sample of which should also be sent to bacteriology. Any firm attachments should be clamped and tied or left alone.

The pancreas can be discerned from peripancreatic tissues often only on the basis of its location and consistency. Resection of the pancreas should be done carefully and only if the CT shows pancreatic parenchymal necrosis.

If necrosis extends deep into the perirenal spaces and this cannot be accessed through the mesocolon, the respective paracolic gutters are opened to remove the debris/necrosis.

After completing the necrosectomy/debridement, the pancreatic bed is irrigated with several liters of normal saline.

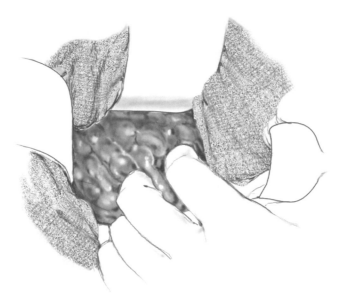

STEP 3   **Drain placement** (A-1, A-2)

Stuffed Penrose drains (often called cigarette drains) made using 3/4-inch Penrose drains stuffed with 2 gauze sponges are used for packing the large, stiff cavity that results after debridement. These drains are introduced into the abdomen through separate stab wounds to the side of the midline incision. The intent of this drain is to fill the cavity and provide compression, rather than strictly to drain the area. The number of drains varies depending on the size of the cavity; in our experience, the number of these drains has ranged from 2 to 12.

In addition, we leave the soft, round Jackson-Pratt, closed suction silicone drains, usually one into each major locale of the debridement cavity.

The stuffed Penrose drains are removed 5–7 days postoperatively. We typically remove one every other day, which allows the cavity to close gradually. Jackson-Pratt drains are removed last when they have no output.

A gastrostomy tube placed at the time of the debridement proves useful in many patients. It prevents the need for a nasogastric tube and can be used eventually for enteric feeding. We do not place jejunostomy tubes routinely .

In patients with cholecystitis, a cholecystectomy can be done at this time if the patient is stable and the degree of inflammation in the right upper quadrant makes it safe. Otherwise, cholecystectomy is better left for a later stage.

The abdomen is closed primarily in routine fashion.

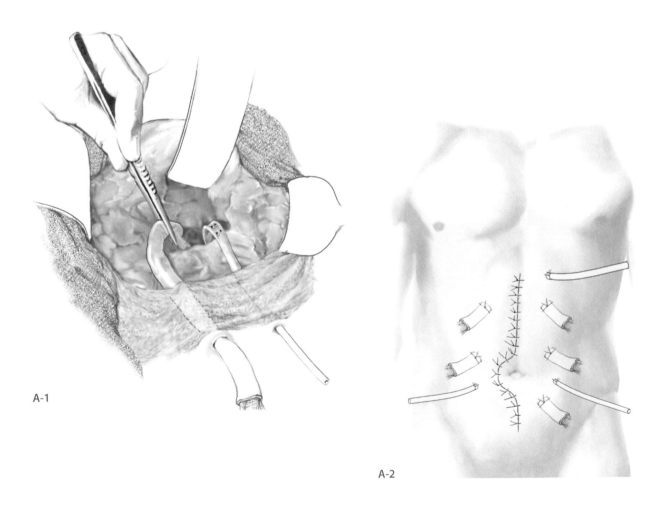

A-1

A-2

Planned Repeated Necrosectomy
Gregory G. Tsiotos, Michael G. Sarr

STEP 1

The operation begins with a systematic, comprehensive, manual and visual exploration of the entire pancreas as well as an exploration to delineate the extent of necrosis in both paracolic gutters, the root of the small bowel mesentery below the transverse mesocolon, and the suprapancreatic retroperitoneal tissues. CT is the guide to locating all areas of necrosis.

Entrance into the lesser omental sac is through the gastrocolic ligament (as opposed to through the transverse mesocolon), as this approach provides superior access to the pancreatic bed not hindered by risking injury to the middle colic or right colic vessels. Although necrosis often presents through the left mesocolon when the pancreatic body and tail are involved or through the right mesocolon when the head and uncinate are involved, any approach from below the mesocolon for a complete pancreatic necrosectomy offers suboptimal exposure and risks inadvertent surgical trauma and incomplete necrosectomy. We believe that exposure via the gastrocolic ligament is especially important for necrosis of the body and tail, except when the necrotizing process involves predominantly the head and uncinate process of the pancreas or when previous pancreatic surgery has obliterated the lesser sac.

Probing the gastrocolic ligament bluntly with a finger will usually identify the cavity containing the necrosis in the lesser sac. Once the finger finds the cavity, the space is unroofed in a controlled fashion, with care to protect the gastroepiploic arcade and vessels in the transverse mesocolon.

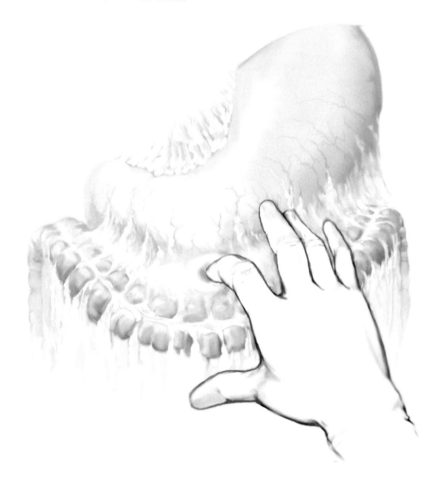

STEP 2

The actual necrosectomy should be carried out by manual, blunt dissection as the technique of choice. Gentle "scooping out" of the putty-like necrosis is sufficient in most cases. Sharp necrosectomy (using knife or scissors) is specifically condemned, especially in the vicinity of the splenic and superior mesenteric veins and in the area of the middle colic vessels. *All* devitalized tissue amenable to blunt debridement should be removed. The initial necrosectomy offers the best possible exposure, and thus every attempt at a complete and safe necrosectomy should be pursued at this time.

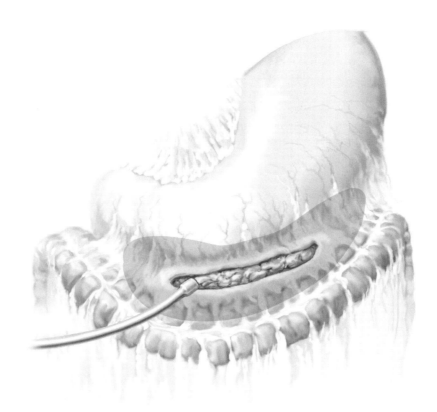

STEP 3

When the necrotic material must be accessed through the gastrocolic ligament, extreme care should be taken to avoid injury to the transverse colon and its mesentery, which is often shrunken, thickened, less immobile, and involved in the obliterated lesser sac region.

When necrotic tissue remains adherent to viable tissue, blunt avulsion or sharp dissection away from the viable tissue may cause bleeding that is difficult to control. These areas will auto-separate from the viable tissue at the time of planned reexploration 2 or more days later. Similarly, inflamed, friable, hypervascular, but viable tissues are not disturbed to minimize blood loss.

During removal of a piece of necrosis, a band or straw-shaped bridge of tissue may span the now defined cavity. Although the tendency is to avulse this persistent bridge of tissue, the surgeon should avoid the urge to do so, because this usually represents a blood vessel, often with persistent flow. Any uncontrolled, active bleeding during necrosectomy may be difficult to control in this inflamed peripancreatic space. Similarly, ligation or suture closure of a major blood vessel will then be subject to pseudoaneurysm formation; the overall goal of the necrosectomy should be to evacuate all necrosis without inducing hemorrhage.

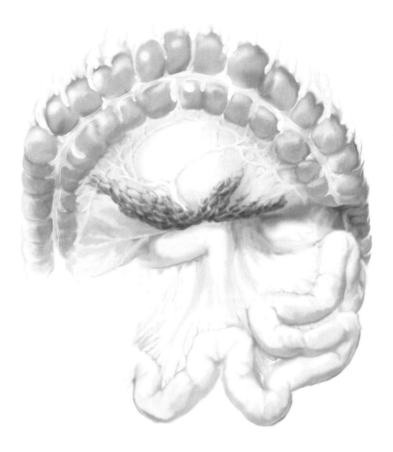

STEP 4

The peritoneum overlying both paracolic gutters should be incised to visualize and expose the retroperitoneal tissues, especially if the CT shows extension of the "inflammation" in these regions; simple palpation can be deceiving as to the presence or absence of peripancreatic fat necrosis, especially in the obese patient. These spaces, if involved, should be unroofed either medially to their colonic mesenteries, or, if more extensive, via a lateral approach with medial mobilization of the colon. The root of the small bowel mesentery and the suprapancreatic area (e.g., periesophageal and periaortic regions) are other locations where the necrotizing process can be concealed as it dissects along the superior mesenteric vessels.

After the necrosectomy, we irrigate the debrided areas extensively to remove devitalized tissue, inflammatory exudate, and residual bacteria using the Water-Pik irrigator (Surgiluv, Model 201, Stryker, Kalamazoo, MI), because it provides a controlled pressure system of blunt, liquid debridement and irrigation.

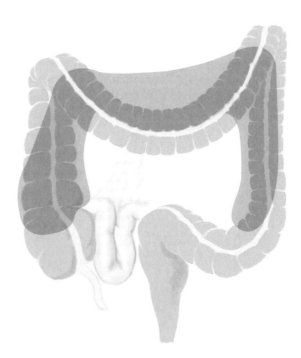

STEP 5

When areas of questionable viability are noted which remain adherent to viable areas, we return the patient to the operating room 2 days later for a repeat operative exploration and necrosectomy under a general anesthesia. In these patients after the initial necrosectomy, the debrided areas are packed with moistened sponges; if exposed, the splenic or superior mesenteric vessels are protected by interposition of a layer of nonadhesive dressing such as Adaptic (Johnson & Johnson, Kalamazoo, MI) or a thin layer of silastic sheeting. Soft, closed-suction drains are positioned *on top* of the gauze packing to evacuate free fluid that might otherwise accumulate and increase intra-abdominal pressure.

Abdominal wall closure proceeds with a zipper sewn to the fascia. This not only speeds opening and closure during any planned operative re-debridements, but also maintains the abdominal domain between debridements, facilitating a delayed primary wound closure and pulmonary ventilation. We specifically avoid sewing the zipper to the skin, because this allows the fascia to retract laterally, making later fascia closure more difficult or impossible. Reoperation is planned for 48 h after the current procedure and proceeds as described above. The zipper is opened and the abdomen fully reexplored in a systematic fashion. Additional necrosectomy and blunt debridement is performed as needed. The process is repeated at 48-h intervals until the necrotizing process has been arrested as evident by cessation of suppuration and absence of necrosis. If at the first necrosectomy a complete necrosectomy is performed as is usually possible when the necrosectomy occurs >21 days after onset of pancreatitis, then the abdomen is closed without planned reexploration.

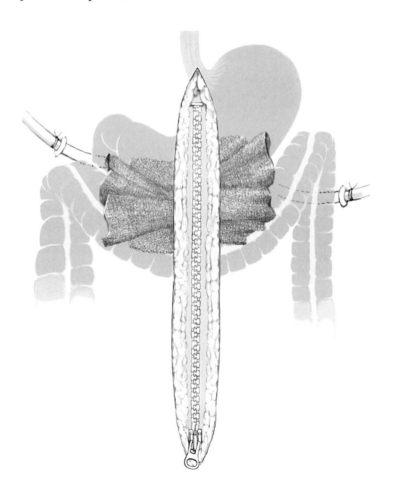

STEP 6

When convinced that all necrotic debris has been removed, the abdomen is closed over drains. We prefer soft, closed-suction silastic drains, which minimize risk of pressure necrosis of adjacent structures. We avoid large stiff "sump" drains with large holes, because with our technique of late (rather than early) first necrosectomy, followed by planned reoperations, only minimal particulate matter remains in the region and large bore drains are unnecessary.

The drains should be positioned away from major vessels and from direct contact with the colon or small bowel. We are very liberal in the number of drains placed, with at least one drain in each anatomic area of necrosis. Drains are routed below the liver and posterior to the hepatic flexure on the right and posterior to the splenic flexure inferior to the lower pole of the spleen on the left. A gastrostomy tube for gastric decompression and a needle catheter jejunostomy for eventual enteral feeding are inserted.

At final closure, the zipper is removed, and the abdominal wall is closed with nonabsorbable suture. The skin remains packed open.

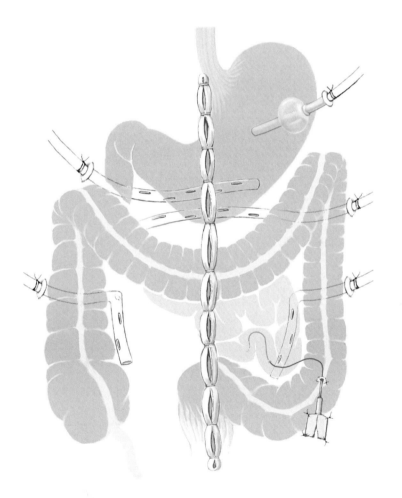

Percutaneous Necrosectomy

C. Ross Carter, Clement W. Imrie

STEP 1   **Access** (A-1, A-2)

Transfer the patient to the Radiology Department for a dual contrast CT of the abdomen with CT-guided puncture and insertion of 8-Fr. drainage catheter.

Sedation vs general anesthetic depends on the degree of organ dysfunction, site of access, and patient selection.

Transfer the patient to the operating room.

The development of minimal access techniques to surgical problems has been limited by technical difficulties. Since the goal of operative necrosectomy is to remove only the necrotic/infected tissues without harming the unaffected tissues, a minimal access approach, when possible, has many advantages.

This operative approach has several specific indications and contraindications. *Specific indication:* The area of necrosectomy must be accessible to percutaneous puncture allowing dilatation of the needle tract. *Specific contraindications:* This technique is not indicated when there is bowel ischemia, perforated viscus (not late fistula), or significant preoperative hemorrhage.

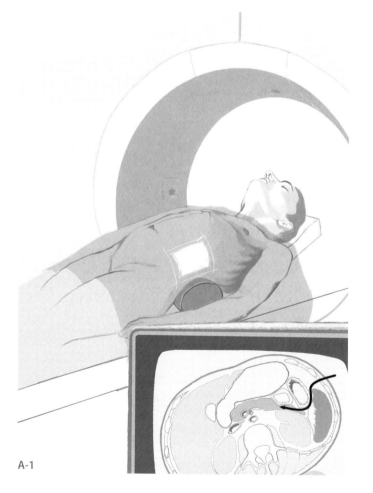

A-1

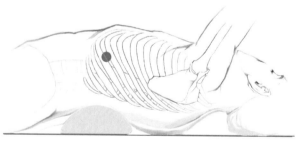

A-2

STEP 2

Preparation of the nephroscope (necrosectoscope) (A-1, A-2)

Attach the suction to a three-way tap.

Use a pressurized irrigation system with warmed fluid only.

The patient should be positioned in the left (or right) lateral position and that side of the upper abdomen raised with a sandbag, to allow horizontal access along the puncture tract.

Use of a "barrier" nephrolithotomy theater drape to collect irrigant fluid is beneficial.

The initial step is to lavage/aspirate the cavity to allow the pus-filled cavity to run clear.

Using soft grasping forceps avoids unnecessary trauma.

General anesthesia is necessary.

Pass a 0.035-mm wire along the 8-Fr. drainage catheter into the cavity.

Exchange the 8-Fr. drainage catheter for a stiffener.

Pass the dilatation balloon along the access tract or dilate the tract using graduated bougies.

Insert a 34-Fr. Amplatz sheath over the largest dilator.

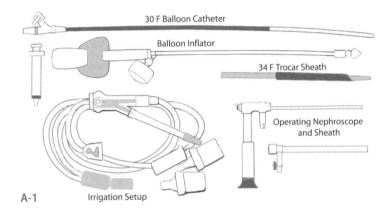

A-1

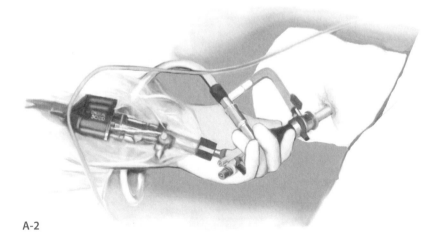

A-2

STEP 3   **Visualization and debridement of necrosis**

Gently insert the nephroscope along the Amplatz sheath to enter the cavity.

Again the initial step is to lavage/aspirate cavity to allow the pus-filled cavity to run clear.

Once devitalized tissue is identified, loose material is removed carefully using forceps.

Use soft grasping forceps to avoid trauma.

Adherent material is left in situ for removal at a subsequent exploration; over zealous debridement may result in major hemorrhage.

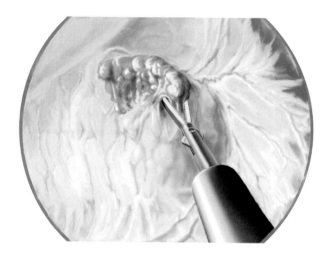

STEP 4

Postoperative management of cavity

Having removed all loose necrotic material, the guide wire stiffener is re-passed along the dilated tract.

A 34-Fr. soft tube drain is passed over the stiffener.

An 8-Fr. umbilical catheter is sutured to the larger drain to allow continuous cavity lavage postoperatively.

Cavity lavage is commenced at 250 ml/h using dialysis fluid via a blood warmer.

A median of three procedures/patient will be required prior to resolution.

Steps 1 and 3 are omitted as the dilatation/access is not required.

The Amplatz sheath is again not required.

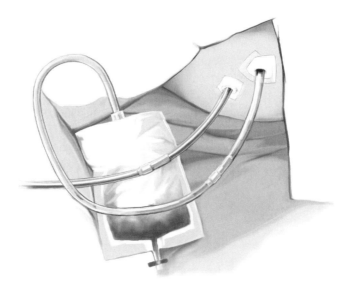

Postoperative Considerations

- Close hemodynamic and respiratory monitoring and support in an ICU
- Appropriate antibiotic and antifungal therapy guided by cultures
- Parenteral nutrition or preferably an elemental enteral diet, especially with extensive pancreatic parenchymal necrosis

Local Postoperative Complications

- Short term:
    - Pancreatic and gastrointestinal fistulae
    - Recurrent peripancreatic abscess
    - Colonic necrosis – abscess/fistula
    - Intra-abdominal hemorrhage
    - Sepsis syndrome
    - Wound infection
- Long term:
    - Endocrine pancreatic insufficiency
    - Exocrine pancreatic insufficiency
    - Incisional hernia
    - Pseudocyst (rare); if present, usually from an isolated remnant or disconnected duct syndrome secondary to complete necrosis of the neck of the pancreas
    - Recurrent pancreatitis (rare)

Tricks of the Senior Surgeon

Open Necrosectomy with Closed Postoperative Lavage

- *Blunt necrosectomy:* necrotic tissue is removed by blunt digital dissection without instruments; use of scissors increases the risk of excising still viable tissue, injuring portal, splenic, or mesocolic vessels, or causing difficult-to-control bleeding.
- *Retroperitoneal necrosis:* Even if the necrotic process in the retroperitoneum extends into the pelvis, blunt digital necrosectomy can be performed via an anterior, supra-colic approach through the lesser sac dissecting inferiorly, following the necrosis.
- *Biliary pancreatitis:* ERC can be performed before necrosectomy in patients with gallstone pancreatitis, clearing the common duct of stones, and thereby only cholecystectomy is performed with exploration of bile duct omitted, reducing the risk of bile duct injury.
- *Diverting ileostomy:* With extension of the necrotic process behind the colon, we often perform a diverting ileostomy to reduce the risk of colonic fistula during the course of disease; intestinal continuity is restored 3 months after discharge.

Necrosectomy and Closed Packing

- Have the recent CT in the operating room. It is your road map to be sure you do not leave collections of necrosis undrained.
- Bleeding inevitably ensues during the debridement. Unless this is copious, finish the debridement before attempting to stop it. It usually stops spontaneously or with the packing.

Planned Repeated Necrosectomy

- Resist operating *early* on patients with necrotizing pancreatitis, even with hemody-namic and metabolic instability. Make every effort to operate as late as possible, even with proof of infected necrosis, provided that the patient remains stable with maximal intensive medical therapy; the necrotizing process will have thus ceased and all viable and devitalized tissue will have defined. In such a case, a single complete necrosectomy and primary abdominal wall closure will be usually enough.
- Operative planning based on the preoperative CT is of paramount importance. *All* areas with fluid collections demonstrated on preoperative CT should be sought for, unroofed, and debrided. Do not rely solely on visual and manual exploration of the peritoneal cavity and the retroperitoneum.
- The initial necrosectomy offers the best possible exposure, and thus every attempt at a complete and safe necrosectomy should be pursued at this time.
- Resist the urge to "debride" a possible "bridge" of tissue traversing the lesser sac cavity after blunt necrosectomy; this "bridge" most probably represents the middle colic vessels.

Percutaneous Necrosectomy

- Use of a "level 1" fluid warmer provides pressurized warm fluid for intraoperative irrigation.
- Be prepared to come back another day or two later rather than be overzealous with the initial or subsequent debridement.
- Significant bleeding may be controlled by balloon tamponade, while laparotomy access and surgical control is obtained.
- Discontinue the procedure if the patient shows signs of cardiovascular instability; resuscitate the patient, lavage the cavity, and come back another day.

Laparoscopic Staging of Periampullary Neoplasms

Kevin C. Conlon, Sean M. Johnston

Introduction

The global concept of preoperative staging of malignancies is to select, as best as possible, those patients who are or are not candidates for operative resection. In the case of periampullary neoplasms, we have good, non-operative "palliation" for patients with non-curable neoplasms. Because a celiotomy for a periampullary neoplasm that proves to be non-resectable is not therapeutic and obligates the patient to an "unnecessary" postoperative recuperation/recovery, preoperative staging laparoscopy can help to select those patients who are at highest chance for potentially curative resection and will prevent celiotomy in most of those with unresectable disease.

Indications and Contraindications

Indications

- Assessment of resectability for:
    - Pancreatic cancer (adenocarcinoma)
    - Distal bile duct cancer
    - Duodenal cancer
    - Ampullary carcinoma
    - Islet cell neoplasms
- Staging of locally advanced disease prior to chemoradiation
- Diagnosis of suspected metastatic disease
- Histologic confirmation of radiologically unresectable disease

Relative Contraindications

- Patient unfit for general anesthesia
- Multiple previous upper abdominal operations
- Intra-abdominal sepsis

Preoperative Investigation and Preparation for Procedure

History:	Jaundice, weight loss, abdominal pain, early satiety
Clinical evaluation:	Signs of jaundice, cachexia, epigastric mass, ascites
Laboratory tests:	Liver function tests (albumin, total protein, bilirubin, alkaline phosphatase, transaminases), coagulation parameters (PT, APTT), urea and electrolytes, full blood count, C-reactive protein, tumor markers (CA19–9, CEA)
Radiological assessment:	Ultrasonography, contrast-enhanced, dynamic, thin-cut CT of the pancreas and liver, in selected patients; endoscopic ultrasonography (EUS), endoscopic retrograde cholangiopancreatography (ERCP), magnetic resonance cholangiopancreatography (MRCP)
Instruments and laparoscopes:	– 30-degree angled laparoscope, either 10 mm or 5mm
	– 5-mm laparoscopic instruments
	– Maryland dissector
	– Blunt tip dissecting forceps
	– Cup-biopsy forceps
	– Atraumatic grasping forceps
	– Liver retractor
	– Scissors
	– 10-mm suction device
	– Laparoscopic ultrasound probe (optional)

Procedure

STEP 1

The patient is positioned supine on the operating table. A warming blanket is placed underneath the patient, who is secured appropriately to the table.

Requirements:

- General anesthesia
- Orogastric tube for stomach decompression
- Urinary catheter (optional)
- Anesthetic equipment on boom or free standing cart

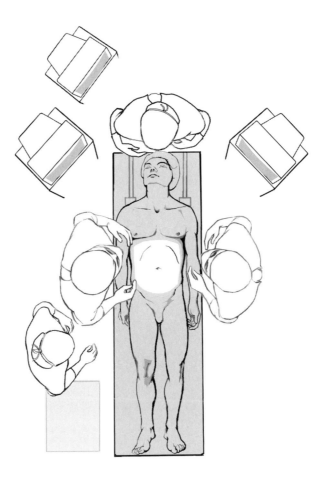

STEP 2   **Trocar placement**

A multiport technique is used. The initial trocar (10-mm blunt port) is placed using
an open cut down usually in the infra-umbilical area. After the skin and subcutaneous
tissue is divided, the fascia is grasped between two forceps and incised with either
a knife or cautery, opening the peritoneum under direct vision. Some form of blunt,
Hassan-type port is inserted, secured in place, and a pneumoperitoneum established
with CO_2 gas. An intraperitoneal pressure of 10–12 mmHg is considered optimal. The
laparoscope is inserted and an initial examination of the peritoneal cavity performed. If
no obvious metastases are seen, further ports are inserted in the right (10 mm and
5 mm) and left (5 mm) upper quadrant along the line of an intended incision.

The 30° angled laparoscope is placed in the umbilical port, with the two 5-mm ports
used for graspers, scissors, and liver retractor. The right lateral 10-mm port is used for
the blunt suction irrigator. This instrument is particularly useful for retraction and
"blunt" palpation. The lateral port is also used for the laparoscopic ultrasonography.

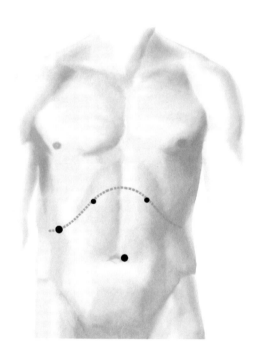

STEP 3

Examination

A systematic examination of the abdominal cavity is performed, which mimics that performed during open exploration. Adhesions if present are divided to facilitate examination. Any peritoneal-based mass is biopsied with a cup biopsy forceps.

The sequence of examination is: (1) peritoneal cavity; (2) right and left lobes of the liver; (3) duodenum and the foramen of Winslow; (4) colonic mesocolon and ligament of Treitz; and (5) gastrohepatic omentum, lesser sac, pancreas, gastric pillar, and hepatic artery.

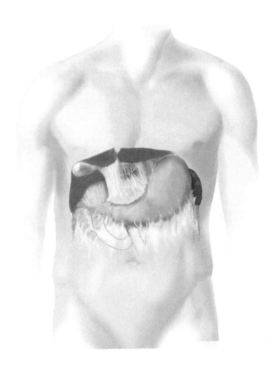

STEP 4   **Abdominal exploration** (A-1, A-2)

After a general inspection of the peritoneal cavity, the patient is tilted approximately 10 degrees head up. Examination of the liver begins with the anterior aspect of the left lateral lobe (segments 2 and 3). Palpation is achieved with the 10-mm and 5-mm instruments. The posterior aspect of the left lateral lobe and the anterior and inferior aspects of the right hepatic lobe are then examined in turn.

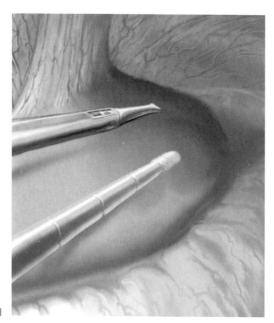

A-1

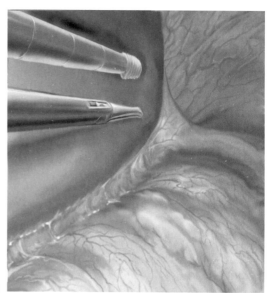

A-2

STEP 5   Inspection of the liver hilus and foramen of Winslow

The right lobe of the liver is elevated with the retractor placed through the left upper quadrant port. The structures of the hepatoduodenal ligament can be dissected out and suspicious nodes biopsied if indicated.

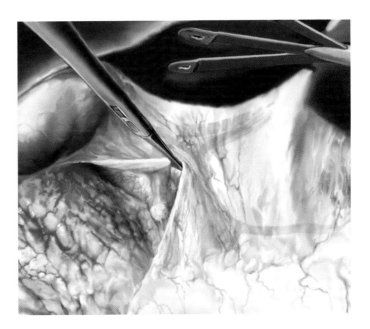

STEP 6   **Examination of the colonic mesocolon** (A-1, A-2)

The patient is now placed in 10 degrees of head down tilt. The omentum and transverse colon are retracted or pushed toward the left upper quadrant. This allows examination of the ligament of Treitz.

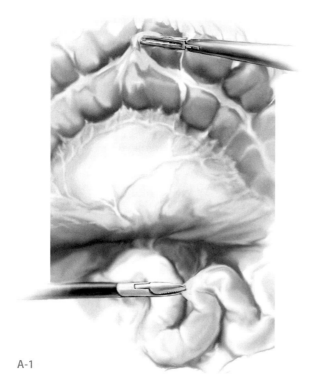

A-1

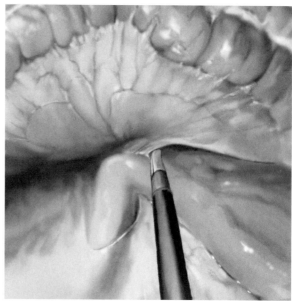

A-2

STEP 7

Examination of lesser sac

The patient is now placed supine. The left lateral lobe of the liver is elevated with a 5-mm retractor placed through the left upper port. The gastrohepatic omentum is grasped, elevated and incised. Care must be taken to identify and preserve an aberrant left hepatic artery if present (A-1).

With the lesser sac opened, suspicious nodes along the left gastric or hepatic arteries can be biopsied if indicated. The neck and body of the pancreas can be examined (A-2).

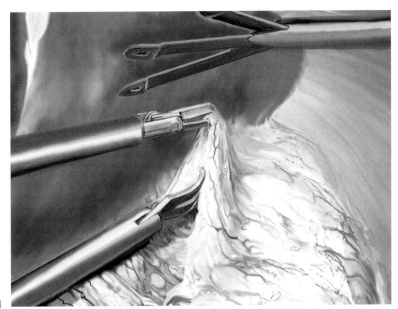

A-1

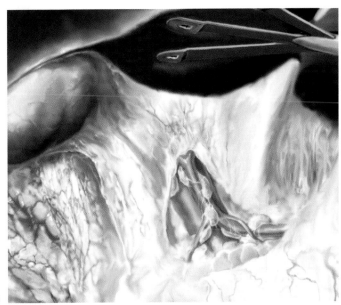

A-2

STEP 8   **Laparoscopic ultrasonography**

The laparoscopic ultrasound probe is inserted through the right lateral port. The examination starts with scanning the left lateral lobe of the liver, examining segments I, II, and III in turn. Examination of the right lobe follows (A-1).

The hepatoduodenal ligament is examined with identification of the common hepatic duct, common bile duct, portal vein, and hepatic arteries (A-2). Visualization of these structures is aided through the use of color flow Doppler. The pancreas is then examined by slowly rotating the head of the transducer. The relationship of the tumor to the pancreatic duct and surrounding peri-pancreatic vessels (portal vein, superior mesenteric vein, superior mesenteric artery) can be determined.

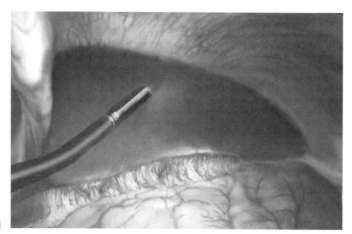

A-1

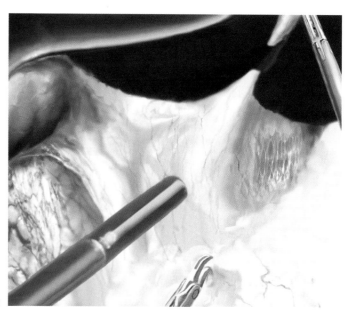

A-2

Postoperative Tests

- This should be an outpatient procedure.
- Laboratory investigation may be unnecessary.

Local Postoperative Considerations

- Monitor for usual problems after laparoscopy – shoulder pain, and infection/hernia at trocar site(s).
- Severe pain or fever should not occur and if present requires an aggressive evaluation for inadvertent injury to an abdominal viscus during the laparoscopic procedure.

Tricks of the Senior Surgeon

- Be patient and move slowly. Metastases are often small and may be missed with a cursory examination.
- Maintain hemostasis; blood absorbs light and obscures the anatomy.
- A single port examination is inadequate. Multiple ports are required for the appropriate exposure to be obtained.
- Mobilization of the duodenum is not required.
- Place the 10-mm port as lateral as possible in the right upper quadrant. This will allow the ultrasound probe to be placed directly at right angles over the hepato-duodenal ligament, making identification of the bile duct/vessels easier.

Distal Pancreatectomy

Richard H. Bell Jr, Erwin W. Denham (Distal Open Pancreatectomy with Splenectomy),
Ronald A. Hinder (Laparoscopic Distal Pancreatectomy)

Introduction

Although distal pancreatectomies for diffuse chronic pancreatitis have gone out of favor, there are still selected situations when a localized, anatomic distal pancreatectomy is indicated. The following two procedures describe open and laparoscopic techniques – each of which may have selected indications/contraindications.

Indications and Contraindications

Indications

- Chronic abdominal pain due to chronic pancreatitis completely or predominantly confined to body/tail of pancreas (e.g., due to post-traumatic/postnecrotic stricture of main pancreatic duct)
- Suspected adenocarcinoma of the body or tail of the pancreas arising in a background of chronic pancreatitis
- Pancreatic ascites from ductal disruption of the body/tail region
- Pancreatic pseudocyst in the distal body/tail region

Contraindications

- Diffuse changes of chronic pancreatitis throughout the gland
- If diffuse changes are present in the gland with predominance of disease in the left gland, distal pancreatectomy *may* occasionally be appropriate (e.g., alcoholic pancreatitis with a left dominant, mid-gland stricture or a complex pseudocyst in the mid/distal pancreas); however, the results are variable
- For *laparoscopic approach:* left-sided sinistral portal hypertension, multiple previous intra-abdominal operations with multiple adhesions

Preoperative Investigation and Preparation for the Procedure

History:	Search for a history of pancreatic trauma and previous/current alcohol abuse, chronic abdominal pain, steatorrhea, diabetes, family history of pancreatitis or pancreatic cancer, and usage of pain medication.
	– If narcotic/alcohol dependency is active, encourage commitment to undergo detoxification in a controlled chemical dependency unit postoperatively.
Clinical evaluation:	Abdominal tenderness or mass, splenomegaly (suspect splenic vein thrombosis)
Laboratory tests:	CBC, glucose, serum calcium, triglycerides
Imaging:	– CT, MRI or EUS: Assess the extent of parenchymal disease (should be confined to body/tail); if splenomegaly and/or gastric varices are present–suspect splenic vein thrombosis.
	– ERCP: Evaluate for a mid pancreatic ductal stricture and an intrapancreatic biliary stricture.
Preoperative considerations:	– If splenectomy is planned, immunize with pneumococcal vaccine, *Haemophilus influenzae* type b vaccine, and meningococcal vaccine 2 weeks preoperatively.
	– Entertain use of an epidural catheter for postoperative pain control (preoperative narcotic dependence is a relative contraindication, because the patient will need systemic levels of the narcotic).
	– DVT prophylaxis with sequential compression devices and/or subcutaneous heparin (check with anesthesia regarding policy on heparin in patients with postoperative epidural analgesia).
	– Prophylactic intravenous antibiotics are given 30 min prior to incision.

Procedures

Distal Open Pancreatectomy with Splenectomy
Richard H. Bell Jr, Erwin W. Denham

STEP 1   **Initial exposure, entering the lesser sac**

Selection of a bilateral subcostal or midline incision depends on the angle of the costal margin; ordinarily, a subcostal incision is preferred.

After full abdominal exploration, self-retaining retractor systems, like the Buckwalter, aid by retracting the costal margin cephalad.

The lesser sac is entered by dissecting the greater omentum off the transverse colon and retracting it rostrally with the stomach.

Ligate and divide the more distal short gastric vessels between the stomach and splenic hilum; higher short gastric vessels are easier to manage once the spleen is mobilized (Step 5). These maneuvers expose the body and tail of the pancreas.

Subsequent dissection is facilitated if the splenic flexure of the colon is fully separated from the omentum and retracted inferiorly.

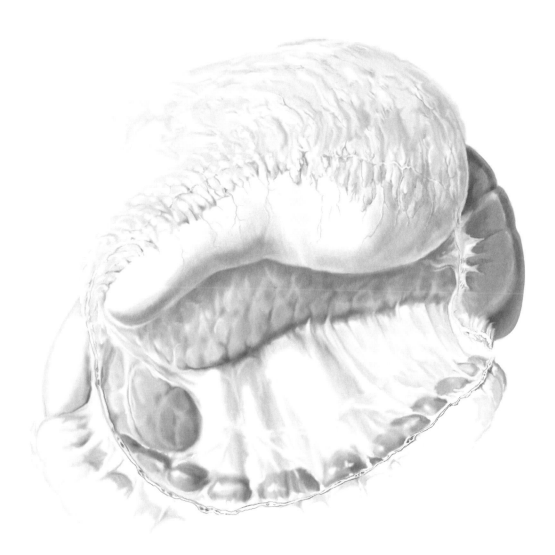

STEP 2   **Identification of the superior mesenteric vein, mobilization of the inferior edge**
                       of the pancreas

The middle colic vein is followed downward to localize the superior mesenteric vein.

   The superior mesenteric vein should be freed below the edge of the pancreas and followed beneath the neck of the pancreas; this maneuver ensures easy division of the neck of the gland later.

   The peritoneum along the inferior border of the pancreas is incised; the body/tail of the pancreas is elevated by gentle sharp dissection behind the gland.

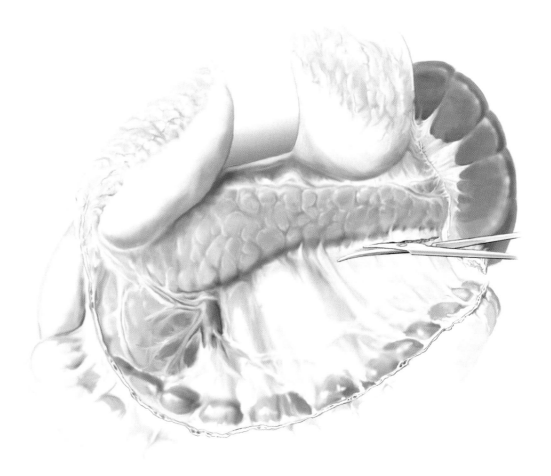

STEP 3

Mobilization of the spleen (A-1, A-2)

The spleen is mobilized anteriorly by dividing the lateral peritoneal attachments.

Splenic attachments to the colon (splenocolic ligament) and diaphragm are then divided.

Residual short gastric vessels from the upper pole of the spleen to the stomach are divided; the stomach is retracted superiorly out of the field, fully exposing the distal pancreas.

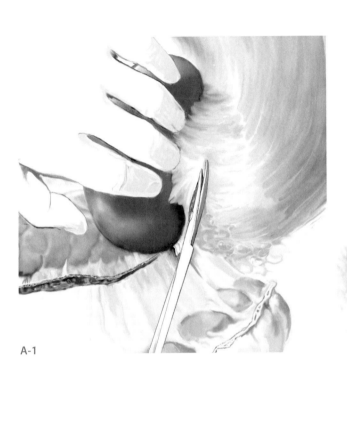

A-1

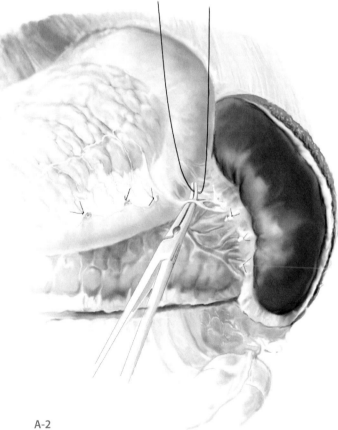

A-2

STEP 4   **Mobilization of the distal pancreas**

The spleen and distal pancreas are mobilized to the patient's right side; it is important to stay between the kidney and tail of pancreas, leaving Gerota's fascia undisturbed posteriorly.

After initial mobilization, the hand enters the retropancreatic space created in Step 3.

Retroperitoneal attachments along the upper border of the pancreas are ligated and divided until the origin of the splenic artery is reached; location of this artery is ascertained by palpation.

The spleen and pancreas are held upward and to the patient's right, so the surgeon can visualize the posterior aspect of the gland and identify the splenic vein as it courses along the back of the gland.

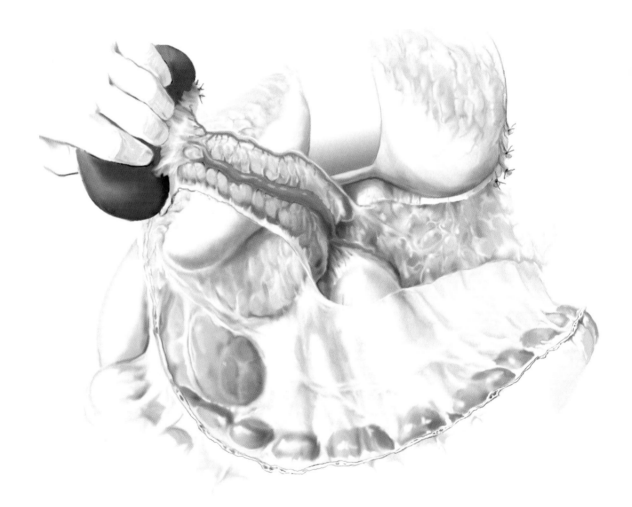

STEP 5

Ligation of the splenic artery

Along the upper border of the pancreas, the splenic artery is isolated near its origin from the celiac axis before it enters the pancreatic substance; here it is suture-ligated proximally with 2-0 suture, ligated distally, and divided. Be certain to fully identify the artery as the splenic artery and to clearly distinguish it from the common hepatic artery.

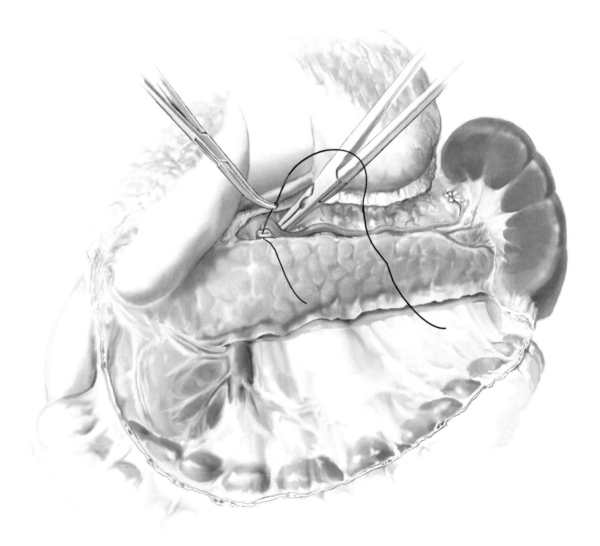

STEP 6   **Isolation/ligation of the splenic vein** (A-1, A-2)

Moving to the inferior and posterior edge of the gland, dissection of the peripancreatic soft tissues continues until the confluence of the splenic vein and superior mesenteric vein (SMV) are visualized.

The inferior mesenteric vein is ligated and divided if it joins the splenic vein directly or if it interferes with ligation of the splenic vein close to the origin with the SMV; this is usually not the case.

Tissues around the entrance of the splenic vein into the SMV are carefully dissected off the vein.

A Satinsky, side-biting vascular clamp is placed on the superior mesenteric–portal vein junction; the splenic end of the splenic vein is tied with 2–0 suture.

The splenic vein is divided between ligature and clamp, being sure to leave the cuff of vein extending beyond the jaws of the clamp.

The proximal end of the splenic vein is oversewn with continuous 5-0 polypropylene suture and the vascular clamp then removed.

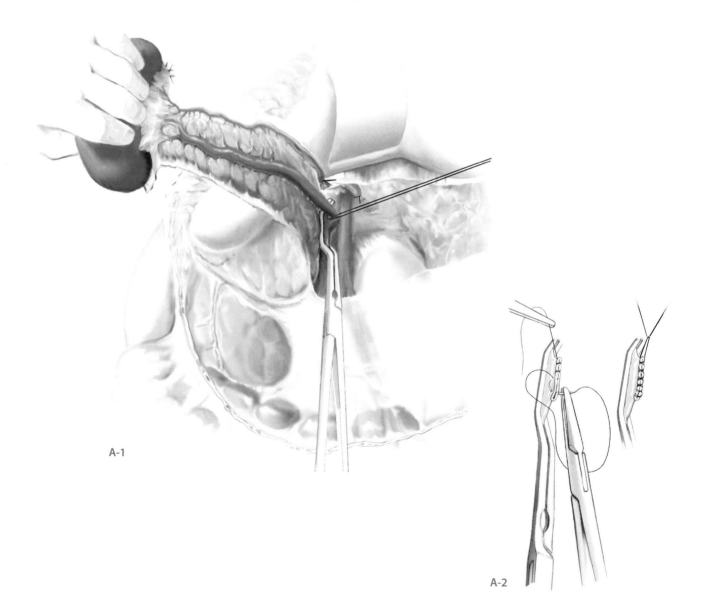

A-1

A-2

STEP 7 **Division of the pancreas**

The neck of the pancreas is divided over the superior mesenteric–portal vein using electrocautery; a large clamp behind the neck of the pancreas protects the vein.

If a neoplasm is suspected, a margin of at least 1 cm to the left of any mass must be maintained and checked with frozen section of the transected margin.

Marginal arteries supplying the pancreas that bleed after the parenchyma is divided are controlled with suture ligatures.

Once the cut edge of the pancreas is hemostatic, the pancreatic duct orifice is identified and ligated with 3-0 polypropylene.

The cut edge of the pancreas is closed with a continuous running suture of 3-0 polypropylene.

Other methods to transed it and "close" the cut edge of the pancreas include using a linear stapler or techniques of tissue welding. A soft, closed-suction drain is placed adjacent to the cut edge of the pancreas and brought out through the left lateral abdominal wall.

The abdominal wall is closed in layers.

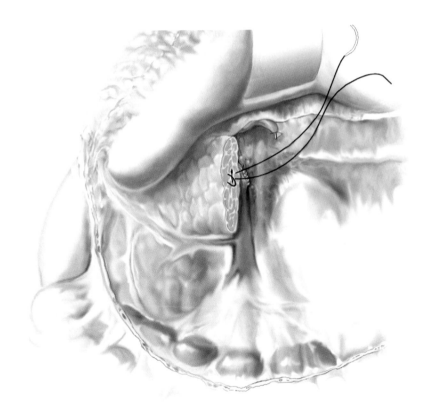

Distal Pancreatectomy with Splenic Preservation

- Preserving the spleen during removal of the body/tail of the pancreas in patients with chronic pancreatitis is difficult; scarring around the splenic vein may make dissection and preservation of the vein difficult and even dangerous.

- If a neoplasm is suspected, the spleen and splenic vessels should not be preserved.

- If the distal pancreatectomy is for pain, there is no suspicion of malignancy, and the splenic vein is patent, an attempt to preserve the spleen is justified.

- The course of the operation is quite different when splenic preservation is the goal.

- After entering the lesser sac, the operation commences with division of the pancreatic neck over the isolated superior mesenteric-portal vein.

- The spleen is not mobilized; the body/tail of the pancreas is dissected from the point of division of the gland toward the spleen by dividing the multiple small branches entering the splenic vein from the pancreatic parenchyma.

- Branches of the splenic artery entering the pancreas are divided individually as dissection progresses to the patient's left.

- Before proceeding with dissection of the body/tail of the gland from the splenic vessels, it is wise to gain control of both the proximal splenic vein near its entrance to the SMV and the splenic artery near its origin; expeditious vascular control can be obtained if bleeding becomes excessive during subsequent dissection.

- Splenic venous branches are controlled best with fine vascular staples or fine ties of 4-0 or 5-0 silk; these vessels are small, delicate, and easily torn.

- The surgeon decides how much blood loss is acceptable when trying to preserve the spleen and should be willing to abandon this approach if necessary.

Laparoscopic Distal Pancreatectomy
Ronald A. Hinder

The advent of minimal access surgery and its technologic advances have made laparoscopic distal pancreatectomy a viable option in selected patients with chronic pancreatitis and other disorders.

STEP 1	**Peritoneal access**

Access to the abdominal cavity is obtained by making an incision below the umbilicus in the midline and establishing a 15-mmHg pneumoperitoneum; the laparoscope is introduced through a 10-mm port

Further ports include right upper and right mid quadrant 5-mm ports in the mid-clavicular line and a 12-mm port in the left lower mid quadrant.

The abdomen is explored laparoscopically for evidence of metastatic disease on the peritoneal surface or within the liver; the spleen is also examined.

The adhesions are divided as needed.

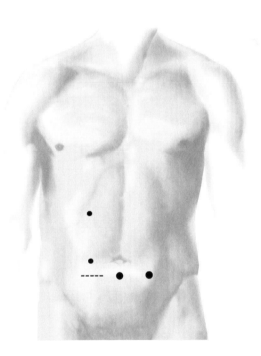

STEP 2

Entering the lesser sac

The gastrocolic omentum is divided using an ultrasonic dissector (harmonic scalpel), allowing access to the lesser sac behind the stomach.

The stomach is retracted rostrally by the assistant, and the lesser sac and anterior surface of the pancreas are explored laparoscopically.

The lesion in the tail of pancreas may then become obvious.

Should the lesion not be obvious, laparoscopic ultrasonography can help localize the site of the lesion.

Laparoscopic ultrasonography should also be used to explore the liver if the possibility of metastasis from the malignant tumor exists.

The posterior peritoneum along the inferior surface of the pancreas is incised toward the spleen.

The pancreas is mobilized gently by lifting it off the posterior, retroperitoneal soft tissues, and the feasibility of laparoscopic resection is confirmed.

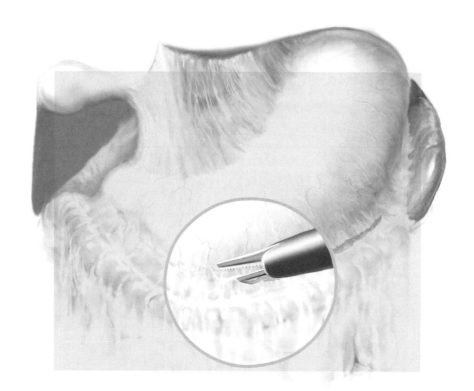

STEP 3   **Hand-assisted technique**

A McBurney incision is made in the right lower quadrant using a muscle-splitting technique; the size of the incision (4–5 cm) should fit snugly around the surgeon's wrist.

The surgeon's hand is introduced into the peritoneum by sliding between the abdominal muscles, keeping a tight fit with the skin around the wrist to prevent leakage of gas; commercially available seals may facilitate this maneuver.

The abdomen is then explored manually.

The hand further dissects the body/tail bluntly, then grasps the pancreas; the stomach is retracted with the back of the hand. This technique involves a medial-to-lateral approach to distal pancreatectomy, with mobilization from the body to tail/spleen, not vice versa.

An ultrasonic dissector facilitates further dissection.

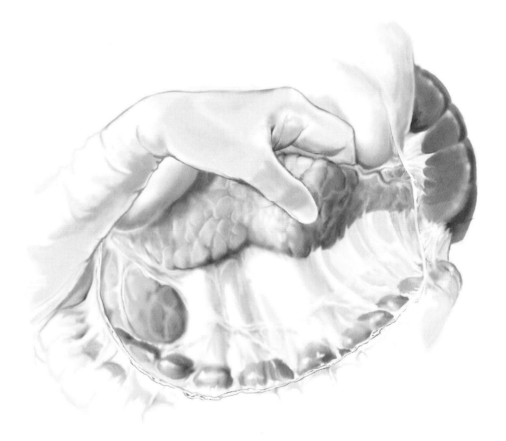

STEP 4

The pancreas is fully dissected into the splenic hilum.

The spleen is mobilized off the retroperitoneum and from attachments to the diaphragm, kidney, and colon by dividing the lienophrenic, lienorenal, and lienocolic ligaments with the ultrasonic dissector; hand manipulation assists these maneuvers.

A sterile specimen bag or sterilized plastic bowel bag inverted over the surgeon's left hand is introduced into the right-sided hand incision and the specimen grasped; as the hand is removed slowly, the bag falls over the specimen, keeping the wound from the surface of the specimen.

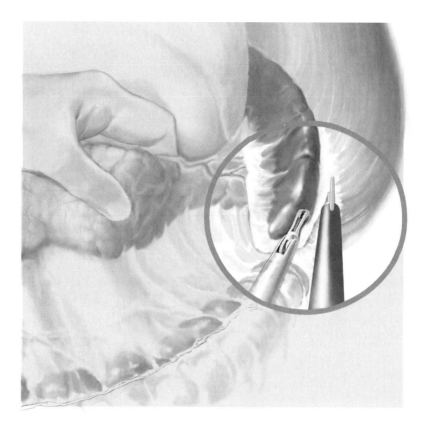

STEP 5

The splenic vein is identified posterior to the pancreas; when possible, the small veins passing to the posterior surface of the pancreas are divided using the ultrasonic dissector when a spleen-preserving resection is contemplated. If it is not possible to separate the vein from the pancreas or for potentially malignant neoplasms, the vein should be resected with the specimen. The vein is ligated either with an intracorporeal knot or a vascular stapler (A-1).

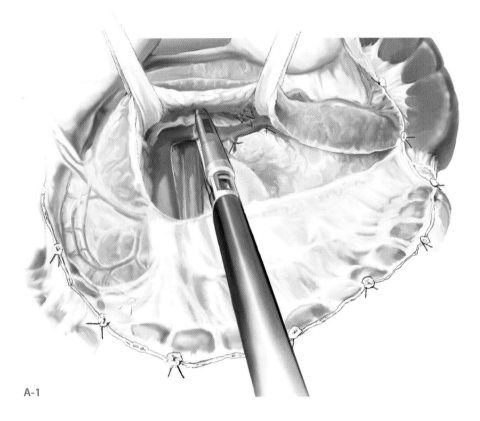

A-1

The splenic artery is identified; it often takes a serpiginous course along the upper border of the pancreas. If a splenectomy is planned, the splenic artery is isolated and divided using the ultrasonic dissector or ligated using intracorporeal knot tying techniques; others divide the splenic artery with a stapler using a vascular load (A-2).

When the spleen is to be preserved, the pancreas is separated from the intact splenic artery and vein using the ultrasonic dissector until the distal pancreas is completely isolated and free of all attachments.

When the spleen is to be removed with the specimen, dissection should proceed outside of these vessels, leaving the splenic artery and vein attached to the tail of the pancreas.

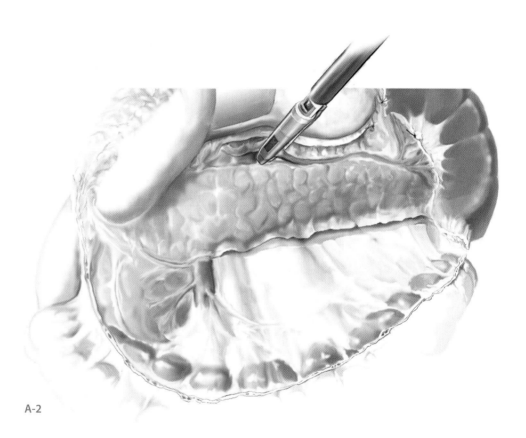

A-2

STEP 6

An Endo GI stapler is passed through the left-sided 12-mm port and fired across the body of the pancreas medial to the pancreas to be resected. Other techniques such as tissue welding may be used to transect the pancreas and "close" the end of the gland.

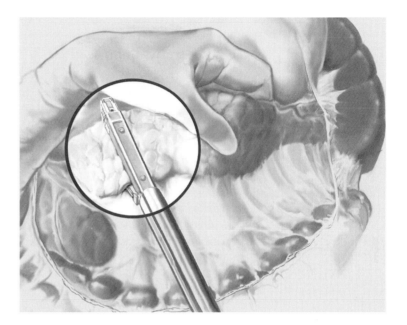

Postoperative Considerations

- Admission to a routine postsurgical ward if the patient is stable
- Nasogastric suction for 24h is optional, usually not necssary
- Liquid diet beginning postoperative day 1; advance as tolerated
- Watch for pancreatic fistula (amylase-rich fluid from drain)
- Discharge 5–6days postoperatively

Local Postoperative Complications

- Short term:
  - Pancreatic leak/fistula from proximal pancreatic remnant
  - Left subphrenic abscess (rule out pancreatic ductal leak)
  - Thrombocytosis secondary to splenectomy
  - Intra-abdominal hemorrhage (especially if splenic vein thrombosis with sinistral portal hypertension is present preoperatively)
- Long term:
  - Diabetes mellitus
  - Maldigestion/malabsorption/steatorrhea or malnutrition from development of exocrine insufficiency secondary to pancreatic parenchymal resection with diseased remaining pancreas

Tricks of the Senior Surgeon

Open Distal Pancreatectomy

- The major intraoperative problems that occur during distal pancreatectomy are injuries to the major veins from excessive traction or incorrect dissection. Early identification of the superior mesenteric vein and development of the tunnel where the superior mesenteric vein passes beneath the pancreas is an important maneuver to be sure of the location of this major venous structure as the dissection proceeds. This allows for rapid division of the pancreatic parenchyma over the vein if necessary to achieve vascular control.
- Because of the risk of vascular injury during distal pancreatectomy, an assortment of vascular clamps should be readily available on the back table; the surgeon should familiarize himself or herself with the selection of clamps before the operation begins.
- Sometimes, a posterior pseudocyst near the tail of the gland close to the splenic hilum or severe chronic inflammation will make it essentially impossible or inadvisable to mobilize the spleen safely from lateral to medial as suggested. In this case, it is sometimes more prudent to try to enter the retropancreatic space more medially, closer to the superior mesenteric vein. If possible, one can establish the proper plane of dissection there and move from medial to lateral behind the pancreas, remembering that the renal vein is at potential risk if the dissection goes too deep. It is important to stay close to the back of the pancreas.
- The spleen is sometimes injured during its mobilization, and it can be tempting to remove the spleen to reduce annoying bleeding. However, the spleen makes a nice "handle" for the distal pancreas and it is best to leave it *in situ* for the remainder of the dissection. Bleeding can often be controlled with a laparotomy pad on the spleen and manual pressure. Another option is to locate and ligate the proximal splenic artery to diminish splenic arterial inflow.

Laparoscopic Distal Pancreatectomy

- Laparoscopic surgery on solid abdominal organs is facilitated greatly by introducing the hand into the abdomen (hand-assisted technique).
- Hand-assisted laparoscopy allows:
  - Manipulation of large organs (colon, stomach, liver, spleen, and pancreas)
  - Control of hemostasis should a vessel bleed significantly during dissection; during distal pancreatectomy, branches of the splenic vein can cause considerable bleeding, controlled easily by pressure of the thumb and not easily controlled by a laparoscopic instrument.
  - Use of proprietary abdominal wall sealing devices is available for hand-assisted laparoscopy but are not mandatory. If the incision in the abdominal wall and muscles is made small enough, introduction of the hand through a small incision easily maintains the pneumoperitoneum. In addition, the abdominal wall can be lifted with the forearm to create extra working space in the abdomen.

Spleen

Robert Padbury

Introduction

Robert Padbury

Total splenectomy has been considered the appropriate management for splenic trauma, diseases, or disease processes that could be modified by splenectomy. This surgical truism has been supported by the belief that the spleen is not essential to life, that mortality is almost universal in non-operated splenic injury and that delayed rupture is a significant danger.

The policy for total splenectomy has been progressively modified by a number of important observations; first, that splenectomy increases the risk of significant septic events and, second, that partial splenectomy or even splenic preservation is possible with low risk to the patient. Major advances in abdominal imaging have contributed significantly to the surgical developments.

Progress has continued with the development of laparoscopic surgery. Initially laparoscopic total splenectomy became a relatively standard procedure, particularly in the non-trauma patient. More recently the concept of partial splenectomy has been successfully used using laparoscopic access. As with other organ systems, laparoscopic surgery served as a stimulus for equipment development, and the benefits of this have been realised in both open and laparoscopic procedures. Particularly valuable in splenic surgery are the endovascular stapling devices.

When considering a patient for splenectomy, decisions regarding the choice of access should take into account the experience and training of the surgeon, as well as the suitability of the patient. The size of the spleen, the nature of the problem and previous abdominal surgery will be factors in the decision. Clearly, appropriate and specific informed consent is mandatory, including a discussion of total splenectomy when a partial procedure is planned.

In this section of the atlas a range of techniques for splenectomy, open and laparoscopic, total and partial, are discussed. Techniques for splenic preservation are described and finally some approaches for splenic cysts are presented.

Open Splenectomy

Scott F. Gallagher, Larry C. Carey, Michel M. Murr

Indications and Contraindications

Indications

- Trauma
- Blood dyscrasias, e.g., idiopathic thrombocytopenic purpura
- Symptomatic relief, e.g., Gaucher's disease, chronic myeloid or lymphatic leukemia
- Splenic cysts and tumors

Contraindications

- No absolute contraindications for splenectomy
- Limited life expectancy and prohibitive operative risk

Contraindications to Laparoscopic Splenectomy

- Previous open upper abdominal surgery
- Uncontrolled coagulation disorder
- Very low platelet count (<20,000/100 ml)
- Massive splenic enlargement, i.e., spleen greater four times normal size or larger
- Portal hypertension

Preoperative Investigation and Preparation

- Imaging studies to estimate the size of the spleen or extent of splenic injury and other abdominal injuries in trauma cases
- Interpretation of bone marrow biopsy, peripheral blood smear, and ferrokinetics in coordination with a hematologist
- Discontinue anticoagulants (such as aspirin, warfarin, clopidogrel and vitamin E)
- Patients routinely given polyvalent pneumococcal vaccine, *Haemophilus influenzae* b conjugate vaccines and meningococcal vaccines on the same day at least 10–14 days prior to splenectomy (given postoperatively in trauma cases)
- Prophylactic antibiotics (cefazolin or cefotetan)
- Perioperative DVT prophylaxis
- Perioperative steroids should be administered to patients on long-term steroid therapy

Procedure

The standard supine position is employed with an optional small roll/bump under the left flank.

The patient should be well secured to the operating table should it become necessary to tilt the table to improve visualization of the operative field.

Mechanical retractors greatly enhance exposure and the primary surgeon should stand on the right side of the patient; the first assistant opposite the surgeon on the left side of the patient.

There are two standard incisions for open splenectomy: a supraumbilical midline or left subcostal with or without midline extension. A midline incision is usually employed in trauma cases.

Examine each patient following induction of anesthesia to estimate the location of the splenic hilum and the tip of the spleen, so the incision location optimizes exposure.

The principle of retraction is that of moving the incision over the operative field.

Two points of retraction include one retractor to gently hold the colon in the lower abdomen and counterretraction to lift the left portion of the incision superiorly and out of the operative field.

The standard order of steps is arranged to minimize blood loss, minimize the size of the spleen and maintain adequate exposure while performing the deepest and most challenging dissection.

Identify the splenic artery near its origin from the celiac axis, which is accessed through the gastrohepatic ligament (A, B).

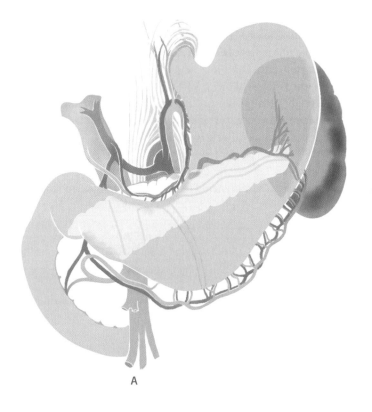

A

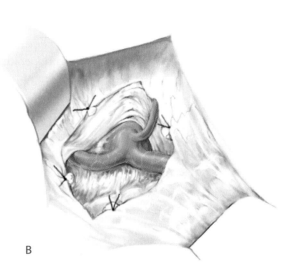

B

STEP 2

Upon entering the peritoneal cavity and again before closing, a thorough search for accessory spleens should be conducted, especially if the indication for splenectomy is hematological.

Open the gastrosplenic ligament through an avascular area and then proceed to dissect the short gastric vessels. These may be secured with hemoclips or ligatures.

The last several vessels in the gastrosplenic ligament are of particular note. These branches are often quite short, so care must be taken to utilize adequate tissue for hemostasis without injuring the greater curvature of the stomach. The LigaSure (R) device, the harmonic/ultrasonic scalpel or a linear stapler can also be utilized for dividing the gastrosplenic ligament as is employed during laparoscopic splenectomy.

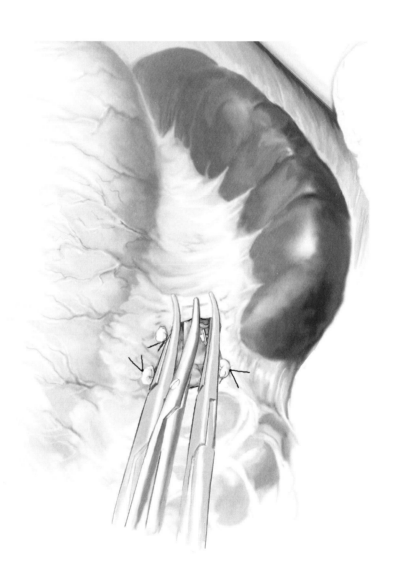

STEP 3   **Dividing the splenic attachments**

While dividing splenic attachments, always attempt to stay closer to the spleen than to
the opposite structure. Proceeding inferiorly along the gastrosplenic ligament typically includes dividing the left gastroepiploic artery. Taking down the splenic flexure
and the splenocolic attachment usually facilitates this dissection (A).

The spleen is then gently and progressively retracted medially with the surgeon's left
hand (B). Using a laparotomy pad under the retracting hand, it is a relatively simple
maneuver for the surgeon to identify the peritoneal attachments and provide exposure with the left index finger. The attachments are divided with curved scissors
proceeding from the inferior pole to the superior pole and then dividing the
splenorenal ligament as the spleen is gradually rotated medially and anteriorly.
Care should be taken with any blunt dissection as the splenic capsule is relatively thin
and even small tears can result in moderate bleeding. Likewise, care should be taken
as proceeding posteriorly around the inferior pole in order to avoid the adrenal
gland.

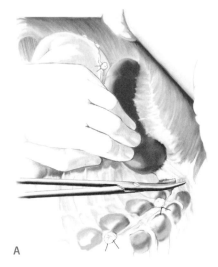

A

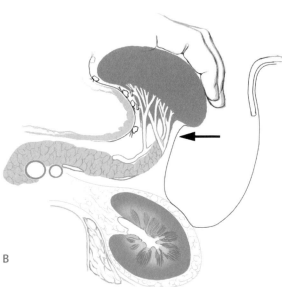

B

| STEP 4 | Control of the splenic hilum |

Once all of the splenic attachments have been divided the splenic hilum can be addressed definitively. Lift the spleen up and out of the retroperitoneum. This maneuver serves to clearly identify and separate the splenic vessels from the tail of the pancreas as shown. Laparotomy pads packed into the retroperitoneum can assist with elevating the spleen into the incision while controlling oozing in the retroperitoneum. With the assistant holding the spleen, the surgeon can separate the tail of the pancreas from the splenic vessels in order to protect the tail of the pancreas prior to dissecting and applying curved clamps. The surgeon divides the splenic artery and vein proximal to their bifurcation between clamps and applies a suture ligature to each after removing the spleen. We first clamp the artery, which is typically anterior to the splenic vein, and then squeeze the spleen in order to promote autotransfusion of splenic blood prior to clamping the vein.

Once the spleen is removed and all of the named vessels have been doubly ligated, the operative field can be inspected for hemostasis. The abdomen is closed with or without a closed suction drain.

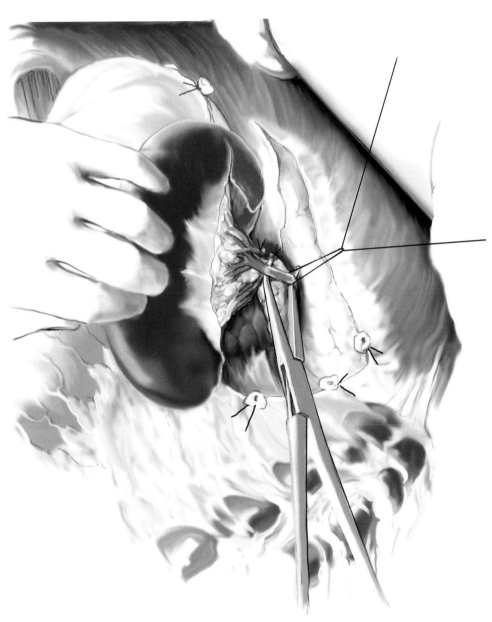

Postoperative Tests

- Monitor in high dependency unit
- Monitor platelets and hemoglobin

Complications

- Bleeding
- Pancreatitis
- Pancreatic fistula
- Colonic or gastric perforation
- Subphrenic abscess
- Wound infection
- Atelectasis
- Left pleural effusion
- Postsplenectomy sepsis
- Thrombocytosis

Tricks of the Senior Surgeon

- If bleeding is excessive and control of the splenic artery has not already been secured, or is not immediately feasible, the splenic artery and veins are easily controlled by gentle pressure applied between the second and third fingers of the surgeon's right hand.
- Control of the splenic artery is most easily accomplished near its origin through the gastrohepatic ligament posterior to the lesser curvature of the stomach (see STEP 1), which is particularly useful during splenorrhaphy.
- Another approach to the splenic hilum is anteriorly which carries increased risk as the splenic vein is immediately posterior to the splenic artery near the hilum and the tail of the pancreas is also intimately associated to the splenic hilum.
- A linear stapler, as with laparoscopic splenectomy, is particularly useful when expeditious division of the hilum is necessary to control hemorrhage.
- For patients in whom difficulty gaining vascular control is anticipated, for those with enormous splenomegaly or those with portal hypertension, splenic artery embolization done immediately prior to the operation can reduce splenic sequestration, congestion and bleeding.
- Early ligation of the splenic artery diminishes blood loss, maximizes the amount of blood in the spleen returning to the patient, decreases the size of the spleen, improves ease of handling, facilitates removal and improves transfusion efficiency of blood products sooner rather than later during the procedure, if necessary.
- Make a thorough search for accessory spleens before and after the spleen is removed, especially when operating for hematological indications. Accessory spleens are found in 15–35% of patients undergoing splenectomy and higher in those with hematological diseases. In order of decreasing frequency, accessory spleens are found in the splenic hilum, the splenorenal ligament, the greater omentum, the retroperitoneum near the tail of the pancreas, and the splenocolic ligament. Less commonly, accessory spleens are found in the mesentery of the small and large intestine, as well as the pelvis, in particular the left ureter and left adnexa, and left gonads.
- Mobilize the splenic flexure and the rest of the colon whenever necessary. Be just as careful protecting the colon and the stomach to prevent injury to either hollow viscus.

Laparoscopic Splenectomy

David I. Watson

For indications, contraindications and preoperative investigations,
see "Open Splenectomy."

STEP 1	**Patient positioning and theatre set-up (A)**

The patient is positioned in the lateral position (left side up) and with the operating
table bent at the level of the patient's waist to flatten the lateral convexity of the patient's
flank. The surgeon and assistant stand facing the patient, with the video monitor sited
opposite.

Port placement (B):

An 11-mm port is placed using an open insertion technique in the left upper quadrant, halfway between the mid-clavicular line and the anterior axillary line, immediately
below the left costal margin. Secondary ports include a 5-mm port in the left mid-axillary line immediately below the costal margin, and a 12-mm port in the left anterior
axillary line also immediately below the costal margin. An additional 5-mm port can
be placed more laterally if necessary (optional). In approximately one-third of cases
the splenic flexure of the colon must be mobilized to provide lateral access for port
placement.

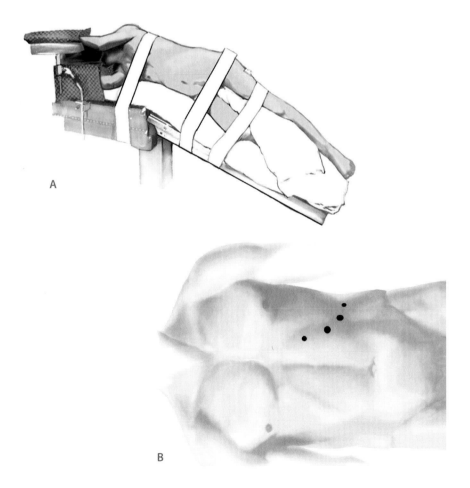

A

B

STEP 2   **Exposure**

No retractors are required. In the lateral position gravity enhances exposure of the
posterior splenic attachments. A blunt ended 5-mm-diameter grasping instrument is
placed through the most medial port is used to manipulate the spleen, lifting it upwards
to expose the hilum, or rotating it towards the midline to expose the posterior attachments. A search for accessory spleens (see "Open Splenectomy," "Tricks of the Senior
Surgeon") should be made before commencing dissection of the spleen, as accessory
spleens are more easily identified at this stage, and they should be removed as soon as
they have been found. Removal later in the procedure can be more difficult.

With the spleen rotated towards the midline, the posterior peritoneal attachments are
divided 5–10 mm away from the splenic capsule using a diathermy hook or ultrasonic
shears. The spleen is progressively mobilized towards the midline, exposing the
"splenic mesentery," which contains the main splenic vessels inferiorly, the short gastric
vessels superiorly, and the tail of the pancreas. For adequate mobilization it is necessary
to divide the posterior splenic attachments up to the left side of the oesophageal
diaphragmatic hiatus superiorly (see "Open Splenectomy," STEP 3). A combination
of gravity and rotation of the spleen displays an avascular fascial plane behind the
splenic mesentery.
It is important to avoid damage to the tail of the pancreas during this dissection.
If bleeding occurs during this step, then dissection is in an incorrect tissue plane.

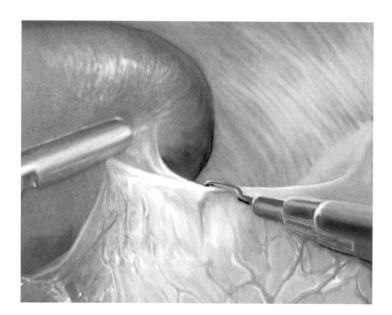

STEP 3   **The vascular attachments are divided next using a 30- or 45-mm endoscopic linear cutting stapler (white cartridge)**

This is applied sequentially across the splenic mesentery commencing inferiorly, and multiple applications of the stapler are required (usually three to five). The stapler is placed adjacent to the splenic capsule at the hilum, to minimize the risk of damaging the pancreatic tail. When applying the stapler, the spleen is lifted up by a blunt instrument passed through the most medial port. With this technique, dissection of individual splenic vessels is not necessary. Furthermore, attempts to dissect individual vessels may result in vessel damage and hemorrhage. If, when sequentially applying the stapler, it becomes apparent that the spleen has not been adequately mobilized superiorly, additional division of the posterior attachments to the upper spleen is then completed to enable final division of the short gastric blood vessels, and complete separation of the spleen from its remaining attachments.

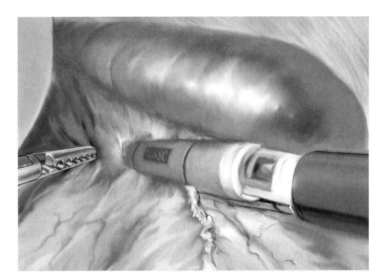

STEP 4   **The spleen is next placed in a large specimen retrieval bag**

An AutoSuture Endocatch II retrieval bag (U.S. Surgical, Norwalk, CT, USA) is positioned underneath the spleen, and then opened so that the spleen drops directly into the bag as the bag is opened. Other specimen bags require additional manipulation to get the spleen into the retrieval bag and are more difficult to use. The neck of the bag is then pulled out through the lateral 12-mm port wound.

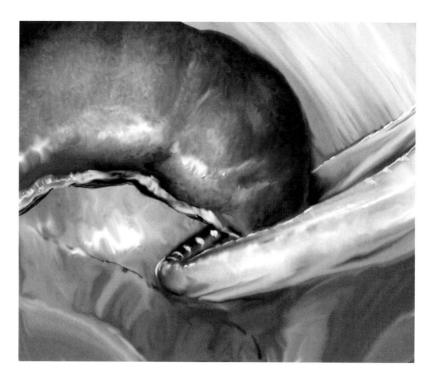

STEP 5

Morcellation of the spleen

The surgeon's index finger is placed inside the bag and through the port wound, to break the spleen into pieces. This is done bimanually with the left hand pushing against the abdominal wall, and the right index finger pushing the spleen against the abdominal wall. Blood released from the broken spleen is then aspirated and an empty sponge holding forceps is used to remove the spleen in pieces. The surgeon must be careful to avoid spillage of splenic material into the abdominal cavity, which can occur if the specimen bag is broken. An alternative method for spleen removal is to remove the spleen intact through a muscle-splitting abdominal incision, usually in the left lower quadrant.

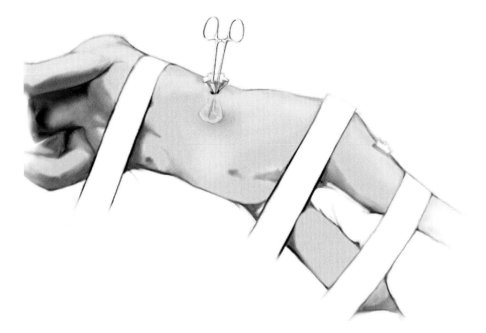

Tricks of the Senior Surgeon

- This procedure is most suitable for spleens which are normal in size or only mildly enlarged. The size of the spleen is best assessed before surgery with patients in the lateral position. If the spleen is easily palpable then it may be too big for laparoscopic dissection of the hilum in the lateral position.

Partial Splenectomy, Open and Laparoscopic

Eric C. Poulin, Christopher M. Schlachta, Joseph Mamazza

Indications and Contraindications

Indications

Trauma
- Selected Class II–III–IV splenic injury with the following:
- Hemodynamic stability
- No evidence of other intra-abdominal organ injury
- No associated head injury
- No coagulopathy
- CT confirmation of isolated splenic injury

Elective
- Resection of non-parasitic cysts
- Hamartomas and other benign splenic tumors
- Inflammatory pseudotumor of the spleen, Type J Gaucher's disease
- Cholesteryl ester storage disease, chronic myelogenous leukemia
- Thalassemia major, spherocytosis, staging of Hodgkin's disease in children

Contraindications
- Inadequate exposure
- Inability to mobilize the spleen and tail of pancreas to the midline
- Inability to leave >25 % of splenic mass for complete splenic function

Indications for Laparoscopic Partial Splenectomy

Still being defined.

Preoperative Investigation and Preparation for the Procedure

See chapter "Open Splenectomy."

Procedure

Planning the partial splenectomy

Assuming that the spleen is appropriately placed for full evaluation and that hemostasis is adequate, the planning for partial splenectomy can start. In trauma cases, it will be dictated by the extent of the injury and in elective cases by the nature of the underlying pathology.

The spleen in the majority of cases can be divided into independent lobes or segments, each with its own terminal blood supply (A, B). The superior pole is supplied by the short gastric vessels and the lower pole by branches of the gastroepiploic artery (up to five) known to anastomose with the inferior polar artery. In addition, most patients, despite possible variations, have two or three major vessels entering the hilum. Therefore there are usually four or five regions or lobes available for partial splenectomy. It is also important to understand that these vessels lie in different supportive ligaments. Vessels to the superior pole (short gastrics) and inferior pole (gastroepiploic branches) rest in the gastrosplenic ligament, whereas the splenic branches proper lie in the splenorenal ligament with the tail of the pancreas.

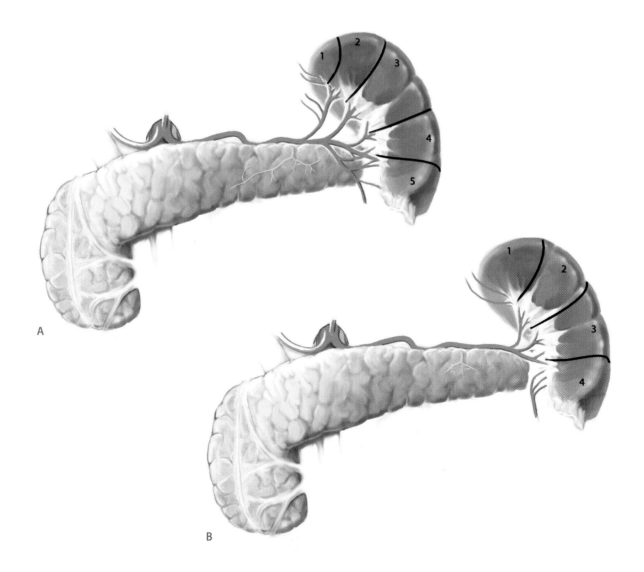

STEP 2

Exposing the entire hilum and ligating appropriate arteries

The next step involves exposure of the entire hilum of the spleen close to the parenchyma. The gastrosplenic and splenorenal ligaments need to be separated while preserving the blood supply to both poles. There is a fairly avascular area of this ligament that needs to be opened between the short gastric vessels to the superior pole and the gastroepiploic branches to the lower pole. This will lead to a complete display of the entire splenic blood supply including both poles.

Selected arterial branches then need to be tediously dissected as close to the spleen parenchyma as possible, noting that the veins are situated posteriorly in close proximity.

The vessels can be doubly ligated, transfixed or clipped. The long slender laparoscopic clip appliers can be used for this step of the procedure. Once the arterial blood supply is controlled, the affected spleen will visibly demarcate rapidly. If the devitalized spleen corresponds to the intended resection, a similar technique is used on the venous side. Access to the venous side can also be achieved from the posterior aspect of the spleen (as indicated in illustration).

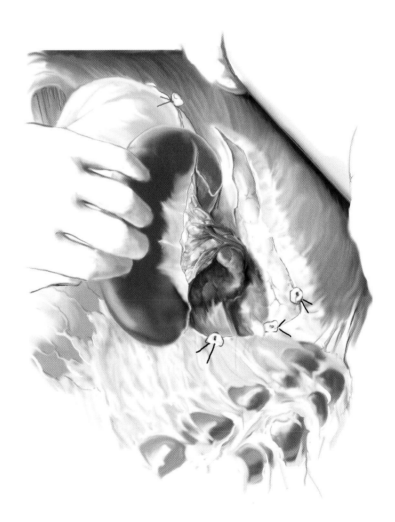

STEP 3   **Incising the splenic capsule and resection**

The capsule of the spleen is incised circumferentially with a scalpel or monopolar cautery, making sure to leave 5 mm of devitalized tissue in situ. The splenic fragments can be transected with a combination of scalpel, scissors or monopolar cautery. When enough residual devitalized tissue is left behind circumferentially, very little hemostasis is required and it can usually be achieved by simple means and topical agents.

The abdomen is closed, with or without a closed suction drain, after complete hemostasis is achieved.

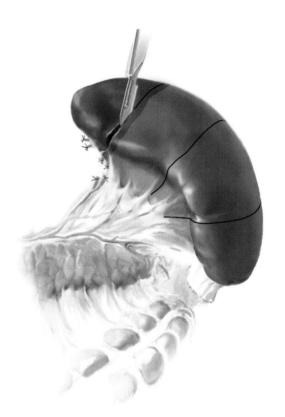

Partial Laparoscopic Splenectomy

STEP 1

Patient positioning, trocar placement and mobilization of the spleen are performed as described in the chapter "Laparoscopic Splenectomy."

Care is taken to leave a 2-cm portion of the splenocolic ligament on the spleen side to allow for easier spleen mobilization. Attention is then given to the gastrosplenic ligament anteriorly. It contains the short gastric arteries to the superior pole and the branches of the gastroepiploic artery (up to five branches) to the lower pole.

This allows definition of the type of splenic blood supply, and the number of splenic branches entering the medial aspect of the hilum, thus helping determine the number of splenic lobes.

Dissecting and Clipping the Appropriate Vessels

Once the surgeon has determined what lobe(s) needs resection, tedious dissection of the involved splenic branch (es) is undertaken and the involved artery (ies) is clipped. This dissection can be performed alternatively from the front or the back of the spleen as the spleen can be mobilized fairly easily. The spleen is allowed to demarcate in the chosen region. Once the devascularized area is found to contain the lesion needing resection, attention is given to the corresponding venous drainage, using a similar technique. Veins are situated closely behind the arteries, except at the level of the penultimate and ultimate branches usually within the spleen, where they can be anterior or posterior.

STEP 2

Resecting, bagging and extracting the specimen:

The capsule of the spleen is then scored with monopolar cautery on coagulating current circumferentially (30–40 W), ensuring that a 5-mm rim of devascularized splenic tissue remains in situ (A). Once the splenic pulp is penetrated, non-crushing intestinal graspers are used to fracture the splenic pulp. A laparoscopic hook and scissors can also be used. If a 5-mm rim of devitalized spleen is left behind, this procedure remains noticeably bloodless. Spot coagulation with monopolar cautery on coagulation or spray current can be used for the remaining hemostasis.

Alternatively the parenchyma can be divided with an endovascular stapler (B).

The specimen is removed as per "laparoscopic splenectomy."

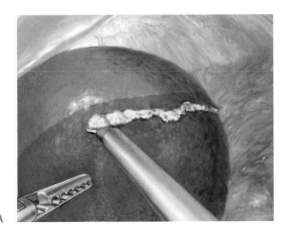

A

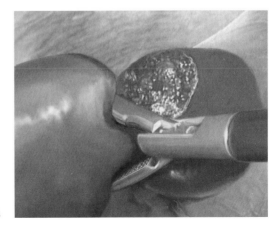

B

Tricks of the Senior Surgeon

- Detailed knowledge of splenic anatomy constitutes the single most important factor that will allow the surgeon to consider all the options available to save splenic parenchyma. There are two patterns of terminal artery branching: *distributed and bundled or magistral* (see STEP 1). Most specimens have two or three terminal branches (superior polar, superior and inferior terminal) determining lobes or segments. Relative avascular planes are identified between lobes and segments. The surgical unit of the spleen is based upon surgically accessible vessels at the hilum.
- The keys to success with partial laparoscopic splenectomy are experience with advanced laparoscopy, case selection, ability to dissect branches of the splenic artery close to the hilum, and foremost the realization that leaving a 5-mm margin of devitalized spleen in situ greatly simplifies homeostasis.
- Specially in the laparoscopic approach, improper use of the cautery can cause iatrogenic injury to the stomach, colon, and pancreas. Structures close to the lower pole in the gastrocolic ligament can be approached aggressively with the cautery, but blind fulguration of fat in the hilum can result in serious bleeding. The instrument should be activated only in proximity to the target organ to avoid arcing and spot necrosis, which may result in delayed perforation and sepsis.
- The role of the assistants is also important in the prevention of complications. In the laparoscopic approach, all instruments, including those handled by assistants, should be moved only under direct vision. Retraction of the liver and stomach and elevation of the spleen require constant concentration to avoid lacerations with subsequent hemorrhage or perforation and jeopardizing the performance of partial splenectomy.

Splenic Preservation and Splenic Trauma

Craig P. Fischer, Frederick A. Moore

Indications and Contraindications

Indications

- Injuries to the spleen, when patients are hemodynamically stable.

Contraindications

- Hemodynamic instability
- Life-threatening concomitant injuries which are likely to cause hemodynamic compromise in the postoperative period, e.g., severe liver injuries or significant pelvic fractures
- Coagulopathy – the most common cause of coagulopathy in this patient group is hypothermia
- Grade V injuries or the pulverized spleen

Preoperative Investigation and Preparation for the Procedure

Clinical Evaluation

- Hemodynamic status, mechanism of injury, other trauma, co-morbidities, age
- Patients who fail non-operative management of blunt splenic injury are usually good candidates for attempted splenic repair. Splenic salvage may also be appropriate when laparotomy is performed for other indications such as penetrating abdominal injury or bowel injury

CT Scan

- *Hemodynamically stable* patients should undergo a CAT scan of the abdomen and pelvis with oral and intravenous contrast.
- Two large bore intravenous catheters should be placed as well as an indwelling urinary catheter and nasogastric tube.

Procedure

STEP 1

Incision – midline

A subcostal incision should not be used in trauma, even if the only suspected injury on preoperative investigations is a splenic injury.

Exposure
See chapter "Open Splenectomy." An initial exploratory laparotomy is performed.

The left upper quadrant should be initially packed with laparotomy pads, then the self-retaining retractor adjusted to facilitate exposure of the left upper quadrant. Gentle pressure on the area of splenic injury with a laparotomy pad will help decrease blood loss.

Mobilization
See splenic mobilization in the chapter "Open Splenectomy."

STEP 2

The lesser sac is entered, somewhat to the left along the greater curvature. The use of an endovascular stapling device will facilitate this step as it is long, and capable of angulation. Generally two applications of a 45-mm stapler will allow rapid, wide access to the lesser sac. The splenic artery superior to the pancreas should be identified and may be temporarily clamped if significant bleeding is encountered (see chapter "Open Splenectomy"). Be sure the artery is dissected away from the pancreas and does not contain arteriosclerotic plaque before clamping.

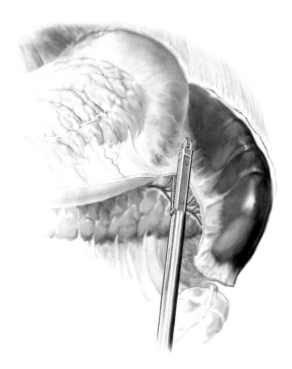

STEP 3

With complete splenic mobilization, the spleen is grasped (A). Again, a laparotomy pad is applied to the area of injury. Initial attempts to control bleeding may include simple hemostatic agents, the use of the argon beam coagulator for surface injuries, and suture ligation for deep parenchymal injuries.

If injury is to a single pole of the spleen, the distal polar branches of the splenic artery may be ligated within the lesser sac, close to the splenic hilum (B). Again, the addition of hemostatic agents and gentle pressure is used.

If initial attempts at hemostasis are unsuccessful, a pledget repair may be used (C, D). The splenic capsule in adults will not hold a stitch – use an appropriate pledget, such as Teflon, felt or autogenous tissue (e.g., posterior rectus sheath). A horizontal mattress technique is used with 3-0 Prolene.

Prior to tying the knots, fibrin glue should be applied to the cleft or site of injury (C).

The use of a spray applicator for the application of fibrin glue is recommended, but not necessary.

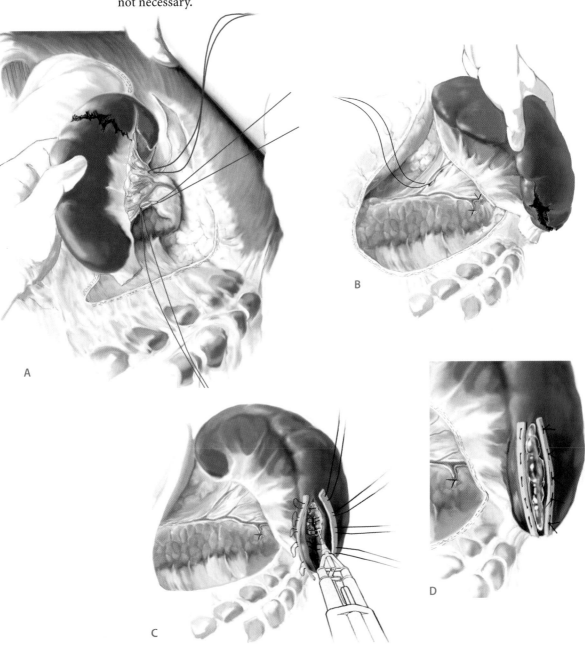

STEP 4

An additional technique that can be used in conjunction with a pledget repair, or alone, is the use of a woven mesh (**A**). A sheet of appropriate material such as polyglycolic acid is obtained and a center cut is made to allow passage of the splenic vessels via the hilum. This technique is particularly useful when capsular injury is encountered. Fibrin sealant should be applied, via an aerosolized technique, to the injured area of the spleen. For the use of a wrap to be successful, all of the short gastric vessels must be ligated to fully mobilize the superior pole and allow for a circumferential application of the wrap. After application of fibrin glue, the woven mesh is closed circumferentially with a running absorbable suture (**B**). Care is taken to ensure the mesh is tightly applied to ensure hemostasis and that an adequate opening is left at the hilum that does not encumber either the splenic artery or vein.

Another technique in splenic salvage is ligation of the splenic artery and vein. This is successful in spleen preserving distal pancreatectomy, and the surgical technique is identical. The splenic artery and vein are ligated en masse with an endovascular stapler. Care must be taken *not to ligate* the short gastric vessels in this case. Additional use of simple hemostatic measures will give a satisfactory result – the spleen will not infarct if the short gastric vessels are left intact.

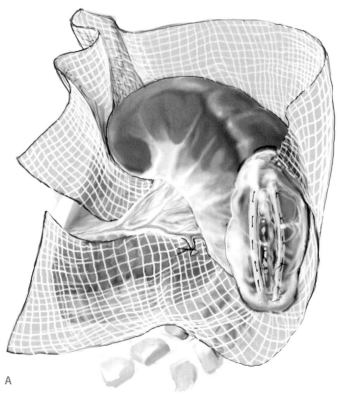

A

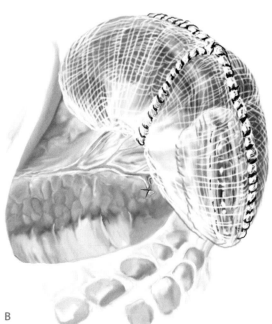

B

Postoperative Tests

See chapter "Open Splenectomy."

Postoperative Complications

See chapter "Open Splenectomy."
- Splenic infarction or splenic abscess is uncommon after splenic repair.
- Postoperative bleeding requiring reexploration. If bleeding (or fresh clot) at site of repair, splenectomy is indicated.

Tricks of the Senior Surgeon

- Do not repair a spleen if it is not bleeding.
- When performing splenic repair early in one's experience, choose the right patient. This generally is a young patient with few other life-threatening injuries.
- Do not accept blood loss while performing the repair – if you cannot quickly stem major hemorrhage, remove the spleen.
- If the patient continues to bleed postoperatively, reoperate promptly.
- When performing ligation of a branch of the splenic artery, or indeed the main artery and splenic vein, do not divide the short gastric vessels.

Laparoscopic Unroofing of Splenic Cysts

Marco Decurtins, Duri Gianom

Indications and Contraindications

Indications

- Nonparasitic cyst >5 cm with and without symptoms
- Nonparasitic cyst <5 cm with symptoms
- Parasitic cyst
- Cyst-related complications (spontaneous or traumatic rupture, abscess formation)
- Neoplastic cysts

Preoperative Investigations/Preparation

- Serological testing for echinococcus

Procedure

STEP 1

Access and insertion of trocars

The patient is positioned in a 45-degree right lateral position. The surgeon and the camera assistant stand at the patient's abdominal side, video-monitor on the opposite site. The first trocar (umbilical, 12 mm) is inserted in an open technique (T1) and the pneumoperitoneum (14 mmHg) is introduced.

Further trocars are inserted under visual control in the left lower abdomen (T2, 10 mm) and in the left midaxillary line just below the costal margin (T3, 10 mm). If needed, additional trocars are placed semicircularly in relation to the spleen (dotted line).

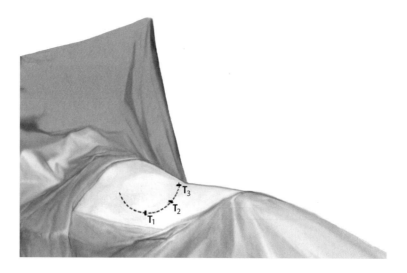

STEP 2

Aspiration of the cyst contents and resection of the cyst wall

The cyst is opened in an avascular region with electrocautery and the contents aspired. The adhesions to the surrounding tissue are dissected and the spleen needs to be completely mobilized as for a laparoscopic splenectomy. Care should be taken with the diaphragmatic adhesions, which can be particularly dense.

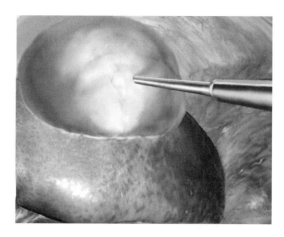

STEP 3

The cyst wall is unroofed using diathermy or harmonic shears until unaffected splenic parenchyma is reached. During the resection of the cyst, meticulous hemostasis is important to prevent impairment of the view. To minimize the risk of recurrence, the largest possible amount of cyst wall should be resected.

The excised tissue is placed in an endoscopic plastic bag and removed.

When technically feasible, an omentum patch is placed in the remaining cyst cavity and the trocar incisions are closed without drainage.

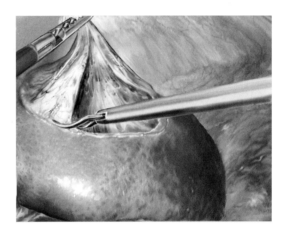

Postoperative Tests

See chapter "Open Splenectomy."

Postoperative Complications

See chapter "Open Splenectomy."
- Cyst recurrence

Tricks of the Senior Surgeon

- Complete mobilization of the spleen prior to resection of the cyst wall is imperative.
- To reduce the risk of bleeding, use dissection with a stapler device in situations where the cyst wall is covered with normal splenic parenchyma. This is especially useful in the region of splenic hilus.
- Use an open approach in parasitic and neoplastic cysts.

Subject Index